Nephrology Essentials

Nephrology Essentials

Editor: Bianca Keaton

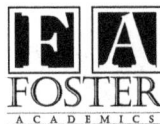

FA
FOSTER
ACADEMICS

www.fosteracademics.com

www.fosteracademics.com

FA
FOSTER
ACADEMICS

Cataloging-in-Publication Data

Nephrology essentials / edited by Bianca Keaton.
    p. cm.
Includes bibliographical references and index.
ISBN 978-1-63242-711-3
1. Nephrology. 2. Kidneys--Diseases. I. Keaton, Bianca.
RC902 .N47 2019
616.61--dc23

Foster Academics,
118-35 Queens Blvd., Suite 400,
Forest Hills, NY 11375, USA

ISBN 978-1-63242-711-3 (Hardback)

Contents

Preface...IX

Chapter 1   **Incidence, Severity and Outcomes of Acute Kidney Injury in Octogenarians following Heart Valve Replacement Surgery**...1
Michael A. Mao, Charat Thongprayoon, YiFan Wu, Vickram Tejwani,
Myriam Vela-Ortiz, Joseph Dearani and Qi Qian

Chapter 2   **Forecasting the Incidence and Prevalence of Patients with End-Stage Renal Disease**...9
Mohamad Adam Bujang, Tassha Hilda Adnan, Nadiah Hanis Hashim,
Kirubashni Mohan, Ang Kim Liong, Ghazali Ahmad, Goh Bak Leong,
Sunita Bavanandan and Jamaiyah Haniff

Chapter 3   **A Study to Inform the Design of a National Multicentre Randomised Controlled Trial to Evaluate if Reducing Serum Phosphate to Normal Levels Improves Clinical Outcomes including Mortality, Cardiovascular Events, Bone Pain or Fracture in Patients on Dialysis**...14
Ramya Bhargava, Philip A. Kalra, Paul Brenchley, Helen Hurst and
Alastair Hutchison

Chapter 4   **Soluble Fas and the−670 Polymorphism of Fas in Lupus Nephritis**.........................26
Juan José Bollain-y-Goytia, Mariela Arellano-Rodríguez,
Felipe de Jesús Torres-Del-Muro, Leonel Daza-Benítez, José Francisco Muñoz-Valle,
Esperanza Avalos-Díaz and Rafael Herrera-Esparza

Chapter 5   **Serum Endocan Levels Associated with Hypertension and Loss of Renal Function in Pediatric Patients after Two Years from Renal Transplant**........................36
Livia Victorino de Souza, Vanessa Oliveira, Aline Oliveira Laurindo,
DelmaRegina Gomes HuarachJ, Paulo Cesar Koch Nogueira,
Luciana de Santis Feltran, José Osmar Medina-Pestana and
Maria do Carmo Franco

Chapter 6   **High Steroid Sensitivity among Children with Nephrotic Syndrome**.......................43
Taiwo Augustina Ladapo, Christopher Imokhuede Esezobor and Foluso Ebun Lesi

Chapter 7   **Comparative Performance of Creatinine-Based Estimated Glomerular Filtration Rate Equations**...49
Maisarah Jalalonmuhali, Ng Kok Peng and Lim Soo Kun

Chapter 8   **Morphological Retrospective Study of Peritoneal Biopsies from Patients with Encapsulating Peritoneal Sclerosis: Underestimated Role of Adipocytes as New Fibroblasts Lineage?**...56
Monika Tooulou, Pieter Demetter, Anwar Hamade, Caroline Keyzer,
Joëlle L. Nortier and Agnieszka A. Pozdzik

Chapter 9   **Management Practice, and Adherence and Its Contributing Factors among Patients with Chronic Kidney Disease at Tikur Anbessa Specialized Hospital**..66
Belayneh Kefale, Yewondwossen Tadesse, Minyahil Alebachew and
Ephrem Engidawork

Chapter 10   **The Clinical Efficacy and Safety of Ertapenem for the Treatment of Complicated Urinary Tract Infections caused by ESBL-Producing Bacteria in Children**..81
Ayse Karaaslan, Eda Kepenekli Kadayifci, Serkan Atici, Gulsen Akkoc,
Nurhayat Yakut, Sevliya Öcal Demir, Ahmet Soysal and Mustafa Bakir

Chapter 11   **Mortality in Patients on Renal Replacement Therapy and Permanent Cardiac Pacemakers**..85
Gabriel Vanerio, Cristina García, Carlota González and Alejandro Ferreiro

Chapter 12   **Factors Predicting Renal Function Outcome after Augmentation Cystoplasty**.................93
Shahbaz Mehmood, Raouf Seyam, Sadia Firdous and
Waleed Mohammad Altaweel

Chapter 13   **Arterial Stiffness and Renal Replacement Therapy: A Controversial Topic**.........................100
Edmundo Cabrera Fischer, Yanina Zócalo, Cintia Galli,
Sandra Wray and Daniel Bia

Chapter 14   **Glycaemic Control Impact on Renal Endpoints in Diabetic Patients on Haemodialysis**...107
Danielle Creme and Kieran McCafferty

Chapter 15   **Decreased Serum 25-hydroxyvitamin D Level Causes Interventricular Septal Hypertrophy in Patients on Peritoneal Dialysis: Cardiovascular Aspects of Endogenous Vitamin D Deficiency**...113
Bennur Esen, Irfan Sahin, Ahmet Engin Atay, Emel Saglam Gokmen,
Ozlem Harmankaya Kaptanogullari, Mürvet Yılmaz, Suat Hayri Kucuk,
Serdar Kahvecioglu and Nurhan Seyahi

Chapter 16   **High Prevalence of Cardiovascular Disease in End-Stage Kidney Disease Patients Ongoing Hemodialysis in Peru: Why should we Care about it?**...........................119
Katia Bravo-Jaimes, Alvaro Whittembury and Vilma Santivañez

Chapter 17   **Clinical Utility of Urinary β2-Microglobulin in Detection of Early Nephropathy in African Diabetes Mellitus Patients**...125
U. E. Ekrikpo, E. E. Effa, E. E. Akpan, A. S. Obot and S. Kadiri

Chapter 18   **Malignancy in Membranous Nephropathy: Evaluation of Incidence**..............................133
Basil Alnasrallah, John F. Collins and L. Jonathan Zwi

Chapter 19   **Association of Poor Social Support and Financial Insecurity with Psychological Distress of Chronic Kidney Disease Patients Attending National Nephrology Unit**...140
Ramya Hettiarachchi and Chrishantha Abeysena

Chapter 20   **Acute Kidney Injury in Diabetes Mellitus**...146
D. Patschan and G. A. Müller

Chapter 21   **Characteristics of the Relationship of Kidney Dysfunction with Cardiovascular Disease in High Risk Patients with Diabetes** 153
Attilio Losito, Loretta Pittavini, Ivano Zampi and Elena Zampi

Chapter 22   **Acute Kidney Injury in Hematopoietic Stem Cell Transplantation** 159
Vinod Krishnappa, Mohit Gupta, Gurusidda Manu, Shivani Kwatra, Osei-Tutu Owusu and Rupesh Raina

Chapter 23   **Pediatric Nephrology and Rheumatology Practice Patterns in Granulomatosis with Polyangiitis: A Midwest Pediatric Nephrology Consortium Study** 171
Cristin D. W. Kaspar, Keia Sanderson, Seza Ozen, Priya S. Verghese, Megan Lo, Timothy E. Bunchman, Scott E. Wenderfer and Jason Kidd

Chapter 24   **Undiagnosed Kidney Injury in Uninsured and Underinsured Diabetic African American Men and Putative Role of Meprin Metalloproteases in Diabetic Nephropathy** 180
Lei Cao, Rashin Sedighi, Ava Boston, Lakmini Premadasa, Jamilla Pinder, George E. Crawford, Olugbemiga E. Jegede, Scott H. Harrison, Robert H. Newman and Elimelda Moige Ongeri

Chapter 25   **Murine Nephrotoxic Nephritis as a Model of Chronic Kidney Disease** 196
M. K. E. Ougaard, P. H. Kvist, H. E. Jensen, C. Hess, I. Rune and H. Søndergaard

Chapter 26   **Contrast-Induced Nephropathy: Update on the use of Crystalloids and Pharmacological Measures** 208
D. Patschan, I. Buschmann and O. Ritter

Chapter 27   **Prevalence of Microalbuminuria in Adult Patients with Sickle Cell Disease** 216
Ahmed M. Alkhunaizi, Adil A. Al-Khatti and Mansour A. Alkhunaizi

Chapter 28   **Matrix Metalloproteinases and Subclinical Atherosclerosis in Chronic Kidney Disease** 221
Andreas Kousios, Panayiotis Kouis and Andrie G. Panayiotou

Chapter 29   **Dialysate White Blood Cell Change after Initial Antibiotic Treatment Represented the Patterns of Response in Peritoneal Dialysis-Related Peritonitis** 232
Pichaya Tantiyavarong, Opas Traitanon, Piyatida Chuengsaman, Jayanton Patumanond and Adis Tasanarong

Permissions

List of Contributors

Index

Preface

Nephrology is a branch of medicine. It studies the functioning of kidneys and their diseases. Some common kidney diseases are kidney stones, acute renal failure and chronic kidney disease. Kidney stones are the solid pieces of material in the urinary tract. They can cause blockage of the ureter which may result in severe pain in the back and abdomen. Acute renal failure is associated with sudden kidney failure or kidney damage that develops within a few hours or a few days. Chronic kidney disease is an illness in which the loss of kidney functioning occurs gradually over a few months or years. This book traces the progress of the field of nephrology and highlights some of its key aspects. It aims to shed light on some of the unexplored aspects and the recent researches in this field. For all those who are interested in nephrology, this book can prove to be an essential guide.

This book unites the global concepts and researches in an organized manner for a comprehensive understanding of the subject. It is a ripe text for all researchers, students, scientists or anyone else who is interested in acquiring a better knowledge of this dynamic field.

I extend my sincere thanks to the contributors for such eloquent research chapters. Finally, I thank my family for being a source of support and help.

Editor

Incidence, Severity, and Outcomes of Acute Kidney Injury in Octogenarians following Heart Valve Replacement Surgery

Michael A. Mao,[1] Charat Thongprayoon,[2] YiFan Wu,[1] Vickram Tejwani,[1] Myriam Vela-Ortiz,[1] Joseph Dearani,[3] and Qi Qian[1]

[1]*Division of Nephrology and Hypertension, Department of Medicine, Mayo Clinic College of Medicine, Rochester, MN 55905, USA*
[2]*Division of Anesthesiology, Mayo Clinic College of Medicine, Rochester, MN 55905, USA*
[3]*Department of Surgery, Mayo Clinic College of Medicine, Rochester, MN 55905, USA*

Correspondence should be addressed to Qi Qian; qian.qi@mayo.edu

Academic Editor: Danuta Zwolinska

Background. The study investigates the occurrence, severity, and outcomes of acute kidney injury (AKI) in octogenarians following heart valve surgery. *Methods.* All patients, age >80 years, not on dialysis and without kidney transplant, undergoing heart valve replacement at Mayo Clinic, Rochester, in the years 2002-2003 were enrolled. AKI was diagnosed based on AKIN criteria. *Results.* 209 octogenarians (88.0% aortic valve, 6.2% mitral valve, 1.0% tricuspid valve, and 4.8% multivalve) with (58.4%) and without CABG were studied. 34 (16.3%) had preexisting CKD. After surgery, 98 (46.8%) developed AKI. 76.5% of the AKI were in Stage 1, 9.2% in Stage 2, and 14.3% in Stage 3. 76.5% CKD patients developed AKI. Length of hospital stay was longer for AKI patients. More AKI patients were discharged to care facilities. Patient survival at 30 days and 1 year for AKI versus non-AKI was 88.8 versus 98.7%, $p = 0.003$, and 76.5 versus 88.3%, $p = 0.025$, respectively. With follow-up of 3.94 ± 0.28 years, Kaplan-Meier analysis showed a reduced survival for AKI octogenarians. Preexisting CKD and large volume intraoperative fluid administration were independent AKI predictors. *Conclusions.* Nearly half of the octogenarians developed AKI after valve replacement surgery. AKI was associated with significant functional impairment and reduced survival.

1. Introduction

Population is aging in the United States and nearly worldwide [1]. The US Census Bureau projects that the very elderly population (age ≥ 80) will grow from 5.8 million (1.8% of the population) in 2012 to 13 million (3.2%) by 2050 [2]. Heart valves are well known to degenerate with aging, affecting up to 13.2% patients age ≥75 years [3]. With limited nonsurgical treatment options for valvular heart diseases and significant clinical morbidity and mortality, it is foreseeable that valve replacement operations will be performed for more elderly in the future [3–7]. With limited organ function reserve, increasing comorbidities, and reduced adaptive capacity, the elderly are at high risk for postoperative complications such as AKI [8]. Aging alone is a significant risk factor for AKI [9], and the severity of AKI is proportional to the poor outcomes including morbidity and mortality [10]. Data on the incidence, severity, and outcomes of AKI in octogenarians undergoing heart valve surgery is, however, scarce [5].

The aim of this study is to determine AKI occurrence, severity, and outcomes in a cohort of octogenarians undergoing valve replacement surgery. We also explore potential predictors for the development of AKI in this cohort.

2. Patients and Methods

2.1. Data Collection and AKI Definitions. The Institutional Review Board approved the study. Between 2002 and 2003, 210 octogenarians with symptomatic cardiac valve disease underwent valve replacement surgery who were not on hemodialysis and without kidney transplant. The Charlson Comorbidity Index at the time of admission was collected for each patient [11]. Survival was censored based on death dates in the institutional records and publically accessible Social Security Death Index http://www.genealogybank.com/gbnk/ssdi/.

Preexisting chronic kidney disease (CKD) was defined based on primary physician's documentation within six months of the surgery. Baseline serum creatinine (s.Cr, in mg/dL) was defined as the s.Cr measurement within three months of the index admission. Estimated GFR was calculated based on the Chronic Kidney Disease Epidemiology Collaboration (CKD-EPI) [12]. The patients were grouped based on their eGFR. One patient who expired intraoperatively was excluded from analysis.

Acute kidney injury (AKI) was defined as an abrupt (within 48 hours) increase in s.Cr ≥ 0.3 mg/dL or s.Cr increase by 50% from baseline within seven days postoperatively. The AKIN urinary criteria were omitted due to incomplete data on urine output [13]. The severity of AKI was determined using s.Cr definitions from the AKIN criteria [13]. The AKIN criteria classify AKI into the following: Stage 1, s.Cr elevation ≥ 1.5 times the baseline s.Cr; Stage 2, ≥ 2 times the baseline s.Cr; Stage 3, ≥ 3 times the baseline s.Cr, s.Cr ≥ 4.0 mg/dL or complete loss of kidney function requiring renal replacement therapy.

Net fluid balance equaled to fluid input minus fluid output (in liters).

2.2. Statistical Analysis. Statistical analysis was performed using JMP version 10.0.0. For categorical variables, Fisher's exact test and Pearson's chi-squared test were utilized. For continuous variables, Student's t-test was applied for comparison between the AKI and non-AKI cohorts. The results are reported as percentage frequencies and means ± standard deviation (SD). p value of <0.05 (two-tailed) was considered significant. Stepwise backward logistic regressions were performed to derive the final multivariate model taking into consideration colinearity, interaction, and number of patients who expressed the outcome of interest. Cox proportional hazard regression modeling was used to compare survival in the two cohorts adjusted for age and comorbidity. Kaplan-Meier analysis was used to compare the long-term survival.

3. Results

3.1. Patient Characteristics. The 209 octogenarians represented 16% of the total patients undergoing valve replacement surgery at Mayo Clinic Rochester in 2002 and 2003. 184 (88.0%) of the 209 underwent aortic valve replacement (AVR), 13 (6.2%) mitral valve replacement (MVR), 2 (1.0%) tricuspid valve replacement (TVR), and 10 (4.8%) combined valve replacement (6 AV-MV, 1 AV-TV, 2 MV-TV, and 1 PV-TV). All but one patient had bioprosthetic replacement valves. Preoperative characteristics of the cohort showed a median age of 84.1 years and a mean Charlson comorbidity score [11] of 2.63 ± 1.76 (Table 1). 127 (60.8%) patients had preexisting hypertension and 35 (16.7%) patients had a prior myocardial infarction. Thirty-four (16.3%) patients had a diagnosis of CKD with a mean s.Cr of 1.7 ± 0.31 mg/dL corresponding to an eGFR of 34.3 ± 10.0 mL/min/BSA,

TABLE 1: Preoperative characteristics of octogenarians.

Baseline characteristics	$N = 209$
Age (year) at surgery, median [range]	84.1 [80.1–93.4]
Males (%)	115 (55.0)
Race (%)	Caucasian 175 (83.7)
	Other: 32 (15.3)
	Black: 1 (0.48)
BMI, mean ± SD	27.7 ± 5.3
HTN (%)	127 (60.8)
Diabetes (%)	40 (19.1)
CKD (%)	34 (16.3)
CHF (%)	167 (79.9)
Prior MI (%)	35 (16.7)
Hyperlipidemia on lipid-lowering agents (%)	104 (49.8)
Charlson Index, mean ± SD	2.63 ± 1.76
Baseline Cr, mean ± SD	1.24 ± 0.30
eGFR, mean ± SD	49.79 ± 12.79
Pre-op EF %, mean ± SD	54.6 ± 14.9

whereas 175 non-CKD patients had s.Cr of 1.15 ± 0.20 mg/dL, eGFR of 52.8 ± 11.0 mL/min/BSA, $p < 0.0001$ (Table 2).

3.2. AKI Occurrence and Severity. Ninety-eight of 209 patients (46.8%) developed postoperative AKI, of which 13 (6.2%) required renal replacement therapy (7 from the CKD group and 6 from the non-CKD group). The majority of AKIs were within AKIN Stage 1 (risk). Patients with preexisting CKD were at higher risk for postoperative AKI, 26 (76.5%) versus 72 (41.1%) in non-CKD, $p = 0.0002$. AKI in CKD patients were more severe, 26.9% versus 9.7% in Stage 3 (Table 2).

Prior studies show that, among octogenarians undergoing AVR, age ≥ 84 years had the highest odds ratio for 6-month mortality [14]. We examined AKI occurrence in octogenarians age <84 and ≥ 84. The eGFR was different, 52.5 mL/min/BSA in those age <84 ($N = 101$) and 47.2 mL/min/BSA in age ≥ 84 ($N = 108$), $p = 0.003$. However, the AKI occurrence between the two age groups did not differ, 44.4 versus 49.5%, $p > 0.05$. The proportion of AKI patients in Stages 1, 2, and 3 was also not different in the two age groups. The 6-month mortality rate was likewise comparable, 12.9 versus 12.0%, $p > 0.05$.

We also compared those with and without concomitant coronary artery bypass grafting (CABG), as previous studies had shown conflicting results on the effect of concomitant CABG on mortality [5, 7, 14]. In our cohort, CABG did not increase postoperative AKI. One-year mortality rate in the two groups was comparable, 13.9% with CABG versus 21.8% without CABG, $p = 0.14$. The number of bypassed vessels did not affect the 30-day, 6-month, or 1-year mortality (data not shown).

3.3. Characteristics of AKI versus Non-AKI Patients. Patient characteristics in AKI and non-AKI were compared. AKI patients tended to have preexisting CKD, prior myocardial

Incidence, Severity, and Outcomes of Acute Kidney Injury in Octogenarians following Heart Valve...

3

TABLE 2: AKI occurrence and severity in CKD and non-CKD patients.

Baseline CKD status	All $n = 209$	CKD $n = 34$	Non-CKD $n = 175$	p value
Presurgery s.Cr, mg/dL	1.24 (0.30)	1.70 ± 0.31	1.15 ± 0.20	<0.0001
Presurgery eGFR	49.8 (12.8)	34.3 ± 10.0	52.8 ± 11.0	<0.0001
Calculated CKD stage[*]				
CKD Stage 1	0	0	0	
CKD Stage 2	45 (21.5)	1 (2.9)	44 (25.1)	0.004
CKD Stage 3a	93 (44.5)	4 (11.8)	89 (50.9)	<0.0001
CKD Stage 3b	57 (27.3)	17 (50.0)	40 (22.9)	0.0011
CKD Stage 4	14 (6.7)	12 (35.3)	2 (1.1)	<0.0001
CKD Stage 5	0	0	0	
Total AKI number (%)	98 (46.8)	26 (76.5)	72 (41.1)	0.0002
Stage 1	75 (76.5)	17 (65.4)	58 (80.6)	
Stage 2	9 (9.2)	2 (7.7)	7 (9.7)	0.0001
Stage 3	14 (14.3)	7 (26.9)[a]	7 (9.7)[b]	

[a]7 of 7 in CKD and [b]6 of 7 in non-CKD required dialysis.
[*]Stratified by eGFR instead of physician's diagnosis of CKD.

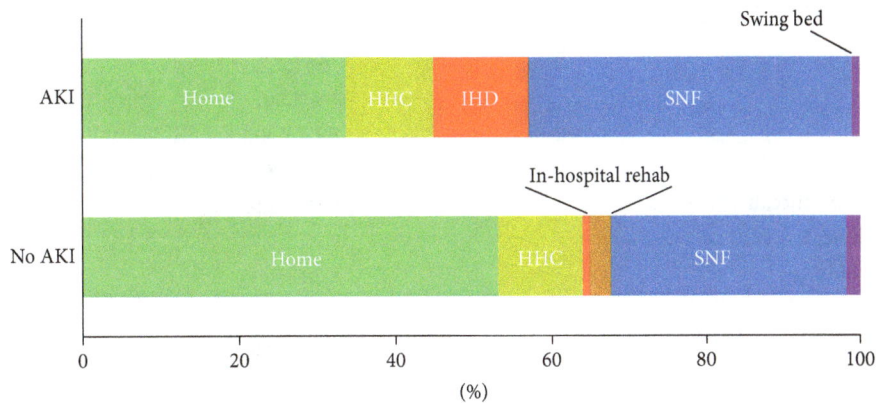

Count	Home	Home health care (HHC)	In-hospital death (IHD)	In-hospital rehab (IHR)	Skilled nursing facility (SNF)	Swing bed	Total
AKI ($n = 98$)	33 (33.7%)	11 (11.2%)	12 (12.2%)	0	41 (41.8%)	1 (1.0%)	98
No AKI ($n = 111$)	59 (53.2%)	12 (10.8%)	1 (0.9%)	3 (2.7%)	34 (30.6%)	2 (1.8%)	111

FIGURE 1: Patient disposition.

infarction, higher Charlson Comorbidity Index, and lower preoperative hemoglobin (Table 3). Intraoperative factors associated with AKI included longer surgical duration, intra-aortic balloon pump use, lower intraoperative nadir hemoglobin, and higher volume of blood transfusion and fluids/saline infusion (Table 3). Additionally, AKI patients were possibly more likely to have a higher BMI and atherosclerotic vascular diseases, although p value did not reach statistical significance.

3.4. Predictors for AKI. Potential AKI predictors in this cohort of octogenarians were explored. Univariate analysis showed prior MI, CKD, higher Charlson Comorbidity Index, lower preoperative hemoglobin, longer surgical duration,

blood transfusion, and intraoperative fluid and saline administration as potential risk factors. Two models of multivariate stepwise backward logistic regression analysis were built. Preexisting CKD (OR 4.87–5.38, 95% CI 2.12–13.6, $p <$ 0.001), intraoperative fluid administration (OR 1.10, CI 1.01–1.21, $p = 0.03$) and intraoperative saline infusion (OR 1.52, CI 1.05–2.24, $p = 0.02$) were shown as independent predictors for AKI (Tables 4(a) and 4(b)).

3.5. Length of Hospital Stay and Disposition. Length of hospital stay (LOS) was longer for AKI patients 14.0 ± 11.7 days versus 9.2 ± 4.2 days for non-AKI patients, $p < 0.0001$. Patient disposition was different in octogenarians with and without AKI (Figure 1, $p = 0.001$). More AKI patients discharged

TABLE 3: Preoperative characteristics and hospital course in AKI and non-AKI octogenarians.

Preoperative characteristics	No AKI, mean ± SD, $n = 111$	AKI, mean ± SD, $n = 98$	p value
Age, median [range]	84.1 ± 2.8 [80.1–93.4]	83.9 ± 2.8 [80.1–92.0]	0.49
Sex, male (%)	57 (51.3)	58 (59.2)	0.26
BMI, kg/m^2	27.1 ± 4.9	28.4 ± 5.7	0.09
HTN (%)	72 (64.9)	55 (56.1)	0.20
Diabetes (%)	18 (16.2)	22 (22.4)	0.25
Hyperlipidemia on lipid-lowering agents (%)	62 (55.9)	42 (42.9)	0.06
Chronic pulmonary disease (%)	19 (17.1)	14 (14.3)	0.58
Preexisting CKD (%)	8 (7.2)	26 (26.5)	<0.0001
Prior myocardial infarction (%)	12 (10.8)	23 (23.5)	0.01
CAD (%)	78 (70.3)	65 (66.3)	0.54
Peripheral vascular, cerebrovascular, or carotid artery disease (%)	29 (26.1)	36 (36.7)	0.10
CHF (%)	94 (84.7)	73 (74.5)	0.07
Charlson Comorbidity Index	2.39	2.91	0.03
Pre-op EF, %	53.7 ± 15.5	55.7 ± 14.3	0.34
Pre-op hemoglobin, g/dL	12.8 ± 1.6	11.9 ± 1.6	0.03
Hospital course			
Surgical duration, min	331.0 ± 82.8	369.1 ± 108.5	0.005
CABG, yes or no (%)	64 (57.7)	58 (59.2)	0.82
IABP (%)	2 (1.80)	9 (9.18)	0.02
Cross clamp time, min	69.7 ± 30.1	69.0 ± 32.3	0.85
CPB, min	96.7 ± 39.3	101.3 ± 43.3	0.42
Net intraoperative fluid balance, L	6.87 ± 2.57	8.12 ± 4.28	0.01
Total intraoperative saline, L	0.90 ± 0.72	1.16 ± 0.95	0.02
Intraoperative hemoglobin, g/dL[a]	8.28 ± 1.04	7.92 ± 1.04	0.01
RBC on operative day, L	0.74 ± 0.63	1.06 ± 1.03	0.008
RBC during hospitalization, L	0.92 ± 0.86	1.54 ± 1.65	0.0007
Length of hospital stay, day	9.2 ± 4.2 ($n = 110$)	14.0 ± 11.7 ($n = 86$)	<0.0001
Discharge creatinine, mg/dL	1.09 ± 0.25	1.46 ± 0.56	<0.0001

[a]The lowest hemoglobin during the operation.

TABLE 4: Multivariate stepwise logistic regression models for predictors of postoperative AKI.

(a) Model number 1

Variables	OR (95% CI)	p value
CHF	0.43 (0.21–0.88)	0.02
CKD	4.87 (2.12–12.3)	<0.001
Intraoperative fluid volume	1.10 (1.01–1.21)	0.03

(b) Model number 2

Variables	OR (95% CI)	p value
CHF	0.43 (0.21–0.87)	0.02
CKD	5.38 (2.34–13.6)	<0.001
Intraoperative saline volume	1.52 (1.05–2.24)	0.02

to skilled nursing facilities (41.8% AKI versus 30.6% non-AKI) and fewer to home (33.7% AKI versus 53.2% non-AKI),

reflecting a higher level of functional impairment in patients with AKI, which is known to be associated with a high long-term mortality rate [15]. The disposition to a swing bed, another hospital adjacent to patient's home, was not different between the AKI and non-AKI groups.

3.6. Renal and Patient Outcomes. Among surviving AKI patients, s.Cr at the time of hospital discharge was higher in AKI patients, 1.46 ± 0.56 mg/dL versus 1.09 ± 0.25 mg/dL in non-AKI patients, $p < 0.0001$. Long-term follow-up for s.Cr values after hospitalization was limited by our hospital being a large referral center. Many patients received their nonsurgical care at local care facilities geographically removed from Mayo Clinic. For those who continued regular nonsurgical follow-up with us, a persistent separation of s.Cr values between the AKI and non-AKI groups was observed (Figure 2(a)).

Early postoperative mortality rates were dramatically different in AKI versus non-AKI octogenarians. In-hospital

TABLE 5: (a) Unadjusted Cox proportional hazard ratio for one-year mortality by AKI stage. (b) Adjusted Cox proportional hazard ratio for one-year mortality by AKI stage.

(a)

AKI stage	HR (95% CI)	p value
No AKI	1	Reference
Stage 1	1.04 (0.4–2.4)	0.92
Stage 2	3.7 (0.8–11.4)	0.08
Stage 3	15.9 (6.9–36.3)	<0.0001

Unadjusted.

(b)

AKI stage	HR (95% CI)	p value
No AKI	1	Reference
Stage 1	1.0 (0.4–2.4)	0.95
Stage 2	3.1 (0.7–10.3)	0.13
Stage 3	13.6 (5.4–33.9)	<0.0001

Adjusted for age and Charlson comorbidity score.

mortality in AKI patients was >10-fold higher than the mortality in non-AKI octogenarians, 12.2% versus 0.9%, p = 0.0003. 30-day postsurgery mortality for AKI group was 10.2% versus 0.9% in non-AKI groups, p = 0.003. For the 13 AKI patients who required dialysis, 46% died within 30 days after surgery, 84.6% died within 1 year, and 92.3% died within 5 years (Figure 2(b)). Only two of the dialysis patients were able to come off dialysis at the time of discharge.

Late postoperative mortality rates were different between AKI and non-AKI octogenarians. AKI patients showed a 1-year mortality of 23.5% versus 11.7% in non-AKI patients, p = 0.02. Figure 2(c) shows 1-year survival in non-AKI and AKI (Stages 1–3) octogenarians. Kaplan-Meier analysis of survival in non-AKI and AKI octogenarians with a mean follow-up of 3.94 ± 4.04 years demonstrates a higher mortality rate in postoperative AKI octogenarians than those without AKI, p = 0.02 (Figure 2(d)).

Unadjusted Cox proportional hazard model showed that AKI Stage 3 was a significant contributor to 1-year patient mortality and AKI Stage 2 was nearly significant (Table 5(a)). Cox proportional hazard model adjusted for age and Charlson comorbidity score showed that AKI Stage 3 independently contributed to the 1-year mortality, HR 13.6, 95% CI: 5.4–33.9, p < 0.0001 (Table 5(b)).

4. Comment

In this study of octogenarians undergoing heart valve replacement surgery, we show that the incidence of postoperative AKI was nearly 50%. Moreover, AKI occurrence is associated with a prolonged hospital stay, increased need for higher level of care following discharge, persistently reduced kidney function, and reduced short-term and long-term patient survival.

Demand for heart valvular surgery in octogenarians is expected to increase as the population ages [3–7, 16]. Studies have shown that valve replacement surgeries have acceptable mortality rates in the very elderly [6, 16]. At Mayo Clinic Rochester, over 16% of valve replacement surgeries in 2002 and 2003 were performed for octogenarians. Although less invasive transcatheter aortic valve implantation (TAVI) has recently been introduced into practice, there has been wide center-to-center variation in the rates of postprocedural complications (AKI, stroke, and mortality), 4.7 to over 20% [17, 18], and the procedure is limited to the aortic valve replacement. Conventional valve surgery remains the standard of care.

Older age and preexisting CKD are major risk factors for AKI [19, 20]. AKI in hospitalized patients tends to progress to end-stage renal failure, especially for the elderly [21], and raises mortality. AKI is known to occur after cardiac surgery and is correlated with mortality [22]. Studies in octogenarians undergoing heart valve replacement have been limited. Available studies examine primarily postoperative mortality; when renal impairments are mentioned, no specific definitions, such as AKIN/RIFLE criteria, were applied [6, 7, 23–25]. The 30-day mortality rates in most studies range from 3.4 to 8.5% after aortic valve replacement [6, 7, 14, 16, 23–28] and 18.2 to 18.5% after mitral valve replacement [5]. One-year mortality ranges from 7.1 to 35%. [6, 7, 14, 25, 28]. The current study, involving all valve replacement surgeries in 209 octogenarians, shows a 30-day mortality of ~5% and 1-year mortality of 17%, roughly in line with previous study results. New to the existing literature is that deaths in this cohort of octogenarians occurred almost exclusively in those with AKI (Table 5(a)). Notably, a small preoperative s.Cr difference of ~0.5 mg/dL between non-CKD and CKD patients reflected an eGFR difference of ~20 mL/min/BSA (from 52.8 to 34.3 mL/min/BSA) and nearly a doubling of AKI occurrence. Moreover, longer follow-up allowed for long-term outcome assessment, showing a persistently poor kidney function and higher mortality among AKI octogenarians.

Predictors for AKI by univariate analysis in this cohort of octogenarians were a higher Charlson Comorbidity Index, preexisting CKD, prior myocardial infarction, preoperative anemia, surgical duration, intraoperative fluid administration, low intraoperative hemoglobin, and blood transfusion. Stepwise multivariate analysis adjusting for relevant univariate risk factors showed that CHF, CKD, total intraoperative fluids, and saline infusion are independent predictors for postoperative AKI in this cohort of octogenarians (Tables 4(a) and 4(b)). Excessive intravenous fluids, especially 0.9% saline, have been associated with the development of postoperative complications and AKI [29–32]. Volume overload in the setting of AKI has been shown to be associated with poor clinical outcomes including mortality [33].

Cox proportional hazard regression was performed to explore survival differences between AKI and non-AKI octogenarians adjusted for age and comorbidity (Table 5). Mortality rates in AKI octogenarians were ~10%, 25%, and 50% in 30 days, 1 year, and 5 years, respectively. Although difficult to make a direct comparison, our results are not inferior to the mortality rates in previous studies inclusive of adult AKI patients of all ages showing in-hospital mortality rates of ~ 20–50% [10, 34, 35]. Among 13 dialysis octogenarians in the current study, 46% died at 30 days after operation. Despite a

(a)

(b)

(c)

(d)

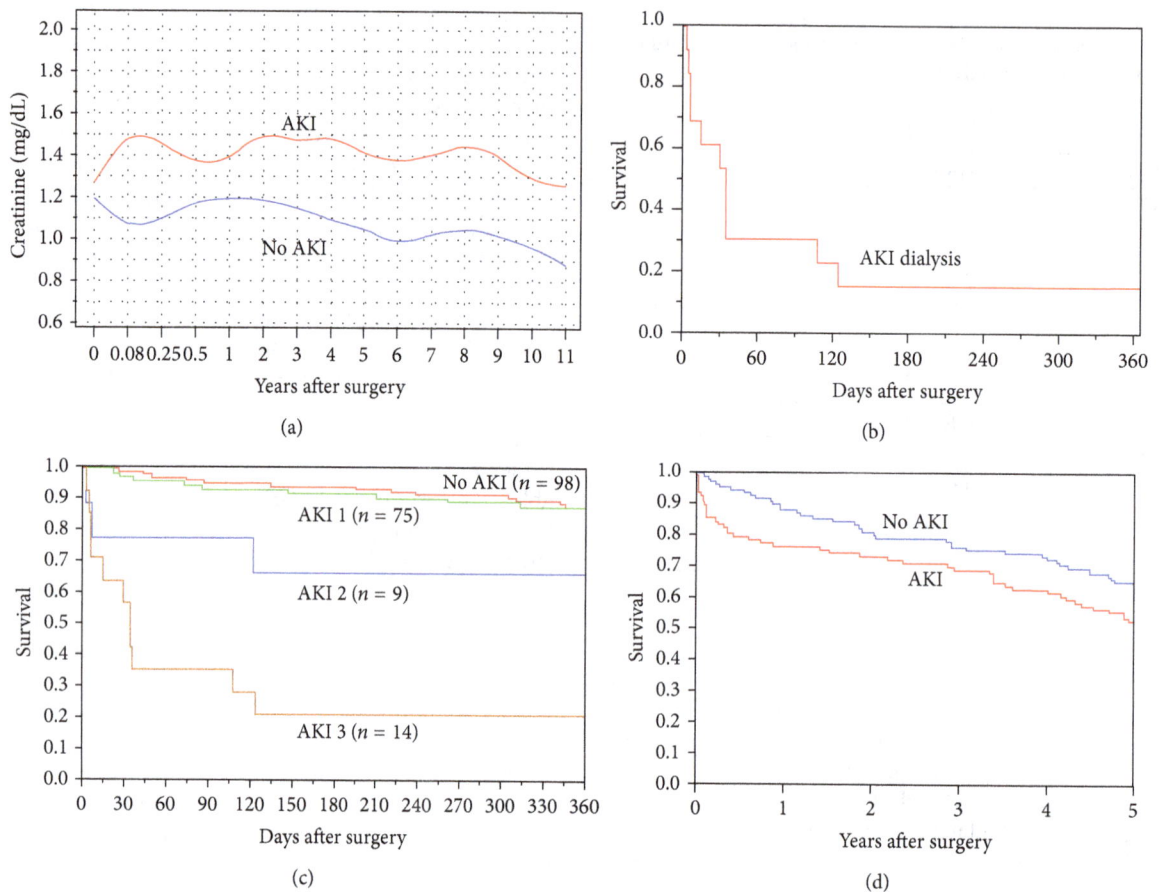

FIGURE 2: Patient survival. (a) Long-term s.Cr in AKI and non-AKI octogenarians. (b) Kaplan-Meier 1-year survival in octogenarians with AKI requiring dialysis ($n = 13$). (c) Kaplan-Meier 1-year survival by AKI Stages versus non-AKI, unadjusted log-rank $p < 0.0001$. (d) Kaplan-Meier survival curves, AKI versus non-AKI patients, log-rank $p = 0.016$. The adjusted[a] HR for AKI 2.02; 95% CI 1.01–4.04, $p = 0.04$.

high mortality rate, it is not inferior to the results generated in nonelderly adult AKI-dialysis patients of 55% [36].

In the current study, concomitant CABG or number of coronary vessels bypassed did not increase the rate of AKI (Table 2) or mortality, consistent with previous studies showing no mortality impact in concomitant CABG to valve surgery [5, 7]. There were, however, also studies showing an increase or decrease in mortality in valve surgery with CABG [14, 23, 24]. Given the limited patient number, our results should be viewed with caution. Further study with larger patient number is necessary.

Florath et al. [14] reported mortality rates of 8.4% at 30 days, 15.2% at 6 months, and 26% at 1 year in octogenarians undergoing AVR. An age >84 years was related to poor survival. We did not find age >84 to have been associated with higher AKI or mortality. This discrepancy could have been due to a small difference in eGFR and similar Charlson Index in our cohorts. Chiappini et al. showed [26] that the predictors for mortality in octogenarians following AVR are poor preoperative EF and heart failure. Our data did not show these being the significant risks for AKI or mortality, although our study patients might be different from theirs. No studies, however, have explored in detail the relationship between post-valve-surgery AKI and patient's outcomes

including disposition, long-term kidney function, and patient survival in octogenarians, as shown in the current study.

Approximately two-thirds of AKI progress to a severe stage [37], which is associated with a further increase in mortality. Nephrology involvement in their care can potentially mitigate progression of AKI and its sequelae. Our results support the early involvement of nephrology in the care of octogenarians with AKI, especially for those with reduced preoperative eGFR and those with a small increase in postsurgery s.Cr (≥ 0.3 mg/dL). In practice, nephrology referral for octogenarian AKI patients has been low at ~20% [38]. That said, confirmatory evidence of the beneficial effects of nephrology involvement should be further studied.

Several limitations in this study should be considered. First, the nature of the observational cohort study limited consistency in the timing of laboratory testing for creatinine and hemoglobin values, which could influence their values. However, surgical patients are unique in that we knew precisely the time of insult (surgery). Furthermore, a single center study prevented large variation in practice and routine blood draws were relatively fixed in time of day. Second, our data were collected in 2002 and 2003, which may not precisely reflect present-day outcomes. However, there has not been a major practice change in valve replacement surgery, and data over an uninterrupted period allowed longitudinal follow-up of patients' outcomes. Third, the majority of our patients are Caucasian, with only one black patient and a few patients of other races, which limits the application of our results to other races. Fourth, AKI patients received more intravenous fluids, which could dilute s.Cr and underestimate AKI severity. However, even with this limitation, we still found significant poor clinical outcomes associated with AKI. Fifth, data on the administration of hydroxyethyl starch (HES) and aprotinin, known to be associated with AKI [39, 40], were not analyzed because these agents were used occasionally and unlikely to have affected the results. Lastly, the association between AKI and poor clinical outcomes could potentially be affected by the preexisting CKD. The strong effect of CKD may hinder the determination of true impact of AKI on patients' outcomes. Nonetheless, severe AKI stood out as an independent risk factor for mortality in our cohort. We believe that even mild-to-moderate degrees of AKI could potentially exert negative impact on patient survival, although the signal may have been overwhelmed by the extraordinarily strong effect of preexisting CKD. Taken together, CKD is a strong reason for increased mortality after AKI, but AKI independently contributed to the poor patient outcomes.

Overall, our data show that octogenarians are able to tolerate heart valve replacement surgery. However, the AKI occurrence rate is substantial and AKI impacts patients' mortality and morbidity. Better patient selection, preoperative preparation, and avoidance of operative risk factors can minimize the AKI risk and adverse consequences.

References

[1] United Nations DoEaSA and Population Division, *World Population Ageing 2013*, United Nations Publication, 2013.

[2] J. M. Ortman, V. A. Velkoff, and H. Hogan, "An aging nation: the older population in the United States," Tech. Rep. P25-1140, United States Census Bureau, 2014.

[3] V. T. Nkomo, J. M. Gardin, T. N. Skelton, J. S. Gottdiener, C. G. Scott, and M. Enriquez-Sarano, "Burden of valvular heart diseases: a population-based study," *The Lancet*, vol. 368, no. 9540, pp. 1005–1011, 2006.

[4] G. Asimakopoulos, M.-B. Edwards, and K. M. Taylor, "Aortic valve replacement in patients 80 years of age and older: Survival and cause of death based on 1100 cases—collective results from the UK heart valve registry," *Circulation*, vol. 96, no. 10, pp. 3403–3408, 1997.

[5] J. Nloga, R. Hénaine, M. Vergnat et al., "Mitral valve surgery in octogenarians: should we fight for repair? A survival and quality-of-life assessment," *European Journal of Cardio-thoracic Surgery*, vol. 39, no. 6, pp. 875–880, 2011.

[6] D. Calvo, I. Lozano, J. C. Llosa et al., "Aortic valve replacement in octogenarians with severe aortic stenosis. Experience in a series of consecutive patients at a single center," *Revista Espanola de Cardiologia*, vol. 60, no. 7, pp. 720–726, 2007.

[7] J. A. Ditchfield, E. Granger, P. Spratt et al., "Aortic valve replacement in octogenarians," *Heart Lung and Circulation*, vol. 23, no. 9, pp. 841–846, 2014.

[8] R. Prêtre and M. I. Turina, "Cardiac valve surgery in the octogenarian," *Heart*, vol. 83, no. 1, pp. 116–121, 2000.

[9] T. Z. Ali, I. Khan, W. Simpson et al., "Incidence and outcomes in acute kidney injury: a comprehensive population-based study," *Journal of the American Society of Nephrology*, vol. 18, no. 4, pp. 1292–1298, 2007.

[10] S. Uchino, R. Bellomo, D. Goldsmith, S. Bates, and C. Ronco, "An assessment of the RIFLE criteria for acute renal failure in hospitalized patients," *Critical Care Medicine*, vol. 34, no. 7, pp. 1913–1917, 2006.

[11] M. E. Charlson, P. Pompei, K. A. Ales, and C. R. MacKenzie, "A new method of classifying prognostic comorbidity in longitudinal studies: development and validation," *Journal of Chronic Diseases*, vol. 40, no. 5, pp. 373–383, 1987.

[12] H. S. Kilbride, P. E. Stevens, G. Eaglestone et al., "Accuracy of the MDRD (Modification of Diet in Renal Disease) study and CKD-EPI (CKD Epidemiology Collaboration) equations for estimation of GFR in the elderly," *American Journal of Kidney Diseases*, vol. 61, no. 1, pp. 57–66, 2013.

[13] R. L. Mehta, J. A. Kellum, S. V. Shah et al., "Acute Kidney Injury Network: report of an initiative to improve outcomes in acute kidney injury," *Critical Care*, vol. 11, no. 2, article R31, 2007.

[14] I. Florath, A. Albert, A. Boening, I. C. Ennker, and J. Ennker, "Aortic valve replacement in octogenarians: identification of high-risk patients," *European Journal of Cardio-Thoracic Surgery*, vol. 37, no. 6, pp. 1304–1310, 2010.

[15] L. Henry, L. Halpin, S. Hunt, S. D. Holmes, and N. Ad, "Patient disposition and long-term outcomes after valve surgery in octogenarians," *Annals of Thoracic Surgery*, vol. 94, no. 3, pp. 744–750, 2012.

[16] T. Langanay, E. Flécher, O. Fouquet et al., "Aortic valve replacement in the elderly: the real life," *Annals of Thoracic Surgery*, vol. 93, no. 1, pp. 70–78, 2012.

[17] M. Rahnavardi, J. Santibanez, K. Sian, and T. D. Yan, "A systematic review of transapical aortic valve implantation," *Annals of Cardiothoracic Surgery*, vol. 1, no. 2, pp. 116–128, 2012.

[18] D. Dvir, J. G. Webb, S. Bleiziffer et al., "Transcatheter aortic valve implantation in failed bioprosthetic surgical valves," *The Journal of the American Medical Association*, vol. 312, no. 2, pp. 162–170, 2014.

[19] K. Nash, A. Hafeez, and S. Hou, "Hospital-acquired renal insufficiency," *American Journal of Kidney Diseases*, vol. 39, no. 5, pp. 930–936, 2002.

[20] C.-Y. Hsu, C. E. McCulloch, D. Fan, J. D. Ordoñez, G. M. Chertow, and A. S. Go, "Community-based incidence of acute renal failure," *Kidney International*, vol. 72, no. 2, pp. 208–212, 2007.

[21] A. Ishani, J. L. Xue, J. Himmelfarb et al., "Acute kidney injury increases risk of ESRD among elderly," *Journal of the American Society of Nephrology*, vol. 20, no. 1, pp. 223–228, 2009.

[22] A. Ishani, D. Nelson, B. Clothier et al., "The magnitude of acute serum creatinine increase after cardiac surgery and the risk of chronic kidney disease, progression of kidney disease, and death," *Archives of Internal Medicine*, vol. 171, no. 3, pp. 226–233, 2011.

[23] K. P. Alexander, K. J. Anstrom, L. H. Muhlbaier et al., "Outcomes of cardiac surgery in patients age ≥ 80 years: results from the national cardiovascular network," *Journal of the American College of Cardiology*, vol. 35, no. 3, pp. 731–738, 2000.

[24] S. J. Melby, A. Zierer, S. P. Kaiser et al., "Aortic valve replacement in octogenarians: risk factors for early and late mortality," *The Annals of Thoracic Surgery*, vol. 83, no. 5, pp. 1651–1657, 2007.

[25] V. H. Thourani, R. Myung, P. Kilgo et al., "Long-term outcomes after isolated aortic valve replacement in octogenarians: a modern perspective," *Annals of Thoracic Surgery*, vol. 86, no. 5, pp. 1458–1465, 2008.

[26] B. Chiappini, N. Camurri, A. Loforte, L. Di Marco, R. Di Bartolomeo, and G. Marinelli, "Outcome after aortic valve replacement in octogenarians," *Annals of Thoracic Surgery*, vol. 78, no. 1, pp. 85–89, 2004.

[27] A. Mortasawi, S. Gehle, M. Yaghmaie et al., "Short and long term results of aortic valve replacement in patients 80 years of age and older," *Herz*, vol. 26, no. 2, pp. 140–148, 2001.

[28] G. Rizzoli, J. Bejko, T. Bottio, V. Tarzia, and G. Gerosa, "Valve surgery in octogenarians: does it prolong life?" *European Journal of Cardio-Thoracic Surgery*, vol. 37, no. 5, pp. 1047–1055, 2010.

[29] N. M. Yunos, R. Bellomo, F. C. Hegarty, D. Story, L. Ho, and M. Bailey, "Association between a chloride-liberal vs chloride-restrictive intravenous fluid administration strategy and kidney injury in critically ill adults," *Journal of the American Medical Association*, vol. 308, no. 15, pp. 1566–1572, 2012.

[30] J. A. Kellum, "Fluid resuscitation and hyperchloremic acidosis in experimental sepsis: improved short-term survival and acid-base balance with Hextend compared with saline," *Critical Care Medicine*, vol. 30, no. 2, pp. 300–305, 2002.

[31] B. A. Cotton, J. S. Guy, J. A. Morris Jr., and N. N. Abumrad, "The cellular, metabolic, and systemic consequences of aggressive fluid resuscitation strategies," *Shock*, vol. 26, no. 2, pp. 115–121, 2006.

[32] B. Brandstrup, H. Tønnesen, R. Beier-Holgersen et al., "Effects of intravenous fluid restriction on postoperative complications: comparison of two perioperative fluid regimens: a randomized assessor-blinded multicenter trial," *Annals of Surgery*, vol. 238, no. 5, pp. 641–648, 2003.

[33] J. Bouchard, S. B. Soroko, G. M. Chertow et al., "Fluid accumulation, survival and recovery of kidney function in critically ill patients with acute kidney injury," *Kidney International*, vol. 76, no. 4, pp. 422–427, 2009.

[34] Y. Fang, X. Ding, Y. Zhong et al., "Acute kidney injury in a chinese hospitalized population," *Blood Purification*, vol. 30, no. 2, pp. 120–126, 2010.

[35] J.-P. Lafrance and D. R. Miller, "Acute kidney injury associates with increased long-term mortality," *Journal of the American Society of Nephrology*, vol. 21, no. 2, pp. 345–352, 2010.

[36] C. V. Thakar, S. Worley, S. Arrigain, J.-P. Yared, and E. P. Paganini, "Improved survival in acute kidney injury after cardiac surgery," *American Journal of Kidney Diseases*, vol. 50, no. 5, pp. 703–711, 2007.

[37] E. A. J. Hoste, G. Clermont, A. Kersten et al., "RIFLE criteria for acute kidney injury are associated with hospital mortality in critically ill patients: a cohort analysis," *Critical Care*, vol. 10, no. 3, article R73, 2006.

[38] T. Ali, A. Tachibana, I. Khan et al., "The changing pattern of referral in acute kidney injury," *QJM*, vol. 104, no. 6, pp. 497–503, 2011.

[39] J. A. Myburgh, S. Finfer, R. Bellomo et al., "Hydroxyethyl starch or saline for fluid resuscitation in intensive car," *The New England Journal of Medicine*, vol. 367, no. 20, pp. 1901–1911, 2012.

[40] D. T. Mangano, I. C. Tudor, and C. Dietzel, "The risk associated with aprotinin in cardiac surgery," *The New England Journal of Medicine*, vol. 354, no. 4, pp. 353–365, 2006.

Forecasting the Incidence and Prevalence of Patients with End-Stage Renal Disease in Malaysia up to the Year 2040

Mohamad Adam Bujang,[1] **Tassha Hilda Adnan,**[1] **Nadiah Hanis Hashim,**[1]
Kirubashni Mohan,[1] **Ang Kim Liong,**[2] **Ghazali Ahmad,**[3] **Goh Bak Leong,**[2,4]
Sunita Bavanandan,[3] **and Jamaiyah Haniff**[5]

[1]*National Clinical Research Centre, Kuala Lumpur, Malaysia*
[2]*Clinical Research Centre, Serdang Hospital, Kajang, Malaysia*
[3]*Department of Nephrology, Kuala Lumpur Hospital, Kuala Lumpur, Malaysia*
[4]*Department of Nephrology, Serdang Hospital, Kajang, Malaysia*
[5]*Malaysian Health Performance Unit, Ministry of Health, Kuala Lumpur, Malaysia*

Correspondence should be addressed to Mohamad Adam Bujang; adam@crc.gov.my

Academic Editor: Tej Mattoo

Background. The incidence of patients with end-stage renal disease (ESRD) requiring dialysis has been growing rapidly in Malaysia from 18 per million population (pmp) in 1993 to 231 pmp in 2013. *Objective.* To forecast the incidence and prevalence of ESRD patients who will require dialysis treatment in Malaysia until 2040. *Methodology.* Univariate forecasting models using the number of new and current dialysis patients, by the Malaysian Dialysis and Transplant Registry from 1993 to 2013 were used. Four forecasting models were evaluated, and the model with the smallest error was selected for the prediction. *Result.* ARIMA (0, 2, 1) modeling with the lowest error was selected to predict both the incidence (RMSE = 135.50, MAPE = 2.85, and MAE = 87.71) and the prevalence (RMSE = 158.79, MAPE = 1.29, and MAE = 117.21) of dialysis patients. The estimated incidences of new dialysis patients in 2020 and 2040 are 10,208 and 19,418 cases, respectively, while the estimated prevalence is 51,269 and 106,249 cases. *Conclusion.* The growth of ESRD patients on dialysis in Malaysia can be expected to continue at an alarming rate. Effective steps to address and curb further increase in new patients requiring dialysis are urgently needed, in order to mitigate the expected financial and health catastrophes associated with the projected increase of such patients.

1. Introduction

End-stage renal disease (ESRD), now termed chronic kidney disease (CKD) stage five is a state of permanent loss of renal function when measured or calculated glomerular filtration rate is less than 15 ml/min permanently. Worldwide, the number of ESRD patients is growing rapidly in developed and developing countries, fueled by aging populations and a pandemic of chronic noncommunicable diseases especially diabetes mellitus and hypertension. Current projections indicate that, by 2030, the global population of ESRD patients living on dialysis may exceed 2 million [1].

In Malaysia, the incidence and prevalence of patients with ESRD has been on an upward trend for the past 20 years. The increase in the dialysis population is attributable to the increasing availability of haemodialysis treatment facilities and easier access to public or subsidised funding, especially in the nongovernmental sector. The 22nd Report of the Malaysian Dialysis and Transplant Registry in 2013 recorded a total of 32,026 patients receiving dialysis treatment, 29,192 on haemodialysis (91%) and 2,834 on peritoneal dialysis (9%) [2]. In 1993, 358 new ESRD patients were treated with dialysis, 2,629 in 2003, while in 2013 the number steeply increased to 6,985. The incidence of patients with ESRD on dialysis was 18 per million population (pmp) in 1993. Subsequently, the numbers doubled from 104 pmp in 2003 to 231 pmp in 2013. The prevalence of patients with ESRD on dialysis was 71 pmp in 1993, rising subsequently more than twofold from 415 pmp in 2003 to 1,059 pmp in 2013 [2].

As the risk of ESRD increases with age, the aging population in Malaysia is expected to have a large impact on the number of incident dialysis patients. A study by Wakasugi et al. observed the trend in the incidence rates of dialysis in Japanese population between 2008 and 2012. The total number of incident dialysis patients was predicted to increase by 12.8% from 36,590 in 2012 to 41,270 in 2025, with higher increment in the oldest age group (≥85 years). Male and female patients were expected to increase by 92.6% and 62.2%, respectively [3].

Looking at the trend in the past 10 years, there is a need to do forecasting studies of ESRD patients to create awareness among the policy makers and the public with regard to the magnitude of the disease. Accurate prediction can be used to facilitate the policy making, decisions on optimal health care allocation and appropriate financial planning and allow for more appropriate use of health care resources for the Malaysian population. This study aims to use time-series techniques on the available historical data to find the best model with the smallest error that can forecast the number of new ESRD patients in Malaysia in the future. Hence, the purpose of this study is to describe the trend of incidence and prevalence of ESRD patients in Malaysia from 1993 to 2013. The study also aims to determine the best univariate forecasting model which produces the smallest root mean squared error (RMSE), mean absolute percentage error (MAPE), and mean absolute error (MAE), subsequently to predict the incidence and prevalence of persons with ESRD up until the year 2040.

2. Methodology

This study was registered and approved by the ethics committee of the National Medical Research Register (NMRR-13-1783-18577). Univariate forecasting modeling was constructed using the new patients (incidence) with a confirmed diagnosis of ESRD on renal replacement therapy (RRT) in Malaysia by year, from 1993 to 2013. The univariate forecasting models were applied since these techniques also generate good forecasts especially when the trend is stable [4]. Four types of time-series analyses methods were assessed, namely, the naive with trend method, the double exponential smoothing method, Holt's method, and autoregressive integrated moving average (ARIMA) modeling method. Forecasting performance is evaluated by estimating the RMSE, MAPE, and MAE and the model with the smallest forecast error was selected to be used in predicting the incidence and prevalence of ESRD up until 2040.

The incidence and prevalence rates of ESRD patients were calculated using population estimates from the Department of Statistics, Malaysia. Meanwhile, based on a previous local study in 2001, the cost of dialysis treatment for each patient was estimated to be RM 30,000 (USD 7,500) per patient, per year [5]. The cost per patient was estimated to be within RM 29,092 to RM 33,642 [5]. The estimated future costs did not incorporate the expected changes due to various factors like changes in foreign exchange rate, consumer price index, changes in the cost of utilities, emoluments, consumables, hardware, pharmaceuticals, and others. The analysis was

conducted using Microsoft Excel and R software (R Development Core Team (2013). R: A language and environment for statistical computing. R Foundation for Statistical Computing, Vienna, Austria. ISBN 3-900051-07-0, URL https://www.R-project.org.).

3. Result

The yearly incidence and prevalence of dialysis patients (haemodialysis and peritoneal dialysis) in Malaysia have been on the increasing trend for the past 20 years. Based on the four types of univariate models measured, the ARIMA modeling which gives the smallest RMSE, MAPE and MAE was selected to be used for predicting the number of new dialysis patients from 2014 to 2040. ARIMA (0, 2, 1) was used for both projection of incidence of dialysis patients (RMSE = 135.50, MAPE = 2.85, and MAE = 87.71) and also prevalence of dialysis patients (RMSE = 158.79, MAPE = 1.29, and MAE = 117.21) (Table 1).

Based on the model selected, the projected number of incidence and prevalence dialysis patients in Malaysia will increase as shown in Figures 1 and 2. The estimated incidence of new dialysis patients in Malaysia in 2020 is 10,208 cases and 19,418 in 2040. Meanwhile, the estimated prevalence is 51,269 and 106,249 cases in 2020 and 2040, respectively. With such projected prevalence, the estimated costs for the treatment are USD 384,517,500 and USD 796,867,500 in the years 2020 and 2040, respectively (Table 2).

4. Discussion

Based on projections made by the Department of Statistics (DOS), Malaysia is expected to reach aging population status by the year 2035, at which point 15 per cent of the total population will be 60 years and older [6]. As the number of older adults is projected to increase dramatically over the next twenty years, this will pose major challenges to our health care systems, as there will be greater healthcare utilization for comorbid conditions among this population [7].

With the rise in conditions such as obesity, diabetes, and hypertension in the middle age population, it is likely that the future prevalence of chronic kidney disease (CKD) will increase further among the elderly. It is a significant concern with both an increasing incidence of treated kidney failure with dialysis and a high prevalence of earlier stages of CKD. CKD is silent and irreversible. If CKD is not detected early or managed properly, the condition will progress to ESRD which will result in the need for renal replacement therapy with either dialysis or kidney transplant. Additionally, ESRD also can lead to mental illnesses such as anxiety and depression which will affect the patients' quality of life [8].

Renal replacement therapy (RRT) in Malaysia has shown an exponential growth since 1990 [9]. The rate of incidence of end-stage renal disease requiring RRT is forecasted to be 3.02 (per 10,000 population) by the year 2020 and to increase further to 3.89 in 2030 and reaching a rate of 4.68 in 2040. There is a projected 1.5-fold increase in overall number of patients on dialysis from 6,985 in 2013 to 10,208 in 2020 and a further 1.5-fold increase to 14,813 in 2030, with a 1.3-fold

TABLE 1: Comparison of forecast error from number of ESRD patients, 1993–2013.

Method	Incidence				Prevalence			
	Parameter	RMSE	MAPE	MAE	Parameter	RMSE	MAPE	MAE
Naive with trend	—	165.12	3.73	116.37	—	195.81	1.81	160.16
Double exponential smoothing	$\alpha = 0.6577$	151.33	5.64	110.87	$\alpha = 0.9999$	205.96	2.72	169.47
Holt	$\alpha = 0.9999$, $\beta = 0.3221$	135.40	3.24	90.26	$\alpha = 0.9999$, $\beta = 0.9999$	199.78	3.09	167.14
ARIMA (0, 2, 1)	—	135.50	2.85	87.71	—	158.79	1.29	117.21

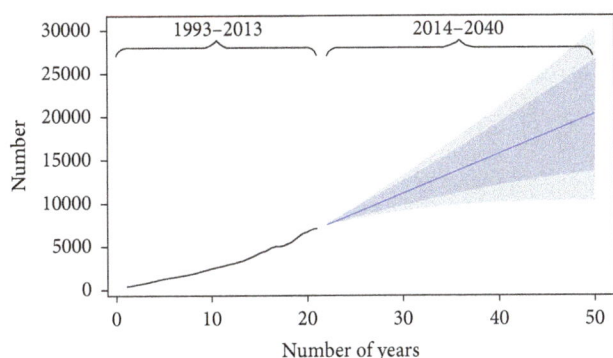

FIGURE 1: Trend and forecast values for incidence of ESRD patients (ARIMA [0, 2, 1]).

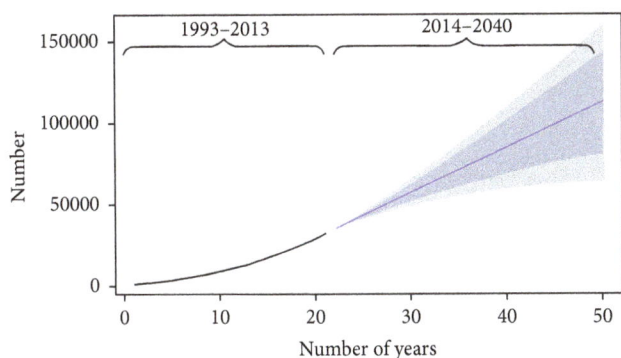

FIGURE 2: Trend and forecast values for prevalence of ESRD patients (ARIMA [0, 2, 1]).

increase to 19,418 in 2040. This is a serious health and economic burden, as patients with ESRD consume a vastly disproportionate amount of financial and human resources.

The cost of CKD to the National Health System in the United Kingdom from the year 2009 to 2010 is estimated to be £1.44 to £1.45 billion, which is about 1.3% of all NHS expenditure in that year. More than half of this amount was spent on RRT, which was provided for 2% of the CKD population [10]. In Malaysia, we projected the costs based on costs estimated by Hooi and colleagues [5]. They estimated the costs were within RM 29,092 to RM 33,642 per patient dialysed at Ministry of Health facilities. By taking average cost of RM 30,000 per patient, the estimated cost incurred to treat all patients with dialysis in the year 2040 is USD 796,867,500

(including new patients at USD 145,635,000) which is more than 10 times compared to the amount in the year 2000. Since the cost was estimated based on year 2001, we postulate that the future cost is higher than what we have estimated due to various factors such as changes in the currency exchange rate, consumer price index, and possibility of the increased costs of the current treatment. Hence, the future costs that is estimated by this study can only become a rough projection to indicate the magnitude and burden of disease.

Careful projections of the demand for dialysis services are important to assist healthcare planners in forecasting the need for equipment, facilities, and personnel [11]. Even so, the setting up of more dialysis centres is not the way to go, as it cannot keep up with the rising need for RRT. More effective prevention, intervention, and early detection programs for renal diseases should be put into place to increase awareness among the public and medical personnel alike.

The health care system should place an emphasis on education and on creating awareness on CKD among the general public. They should be aware of the comorbid conditions that lead to CKD and should learn to adapt lifestyle changes to manage their health properly. Medical professionals should be trained adequately and expanded surveillance and screening systems for chronic diseases made available and easily accessible. The Disease Control Priorities Project offers recommendations on these measures, supporting the establishment of international centers of excellence for CKD that can work in tandem with centers of cardiovascular diseases (CVD) and diabetes [12]. Also, there are collaborations between the International Society of Nephrology and Kidney Disease Improving Global Outcomes with societies such as the International Diabetes Federation (IDF), WHO, and the World Bank to influence global and national health decision-making with regard to the growing burden of CKD and chronic diseases [13, 14].

On a larger scale, there needs to be better alignment of disease funding with burden of disease, transparency of projects, and data availability and better sharing of knowledge with more concerted activities to address the problem of chronic kidney disease (CKD) [15]. More specific cost-effective strategies need to be implemented to cope with the rising demand for RRT. Specific interventions may be used, for example, the increased use of angiotensin-converting enzyme inhibitors and angiotensin receptor type 2 antagonists to slow the rate of decline in renal function [16]. In diabetics, glycaemic control may be improved with the use of newer

TABLE 2: Estimated cost to treat patients with ESRD in year 2000 to 2040.

Year	Est. pop. (in '000)	Incidence				Prevalence			
		Number	Rate (per 10,000 pop.)	Est. cost (RM mil)	Est. cost (USD mil)	Number	Rate (per 10,000 pop.)	Est. cost (RM mil)	Est. cost (USD mil)
2000	23,494.90	1,853	0.79	55.59	13.90	6,702	2.85	201.06	50.27
2005	26,045.50	3,167	1.22	95.01	23.75	13,356	5.13	400.68	100.17
2010	28,588.60	5,305	1.86	159.15	39.79	23,709	8.29	711.27	177.82
2015[a]	31,186.10	7,906	2.54	237.18	59.30	37,524	12.03	1,125.72	281.43
2020[a]	33,782.40	10,208	3.02	306.24	76.56	51,269	15.18	1,538.07	384.52
2025[a]	36,022.70	12,511	3.47	375.33	93.83	65,014	18.05	1,950.42	487.61
2030[a]	38,062.20	14,813	3.89	444.39	111.10	78,759	20.69	2,362.77	590.69
2035[a]	39,879.30	17,116	4.29	513.48	128.37	92,504	23.20	2,775.12	693.78
2040[a]	41,503.10	19,418	4.68	582.54	145.64	106,249	25.60	3,187.47	796.87

Est. = estimated; pop. = population.
a estimates number of cases from the selected model (ARIMA [0, 2, 1]).
Each ESRD patient is estimated to incur cost for RM 30,000 (on estimated rate of 1.00 USD = 4.00 MYR).
Source of estimated population from Department of Statistics, Malaysia.

antidiabetics agents, thus lowering the rate of renal loss. Furthermore, antismoking initiatives may also help slow the progression of chronic kidney disease to ESRD [17].

With these efforts in place, we can perhaps better respond to the challenging burden of CKD and the rising need for RRT in the country. As for conclusions, the predicted number of incidence and prevalence of dialysis patients in Malaysia seem to be increasing over the years until 2040. The number of patients commencing dialysis in Malaysia is predicted to be more than tripled, from 32,026 in 2013 to 106,249 in 2040 (including new patients from 6,985 in 2013 to 19,418 in 2040). The pmp of new dialysis patients in Malaysia is estimated to increase by almost twofold; from 231 pmp in 2013 to 467 pmp in 2040. In view of these trends especially with the trend of aging population in the country [7], there is a need for more targeted, unified, and coordinated efforts to better manage the issues that may arise from this pattern.

The limitation of study is that the univariate forecasting model was used. Therefore, this model did not incorporate other important factors such as age, prevalence of comorbidities (i.e., diabetes mellitus and hypertension), and lifestyle factors. Most of these data are difficult to be retrieved; hence, applying a univariate forecasting model especially for stable time-series pattern is necessary. The forecasted incidence is assumed to be true based on historical data when there is no change in the populations' behavior and no specific interventions have been made. However, with public awareness and lifestyle changes with effective changes in healthcare management, it is possible that in the future the true incidence and prevalence will be lower than what has been estimated.

Ethical Approval

This study was registered and approved by the ethics committee of the National Medical Research Register.

Acknowledgments

The authors thank the Director General of Ministry of Health for the permission to publish this manuscript and the National Renal Registry, Malaysia, especially Lee Day Guat for their contribution and data sharing.

References

[1] L. A. Szczech and I. L. Lazar, "Projecting the United States ESRD population: issues regarding treatment of patients with ESRD," *Kidney International, Supplement*, vol. 66, no. 90, pp. S3–S7, 2004.

[2] The National Renal Registry, "22nd Report of the Malaysian Dialysis and Transplant Registry 2014," 2015.

[3] M. Wakasugi, J. J. Kazama, and I. Narita, "Anticipated increase in the number of patients who require dialysis treatment among the aging population of Japan," *Therapeutic Apheresis and Dialysis*, vol. 19, no. 3, pp. 201–206, 2015.

[4] M. A. Bujang, T. H. Adnan, P. Supramaniam, A. M. Abd Hamid, and J. Haniff, "Prediction number of deaths by occurrence in Malaysia: a comparison between simple linear regression model and holt's linear trend model," *Statistics Malaysia—Journal of the Department of Statistics, Malaysia*, vol. 2, pp. 25–37, 2009.

[5] L. S. Hooi, T. O. Lim, A. Goh et al., "Economic evaluation of centre haemodialysis and continuous ambulatory peritoneal dialysis in Ministry of Health hospitals, Malaysia," *Nephrology*, vol. 10, no. 1, pp. 25–32, 2005.

[6] Department of Statistics Malaysia, "Population Quick Info. Department of Statistics," http://pqi.stats.gov.my/searchBI.php.

[7] M. A. Bujang, A. M. Abdul Hamid, N. A. Zolkepali, N. M. Hamedon, S. S. Mat Lazim, and J. Haniff, "Mortality rates by specific age group and gender in Malaysia: trend of 16 years, 1995–2010," *Journal of Health Informatics in Developing Countries*, vol. 6, no. 2, pp. 521–529, 2012.

[8] M. A. Bujang, R. Musa, W. J. Liu, T. F. Chew, C. T. S. Lim, and Z. Morad, "Depression, anxiety and stress among patients with dialysis and the association with quality of life," *Asian Journal of Psychiatry*, vol. 18, pp. 49–52, 2015.

[9] L. S. Hooi, H. S. Wong, and Z. Morad, "Prevention of renal failure: the Malaysian experience," *Kidney International, Supplement*, vol. 67, no. 94, pp. S70–S74, 2005.

[10] M. Kerr, B. Bray, J. Medcalf, D. J. O'Donoghue, and B. Matthews, "Estimating the financial cost of chronic kidney disease to the NHS in England," *Nephrology Dialysis Transplantation*, vol. 27, no. 3, pp. iii73–iii80, 2012.

[11] R. R. Quinn, A. Laupacis, J. E. Hux, R. Moineddin, M. Paterson, and M. J. Oliver, "Forecasting the need for dialysis services in Ontario, Canada to 2011," *Healthcare Policy*, vol. 4, no. 4, pp. e151–e161, 2009.

[12] D. Jamison, W. Mosley, and A. Measham, *Disease Control Priorities in Developing Countries*, World Bank, Washington, DC, USA, 2006.

[13] R. C. Atkins, "The epidemiology of chronic kidney disease," *Kidney International, Supplement*, vol. 67, no. 94, pp. S14–S18, 2005.

[14] K. Iseki, "Metabolic syndrome and chronic kidney disease: a Japanese perspective on a worldwide problem," *Journal of Nephrology*, vol. 21, no. 3, pp. 305–312, 2008.

[15] R. A. Nugent, S. F. Fathima, A. B. Feigl, and D. Chyung, "The burden of chronic kidney disease on developing nations: a 21st century challenge in global health," *Nephron—Clinical Practice*, vol. 118, no. 3, pp. c269–c277, 2011.

[16] American Diabetes Association, "Standards of medical care for patients with diabetes mellitus, position Statement. Clinical practice recommendations (2001)," *Diabetes Care*, vol. 24, pp. S33–S43, 2001.

[17] R. H. Grimm Jr., K. H. Svendsen, B. Kasiske, W. F. Keane, and M. M. Wahi, "Proteinuria is a risk factor for mortality over 10 years of follow-up. MRFIT Research Group. Multiple Risk Factor Intervention Trial," *Kidney International. Supplement*, vol. 63, pp. S10–S14, 1997.

A Study to Inform the Design of a National Multicentre Randomised Controlled Trial to Evaluate If Reducing Serum Phosphate to Normal Levels Improves Clinical Outcomes including Mortality, Cardiovascular Events, Bone Pain, or Fracture in Patients on Dialysis

Ramya Bhargava,[1,2] **Philip A. Kalra,**[3,4] **Paul Brenchley,**[1,2]
Helen Hurst,[2] **and Alastair Hutchison**[1,2]

[1]*Institute of Cardio-Vascular Sciences, Faculty of Medical and Human Sciences, University of Manchester, Manchester M13 9PL, UK*
[2]*Manchester Royal Infirmary, Central Manchester University Hospitals NHS Foundation Trust,*
 Manchester Academic Health Science Centre, Manchester M13 9WL, UK
[3]*Salford Royal Hospitals NHS Foundation Trust, Salford M6 8HD, UK*
[4]*Institute of Population Studies, Faculty of Medical and Human Sciences, University of Manchester, Manchester M13 9PL, UK*

Correspondence should be addressed to Ramya Bhargava; ramya.bhargava@cmft.nhs.uk

Academic Editor: Danuta Zwolinska

Background. Retrospective, observational studies link high phosphate with mortality in dialysis patients. This generates research hypotheses but does not establish "cause-and-effect." A large randomised controlled trial (RCT) of about 3000 patients randomised 50 : 50 to lower or higher phosphate ranges is required to answer the key question: does reducing phosphate levels improve clinical outcomes? Whether such a trial is technically possible is unknown; therefore, a study is necessary to inform the design and conduct of a future, definitive trial. *Methodology.* Dual centre prospective parallel group study: 100 dialysis patients randomized to lower (phosphate target 0.8 to 1.4 mmol/L) or higher range group (1.8 to 2.4 mmol/L). Non-calcium-containing phosphate binders and questionnaires will be used to achieve target phosphate. Primary endpoint: percentage successfully titrated to required range and percentage maintained in these groups over the maintenance period. Secondary endpoints: consent rate, drop-out rates, and cardiovascular events. *Discussion.* This study will inform design of a large definitive trial of the effect of phosphate on mortality and cardiovascular events in dialysis patients. If phosphate lowering improves outcomes, we would be reassured of the validity of this clinical practice. If, on the other hand, there is no improvement, a reassessment of resource allocation to therapies proven to improve outcomes will result.

1. Background

Dialysis requires more "self-management" than any other medical treatment to control risk factors associated with increased mortality. A patient starting dialysis, aged 60 years, may be informed that they have a 50% chance of surviving five years [1], but observational studies suggest this can be improved by controlling intake of fluids, salt, fat, phosphate, and potassium, attending regularly for dialysis, monitoring blood pressure, cholesterol, phosphate, and haemoglobin, and taking prescribed medication to control these factors, plus weekly injections to improve haemoglobin [2]. Few people are able to understand and manage all aspects simultaneously, and their relative importance is unknown. Meaningful discussion between clinician and patient about these issues, and phosphate control in particular, is currently not possible and unsurprisingly adherence to prescribed regimens is poor [3, 4]. We will address the significance of one risk factor for mortality in dialysis patients—serum phosphate—to facilitate and inform future patient-clinician discussions and enhance the shared decision making process.

The normal serum phosphate is 0.8 to 1.4 mmol/L. Serum phosphate increases in chronic kidney disease and by the time the patients are on dialysis, high serum phosphate is found in more than 40% of dialysis patients and is linked with a 40–100% increased mortality risk in retrospective, observational studies [5, 6]. Opinion-based serum phosphate of less than 1.7 mmol/L is the target for treatment in dialysis patients [7]. 27 observational studies were included in a meta-analysis which examined the relationship between dysregulated mineral metabolism and all-cause or cardiovascular mortality or cardiovascular events in patients with chronic kidney disease (CKD) or end-stage renal disease (ESRD, which is when they need to start dialysis treatment) [8]. Though there were limitations in the analysis noted by the authors due to the low number of studies included and the quality of the data obtained from them, a greater risk of all-cause and cardiovascular mortality was seen with elevated phosphate concentrations. The Dialysis Outcomes and Practice Patterns Study (DOPPS), a prospective cohort study in 25,588 patients with ESRD receiving haemodialysis, showed an increased risk of cardiovascular mortality with serum phosphate concentrations of 5.1–5.5 mg/dL (1.6–1.78 mmol/L) and an increase in all-cause mortality at serum concentrations over 6.0 mg/dL (1.94 mmol/L) [9]. It is recognised that such studies are useful for generating research hypotheses but cannot definitively establish "cause/effect" relationships. Consequently it is believed important to control phosphate, but whether this improves patient outcomes remains unknown, since no randomised interventional trials have been undertaken.

Dietary control and dialysis are insufficient to normalise phosphate, and tablets are required to bind phosphate in the gut. Binders make phosphate insoluble, preventing absorption from the intestinal lumen. The available phosphate binders can be broadly classified into calcium containing phosphate binders like calcium carbonate and calcium acetate and non-calcium containing binders like lanthanum (Fosrenol—trade name) and sevelamer (Renvela and Renagel—trade names for sevelamer carbonate and sevelamer hydrochloride, resp.) and aluminium containing and iron containing phosphate binders. This classification is important because several small interventional randomised controlled trials have looked at difference in clinical outcomes between calcium containing phosphate binders and the common non-calcium containing ones like lanthanum and sevelamer. Jamal et al. published a meta-analysis of 11 such studies, 9 of them in dialysis patients, and compared outcomes between patients with chronic kidney disease taking calcium-based phosphate binders and those taking non-calcium-based binders. They concluded that non-calcium-based phosphate binders were associated with a decreased risk of all-cause mortality compared with calcium-based phosphate binders in patients with chronic kidney disease [10]. Multiple clinical trials have further shown an increase in coronary artery calcification with calcium-based binders

compared to non-calcium-based binders [11–18]. There is an increasing acceptance among clinicians that calcium containing phosphate binder is not optimum therapy and has resulted in greater use of non-calcium containing binders which are ten times more expensive than the calcium containing binders.

A study of patients' perspectives of phosphate binding medication identified gaps in understanding of the concept of phosphate control and the role of medication [3, 19]. Even when binders are taken correctly, achieving normal phosphate levels is difficult, and more than 25% of patients remain above the current opinion-based target range of 1.1–1.7 mmol/L, and more than 40% are above the true normal limit of 1.4 mmol/L [20, 21]. Despite the publication of multiple guidelines, there is a significant gap between the recommendations and the serum phosphate concentrations achieved by patients in clinical practice [22]. The important contributing causes to the lack of effective phosphate control are nonadherence to a low phosphate diet and to phosphate binder medication [23]. Despite the investment in expensive binder medication (up to £3,000 per patient/per annum, 30% of the 27000 prevalent dialysis patients in UK [24], works out to more than £24 m per annum) and large pill burden (up to 15 pills with meals daily in some cases) with significant gastrointestinal side-effects [25], we do not know if lowering serum phosphate is of benefit [26]. A review of all available evidence by the international "Kidney Disease Improving Global Outcomes (KDIGO)" expert group [7] concluded, "*the extensive review... exposed significant gaps in our knowledge... robust studies of a large sample size addressing the following issues should be given priority: Does lowering phosphate... improve clinical outcomes including mortality?*" Our trial will examine the feasibility of conducting such a study of large sample size, which we hope will ultimately answer the questions posed by KDIGO.

2. Methods/Design

2.1. Primary Endpoint. The primary endpoint is the percentage of study participants achieving, and being maintained within, the higher and lower target ranges for phosphate, over the duration of the maintenance phase of the study.

2.2. Secondary Endpoints. The secondary endpoints are the following:

(1) Percentage of Greater Manchester kidney physicians agreeing to enter patients into a study which includes a "higher range" group.

(2) Percentage of eligible invited participants willing to be randomised into a study which includes a "higher range" group.

(3) Percentage of participants achieving consistent control of serum phosphate in each group over a 10-month maintenance period.

(4) Drop-out rate from the study due to adverse events, kidney transplantation, intercurrent illness, and death. These numbers will inform the power calculation for the larger national study.

(5) Pill burden per participant required to control serum phosphate.

(6) Adherence to therapy.

(7) Number of participants willing to participate in "Communicare" patient support programme.

(8) Mean symptom score assessed by Pittsburgh Dialysis Symptoms Index.

(9) Incidence of major vascular events, defined as non-fatal myocardial infarction or any cardiac death, any stroke, or any arterial revascularisation excluding dialysis access procedures (expected mortality of around 14% per annum in patients on dialysis).

2.3. Design. The design is a dual-centre, pan-Manchester prospective randomised parallel group study, with titration to target (2 months) and maintenance phase (10 months).

2.4. Total Number of Participants Planned. The total number of participants planned is 100 at randomisation (up to 300 at consent).

2.5. Setting. The study will be conducted across two large renal units in Greater Manchester which cover a population of about 3.2 million. Prevalent dialysis patients will be recruited from the renal units and their associated satellite dialysis units which give a target dialysis population of about 1100 patients with 900 patients on haemodialysis.

2.6. Ethics, Informed Consent, and Safety. Documented approval has been obtained from appropriate ethics committee and the CMFT Research and Development Department. The study conforms to International Conference on Harmonization of good clinical practice guidelines and with the Declaration of Helsinki. Written informed consent will be obtained from each patient before any study-specific procedure takes place. Participation in the study and date of informed consent of patients will be documented appropriately in each patient's files. Safety Monitoring Committee is in place to review SAEs as is Trial Steering Committee to review progress and Trial Management Committee to oversee the conduct of the trial.

2.6.1. Identifying Participants. The medical records of all the dialysis patients in the Greater Manchester area will be accessed by the study personnel that are also a part of the direct care team (some study personnel will be members of the direct care team). A retrospective screening of their previous serum phosphate levels (which would have been done as part of their routine monthly blood tests) will be completed. Patients with a mean level of >1.4 mmol/L over the past 3 months, and taking an oral phosphate binder, will be identified and flagged up.

2.6.2. Inclusion Criteria. Inclusion criteria are as follows:

(1) Male and female patients aged 30 years or above, on dialysis for at least 6 months (to ensure no recovery of renal function), and under the supervision across pan-Manchester sites. Patients less than 30 years of age have a low rate of vascular events and will not be recruited.

(2) Serum phosphate level of 1.7 mmol/L or greater after wash-out (discontinuation) of previous phosphate binding medication.

(3) Able to achieve Renal Association standards for quality of dialysis on the most recent test of dialysis efficacy. This would be a urea reduction ratio of 65%.

(4) Able to communicate in English because "Communicare" package (the package is explained in Treatments) is currently available only in English.

(5) Able to consent.

2.6.3. Exclusion Criteria. Exclusion criteria are as follows:

(1) Living donor renal transplant planned in the next 12 months.

(2) Serum parathyroid hormone greater than 800 pg/mL (85 pmol/L) on 2 consecutive 2- or 3-monthly blood tests. Such patients probably have uncontrolled hyperparathyroidism which adversely influences serum phosphate levels and needs treatment in its own right.

(3) Known intolerance of both oral sevelamer and lanthanum carbonate.

(4) Medical history that might limit the individual's ability to take the trial treatments for the duration of the study (e.g., history of cancer other than non-melanoma skin cancer or recent history of alcohol or substance misuse).

Figure 1 shows the outline of recruitment and randomisation.

2.7. Estimated Timeline. The trial is estimated to run over a period of 24 months. The duration of the study for each participant will be 13 months. Figure 1 illustrates the timeline for each participant in the study.

2.8. Treatments. Prior to randomisation, the number of potentially eligible participants will be identified (medical records) and each will be sent the Participant Information Sheet with an invitation to attend a screening clinic appointment. Written informed consent will be sought from those who attend the appointment and are willing to participate (−3 weeks). The ratio of "eligible" to "willing" will be recorded. Consenting participants will complete the "Pittsburgh Dialysis Symptom Index" [27] to identify baseline symptom score. They will undergo an assessment of adherence at baseline using modified Basel Assessment of Adherence Scale for ImmunoSuppressives (BAASIS). Patients whose average serum phosphate is more than or equal to 1.7 mmol/L despite ongoing therapy with phosphate binders will be randomised. Patients whose average serum phosphate is less than 1.7 mmol/L, and who are taking phosphate binders, will enter a 3- to 5-week "wash-out" period from their previous phosphate binder and receive standard dietary advice

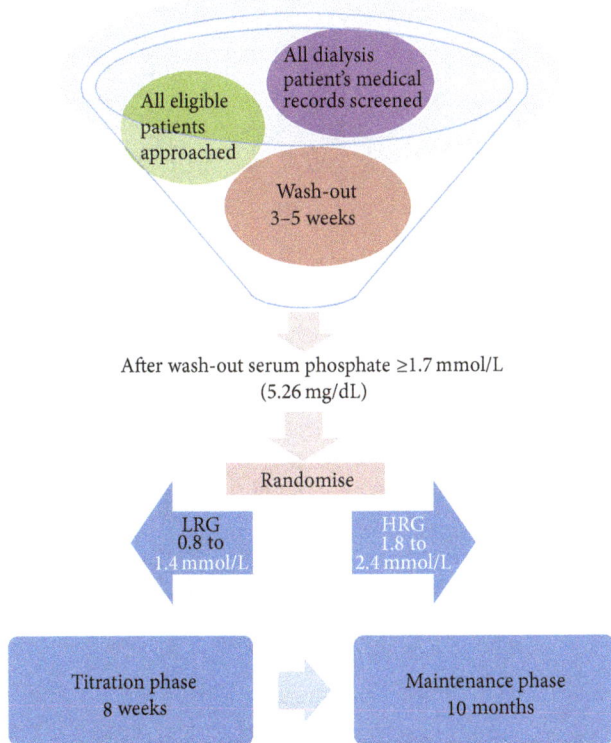

After wash-out serum phosphate ≥1.7 mmol/L
(5.26 mg/dL)

Randomise

LRG
0.8 to
1.4 mmol/L

HRG
1.8 to
2.4 mmol/L

Titration phase
8 weeks

Maintenance phase
10 months

FIGURE 1: Recruitment and randomisation.

from a renal dietician. Serum lipids will be measured and treated according to UK Renal Association guidelines with a statin and/or ezetimibe [28]. Equivalent lipid levels would be required in the larger definitive trial to exclude the possibility of this influencing mortality. This is because two non-calcium containing phosphate binders, sevelamer and colestilan (Bindren—trade name), also reduce serum cholesterol [29]. Sevelamer has been observed to reduce absorption of advanced glycated end-products, bacterial toxins, and bile acids, suggesting that it may reduce inflammatory, oxidative, and atherogenic stimuli in addition to its lowering of serum phosphate [30]. Provided that serum phosphate level rises to greater than or equal to 1.7 mmol/L after wash-out, each participant will be randomised to either the lower range (LRG) or higher range (HRG) phosphate group. Participants with phosphate of less than 1.7 mmol/L after wash-out will not continue the study. This minimises the possibility of an individual being randomised to HRG but whose phosphate level will not reach 1.7 mmol/L.

Those randomised to LRG will undergo a stepped approach to aid achievement of the lower range phosphate target. The treatment for each study visit is summarised in Table 1.

2.8.1. Communicare Package. During each of their dialysis sessions in the first week after randomisation, participants will be given access to, and encouraged to utilise, the "Communicare" online patient adherence support programme. This comprises a patient questionnaire, developed by the London School of Behavioural Science, which highlights individual patient information needs and concerns related to taking phosphate binding medication. Questionnaire results give participants access to online tailored, personalised (but reproducible and standardised) information or "Info Bytes" to help address the concerns they have about taking phosphate binding medication. The package also provides training for the study staff to enable them to discuss phosphate control knowledgeably with participants. There is a paper version of the "Communicare" package which can also be used.

The LRG participants will be able to access the Communicare online support programme at any time but will be specifically encouraged to do so again during dialysis session in month 4 and month 8.

2.8.2. Oral Phosphate Binders. They will recommence oral phosphate binding medication with either lanthanum carbonate or sevelamer (either carbonate or hydrochloride), titrated on a weekly basis with meals to achieve serum phosphate of 0.8 to 1.4 mmol/L in 8 weeks' time.

Since sevelamer reduces serum lipid levels, those individuals taking a statin for cholesterol reduction may require dose adjustment. The dose adjustment of statin will be completed by the study clinicians according to their clinical judgement, with a view to maintaining the serum cholesterol according to the standards set by the Renal Association.

2.8.3. Assessment of Adherence. Adherence will be assessed by the modified BAASIS questionnaire [31, 32]. This is a validated questionnaire which we have modified to reflect phosphate binders instead of immunosuppressants. It comprises 4 questions which the patient answers once every 4 weeks. This questionnaire has been validated in kidney transplant patients [33] on immunosuppressive medications and in HIV patients who are on antiretroviral medications. Both of these groups need to take their medications on a regular timely basis. This criterion applies to the administration of phosphate binders which need to be taken regularly and with each meal to be effective.

All patients will have their adherence assessed at baseline; only the patients randomised to the LRG will continue to have their adherence assessed once every 4 weeks.

Those randomised to HRG will recommence oral phosphate binding medication in the weeks following randomisation, with either lanthanum carbonate or sevelamer, titrated on a weekly basis to achieve a serum phosphate level of 1.8–2.4 mmol/L. We anticipate that some will require no phosphate binding medication to achieve this. The treatment for each study visit is summarised in Table 2.

The participants will have a range of licensed phosphate binding medication to choose from—chewable tablets (lanthanum—Fosrenol), tablets to be swallowed (sevelamer—Renvela, Renagel), and granules that can be mixed with water and consumed (Fosrenol, Renvela)—as first-line therapy. Changes to the phosphate binders and the cholesterol medications during the study will be documented in a drug dosing diary which will be carried by the patient.

Phosphate in all participants will be monitored on a monthly basis from week 8 onwards, with medication

TABLE 1: LRG—treatment for each study visit.

Visit number	Trial timeline/study visits	Blood tests (renal/liver profiles/cholesterol)	Blood test (PTH) + extra sample	Dietician advice	Pittsburgh Dialysis Symptoms Index	Communicare package	BAASIS	Other events
0	−6 weeks to −3 weeks							Potential participants identified from patient records Contact made; PIS provided
1	−3 weeks			✓				Consent Washout period commences
2	Randomisation week 0	✓	✓			✓		Randomisation Commence oral phosphate binding trial medication— sevelamer or lanthanum
3	1 week after randomisation	✓						Titrate trial medication and statins Discuss symptoms
4	2 weeks after randomisation	✓						Titrate trial medication and statins Discuss symptoms
5	3 Weeks after randomisation	✓						Titrate trial medication and statins Discuss symptoms
6	4 weeks after randomisation	✓					✓	Titrate trial medication and statins Discuss symptoms
7	5 weeks after randomisation	✓						Titrate trial medication and statins Discuss symptoms
8	6 weeks after randomisation	✓						Titrate trial medication and statins Discuss symptoms
9	7 weeks after randomisation	✓						Titrate trial medication and statins Discuss symptoms
10	8 weeks after randomisation	✓	✓				✓	Review medical history Discuss symptoms Titrate trial medication and statins if necessary
11	12 weeks after randomisation	✓				✓	✓	Review medical history Discuss symptoms Titrate trial medication and statins if necessary
12	16 weeks after randomisation	✓					✓	Review medical history Discuss symptoms Titrate trial medication and statins if necessary
13	20 weeks after randomisation	✓	✓		✓		✓	Review medical history Discuss symptoms Titrate trial medication and statins if necessary
14	24 weeks after randomisation	✓					✓	Review medical history Discuss symptoms Titrate trial medication and statins if necessary

TABLE 1: Continued.

Visit number	Trial timeline/study visits	Blood tests (renal/liver profiles/cholesterol)	Blood test (PTH) + extra sample	Dietician advice	Pittsburgh Dialysis Symptoms Index	Communicare package	BAASIS	Other events
15	28 weeks after randomisation	Y				Y	Y	Review medical history / Discuss symptoms / Titrate trial medication and statins if necessary
16	32 weeks after randomisation	Y	Y				Y	Review medical history / Discuss symptoms Titrate trial medication and statins if necessary
17	36 weeks after randomisation	Y					Y	Review medical history / Discuss symptoms / Titrate trial medication and statins if necessary
18	40 weeks after randomisation	Y					Y	Review medical history / Discuss symptoms / Titrate trial medication and statins if necessary
19	44 weeks after randomisation	Y	Y				Y	Review medical history / Discuss symptoms / Titrate trial medication and statins if necessary
20	48 weeks after randomisation	Y					Y	Review medical history / Discuss symptoms / Titrate trial medication and statins if necessary
21	52 weeks after randomisation	Y					Y	Review medical history / Discuss symptoms / Patient's involvement in the trial ends

TABLE 2: HRG—treatment for each study visit.

Visit number	Trial timeline	Blood tests (renal/liver/cholesterol)	Blood test (PTH) + extra sample	Dietician advice	Pittsburgh Dialysis Symptoms Index	Other events
0	−6 weeks to −3 weeks					Potential participants identified from patient records Contact made; PIS supplied
1	−3 weeks			✓		Consent Washout period commences
2	Randomisation week 0	✓	✓			Randomisation Commence oral phosphate binding trial medication—sevelamer or lanthanum
3	1 week after randomisation	✓				Titrate trial medication and statins Discuss symptoms
4	2 weeks after randomisation	✓				Titrate trial medication and statins Discuss symptoms
5	3 weeks after randomisation	✓				Titrate trial medication and statins Discuss symptoms
6	4 weeks after randomisation	✓				Titrate trial medication and statins Discuss symptoms
7	5 weeks after randomisation	✓				Titrate trial medication and statins Discuss symptoms
8	6 weeks after randomisation	✓				Titrate trial medication and statins Discuss symptoms
9	7 weeks after randomisation	✓				Titrate trial medication and statins Discuss symptoms
10	8 weeks after randomisation	✓	✓			Review medical history Discuss symptom Titrate trial medication and statins if necessary
11	12 weeks after randomisation	✓				Review medical history Discuss symptoms Titrate trial medication and statins if necessary
12	16 weeks after randomisation	✓				Review medical history Discuss symptoms Titrate trial medication and statins if necessary
13	20 weeks after randomisation	✓	✓		✓	Review medical history Discuss symptoms Titrate trial medication and statins if necessary
14	24 weeks after randomisation	✓				Review medical history Discuss symptoms Titrate trial medication and statins if necessary

TABLE 2: Continued.

Visit number	Trial timeline	Blood tests (renal/liver/cholesterol)	Blood test (PTH) + extra sample	Dietician advice	Pittsburgh Dialysis Symptoms Index	Other events
15	28 weeks after randomisation	✓				Review medical history Discuss symptoms Titrate trial medication and statins if necessary
16	32 weeks after randomisation	✓	✓			Review medical history Discuss symptoms Titrate trial medication and statins if necessary
17	36 weeks after randomisation	✓				Review medical history Discuss symptoms Titrate trial medication and statins if necessary
18	40 weeks after randomisation	✓				Review medical history Discuss symptoms Titrate trial medication and statins if necessary
19	44 weeks after randomisation	✓	✓			Review medical history Discuss symptoms Titrate trial medication and statins if necessary
20	48 weeks after randomisation	✓				Review medical history Discuss symptoms Titrate trial medication and statins if necessary
21	52 weeks after randomisation	✓				Review medical history Discuss symptoms Patient's involvement in the trial ends

adjustments as necessary to maintain results within range. All haemodialysis patients have blood taken routinely for biochemical and haematological measurements on a monthly basis; attempts will be made to ensure that the study blood tests coincide with the routine monthly blood tests; this ensures a reduction in the number of additional blood tests required by this study during the maintenance phase.

A blood sample will be collected at the consent visit, at randomisation, and every 12 weeks thereafter to measure the serum level of parathyroid hormone (PTH). All dialysis patients have this blood test once every three months as part of routine clinical care. Efforts will be made to ensure that the study blood test coincides with their routine test to minimise the number of extra blood tests.

Participants will be asked to gift an extra 5 mL of blood with every blood sample collected for parathyroid hormone. This will be stored in the biobank at the Renal Research Laboratories, Manchester Royal Infirmary, for future biomarker analysis. All participants will complete the Pittsburgh Dialysis Symptoms Index [27] again at month 6 and month 12 (study end).

Oral vitamin D dosage will be altered if necessary to ensure good control of serum calcium PTH [7].

2.9. Drug Dosing. All participants will be given a choice of phosphate binders to use. They will be commenced on one of the two non-calcium containing phosphate binders determined by their preference (chewable, swallowed, and granules). The dosage of the medication will be increased once a week during the titration phase. The target will be to achieve the desired range of serum phosphate. The changes to drugs and dosages done as part of the study will be recorded in a drug dosing diary which the patient will carry.

2.10. Dosing Schedule in the LRG (0.8 to 1.4 mmol/L). Phosphate binders are prescribed in daily doses divided according to the estimated phosphate content of the meals. For some patients, this is three equal doses, whilst for others it might be two different daily doses. Standard practice is for this advice to be given by the prescribing physician or by a renal dietician.

The dosing schedule shown in Table 3 is only a guide and the phosphate binders can be dosed according to clinician judgement.

2.11. Dosing Schedule in the HRG (1.7 to 2.4 mmol/L). It is expected that many patients in the HRG will not require a phosphate binder. However, at any stage during the study,

TABLE 3: Dosing schedule in the LRG.

Titration step	Renvela	Renagel	Fosrenol	Other phosphate binder (sevelamer if previously on lanthanum and vice versa)
1	2.4 g per day in divided doses	2.4 g per day in divided doses	1.5 g per day in divided doses	
2 (increase if needed)	4.8 g per day in divided doses	4.8 g per day in divided doses	2.0 g per day in divided doses	
3 (increase if needed)	7.2 g per day in divided doses	7.2 g per day in divided doses	2.5 g per day in divided doses	
4 (increase if needed)	9.6 g per day in divided doses	9.6 g per day in divided doses	3 g per day in divided doses	
6 (if needed)	Continue at 9.6 g per day	Continue at 9.6 g per day	Continue at 3 g per day	Commence on week 3 dose
7 (increase if needed)	Continue at 9.6 g per day	Continue at 9.6 g per day	Continue at 3 g per day	Commence on week 4 dose

oral non-calcium containing phosphate binder will be introduced if the serum phosphate level exceeds the upper limit of 2.4 mmol/L. The intention would be to reduce and stabilise the phosphate level within the specified range of 1.7–2.4 mmol/L.

Table 4 outlines the titration regime, but if a patient's serum phosphate exceeds 2.4 mmol/L for the first time during, for example, week 4, then they should commence titration at that point. Therefore this table describes "titration steps" rather than study weeks.

The participants in both of the groups are allowed to switch their phosphate binding medication at any stage in the study to one of the other non-calcium containing formulations. They will then be changed to their trial phosphate binding medication of choice at a dose determined by the trial physicians. The target is to achieve the desired range of serum phosphate with a dose and combination that is convenient to the patient in order to encourage adherence. The dose of the study medications can be altered to maintain the serum phosphates in the desired range in the maintenance period on a monthly basis, according to the discretion of the study clinicians. Each change will be documented and recorded.

2.12. Sample Size. No formal sample size calculation has been conducted given the exploratory and evaluative nature of the study. We will randomise 100 patients in total to the "lower range" group and "higher range" group. Assuming an overall attrition rate of 25% at 12 months, 75 patients will "complete" the data-monitoring period. This will be sufficient to allow the monitoring of logistical aspects of this study (such as recruitment, randomisation, and attrition).

2.13. Statistical Analysis and Data Collection. The analysis of this study will be largely descriptive. Detailed statistical evaluation will not be undertaken, and therefore the sample size is chosen to be representative of the Manchester dialysis population (1100 in total). It will be large enough to address the outcome measures but small enough to facilitate timely recruitment and follow-up.

We will be able to

(1) estimate a confidence interval for the proportion of patients achieving consistent control of serum phosphate in each group,

(2) estimate the major cardiovascular event (including death) rate and a confidence interval for this parameter,

(3) observe and record time-to-event data.

These calculations will help to inform the sample size calculation for a multicentre randomised controlled trial, for which mortality and cardiovascular event rate are expected to be the primary outcome measures but only if sufficient events are observed. We will also monitor and summarise recruitment and attrition rates and collect data on reasons for study withdrawal.

Table 5 gives a list of assessment measures used for the different endpoints in the study.

3. Discussion

This study will inform design of a large definitive trial of the effect of phosphate on mortality and cardiovascular events in dialysis patients, starting 2016/17. If reduction of phosphate improves life expectancy, then both clinicians and patients will be better informed and will be able to address this issue more certainly and appropriately, despite current drawbacks of phosphate binding medication. The time, inconvenience, and expense associated with phosphate control would be justified. If there is no benefit to reducing phosphate to a prespecified range, then patients may be relieved of the burden of excessive binding medication and side-effects. Savings from reduced prescriptions could be redirected to develop other methods believed to improve patients' quality and quantity of life, for example, increased provision of home dialysis therapies, with benefits to NHS capital/revenue expenditure. A study which could definitively show a cause-effect relationship between serum phosphate

TABLE 4: Dosing schedule in the HRG.

Titration step	Renvela	Renagel	Fosrenol
1 if serum phosphate >2.4 mmol/L	1.6 g per day in divided doses	1.6 g per day in divided doses	500 mg per day
2 if serum phosphate >2.4 mmol/L	2.4 g per day in divided doses	2.4 g per day in divided doses	1.0 g per day in divided doses
3 if serum phosphate >2.4 mmol/L	3.2 g per day in divided doses	3.2 g per day in divided doses	1.5 g per day in divided doses
4 if serum phosphate >2.4 mmol/L	4.0 g per day in divided doses	4.0 g per day in divided doses	2.0 g per day in divided doses
6 (increase if needed)	4.8 g per day in divided doses	4.8 g per day in divided doses	2.5 g per day in divided doses
7 (increase if needed)	5.6 g per day in divided doses	5.6 g per day in divided doses	3.0 g per day in divided doses

TABLE 5: Measuring trial endpoints.

Outcome measures	Assessment
Percentage of Greater Manchester kidney physicians agreeing to enter patients into a study which includes a "higher range" group	Survey of the nephrology consultants in the Greater Manchester area
Percentage of eligible invited patients willing to be randomised into a study which includes a "higher range" group	Log of all eligible patients in the Greater Manchester area to be maintained
Percentage of patients achieving consistent control of serum phosphate in each group over a 10-month maintenance period	This information will be obtained from the trial database
Drop-out rate from the study due to adverse events, kidney transplantation, intercurrent illness, and death; these numbers will inform the power calculation for the larger national study	This information will be obtained from the trial database
Pill burden per patient to control serum phosphate	The total number of phosphate binding medications needed in every patient to achieve the desired range of serum phosphates will be calculated
Adherence with therapy	BAASIS once every 4 weeks
Willingness of subjects to participate in Communicare patient support programme	The number of patients willing to use the package will be documented
Mean symptom score assessed by Pittsburgh Dialysis Symptoms Index	This will be done at the beginning, midway, and the end of the study
Incidence of major vascular events, defined as nonfatal myocardial infarction or any cardiac death, any stroke, or any arterial revascularisation excluding dialysis access procedures	This information will be captured on the CRF and transferred to the trial database

levels and clinical outcomes like mortality and cardiovascular events will be a game-changer in the management of dialysis patients.

Authors' Contribution

Dr. Ramya Bhargava has written the draft protocol and generated all paperwork related to the study including the protocol, PIS, GP letter, consent form, and drug diaries. She has been instrumental in setting up the study by applying for and obtaining approvals from the regional ethics committee and from the two sites involved in the study. She coordinates with the Manchester Academy of Health Sciences Clinical Trials Unit, the designated monitors for the study. She further organises and keeps minutes of the meetings of the committees involved in the conduct of the study. She makes sure the patients provide consent, reviews blood results, and doses the phosphate binder medication. She was instrumental in setting up the Greater Manchester Kidney Patient Research Advisory Group (GMKPRAG) which enabled the Public

and Patient Involvement (PPI) which is a very important aspect of the study. Professor Philip Kalra is the principal investigator at one of the sites of the study. He has made substantial contributions to conception and design of the study. He has revised the paper critically for important intellectual content and has given approval of the version to be published. Professor Paul Brenchley has contributed to the GMKPRAG meetings and has revised the paper. Dr. Helen Hurst continues to coordinate meetings of the GMKPRAG and has contributed to the study protocol. She has critically reviewed the paper and made valuable suggestions. Professor Alastair J. Hutchison is the CI. He has designed the study and obtained funding from the National Institute of Health Research-Research for Patient Benefit (NIHR-RfPB) through competitive funding. He holds an internationally acclaimed track record for research in CKD-MBD and is an active member of the UK Kidney Research Council and of the KDIGO CKD-MBD group. He is a member of the GMKPRAG which is a very important aspect of the RfPB stream of funding. He has ensured involvement of all the nephrology consultants in

Greater Manchester. He has ensured adequate nursing and administrative support for the smooth conduct of the study. He has edited all the study-related paperwork and will edit all the publications ensuing from the study.

Acknowledgments

This research was funded by National Institute of Health Research-The Collaboration for Leadership in Applied Health Research and Care and by National Institute of Health Research-Research for Patient Benefit (Grant no. PB-PG-0711-25112). The research was facilitated by the Manchester Biomedical Research Centre and the NIHR Greater Manchester: Clinical Research Network.

References

[1] M. Wagner, D. Ansell, D. M. Kent et al., "Predicting mortality in incident dialysis patients: an analysis of the United Kingdom renal registry," *American Journal of Kidney Diseases*, vol. 57, no. 6, pp. 894–902, 2011.

[2] B. Wikström, S. H. Jacobson, J. Bragg-Gresham, M. Eichleay, R. Pisoni, and F. Port, "Dialysis outcomes and practice patterns study estimate of patient life-years attributable to modifiable haemodialysis practices in Sweden," *Scandinavian Journal of Urology and Nephrology*, vol. 44, no. 2, pp. 113–120, 2010.

[3] C. Karamanidou, J. Clatworthy, J. Weinman, and R. Horne, "A systematic review of the prevalence and determinants of non-adherence to phosphate binding medication in patients with end-stage renal disease," *BMC Nephrology*, vol. 9, no. 1, article 2, 2008.

[4] Y.-W. Chiu, I. Teitelbaum, M. Misra, E. M. de Leon, T. Adzize, and R. Mehrotra, "Pill burden, adherence, hyperphosphatemia, and quality of life in maintenance dialysis patients," *Clinical Journal of the American Society of Nephrology*, vol. 4, no. 6, pp. 1089–1096, 2009.

[5] G. A. Block, T. E. Hulbert-Shearon, N. W. Levin, and F. K. Port, "Association of serum phosphorus and calcium x phosphate product with mortality risk in chronic hemodialysis patients: a national study," *The American Journal of Kidney Diseases*, vol. 31, no. 4, pp. 607–617, 1998.

[6] G. A. Block, P. S. Klassen, J. M. Lazarus, N. Ofsthun, E. G. Lowrie, and G. M. Chertow, "Mineral metabolism, mortality, and morbidity in maintenance hemodialysis," *Journal of the American Society of Nephrology*, vol. 15, no. 8, pp. 2208–2218, 2004.

[7] Kidney Disease: Improving Global Outcomes (KDIGO) CKD-MBD Work Group, "KDIGO clinical practice guideline for the diagnosis, evaluation, prevention, and treatment of Chronic Kidney Disease-Mineral and Bone Disorder (CKD-MBD)," *Kidney International. Supplement*, no. 113, pp. S1–S130, 2009.

[8] A. Covic, P. Kothawala, M. Bernal, S. Robbins, A. Chalian, and D. Goldsmith, "Systematic review of the evidence underlying the association between mineral metabolism disturbances and risk of all-cause mortality, cardiovascular mortality and cardiovascular events in chronic kidney disease," *Nephrology Dialysis Transplantation*, vol. 24, no. 5, pp. 1506–1523, 2009.

[9] F. Tentori, M. J. Blayney, J. M. Albert et al., "Mortality risk for dialysis patients with different levels of serum calcium, phosphorus, and PTH: the Dialysis Outcomes and Practice Patterns Study (DOPPS)," *American Journal of Kidney Diseases*, vol. 52, no. 3, pp. 519–530, 2008.

[10] S. A. Jamal, B. Vandermeer, P. Raggi et al., "Effect of calcium-based versus non-calcium-based phosphate binders on mortality in patients with chronic kidney disease: an updated systematic review and meta-analysis," *The Lancet*, vol. 382, no. 9900, pp. 1268–1277, 2013.

[11] G. M. Chertow, P. Raggi, J. T. McCarthy et al., "The effects of sevelamer and calcium acetate on proxies of atherosclerotic and arteriosclerotic vascular disease in hemodialysis patients," *The American Journal of Nephrology*, vol. 23, no. 5, pp. 307–314, 2003.

[12] G. M. Chertow, S. K. Burke, and P. Raggi, "Sevelamer attenuates the progression of coronary and aortic calcification in hemodialysis patients," *Kidney International*, vol. 62, no. 1, pp. 245–252, 2002.

[13] D. Russo, I. Miranda, C. Ruocco et al., "The progression of coronary artery calcification in predialysis patients on calcium carbonate or sevelamer," *Kidney International*, vol. 72, no. 10, pp. 1255–1261, 2007.

[14] J. Braun, H.-G. Asmus, H. Holzer et al., "Long-term comparison of a calcium-free phosphate binder and calcium carbonate—phosphorus metabolism and cardiovascular calcification," *Clinical Nephrology*, vol. 62, no. 2, pp. 104–115, 2004.

[15] D. V. Barreto, F. D. C. Barreto, A. B. de Carvalho et al., "Phosphate binder impact on bone remodeling and coronary calcification—results from the BRiC study," *Nephron Clinical Practice*, vol. 110, no. 4, pp. c273–c283, 2008.

[16] W. Qunibi, M. Moustafa, L. R. Muenz et al., "A 1-year randomized trial of calcium acetate versus sevelamer on progression of coronary artery calcification in hemodialysis patients with comparable lipid control: the Calcium Acetate Renagel Evaluation-2 (CARE-2) Study," *American Journal of Kidney Diseases*, vol. 51, no. 6, pp. 952–965, 2008.

[17] W. N. Suki, "Effects of sevelamer and calcium-based phosphate binders on mortality in hemodialysis patients: results of a randomized clinical trial," *Journal of Renal Nutrition*, vol. 18, no. 1, pp. 91–98, 2008.

[18] T. Takei, S. Otsubo, K. Uchida et al., "Effects of sevelamer on the progression of vascular calcification in patients on chronic haemodialysis," *Nephron Clinical Practice*, vol. 108, no. 4, pp. c278–c283, 2008.

[19] R. Parham, S. Riley, A. Hutchinson, and R. Horne, "Patients' satisfaction with information about phosphate-binding medication," *Journal of Renal Care*, vol. 35, supplement 1, pp. 86–93, 2009.

[20] L. Webb, A. Casula, R. Ravanan, and C. R. V. Tomson, "UK Renal Registry 12th Annual Report (December 2009): chapter 5: demographic and biochemistry profile of kidney transplant recipients in the UK in 2008: national and centre-specific analyses.," *Nephron. Clinical practice*, vol. 115, supplement 1, pp. c69–102, 2010.

[21] C. R. V. Tomson, "UK Renal Registry 12th Annual Report (December 2009): chapter 1 summary of findings in the 2009 UK Renal Registry Report," *Nephron. Clinical Practice*, vol. 115, supplement 1, pp. c1–c2, 2010.

[22] N. D. Toussaint, E. Pedagogos, J. Beavis, G. J. Becker, K. R. Polkinghorne, and P. G. Kerr, "Improving CKD-MBD management in haemodialysis patients: barrier analysis for implementing

better practice," *Nephrology Dialysis Transplantation*, vol. 26, no. 4, pp. 1319–1326, 2011.

[23] A. Covic and A. Rastogi, "Hyperphosphatemia in patients with ESRD: assessing the current evidence linking outcomes with treatment adherence," *BMC Nephrology*, vol. 14, article 153, 2013.

[24] C. Shaw, R. Pruthi, D. Pitcher, and D. Fogarty, "UK renal registry 15th annual report: chapter 2 UK RRT prevalence in 2011: National and centre-specific analyses," *Nephron. Clinical Practice*, vol. 123, supplement 1, pp. 29–54, 2013.

[25] A. J. Hutchison, C. P. Smith, and P. E. C. Brenchley, "Pharmacology, efficacy and safety of oral phosphate binders," *Nature Reviews Nephrology*, vol. 7, no. 10, pp. 578–589, 2011.

[26] T. Isakova, O. M. Gutierrez, Y. Chang et al., "Phosphorus binders and survival on hemodialysis," *Journal of the American Society of Nephrology*, vol. 20, no. 2, pp. 388–396, 2009.

[27] S. D. Weisbord, L. F. Fried, R. M. Arnold et al., "Development of a symptom assessment instrument for chronic hemodialysis patients: the Dialysis Symptom Index," *Journal of Pain and Symptom Management*, vol. 27, no. 3, pp. 226–240, 2004.

[28] C. Baigent, M. J. Landray, C. Reith et al., "The effects of lowering LDL cholesterol with simvastatin plus ezetimibe in patients with chronic kidney disease (Study of Heart and Renal Protection): a randomised placebo-controlled trial," *The Lancet*, vol. 377, no. 9784, pp. 2181–2192, 2011.

[29] A. Rastogi, "Sevelamer revisited: pleiotropic effects on endothelial and cardiovascular risk factors in chronic kidney disease and end-stage renal disease," *Therapeutic Advances in Cardiovascular Disease*, vol. 7, no. 6, pp. 322–342, 2013.

[30] H. E. Bays, R. B. Goldberg, K. E. Truitt, and M. R. Jones, "Colesevelam hydrochloride therapy in patients with type 2 diabetes mellitus treated with metformin: glucose and lipid effects," *Archives of Internal Medicine*, vol. 168, no. 18, pp. 1975–1983, 2008.

[31] P. Schäfer-Keller, J. Steiger, A. Bock, K. Denhaerynck, and S. De Geest, "Diagnostic accuracy of measurement methods to assess non-adherence to immunosuppressive drugs in kidney transplant recipients," *The American Journal of Transplantation*, vol. 8, no. 3, pp. 616–626, 2008.

[32] F. Dobbels, L. Berben, S. De Geest et al., "The psychometric properties and practicability of self-report instruments to identify medication nonadherence in adult transplant patients: a systematic review," *Transplantation*, vol. 90, no. 2, pp. 205–219, 2010.

[33] A. O. Doesch, S. Mueller, M. Konstandin et al., "Increased adherence after switch from twice daily calcineurin inhibitor based treatment to once daily modified released tacrolimus in heart transplantation: a pre-experimental study," *Transplantation Proceedings*, vol. 42, no. 10, pp. 4238–4242, 2010.

Soluble Fas and the−670 Polymorphism of Fas in Lupus Nephritis

Juan José Bollain-y-Goytia,[1] **Mariela Arellano-Rodríguez,**[1]
Felipe de Jesús Torres-Del-Muro,[1] **Leonel Daza-Benítez,**[2]
José Francisco Muñoz-Valle,[3] **Esperanza Avalos-Díaz,**[1] **and Rafael Herrera-Esparza**[1]

[1] *Laboratorios de Inmunología y Biología Molecular, UA Ciencias Biológicas, Universidad Autónoma de Zacatecas,
98040 Zacatecas, ZAC, Mexico*
[2] *Unidad Médica de Alta Especialidad (UMAE) HPG No. 48, Instituto Mexicano del Seguro Social (IMSS), 37320 León, GTO, Mexico*
[3] *Instituto de Investigación en Ciencias Biomédicas, Centro Universitario de Ciencias de la Salud, Universidad de Guadalajara,
45178 Guadalajara, JAL, Mexico*

Correspondence should be addressed to Rafael Herrera-Esparza; rafael.herreraesparza@gmail.com

Academic Editor: Danuta Zwolinska

This study was performed to clarify the role of soluble Fas (sFas) in lupus nephritis (LN) and establish a potential relationship between LN and the −670 polymorphism of Fas in 67 patients with systemic lupus erythematosus (SLE), including a subset of 24 LN patients with proteinuria. Additionally, a group of 54 healthy subjects (HS) was included. The allelic frequency of the −670 polymorphism of Fas was determined using PCR-RFLP analysis, and sFas levels were assessed by ELISA. Additionally, the WT-1 protein level in urine was measured. The Fas receptor was determined in biopsies by immunohistochemistry (IHC) and *in situ* hybridization (FISH) and apoptotic features by TUNEL. *Results.* The −670 Fas polymorphism showed that the G allele was associated with increased SLE susceptibility, with an odds ratio (OR) of 1.86. The sFas was significantly higher in LN patients with the G/G genotype, and this subgroup exhibited correlations between the sFas level and proteinuria and increased urinary WT-1 levels. LN group shows increased expression of Fas and apoptotic features. In conclusion, our results indicate that the G allele of the −670 polymorphism of Fas is associated with genetic susceptibility in SLE patients with elevated levels of sFas in LN with proteinuria.

1. Introduction

Systemic lupus erythematosus (SLE) is a systemic autoimmune disease characterized by the production of autoantibodies and multiorgan involvement, including kidney damage in 60% of patients [1, 2]. Antinuclear antibodies (ANAs) are the hallmark of SLE, and specific anti-Sm, anti-dsDNA, anti-nucleosome, anti-Clq, and anti-GBM antibodies have been associated with LN [3–5].

Renal involvement is a serious complication of SLE because it can lead to high rates of morbidity and mortality [6]. The diagnosis of glomerulonephritis is suspected when proteinuria and urinary sediment alteration are accompanied by arterial hypertension. These data may predict kidney involvement, although renal biopsy remains the gold standard for the diagnosis and classification of LN. In particular, histological analysis can be used to identify the lesion and progression stages of renal disease according to the activity and chronicity index. However, despite the benefits of renal biopsy, this is an invasive procedure that requires an exhaustive review by a skilled pathologist; therefore, alternative biomarkers to identify renal disease are urgently needed [7]. Currently and traditionally used urinary biomarkers include proteinuria >0.5 g/L, alterations in renal ultrasound results, and changes in the rate of glomerular filtration, indicating the degree of renal function. Recently, additional urinary biomarkers have been used to predict renal damage, including markers of urinary podocytes, such as the transcription factor Wilm's tumor 1 (WT-1) [8].

Genetic susceptibility to SLE involves certain major histocompatibility complex class II (MHC II) alleles, such as HLA-DRB1*0301 and DRB1*1501 [9]. In addition, polymorphisms in genes encoding the cytokines interleukin-10 (IL-10), IL-6, tumor necrosis factor-α (TNF-α), and interferon-γ (IFN-γ) have been associated with SLE. Therefore, these polymorphisms could confer different degrees of susceptibility according to the ethnic group [10–12]. Additionally, mutations in cytokine receptors and costimulatory molecules, such as CD28/B7 [13], and polymorphisms in genes associated with apoptosis, such as Fas, FasL, and Bcl-2, have been implicated in disease pathogenesis [14]. Accordingly, SLE is a polygenic disease in which different genes may be associated with different SLE disease subsets, including the nephritogenic phenotype.

Polymorphisms in the GMCP-1 gene were previously shown to be associated with increased susceptibility to SLE in a Mexican mestizo population [15, 16]. Additionally, the −1149 G/T polymorphism of the prolactin promoter has been correlated with the production of anti-DNA antibodies [17]. In contrast, the −653 G/A NRF-2 (erythroid nuclear factor-2) polymorphism does not increase SLE susceptibility during childhood, although such polymorphisms may be associated with LN [18].

The role of apoptosis in SLE has been intensively studied, and the Fas/CD95/Apo-1 gene has been mapped to the 10q 24.1 region. This gene consists of nine exons and eight introns as well as the promoter responsible for allelic variations in Fas, which can also modify the transcriptional rate. For example, if a guanine (G) is replaced by an adenine (A) at position −670, the resulting polymorphism increases the binding affinity of the transcription factor STAT-1 for the interferon gamma-activated sequence (GAS), which in turn alters the transcription rate of the Fas receptor [19]. Another polymorphism of Fas at position 297, with the presence of a C allele, is associated with SLE development in the Japanese population; interestingly, this polymorphism does not increase the risk for SLE in the Italian population [20].

The Fas receptor exists in two forms; one form is anchored to the plasma membrane, whereas the other is soluble (sFas). The latter form is highly regulated at the transcriptional level [21, 22]. sFas plays a role as an antiapoptotic molecule that blocks FasL or sFasL binding, and its concentration in the serum of healthy subjects is independent of gender and age [23]. Additionally, in clinical practice, sFas has been defined as a marker of inflammation related to endothelial dysfunction in chronic renal diseases [24–26]. In SLE, sFas levels are increased due to a deletion in exon 6 [21, 23, 27], although knowledge about its participation in LN is lacking.

The present study was performed to assess the possible role of the −670 Fas polymorphism in LN and address the issue of whether increased levels of sFas are related to podocyte damage, proteinuria, and autoantibody production.

2. Materials and Methods

2.1. Biological Samples. This cross-sectional study of cases and controls analyzed the −670 polymorphism of Fas in a mestizo group of SLE patients living in the north-central region of Mexico. The mean age of the subjects was 41.2 ± 22.1 years, and all patients met the American College of Rheumatology (ACR) criteria for SLE classification [28] (females 79.6% and males 20.3%).

The SLE group was divided into two subsets. This first group lacked evidence of renal involvement, tested positive for ANAs (80%) or anti-dsDNA antibodies (*Crithidia luciliae*) (7.14%), and showed negative or irrelevant levels of proteinuria (mean level of 0.116 g/L). The second group had LN with proteinuria levels higher than 0.5 g/L and displayed a positive ANA test result (90%) and a high prevalence of anti-dsDNA antibodies (67%). Additionally, a control group was included, consisting of 54 healthy subjects (HS) without evidence of autoimmune disease. This group was 84.31% female and 15.6% male with an average age of 34.3 ± 14.51 years, and all HS tested negative for ANAs, anti-dsDNA antibodies, and proteinuria. This study was performed according to the principles of the Declaration of Helsinki and was approved by the ethics committees of our institutions. After providing detailed information, signed informed consent was obtained from the patients and controls.

2.2. Blood Collection. Peripheral blood was collected in Vacutainer 7.2 mg K2 EDTA tubes and used for DNA extraction; simultaneously, tubes without anticoagulant were used to obtain serum.

2.3. Autoantibodies. ANA measurements were performed by immunofluorescence (IF) using HEp-2 cells and anti-DNA antibodies by *Crithidia luciliae* (Immuno Concepts NA, Ltd., Sacramento, CA). The following antibody specificities were quantified by enzyme-linked immunosorbent assay (ELISA): anti-Ro-60 (EA 1595-9601 G), anti-La-48 (EA 1597-9601 G), anti-nRNP/Sm (EA 1591-9601 G), and antiglomerular basement membrane (GBM) (EA 1251-9601 G), according to the manufacturer's recommendations (Euroimmun US Inc.).

2.4. Soluble Fas. sFas levels were determined using a commercial ELISA kit (Quantikine Human sFAS/TNFRSF6 R&D System, Abingdon, UK), and the optical density (OD) was measured at 450 nm using an ELISA plate reader (Multiskan FC, Thermo Scientific). The sFas concentration was expressed in ρg/mL according to the curves obtained from the standards.

2.5. Restriction Fragment Length Polymorphism (PCR-RFLP) Analysis. The −670 polymorphism of the Fas receptor was analyzed using PCR-RFLP analysis, as previously reported [19]. DNA from peripheral blood was extracted using Miller's modified technique [29]. The PCR reaction was performed using Taq DNA polymerase (Platinum High Fidelity from Invitrogen, Life Technologies) as follows. First, $1\,\mu$g of DNA was placed in an Eppendorf tube with a reaction mixture containing 0.2 mM of the sense (5′-CTACCTAAGAGCTA-TCTACCGTTC-3′) and antisense (5′-GGCTGTCCATG-TTGTTGGCTGC-3′) oligonucleotides; then, 5 μL of 10X high fidelity PCR buffer, 25 μL of 2X nucleotides, 2 μL of 50 mM $MgSO_4$, and 0.2 μL of Taq enzyme mixture were incubated at 4°C and adjusted to a final volume of 50 μL with H_2O (GIBCO Ultrapure). The PCR reaction was performed in a Perkin Elmer 2400 thermocycler using 35 cycles at the following conditions: 94°C for 2 min, 94°C for 30 s, 58°C for 30 s, and 72°C for 30 s. A final reaction extension was performed at 72°C for 10 min. PCR products were digested at 37°C for 1 h with the restriction enzyme Mva-I (Cat. number 11288075001, Roche Diagnostics, Indianapolis, USA), and 10 μL of digested and undigested PCR products was separately run in a 2% agarose gels using 1X TAE buffer for 40 min at 80 volts; the gels were then stained with ethidium bromide. A DNA ladder was used (1 Kb Plus DNA Ladder of Invitrogen), and the gels were analyzed using the Carestream Molecular Imaging Software, version 5.0.

2.6. Fas Expression Was Determined in Renal Biopsies by Immunohistochemistry (IHC) and by In Situ Hybridization (FISH)

2.6.1. Preparation of Fas Fluorescent Probes. Fluorescent-labelled PCR-derived probes were synthesized by PCR using a random-primed λgt11-human spleen library as a template (Clontech, Palo Alto, CA, USA), using the following oligonucleotides: Fas forward 5′-GGT GGG TTA CAC TGG TTT ACA-3′ and backward 5′-GTG CTA CTC CTA ACT GTG AC-3′ [30]. The PCR reaction was done by incubation of 1 μg of template with 25 μM of nucleotides 2X dNTP, 100 μM fluoro-Red-labelled-UTP (Amersham Biosciences, Buckingham, UK), and 0.2 μM of the aforementioned primers mixed with 0.5 U/50 μL of DNA polymerase (Platinum Taq DNA polymerase High Fidelity of Invitrogen Life Technology Ltd, Carlsbad, CA USA). The reaction tubes containing 50 μL of the sample mixture were amplified in a thermocycler (PerkinElmer, GeneAmp PCR system 2400) using 30 cycles (94°C for 2 min, 48°C for 2 min, and 72°C for 1.4 min). At the end of the PCR, the amplicates were electrophoresed in 0.8% agarose. The internal fluorescent red labeling of the PCR products was observed under ultraviolet light as reed bands in agarose gels lacking in ethidium bromide.

2.6.2. In Situ Hybridization. Slides containing 4 μm sections of renal tissues were incubated with 0.02 M HCl, permeabilized with 0.01% Triton X-100/PBS-DEPC, and washed in cold 20% acetic acid. Probes were adjusted to 50 ng/mL in 1 : 1 hybridization buffer: formamide and were applied individually to the tissues. Tissues were prehybridized at 90°C for 3 min, followed by hybridization at 37°C for 24 hrs, and were washed in SSC 2X buffer. In addition, following the washes some slides were counterstained with 4′,6-Diamidine-2′-phenylindole dihydrochloride (DAPI) [31]. Finally, the slides were mounted and evaluated under confocal microscope. The intensity of the color red obtained by FISH was analyzed in the software Image-Pro Plus Versión 7.0. (Media Cybernetics, USA).

2.7. Biopsies. Tissues were from patients with LN and control biopsies obtained during necropsy of individuals who died in a car accident, after obtaining written consent from their families. In all the patients, kidney biopsies were performed percutaneously, and a segment of each biopsy was stained for hematoxylin and eosin (H and E) and evaluated under light microscopy. The biopsies were classified according to the ISN/RPS 2004 classification of LN [32].

2.8. Immunohistochemistry. The Fas receptor was detected by IHC on 4 μm thick sections of renal tissues mounted on microscope slides. The specimens were dewaxed, permeabilized with 0.01% Triton X-100/phosphate buffered saline (PBS), and then washed thrice with PBS. Endogenous peroxidase was blocked for 10 minutes with 3% H_2O_2 dissolved in methanol. After an additional wash, the tissues were incubated for 12 hours with a monoclonal anti-APO-1 (DAKO) and diluted 1:100 in 10% FBS-PBS, the tissues were then washed in several changes of PBS, and the bound antibodies were identified with HRP-goat anti-mouse IgG (Zymed, Laboratories Inc., San Francisco, CA). The color reaction was induced by 3,3′-diaminobenzidine-0.06% H_2O_2 (Sigma, St. Louis, MO), and the reaction was stopped with 0.5 M sulfuric acid. The slides were then examined under a light microscope. The assays were performed in triplicate and evaluated by two pathologists in a blinded fashion. The intensity of the color reaction obtained by IHC was analyzed in the software Image-Pro Plus Versión 7.0. (Media Cybernetics, USA).

2.9. Other Parameters. Proteinuria was measured using the conventional dry chemistry method. The level of the WT-1 podocyte marker was measured by ELISA in urine collected over a 24 h period using a previously described method [8]. Apoptotic features were detected by TUNEL (Roche Molecular Biochemical's. Penzberg, Germany).

2.10. Statistical Analysis. Differences in the measured parameters between different groups were evaluated by analysis of variance (ANOVA) tests with Tukey's and Pearson's correlations. GraphPad Prism version 17 was used for analysis, and P values < 0.05 were considered significant.

3. Results

3.1. The −670 Fas Polymorphism in SLE. After the PCR reaction, the products were digested to obtain the polymorphic fragments. The A/A genotype was identified as a 232-base pair (bp) band, the G/G genotype appeared as a 188 bp band, and the heterozygous A/G variant appeared as a doublet of the 188 bp and 232 bp bands, as shown in Figure 1. The A and G allelic frequencies were 0.41 and 0.45, respectively. These results indicated that the Fas G allele was associated with susceptibility to SLE, with odds ratios (ORs) of 1.86 ($P = 0.03$) and 2.23 ($P = 0.05$) for the dominant and recessive models, respectively (Table 1).

3.2. Soluble Fas Is Increased in Lupus Nephritis. The sFas level was slightly elevated in the LN subset with the G/G genotype compared to SLE patients without LN (Figure 2).

TABLE 1: Genotype and alleles frequencies of the −670 A/G Fas polymorphism in SLE and LN patients and HS.

	SLE ($n = 43$) % (n)	LN ($n = 24$) % (n)	HS ($n = 54$) % (n)	P value
Genotype				
A/A	33 (14)	29 (7)	52 (28)	[§,&]$P = 0.22$
A/G	30 (13)	38 (9)	22 (12)	
G/G	37 (16)	33 (8)	26 (14)	
Allele				
A	48 (41)	48 (23)	63 (68)[§]	[§,&]$P = 0.03$*
G	52 (45)[&]	52 (25)	37 (40)	OR = 1.86 95% CI = 1.007–3.45
A/A + **A**/G	63 (27)	67 (16)	74 (40)	
GG	37 (16)	33 (8)	26 (14)	$P = 0.23$
AA	33 (14)	29 (7)	52 (28)[Φ]	$P = 0.05$*
A/G + G/G	67 (29)[φ]	71 (17)	48 (26)	OR = 2.23 95% CI = 0.90–5.6

LN: lupus nephritis; SLE: systemic lupus erythematosus; HS: healthy subjects; [§]HS versus SLE; [&]SLE versus HS; [Φ]HS versus SLE; [φ]SLE versus HS. *A P value <0.05 is significant.

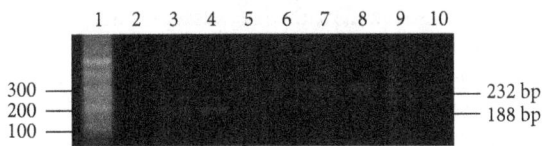

FIGURE 1: Electrophoresis of PCR products in patients and controls. The polymorphic fragments A/A resulted in a 232 bp band, the G/G fragment resulted in a 188 bp band, and the A/G variation resulted in a doublet of the 188 bp and 232 bp bands on a 2% agarose gel.

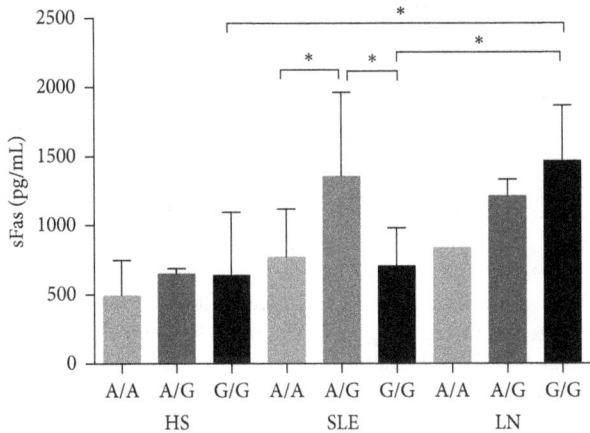

FIGURE 3: sFas concentration according to −670 Fas genotype. The sFas concentrations in patients with the A/A and G/G genotypes were not significantly different. In contrast, the sFas concentration in patients with the A/G genotype was different compared to other genotypes. *$P < 0.05$.

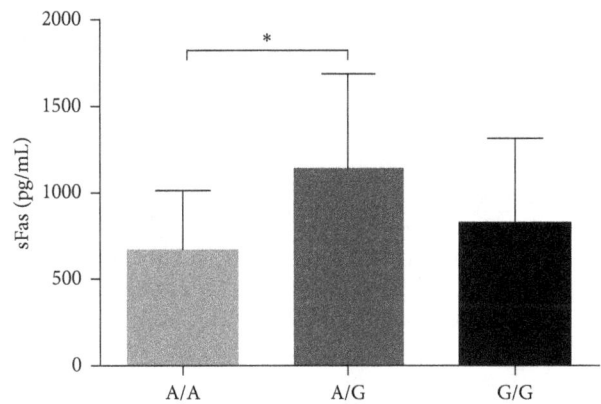

FIGURE 2: The sFas concentration according to −670 Fas genotype in LN and SLE patients and HS. The concentration of sFas was increased in LN patients with the G/G genotype and was significantly different from patients with SLE. *$P < 0.05$.

3.3. Association between sFas and the −670 Fas Polymorphism.

To address the question of whether sFas is associated with the −670 polymorphism of the Fas receptor, the sFas levels in the serum were compared between the A/A, A/G, and G/G genotypes. The average concentration of sFas for the A/A

genotype was 668.99 ± 344.04 ρg/mL, whereas the concentration for the A/G genotype was $1,140.17 \pm 559.89$ ρg/mL, and this difference between genotypes was significant ($P < 0.05$). In contrast, the G/G genotype showed a mean concentration of 828.06 ± 486.78 ρg/mL, and this value was not significantly different compared to the A/A or A/G genotype (Figure 3).

3.4. sFas Is Increased and Correlated with Autoantibodies and Proteinuria.

The concentration of sFas was increased regardless of the age of the SLE patients, with a mean value of 845.84 ± 444.66 ρg/mL, whereas this concentration was $1,342.997 \pm 337.10$ ρg/mL in LN subjects. When these values were compared to those of the HS (630.44 ± 385.34 ρg/mL), there was a significant difference ($P < 0.001$) (Figure 4).

3.5. Fas Protein and mRNA Is Expressed in Glomerulus.

The lupus nephritis biopsies included were 14 that had Class

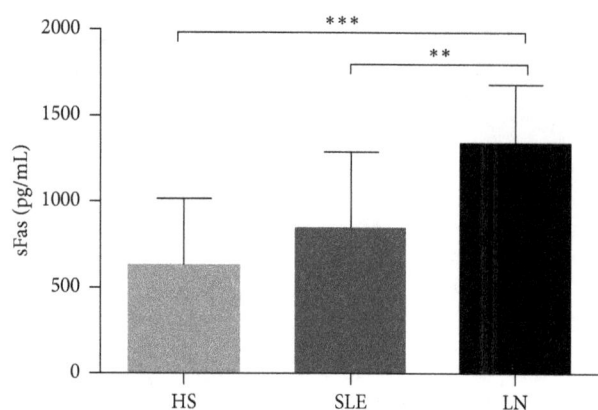

FIGURE 4: The sFas level in the serum of SLE and LN patients and HS. The concentration of sFas was increased in patients with LN. $^{**}P < 0.01$; $^{***}P < 001$.

TABLE 2: Biomarkers in HS and lupus nephritis.

Group	HS	LN	P value
sFas ρg/mL	630.44 ± 385.34	1,342.99 ± 337.10	0.001
mRNA Fas	13.73 ± 1.805	18.68 ± 0.915	0.006
Protein Fas	171.51 ± 8.468	221.53 ± 7.642	0.007
Apoptotic cells	23.496 ± 1.283	32.059 ± 5.800	0.01

sFas: soluble Fas, HS: healthy subjects, LN: lupus nephritis. Significance $P <$ 0.05.

4. Discussion

In the present investigation, the −670 polymorphism of the promoter region of the Fas gene was analyzed. We also sought to determine whether the association between LN and sFas levels is associated with the −670 Fas polymorphism. Finally, we evaluated whether these factors are associated with the lupus nephritis susceptibility in the Mexican mestizo population.

The present results suggest that the G allele of the Fas promoter is associated with SLE susceptibility (OR, 1.86). Second, an increased serum level of sFas was detected in LN patients with the G/G and A/G −670 genotypes. Third, this increase in sFas among LN patients with proteinuria and podocyturia, suggests that the increase in the sFas level may be transcriptionally regulated, and it is associated to the G/G and A/G genotypes. Fourth, the broad expression of Fas receptor in LN biopsies correlated with apoptotic features.

Associations between the A/G −670 Fas polymorphism and autoimmune diseases, such as type 1 diabetes, multiple sclerosis, Sjögren's syndrome, rheumatoid arthritis (RA), and SLE, have been described [19, 33, 34, 46]. Nevertheless, it remains unclear how this polymorphism participates in LN pathogenesis.

The present results suggest that the genotype and allelic frequency of the G allele of the Fas −670 polymorphism are associated with SLE in Mexican mestizo patients; therefore, this genotype may confer susceptibility to SLE. We should note that the studied population lives in the north-central area of Mexico, and our results differ with those reported in Japanese SLE patients in which the A allele was associated with SLE development [43]. However, these results suggest that the Fas promoter partially contributes to the pathogenesis of SLE [33]. Other studies in India have reported the association between SLE and the −670 Fas polymorphism [37], and the allelic differences with the present work seem to be due to the mixed ethnic groups present in the Mexican mestizo population [47].

Our results agree with other reports showing that the −670 polymorphism is associated with certain ANA specificities, which is in agreement with a report on Korean SLE patients [44]. Taking into account the fact that different genes participate in SLE, transcriptional regulation of the Fas receptor in SLE seems to be activated by IFN-γ [43].

Regarding the possible association between the −670 polymorphism and sFas levels, we found that sFas levels were increased in LN patients with the A/G and G/G genotypes, which is in agreement with previous reports [33, 37, 43].

IV and 10 with Class III. Patients with Class IV nephritis displayed the highest activity and chronicity scores, while control kidneys had no histological evidence of renal disease (Figures 5 and 6).

3.6. The Fas Protein Expression Was Increased in Lupus Nephritis. The LN biopsies broadly expressed the Fas receptor, which was mainly detected along the tubules, in glomerular endothelial cells and in the mesangium. Although HS biopsies showed similar distributions of Fas, their staining intensities were lower (Figure 7). Additionally, the color intensity was measured by an image analyzer program, and values were expressed as sum of intensities in pixels is one hundred fields. Using this approach, significant differences of Fas between HS and LN were observed (Figure 8).

3.7. Apoptotic Cell in Glomeruli. An increase in values obtained by apoptotic cells in LN was observed, and significant differences between HS and LN were observed (Figure 9 and Table 2).

Additionally, there was a significant difference between the SLE and LN subsets (P < 0.01) (Figure 10). LN subjects demonstrated a positive ANA test (90%) and a high prevalence of anti-dsDNA antibodies (67%); this result was in contrast with the SLE group without nephritis, which showed an ANA level of 80% with anti-dsDNA antibodies in only 7.14% of cases. Thus, we next sought to determine whether sFas in LN is associated with a high prevalence of autoantibodies, including anti-DNA antibodies, and proteinuria. To this end, a Pearson's correlation analysis was performed, and as expected, a significant correlation among proteinuria, podocyturia (as measured by WT-1), and the levels of anti-dsDNA and anti-Ro-60 antibodies was observed in the LN subset. However, there was a lack of correlation with anti-nRNP/Sm and anti-La-48 autoantibodies (Table 3).

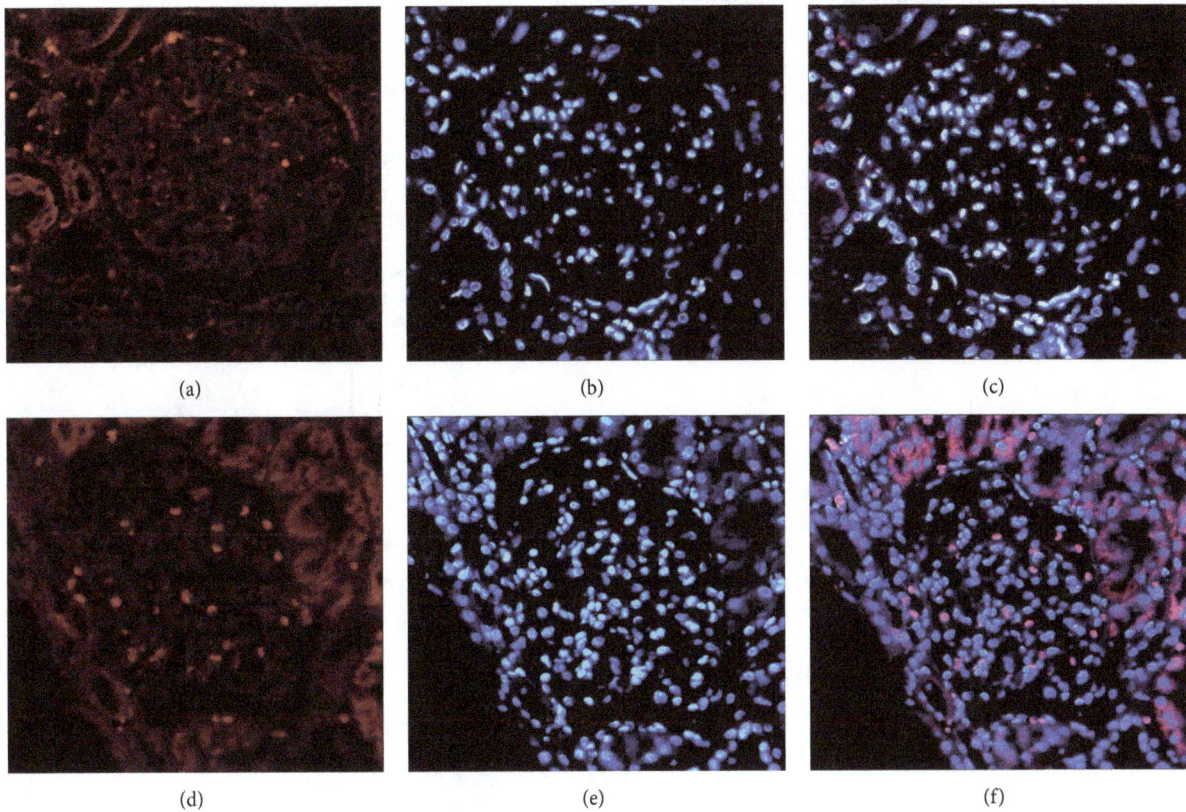

(a) (b) (c)

(d) (e) (f)

FIGURE 5: The expression of mRNA Fas receptor in renal tissue of LN patients and HS by FISH. The upper panel (a), (b), and (c) shows the HS tissue, and the lower panel (d), (e), and (f) shows a representative LN. (a) and (d) Expression of the mRNA Fas receptor (red). (b) and (e) Staining in blue by DAPI. (c) and (f) show the overlapping (pink).

TABLE 3: Correlation between sFas levels and markers of disease in LN patients.

	Proteinuria ≥ 0.5 g/L	WT-1	anti-Ro-60	anti-dsDNA	anti-MBG	nRNP/Sm	anti-La-48
sFas	$r = 0.864$	$r = 0.718$	$r = 0.659$	$r = 0.593$	$r = 0.276$	$r = 0.522$	$r = -0.372$
	$P = 0.01^*$	$P = 0.004^{**}$	$P = 0.05^*$	$P = 0.032^*$	$P = 0.440$	$P = 0.150$	$P = 0.324$

*Correlation is significant at the 0.05 level (two-tailed).
**Correlation is significant at the 0.01 level (two-tailed).

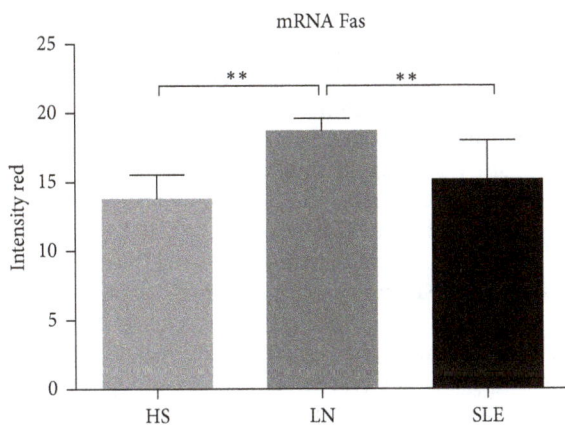

FIGURE 6: Expression the mRNA Fas receptor in renal tissue of SLE, LN patients, and HS. Difference between LN with other groups was significant. $^{**}P < 0.006$.

The meta-analysis studies related with Fas −670 A/G polymorphism show that such genotype confers susceptibility to SLE in Asian population (Table 4) [33, 34]. We should note that these studies do not include any Latin America country; this is the first study on the Fas −670 polymorphism in a population of north-central area of Mexico, as depicted in Table 4, that compares our results with other reports [33, 34, 37, 40, 43, 44, 47]. The studies on the association between Fas −670 A/G polymorphism and SLE produced controversial results; it may be because of the clinical heterogeneity, different ethnicities, and real genetic heterogeneity. Another possible explanation is the small sample size; nevertheless our results agree with other reports showing the association between the Fas −670 G allele carrier and SLE [33]. The association of functional polymorphisms in the promoter of Fas with SLE susceptibility has been a controversial issue. Therefore different single-nucleotide polymorphisms have been identified in the promoter region of Fas; one of

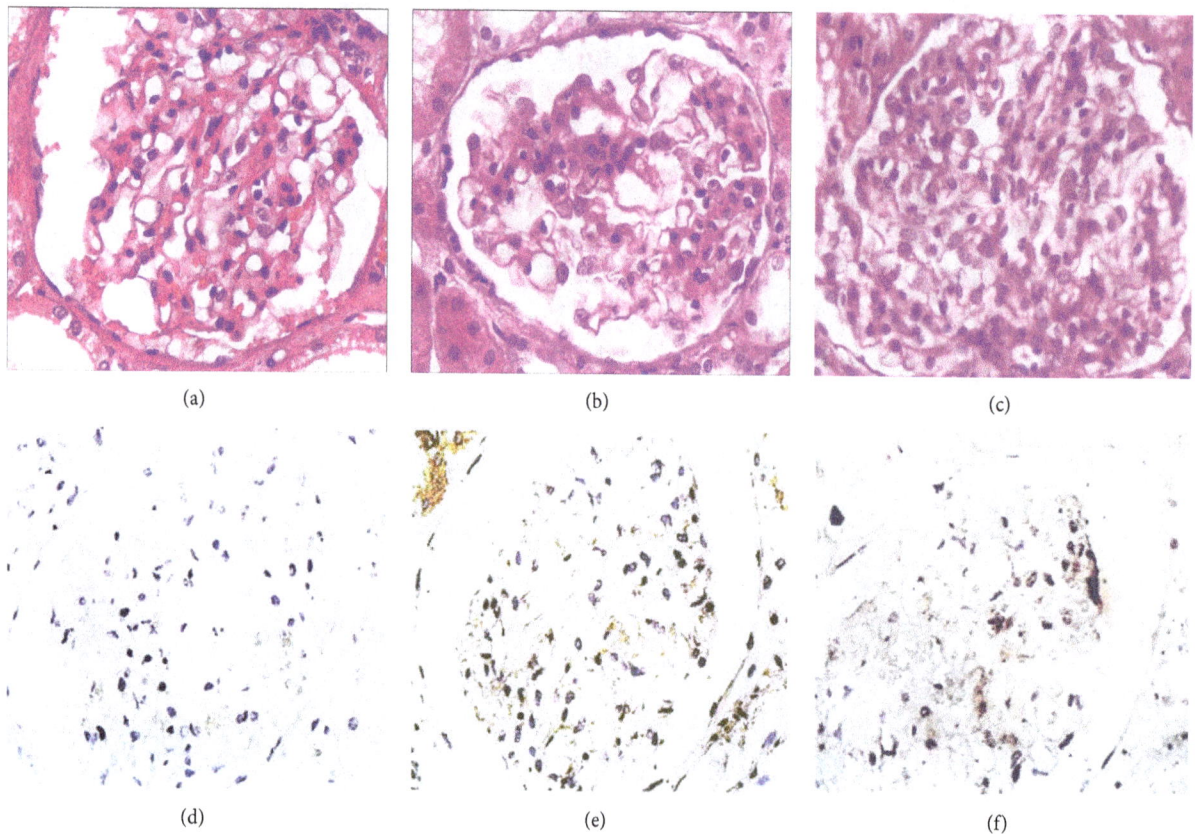

(a)
(b)
(c)
(d)
(e)
(f)

FIGURE 7: The expression of Fas receptor in renal tissue of LN patients and HS by IHC. Superior panel stained by H and E. Inferior panel, IHC for Fas. (a) and (d) HS biopsies; (b), (c), (e), and (f) show a representative of LN. (b) and (e) LN Class-IV. (c) and (f) LN Class-III.

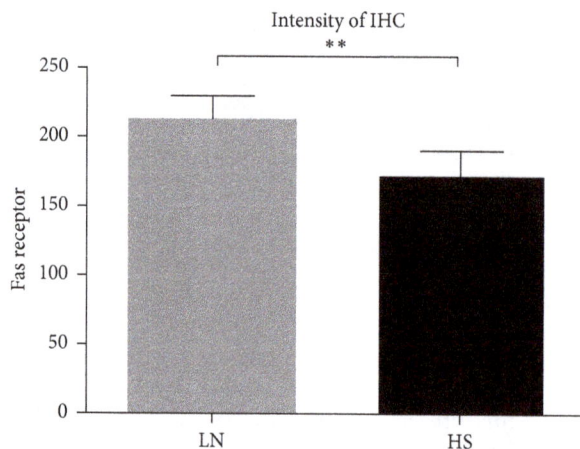

FIGURE 8: Expression of Fas receptor in renal tissue of LN patients and HS. The expression of Fas was increased in patients with LN ($^{**}P < 0.007$).

them is the substitution of A to G at position −670, which theoretically affect the binding ability of the GAS binding protein to the nuclear transcription element STAT-1; this genotype decreases the promoter activity and consequently the Fas-expression. Regarding the two forms of Fas receptor, we should note that both normal Fas and the sFas transcripts are derived by the same gene promoter; in the case of sFas transcript it results from an alternative splicing that truncates the transcript and results in a protein that lacks intracellular and transmembrane domains (sFas). In theory the increase of the sFas level might antagonize the Fas-FasL apoptotic pathway [48]; nevertheless and taking into account our results, the mRNA of Fas as well as the Fas protein was fully expressed at glomerular level as our FISH and immunohistochemistry assays demonstrated; furthermore the Fas pathway was functional because we were able to demonstrate correlation between Fas receptor expression and apoptotic features of lupus nephritis patients as the TUNEL assays demonstrated; another alternative explanation for sFas increasing in LN patients could be secondary to the local inflammatory process. In this scenario the matrix metalloproteinases (MMP) are produced and are related with renal dysfunction; therefore MMP associates to proliferating events at glomerular level, and therefore enhanced MMP activity in lupus nephritis patients as well as in experimental models has been reported [49], interestingly MMP can digest part of the extracellular domain of Fas receptor [26] increasing the sFas levels; it might be the case of our findings in lupus nephritis patients, as we observed in patients with active renal disease, and previously the association of high levels of sFas in patients with kidney damage by lupus was reported [35, 50, 51].

Additionally, another study related with Fas −1377 polymorphism in SLE patients shows an increase in the rate of Fas

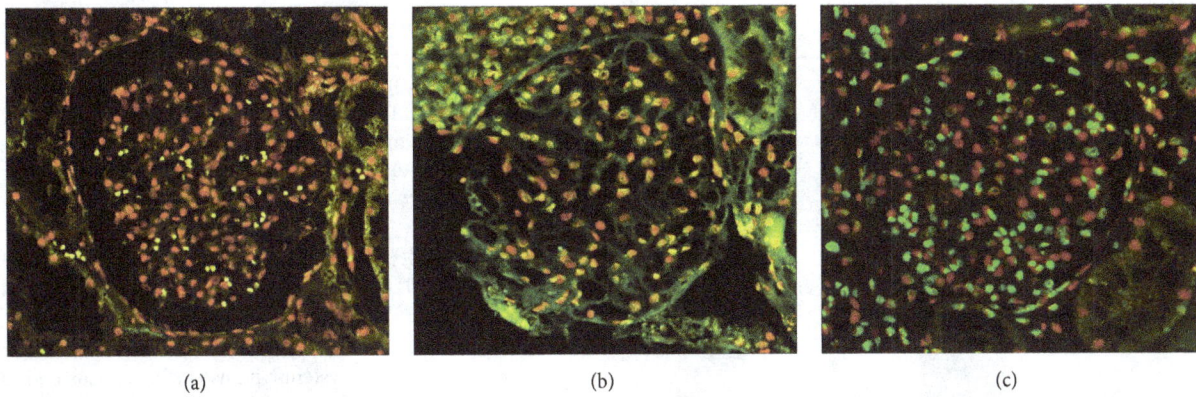

FIGURE 9: TUNEL assays in renal tissue of LN patients and HS. Positive apoptotic cell exhibited nuclei tagged in green. (a) HS biopsies. (b) and (c) show a representative of LN. The nuclei of nonapoptotic cell were red-tagged.

TABLE 4: Characteristics of the individual studies of the −670 (A/G) Fas polymorphism in SLE and sFAS adapted from [33, 34].

Studies	Years	Country	sFas levels ρg/mL SLE/controls	Numbers SLE/controls	A alleles (%) SLE/controls	Association P value
Hatef et al. [35]	2013	Iran	409.38/168 $P = 0.03$	32/46	ND	ND
Moudi et al. [36]	2013	Iran	ND	106/149	58/49	0.03
Pradhan [37]	2012	India	4771.5/1131.4 $P = $ ND	70/70	58/42	0.001
Molin et al. [38]	2012	Germany	ND	46/96	37/11.5	0.001
Man et al. [39]	2012	China	ND	552/718	61.1/58.1	NS
Araste et al. [40]	2010	Iran	158.1/48.7 $P = 0.001$	249/212	51.6/49.5	NS
Sahebari et al. [25]	2010	Iran	372.2/190.3 $P = 0.001$	114/50	ND	ND
Mahfoudh et al. [41]	2007	Tunisia	0/3,200	0/170	0/57	ND
Xu et al. [42]	2004	China	ND	103/110	NS	NS
Kanemitsu et al. [43]	2002	Japan	ND	109/140		0.004
Lee et al. [44]	2001	Korea	ND	87/86	NS	NS
Al-Maini et al. [45]	2000	United Arab Emirates	600/260 $P = 0.0001$	39/22	ND	ND
Huang et al. [19]	1997	Australia	ND	79/86	NS	NS
Jodo et al. [21]	1997	Japan	870/220 $P = 0.001$	77/40	ND	ND
Present study	2014	Mexico	1094.41/630.44 $P = 0.001$	67/54	48/63	0.03

sFas: soluble Fas, SLE: systemic lupus erythematosus, ND: undetermined, NS: not significant.

transcription, which may increase the number of apoptotic cells, resulting in a deficiency in the clearing of apoptotic bodies. These cells undergo secondary necrosis, releasing intracellular antigens that break down immune tolerance, resulting in autoimmunity and tissue damage that affects natural filters, such as the kidneys. In the present study, we demonstrate that increased levels of sFas correlate with the presence of autoantibodies and proteinuria due to podocyte damage, and our results confirm previous reports [25].

Finally, we observed a higher sFas concentration in SLE patients with greater proteinuria, reflecting podocyte damage according to the increased levels of the urinary biomarker WT-1. As a result, sFas may be used as an alternate biomarker in patients with LN, as these levels may predict damage to the ultrafiltration glomerular unit. In conclusion, the present study indicates that the G allele of the Fas −670 polymorphism is associated with genetic susceptibility to SLE as well as increased levels of sFas in patients with LN.

Conflict of Interests

The authors declare that there is no conflict of interests regarding the publication of this paper.

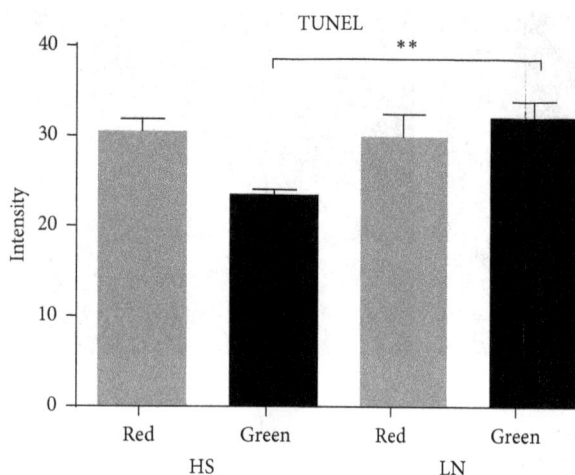

FIGURE 10: TUNEL assays in renal tissue of LN patients and HS. The intensity green belongs to glomerular apoptotic cells in LN biopsies, the red color belongs to nonapoptotic cells. $^{**}P < 0.008$.

Acknowledgment

This work was partially supported by Grant PROMEP UAZ-CA-5 Autoinmunidad (R. Herrera-Esparza) and by CONACYT-FOMIX grant ZAC-09-C01-122342 (E. Avalos-Díaz and J. J. Bollain-y-Goytia). Article processing charges were supported by PIFI 2013, area of Health Sciences.

References

[1] D. P. D'Cruz, M. A. Khamashta, and G. R. Hughes, "Systemic lupus erythematosus," *The Lancet*, vol. 369, no. 9561, pp. 587–596, 2007.

[2] J. H. M. Berden, "Lupus nephritis: consequence of disturbed removal of apoptotic cells?" *The Netherlands Journal of Medicine*, vol. 61, no. 8, pp. 233–238, 2003.

[3] K. Miyake, M. Akahoshi, and H. Nakashima, "Th subset balance in lupus nephritis," *Journal of Biomedicine and Biotechnology*, vol. 2011, Article ID 980286, 7 pages, 2011.

[4] R. W. Read, "Clinical mini-review: systemic lupus erythematosus and the eye," *Ocular Immunology and Inflammation*, vol. 12, no. 2, pp. 87–99, 2004.

[5] C. Hanrotel-Saliou, I. Segalen, Y. Le Meur, P. Youinou, and Y. Renaudineau, "Glomerular antibodies in lupus nephritis," *Clinical Reviews in Allergy & Immunology*, vol. 40, no. 3, pp. 151–158, 2011.

[6] Y. Iwata, K. Furuichi, S. Kaneko, and T. Wada, "The role of cytokine in the lupus nephritis," *Journal of Biomedicine and Biotechnology*, vol. 2011, Article ID 594809, 7 pages, 2011.

[7] S. Torabinejad, R. Mardani, Z. Habibagahi et al., "Urinary monocyte chemotactic protein-1 and transforming growth factor-β in systemic lupus erythematosus," *Indian Journal of Nephrology*, vol. 22, no. 1, pp. 5–12, 2012.

[8] J. J. Bollain-Y-Goytia, M. González-Castañeda, F. Torres-del-Muro et al., "Increased excretion of urinary podocytes in lupus nephritis," *Indian Journal of Nephrology*, vol. 21, no. 3, pp. 166–171, 2011.

[9] M. M. A. Fernando, C. R. Stevens, P. C. Sabeti et al., "Identification of two independent risk factors for lupus within the MHC in United Kingdom families," *PLoS Genetics*, vol. 3, no. 11, article e192, 2007.

[10] A. W. Gibson, J. C. Edberg, J. Wu, R. G. J. Westendorp, T. W. J. Huizinga, and R. P. Kimberly, "Novel single nucleotide polymorphisms in the distal IL-10 promoter affect IL-10 production and enhance the risk of systemic lupus erythematosus," *The Journal of Immunology*, vol. 166, no. 6, pp. 3915–3922, 2001.

[11] M. Linker-Israeli, D. J. Wallace, J. Prehn et al., "Association of IL-6 gene alleles with systemic lupus erythematosus (SLE) and with elevated IL-6 expression," *Genes and Immunity*, vol. 1, no. 1, pp. 45–52, 1999.

[12] A. G. Wilson, C. Gordon, F. S. di Giovine et al., "A genetic association between systemic lupus erythematosus and tumor necrosis factor alpha," *European Journal of Immunology*, vol. 24, no. 1, pp. 191–195, 1994.

[13] M. Matsushita, N. Tsuchiya, T. Oka, A. Yamane, and K. Tokunaga, "New polymorphisms of human CD80 and CD86: lack of association with rheumatoid arthritis and systemic lupus erythematosus," *Genes and Immunity*, vol. 1, no. 7, pp. 428–434, 2000.

[14] T. Kojima, T. Horiuchi, and H. Nishizaka, "Analysis of fas ligand gene mutation in patients with systemic lupus erytematosus," *Arthritis and Rheumatism*, vol. 43, no. 1, pp. 135–139, 2000.

[15] G. Lima, E. Soto-Vega, Y. Atisha-Fregoso et al., "MCP-1, RANTES, and SDF-1 polymorphisms in Mexican patients with systemic lupus erythematosus," *Human Immunology*, vol. 68, no. 12, pp. 980–985, 2007.

[16] R. Velázquez-Cruz, L. Orozco, F. Espinoza-Rosales et al., "Polimorfismo PDCD-1 al inicio de la infancia y su asociación con lupus eritematoso sistémico," *European Journal of Human Genetics*, vol. 15, no. 3, pp. 336–341, 2007.

[17] E. Montoya-Díaz, H. Cervera-Castillo, L. Chávez-Sánchez et al., "Prolactin promoter polymorphism (-1149 G/T) is associated with ANTI-DNA antibodies in Mexican patients with systemic lupus erythematosus," *Immunological Investigations*, vol. 40, no. 6, pp. 614–626, 2011.

[18] E. J. Córdova, R. Velázquez-Cruz, F. Centeno, V. Baca, and L. Orozco, "The NRF2 gene variant, -653G/A, is associated with nephritis in childhood-onset systemic lupus erythematosus," *Lupus*, vol. 19, no. 10, pp. 1237–1242, 2010.

[19] Q. R. Huang, D. Morris, and N. Manolios, "Identification and characterisation of polymorphisms in the promoter region of the human Apo-1/Fas (CD95) gene," *Molecular Immunology*, vol. 34, no. 8-9, pp. 577–582, 1997.

[20] I. Cascino, C. Ballerini, S. Audino et al., "Fas gene polymorphisms are not associated with systemic lupus erythematosus, multiple sclerosis and HIV infection," *Disease Markers*, vol. 13, no. 4, pp. 221–225, 1998.

[21] S. Jodo, S. Kobayashi, N. Kayagaki et al., "Serum levels of soluble Fas/APO-1 (CD95) and its molecular structure in patients with systemic lupus erythematosus (SLE) and other autoimmune diseases," *Clinical and Experimental Immunology*, vol. 107, no. 1, pp. 89–95, 1997.

[22] S. Kamihira and Y. Yamada, "Soluble Fas (APO-1/CD95) isoform in adult T-cell leukemia," *Leukemia and Lymphoma*, vol. 41, no. 1-2, pp. 169–176, 2001.

[23] A. Tomokuni, T. Aikoh, T. Matsuki et al., "Elevated soluble Fas/APO-1 (CD95) levels in silicosis patients without clinical symptoms of autoimmune diseases or malignant tumours," *Clinical and Experimental Immunology*, vol. 110, no. 2, pp. 303–309, 1997.

[24] H. Sano, K. Asano, S. Minatoguchi et al., "Plasma soluble Fas and soluble Fas ligand in chronic glomerulonephritis," *Nephron*, vol. 80, no. 2, pp. 153–161, 1998.

[25] M. Sahebari, M. Reza, Z. Rezaieyazdi, M. Abbasi, B. Abbasi, and M. Mahmoudi, "Correlation between serum levels of soluble fas ((CD95)/Apo 1) with disease activity in systemic lupus erythematosus patients in Khorasan," *Archives of Iranian Medicine*, vol. 13, no. 2, pp. 135–142, 2010.

[26] K. Musia and D. Zwolińska, "Matrix metalloproteinases and soluble Fas/FasL system as novel regulators of apoptosis in children and young adults on chronic dialysis," *Apoptosis*, vol. 16, no. 7, pp. 653–659, 2011.

[27] I. Cascino, G. Papoff, A. Eramo, and G. Ruberti, "Soluble Fas/Apo-1 splicing variants and apoptosis," *Frontiers in Bioscience*, vol. 1, no. 1, pp. d12–d18, 1996.

[28] E. M. Tan, A. S. Cohen, J. F. Fries et al., "The 1982 revised criteria for the classification of systemic lupus erythematosus," *Arthritis & Rheumatism*, vol. 25, no. 11, pp. 1271–1277, 1982.

[29] S. A. Miller, D. D. Dykes, and H. F. Polesky, "A simple salting out procedure for extracting DNA from human nucleated cells," *Nucleic Acids Research*, vol. 16, no. 3, p. 1215, 1988.

[30] A. K. Vaishnaw, J. R. Orlinick, J.-L. Chu, P. H. Krammer, M. V. Chao, and K. B. Elkon, "The molecular basis for apoptotic defects in patients with CD95 (Fas/Apo-1) mutations," *Journal of Clinical Investigation*, vol. 103, no. 3, pp. 355–363, 1999.

[31] I. Badillo-Almaráz, L. Daza, E. Avalos-Díaz, and R. Herrera-Esparza, "Glomerular expression of Fas ligand and Bax mRNA in lupus nephritis," *Autoimmunity*, vol. 34, no. 4, pp. 283–289, 2001.

[32] J. J. Weening, V. D. D'Agati, M. M. Schwartz et al., "The classification of glomerulonephritis in systemic lupus erythematosus revisited," *Journal of the American Society of Nephrology*, vol. 15, no. 2, pp. 241–250, 2004.

[33] Y. H. Lee, S.-C. Bae, S. J. Choi, J. D. Ji, and G. G. Song, "Associations between the FAS -670 A/G and -1,377 G/A polymorphisms and susceptibility to autoimmune rheumatic diseases: a meta-analysis," *Molecular Biology Reports*, vol. 39, no. 12, pp. 10671–10679, 2012.

[34] N. Xiang, X.-M. Li, G.-S. Wang, J.-H. Tao, and X.-P. Li, "Association of Fas gene polymorphisms with systemic lupus erythematosus: a meta-analysis," *Molecular Biology Reports*, vol. 40, no. 1, pp. 407–415, 2013.

[35] M. R. Hatef, M. Sahebari, Z. Rezaieyazdi, M. R. Nakhjavani, and M. Mahmoudi, "Stronger correlation between interleukin 18 and soluble fas in lupus nephritis compared with mild lupus," *ISRN Rheumatology*, vol. 2013, Article ID 850851, 6 pages, 2013.

[36] B. Moudi, S. Salimi, F. F. Mashhadi et al., "Association of FAS and FAS ligand genes polymorphism and risk of systemic lupus erythematosus," *The Scientific World Journal*, vol. 2013, Article ID 176741, 6 pages, 2013.

[37] V. D. Pradhan, "APO1/F as promoter polymorphism in systemic lupus erythematosus (SLE): significance in clinical expression of the disease," *The Journal of the Association of Physicians of India*, vol. 60, no. 9, pp. 34–37, 2012.

[38] S. Molin, E. H. Weiss, T. Ruzicka, and G. Messer, "The FAS/cd95 promoter single-nucleotide polymorphism -670 A/G and lupus erythematosus," *Clinical and Experimental Dermatology*, vol. 37, no. 4, pp. 425–427, 2012.

[39] M. Man, Y. Quian, C. Chen et al., "Association of FAS gene polymorphism with systemic lupus erythematosus: a case-control study and meta-analysis," *Experimental and Therapeutic Medicine*, vol. 4, no. 3, pp. 497–502, 2012.

[40] J. M. Araste, E. K. Sarvestani, E. Aflaki, and Z. Amirghofran, "Fas gene polymorphisms in systemic lupus erythematosus and serum levels of some apoptosis-related molecules," *Immunological Investigations*, vol. 39, no. 1, pp. 27–38, 2010.

[41] W. Mahfoudh, B. Bel Hadj Jrad, A. Romdhane, and L. Chouchane, "A polymorphism in FAS gene promoter correlated with circulating soluble FAS levels," *International Journal of Immunogenetics*, vol. 34, no. 3, pp. 209–212, 2007.

[42] A. P. Xu and P. D. Yin, "Association of Fas promoter -670 polymorphism with systemic lupus erythematosus in southern Chinese," *Chinese Journal of Pathophysiology*, vol. 20, no. 1, pp. 1819–1822, 2004.

[43] S. Kanemitsu, K. Ihara, A. Saifddin et al., "A functional polymorphism in Fas (CD95/APO-1) gene promoter associated with systemic lupus erythematosus," *Journal of Rheumatology*, vol. 29, no. 6, pp. 1183–1188, 2002.

[44] Y. H. Lee, Y. R. Kim, J. D. Ji, J. Sohn, and G. G. Song, "Fas promoter -670 polymorphism is associated with development of anti-RNP antibodies in systemic lupus erythematosus," *Journal of Rheumatology*, vol. 28, no. 9, pp. 2008–2011, 2001.

[45] M. H. Al-Maini, J. D. Mountz, H. A. Al-Mohri et al., "Serum levels of soluble Fas correlate with indices of organ damage in systemic lupus erythematosus," *Lupus*, vol. 9, no. 2, pp. 132–139, 2000.

[46] W. B. Aleya, I. Sfar, L. Mouelhi et al., "Association of Fas/Apo1 gene promoter (-670 A/G) polymorphism in Tunisian patients with IBD," *World Journal of Gastroenterology*, vol. 15, no. 29, pp. 3643–3648, 2009.

[47] I. Silva-Zolezzi, A. Hidalgo-Miranda, J. Estrada-Gil et al., "Analysis of genomic diversity in Mexican Mestizo populations to develop genomic medicine in Mexico," *Proceedings of the National Academy of Sciences of the United States of America*, vol. 106, no. 21, pp. 8611–8616, 2009.

[48] L. Lima, A. Morais, F. Lobo, F. M. Calais-da-Silva, F. E. Calais-da-Silva, and R. Medeiros, "Association between FAS polymorphism and prostate cancer development," *Prostate Cancer and Prostatic Diseases*, vol. 11, no. 1, pp. 94–98, 2008.

[49] A. A. Tveita, O. P. Rekvig, and S. N. Zykova, "Glomerular matrix metalloproteinases and their regulators in the pathogenesis of lupus nephritis," *Arthritis Research and Therapy*, vol. 10, no. 6, pp. 229–237, 2008.

[50] E. Tinazzii, A. Puccetti, R. Gerli et al., "Serum DNase I, soluble Fas/FasL levels and cell surface Fas expression in patients with SLE: a possible explanation for the lack of efficacy of hrDNase I treatment," *International Immunology*, vol. 21, no. 3, pp. 237–243, 2009.

[51] J. H. Hao, D. Q. Ye, G. Q. Zhang et al., "Elevated levels of serum soluble Fas are associated with organ and tissue damage in systemic lupus erythematosus among Chinese," *Archives of Dermatological Research*, vol. 297, no. 7, pp. 329–332, 2006.

Serum Endocan Levels Associated with Hypertension and Loss of Renal Function in Pediatric Patients after Two Years from Renal Transplant

Livia Victorino de Souza,[1] Vanessa Oliveira,[1] Aline Oliveira Laurindo,[1]
DelmaRegına Gomes Huarachı,[2] Paulo Cesar Koch Nogueira,[2] Luciana de Santis Feltran,[1]
José Osmar Medina-Pestana,[1] and Maria do Carmo Franco[1]

[1]*Nephrology Division, School of Medicine, Federal University of São Paulo, São Paulo, SP, Brazil*
[2]*Pediatrics Department, School of Medicine, Federal University of São Paulo, São Paulo, SP, Brazil*

Correspondence should be addressed to Maria do Carmo Franco; mariadocarmo.franco@gmail.com

Academic Editor: Laszlo Rosivall

Endocan is an important biomarker of inflammation and endothelial dysfunction that increases in association with several chronic diseases. Few published data have described the role of endocan in pediatric renal transplant (RT) patients. We evaluated the endocan concentrations in 62 children who underwent renal transplantation and assessed their relationships with the patients' blood pressure and loss of renal function. The endocan levels were significantly elevated in the pediatric RT patients who had hypertension and a loss of renal function. We determined positive correlations between the endocan concentrations and the hemodynamic variables (systolic blood pressure: $r = 0.416$; $P = 0.001$; pulse pressure: $r = 0.412$; $P = 0.003$). The endocan levels were inversely correlated with the estimated glomerular filtration rate ($r = -0.388$; $P = 0.003$). An endocan cutoff concentration of 7.0 ng/mL identified pediatric RT patients who had hypertension and a loss of renal function with 100% sensitivity and 75% specificity. In conclusion, the endocan concentrations were significantly elevated in pediatric RT patients who had both hypertension and a loss of renal function. The correlations between the endocan levels and the hemodynamic variables and the markers of renal function strengthen the hypothesis that it is an important marker of cardiorenal risk.

1. Introduction

Renal transplantation is one of the most effective options for the treatment of chronic renal failure in children [1, 2]. Children who receive renal transplants (RTs) have better survival rates than children who undergo dialysis [3]. In addition, these children show improvements in the quality of their lives and their life expectancies [3, 4].

Despite a positive prognosis, concerns continue to exist about the progressive loss of renal function and the development of cardiometabolic diseases among pediatric RT recipients [5–7]. The findings from several studies have demonstrated that hypertension (HT) is a major cardiovascular comorbidity that can follow renal transplantation in pediatric patients [8–11], and the prevalence of HT among these

patients ranges from 60% to 90% [8]. Some investigators have verified that the development or the persistence of HT during the posttransplant period is an important risk factor that is associated with graft loss and survival [8–11]. Indeed, a negative association between HT and the glomerular filtration rate (GFR) was determined after renal transplantation in children [9]. While several factors may explain this association, the underlying mechanism remains unclear. It is possible that posttransplant HT together with donor and recipient factors, including the time on dialysis, immunosuppressive therapy, the timing of the transplantation, and the donor's age, converge to negatively impact upon the GFR.

The findings from recent research indicate that endocan could be an important predictive marker of arterial HT and renal failure [12–14]. Endocan is a soluble dermatan sulfate proteoglycan that is expressed by the human endothelial cells that are present in many different vascular beds [15, 16]. Its expression is regulated by inflammatory cytokines that induce the upregulation of endocan messenger ribonucleic acid, and the molecule is subsequently released by the endothelial cells [17]. Several reports indicate that the endocan concentrations negatively impact upon the severity of illnesses and the clinical outcomes [14, 18, 19]. The purpose of this study was to analyze the endocan concentrations in pediatric patients during the 6–24-month period after renal transplantation. We also assessed the relationships between the endocan levels and the patients' blood pressure and loss of renal function.

2. Methods

This study was conducted at the Renal Transplant Unit of the Nephrology Division from Kidney & Hypertension Hospital (Federal University of São Paulo; UNIFESP-EPM, São Paulo, Brazil) on pediatrics patients, who were recruited between August 2013 and July 2014. The study was carried out on 62 RT children (43 boys and 19 girls). Inclusion criteria were as follows: RT patients of either sex; patients who were between 6 and 24 months after transplant. On the other hand, patients were excluded for the following reasons: presence of systemic infection or acute rejection clinically diagnosed and biopsy proven. None of the children who underwent renal transplant received vitamin D supplementation. All patients provided a blood sample, which was collected in the morning, following an overnight fast. After that, the body weight and height were measured using a standard balance beam scale. The local ethics committee approved the study protocol *(Protocol Number: 354.875)*. All parents and children signed written informed consent/assent forms.

2.1. Measurement of Blood Pressure Levels. Systolic (SBP) and diastolic (DBP) blood pressure were measured with appropriate cuff size by auscultation after the child was seated for 10 min. We defined HT in accordance with the Fourth National Task Force on High Blood Pressure in Children and Adolescents [20]. An HT diagnosis was established when three or more assessments of the SBP and/or the DBP on different days over a 21-day interval were above the 95th percentiles at 6 months after transplant. We calculated the pulse pressure (PP) using the following formula: PP = SBP − DBP.

2.2. Renal Function Assay. The serum creatinine (sCr) levels were measured using an automated picric acid assay and a Hitachi 717 analyzer in accordance with the manufacturers' instructions. The estimated GFR (eGFR) was determined based on the sCr levels using the Bedside Schwartz equation, as follows: (eGFR = $0.413 \times$ height (cm)/Scr [mg/dL] = mL/min/1.73 m^2) [21].

2.3. Endocan Measurement. The serum endocan levels were measured using a magnetic bead-based immunoassay kit (HCVD1MAG-67K–1 Plex; Merck Millipore, Billerica, MA, USA), according to the manufacturer's protocol. The assay's concentration range was 0.02–9.6 ng/mL. The intra-assay and

interassay coefficients of variation for the endocan assay were <2.43% and <5.57%, respectively. Neither significant cross-reactivity nor interference between human endocan and the breakdown product, which is a p14 peptide fragment, has been reported.

2.4. Statistical Analysis. The categorical variables are presented as the frequencies and the percentage distributions. The continuous variables were assessed for normality before the data were analyzed, and they are summarized as the means, standard deviations, and the 95% confidence intervals (CIs). The analyses were performed by stratifying the pediatric RT patients according to the chronic kidney disease (CKD) cutoff point, namely, an eGFR of <60 mL/min/1.73 m^2, and the presence or absence of HT [20, 22]. To examine the effects of HT and CKD on the endocan levels, we performed a two-way analysis of variance (ANOVA) followed by pairwise multiple comparisons using the Bonferroni test that examined the significance of the main effect and/or the interactions between HT and CKD. Correlations between the continuous variables were determined using Pearson's correlation coefficient. Furthermore, logistic regression analyses were performed. Variables that showed a tendency towards a correlation and had a value of $P < 0.20$ in the univariate model were included in the multivariate analysis. A receiver operating characteristic (ROC) curve was applied to identify the best endocan cutoff point. All of the statistical tests were two-tailed, and the significance level was set at $P < 0.05$. The statistical analyses were performed using IBM®SPSS® software (Version 22, IBM Corporation, Armonk, NY, USA).

3. Results

Our study cohort comprised 62 pediatric RT patients, and 67% of the patients were boys. The mean age of the recipients at transplantation was 12.8 years (range: 3–17 years), and the mean age of the donors was 12.7 years (range: 2–43 years). Six of the donors were adults and 56 donors were younger than 18 years of age. The causes of renal failure were defined as uropathy in 22.6% and glomerulonephritis in 17.7% of the patients, and the etiologies were undetermined or the renal failure was associated with other causes in 59.7% of the RT patients (Table 1). After renal transplantation, 29 of 62 (46.8%) children had CKD, which was defined as an eGFR < 60 mL/min/1.73 m^2. HT was detected in 44 of the children before renal transplantation, and HT persisted in 29 of the children after transplantation. Sixteen children had both HT and CKD after renal transplantation, and 20 children had neither HT nor CKD. Seventeen children (26%) were given steroid-free immunosuppressive therapy and seven children (25%) were given single agent antihypertensive therapy that comprised calcium channel blockers (CCBs). Demographic, anthropometric, and clinical data are presented in Tables 1 and 2.

The mean endocan concentration was 12.2 ng/mL (range: 4.3–15.4 ng/mL), and there was no significant difference between the genders with respect to the endocan concentration ($P = 0.252$). There were no correlations between

TABLE 1: Clinical characteristics of the study population at renal transplant.

Characteristic	
Age at transplantation (years)	12.8 (3.51) (11.9–13.8)
Male gender	43 (69)
Causes of chronic kidney disease	
Glomerulonephritis	11 (17.7)
Uropathy	14 (22.6)
CAKUT	10 (16)
Recurrent urinary tract infections	2 (3)
Hemolytic-uremic syndrome	2 (3)
Multicystic dysplastic kidney	2 (3)
Nephropathic cystinosis	1 (1.6)
Undetermined cause	20 (33.1)
Mode of dialysis	
CAPD	16 (26)
HD	35 (56)
CAPD + HD	6 (10)
No dialysis	5 (8)
Time on chronic dialysis (months)	15.8 (9.66) (12.9–18.7)
Preexisting hypertension	44 (55)
Deceased donor	60 (96.8)
Male donor	40 (66)
Donor age	12.7 (8.7) (10.3–15.1)
Acute rejection	9 (15)
Delayed graft function	22 (36)
Cold ischemia time (min)	1265.6 (360.8) (1158.4–1372.7)
Renal artery stenosis	2 (3.2)

Data are reported as number with percent in parentheses or mean with standard deviation and 95% confidence interval in parentheses. CAKUT: congenital anomalies of the kidney and the urinary tract; HD: hemodialysis; CAPD: continuous ambulatory peritoneal dialysis.

TABLE 2: Characteristics of the study population after transplantation.

Characteristic	
Age (years)	14.5 (3.3) (13.6–15.4)
Height (cm)	149.5 (16.6) (144.9–154.1)
Weight (Kg)	45.5 (16.2) (41.0–49.6)
BMI (Kg/m^2)	19.9 (4.5) (18.6–21.2)
SBP (mmHg)	125 (13.5) (121–128)
DBP (mmHg)	83 (12.4) (80–87)
PP (mmHg)	42 (13.2) (38–45)
sCr (mg/dL)	1.01 (0.28) (0.93–1.09)
eGFR (mL/min/1.73 m^2)	64.3 (17.6) (59.4–69.2)
Endocan (ng/mL)	12.5 (4.2) (11.3–13.6)
Immunosuppressive therapy	
TAC + MMF + AZA	5 (8)
AZA + MMF	12 (18)
PRED + AZA + CSA	4 (6)
PRED + TAC + AZA	32 (53)
PRED + TAC	9 (15)
Antihypertensive therapy	
ACE-I + CCBs	4 (14)
ACE-I + ARBs	5 (18)
ARBs + CCBs + β-blockers	4 (14)
Diuretics + CCBs + β-blockers	8 (29)
CCBs	7 (25)

Data are reported as number with percent in parentheses or mean with standard deviation and 95% confidence interval in parentheses. BMI: body mass index; SBP: systolic blood pressure; DBP: diastolic blood pressure; PP: pulse pressure; sCr: serum creatinine; eGFR: glomerular filtration rate estimated by creatinine; TAC: tacrolimus; MMF: mycophenolate mofetil; AZA: azathioprine; CSA: cyclosporine A; PRED: prednisone; ACE-I: ACE inhibitors; CCBs: calcium channel blockers; ARBs: angiotensin receptor blockers.

the endocan levels and age ($r = 0.120$; $P > 0.05$) or the body mass index (BMI) ($r = 0.107$; $P > 0.05$). We found positive correlations between the endocan levels and the SBP ($r = 0.416$; $P = 0.001$) and the PP ($r = 0.412$; $P = 0.003$) (Figures 1(a) and 1(b)). These correlations remained significant after adjusting for gender, age, BMI, and the time on chronic dialysis (SBP: $r = 0.333$; $P = 0.018$ and PP: $r = 0.358$ and $P = 0.011$). The serum endocan levels did not change significantly when immunosuppressive or antihypertensive agents were administered (both $P > 0.05$). Inverse correlations were detected between the eGFR and the SBP ($r = -0.274$; $P = 0.037$) and the PP ($r = -0.281$; $P = 0.032$). Interestingly, endocan levels were inversely correlated with the eGFR ($r = -0.388$; $P = 0.003$).

The two-way ANOVA revealed the significant effects of HT ($F = 5.989$; $P = 0.017$) and CKD ($F = 25.959$; $P < 0.001$) on the serum endocan concentrations (Figure 2(a)). Pediatric

RT patients with HT and CKD ($n = 16$) had a significantly higher mean serum endocan concentration (15.4 ng/mL; 95% CI: 13.8–17.2) compared with that in the pediatric RT patients who did not have either of these conditions ($n = 20$) (8.9 ng/mL; 95% CI: 7.4–10.5) ($P < 0.001$) and the mean serum endocan concentration in those with HT only ($n = 13$) (10.8 ng/mL; 95% CI: 8.9–12.6) ($P = 0.002$). There was no significant difference with respect to the mean serum endocan concentration between the pediatric RT patients with HT and CKD and those with CKD only ($n = 13$) (13.1 ng/mL; 95% CI: 11.2–14.9) ($P = 0.342$) (Figure 2(b)). The mean serum endocan concentration in the pediatric RT

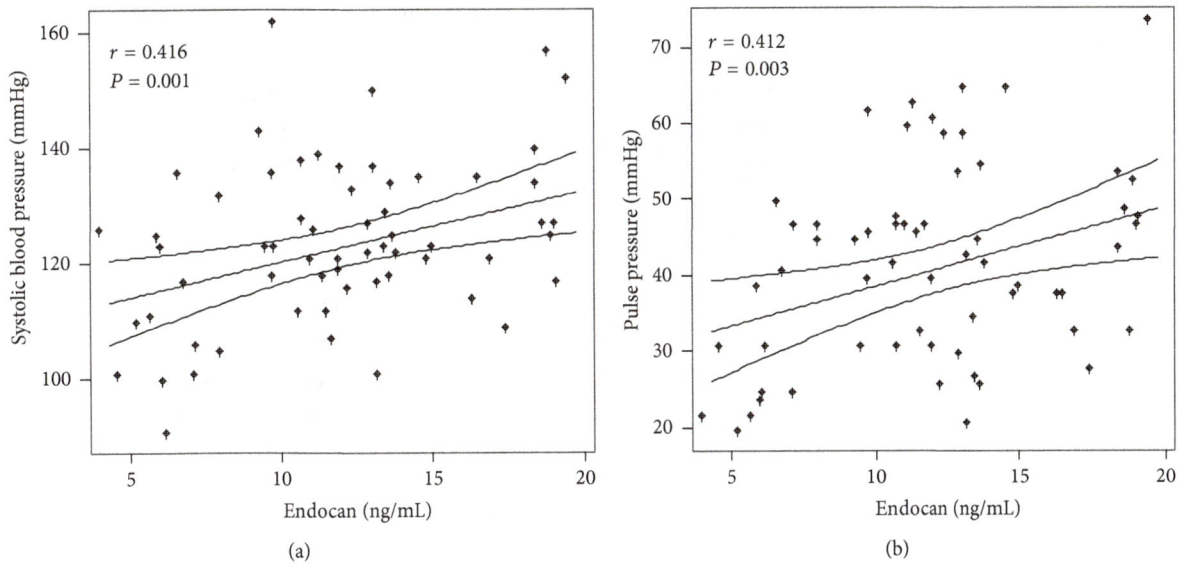

(a)   (b)

FIGURE 1: Scatter plots showing the correlations between endocan with (a) systolic blood pressure ($r = 0.416$; $P = 0.001$) and endocan with (b) pulse pressure ($r = 0.412$; $P = 0.003$). The lines represent the weighted regression with its 95% confidence interval. Statistical analysis: Pearson's correlation method.

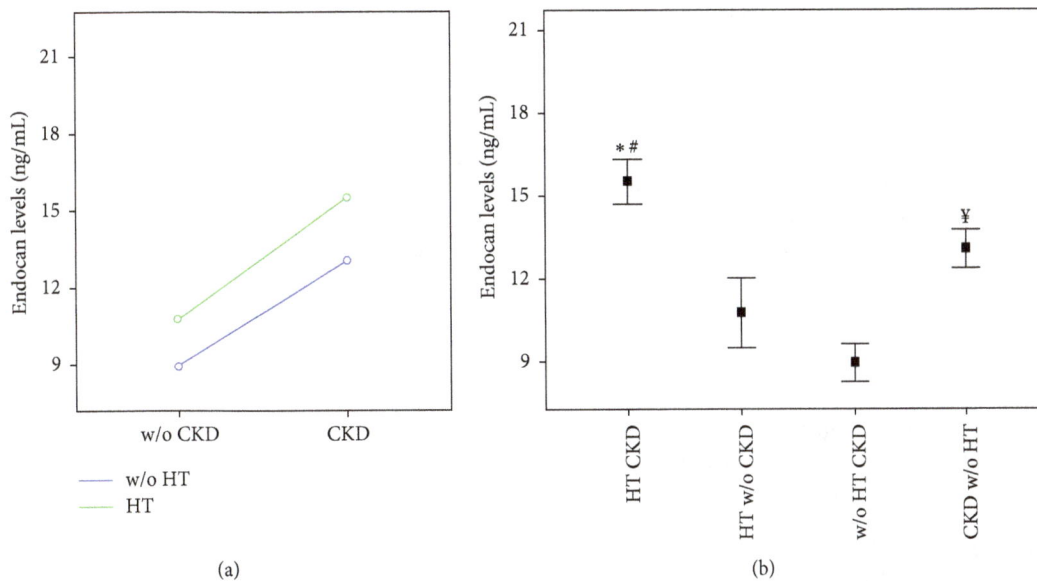

(a)   (b)

FIGURE 2: (a) Interaction plot of the mean endocan levels in RT children ($n = 62$) according to presence or not of the hypertension (HT) and/or chronic kidney disease (CKD). Statistical analysis: two-way analysis of variance (ANOVA) method. (b) Changes in the endocan levels in RT children with both HT and CKD (HTCKD; $n = 16$), with HT without CKD (HT w/o CKD; $n = 13$), with CKD without HT (CKD w/o HT, $n = 13$), and without both conditions (w/o HTCKD; $n = 20$). The bars indicate standard error of mean. Statistical analysis: two-way analysis of variance (ANOVA) followed by pairwise multiple comparison (Bonferroni test) method. $^{*}P < 0.001$ versus w/o HTCKD; $^{#}P = 0.002$ versus HT w/o CKD; $^{¥}P = 0.007$ versus w/o HTCKD.

patients with only CKD was significantly higher compared with that in the pediatric RT patients who did not have HT or CKD ($P = 0.007$) (Figure 2(b)).

We performed logistic regression analyses to identify the risk factors associated with HT and the loss of renal function in the pediatric RT patients. The univariate analysis showed that donor age, a male donor, the PP, and the use of prednisone tended to be associated with these dependent

variables ($P < 0.20$) (Table 3). The endocan levels were independently associated with the presence of HT and the loss of renal function in the pediatric RT patients (Table 3). The multivariate logistic regression analysis determined that only the endocan levels were independently associated with the presence of HT and the loss of renal function in our study population (Table 3). The ROC curve analysis demonstrated that an endocan cutoff concentration of 7.0 ng/mL could

TABLE 3: Logistic regression analysis for the presence of hypertension and chronic kidney disease (CKD) in RT children.

Variables	Univariate regression Analysis OR (95% CI)	P value	Multivariate regression Analysis OR (95% CI)	P value
Age (per years)	1.110 (0.884–1.395)	0.369		
Male gender (no/yes)	1.333 (0.269–5.606)	0.725		
BMI (per Kg/m²)	1.066 (0.902–1.260)	0.456		
Pulse pressure (mmHg)	1.084 (1.015–1.157)	0.016	1.079 (0.969–1.202)	0.166
Endocan (per ng/mL)	1.855 (1.187–2.898)	0.007	2.070 (1.097–3.907)	0.035
Donor age (per year)	0.832 (0.708–0.978)	0.086	0.839 (0.659–1.085)	0.317
Male donor (no/yes)	1.367 (0.860–1.767)	0.176	1.317 (0.448–4.577)	0.399
Preexisting hypertension (no/yes)	4.437 (0.449–9.723)	0.224		
Chronic dialysis (per months)	1.021 (0.932–1.120)	0.652		
Delayed graft function (no/yes)	1.592 (0.382–6.625)	0.523		
Cold ischemia time (per min)	1.048 (0.258–4.256)	0.948		
Prednisone (no/yes)	1.640 (0.168–2.436)	0.198	1.486 (0.743–5.987)	0.567
Tacrolimus (no/yes)	2.213 (0.467–7.238)	0.298		
Mycophenolate mofetil (no/yes)	1.201 (0.221–5.521)	0.833		
Azathioprine (no/yes)	0.400 (0.109–1.254)	0.251		

Data are reported as odds ratio (OR) and 95% confidence interval (95% CI).

identify pediatric RT patients with both HT and the loss of renal function with a sensitivity of 100% and a specificity of 75% (area under the curve: 0.894; standard error: 0.053; 95% CI: 0.790–0.998; $P < 0.001$) (Figure 3).

4. Discussion

The main finding of present study is that serum endocan levels were significantly elevated in RT children with both HT and loss of renal function and that the serum endocan concentration was an independent predictor of the presence of HT and a loss of renal function in pediatric RT patients, after adjusting for multiple confounders. In addition, we found positive correlation of endocan with SBP and pulse pressure, and the serum levels of this biomarker were inversely correlated with eGFR among RT children.

Endocan is a soluble proteoglycan that is detected in the blood and is expressed by endothelial cells of the vasculature, lung, and kidney [16, 17]. There is strong evidence to support its role in several chronic diseases and that suggests that it is an important biomarker of endothelial function [13, 18, 19]. The findings from a recent study showed that patients with type 2 diabetes who had microalbuminuria had lower endocan levels [23], and the investigators suggested that higher levels of endocan may be present in the early phase of diabetic nephropathy and that the levels of endocan decline as the disease progresses [23]. To date, few studies have evaluated the role of the endocan levels in RT patients. The findings from a study by Li et al. [24] showed that the circulating endocan level could be used as a marker of acute rejection in RT patients. In another report, high levels of endocan were

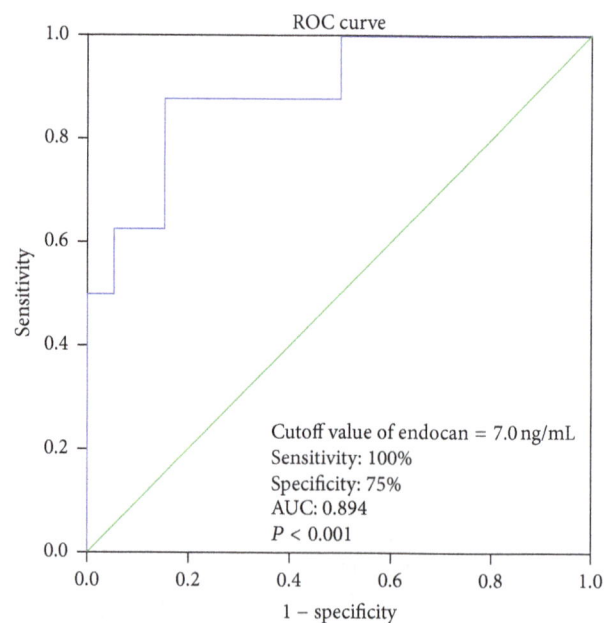

FIGURE 3: Receiver operating characteristic (ROC) curve of endocan levels predicting presence of both hypertension and loss renal function in RT children.

correlated with different stages of the CKD in RT patients [25]. These authors also observed that GFR loss was greater in the group with higher serum endocan levels [25]. In addition, negative correlations have been described between the endocan levels and the eGFR and endothelial function in patients with CKD who had not undergone hemodialysis or peritoneal dialysis [13]. Our results concur with and extend the findings from these studies, and they link high endocan levels with HT and GFR reductions in RT patients. Another interesting finding was the positive association between the endocan levels and the PP. Furthermore, we found that pediatric RT patients who had HT and a loss of renal function also had higher PPs compared with the pediatric RT patients who did not have these conditions. The PP elevations observed in these children might indicate the presence of arterial stiffness that leads to adverse cardiovascular outcomes. The impairment of the elastic properties of the vasculature is widely regarded as a factor that could contribute to the development and/or the persistence of HT and CKD progression [26]. Interestingly, endocan is involved in the development of vascular tissue under physiological and pathological conditions [27–30]. An important consideration is that treatment with antihypertensive and/or immunosuppressive agents may have an effect on the endocan levels. Some drugs, including angiotensin II receptor blockers, tacrolimus, and CCBs, promote alterations in endothelial function that could also influence the circulating endocan levels [31, 32]. In the current study, there were no significant changes in the serum endocan levels that were associated with the administration of immunosuppressive or antihypertensive therapy. Therefore, therapeutic scheme in the RT patient should be taken into account which makes the interpretation of endocan data among these patients even more difficult.

Some mechanisms could explain the high endocan levels in the pediatric RT patients with HT and the loss of renal function. The findings from recent studies have shown links between the endocan levels and endothelial dysfunction and inflammation [13, 18, 19]. Endocan is expressed by the endothelium, and in response to endothelial damage or the presence of inflammatory cytokines, including tumor necrosis factor-alpha and interleukin-1 beta, the endothelial cells upregulate the expression and secretion of endocan [15–17]. Endocan may stimulate the proliferation and migration of vascular smooth muscle cells [33]. Since endothelial dysfunction and inflammatory factors are associated with the development of HT and other cardiovascular diseases in RT patients, it is possible that the presence of these conditions could, at least in part, reflect the processes that were involved in increasing the endocan levels in our study population. Moreover, the increase in the endocan levels in patients with CKD may be a consequence of a reduction in its renal clearance [13]. We did not collect urine samples from the patients in the present study; therefore, we could not compare the fractional excretions of endocan in the pediatric RT patients. However, based on data recently reported in the literature, the high endocan levels in the pediatric RT patients do not appear to have been caused by reductions in the renal clearance of endocan, which results in high concentrations of endocan in the plasma [31]. Endocan is a negatively charged 50 kDa proteoglycan; therefore, under physiological conditions it cannot pass through the glomerular filtration barrier [17, 31]. Indeed, recent study found that endocan was undetectable or was present at very low levels in urine samples from healthy individuals [31]. The same investigators also found that both the plasma and the urinary concentrations of endocan were high in patients with immunoglobulin A nephropathy, which suggests that the presence of glomerular injury that involves the disruption of the basement membrane in patients with pathological renal conditions could promote endocan excretion into the urine [31]. Thus, more knowledge about renal handling of endocan is required to help us understand the mechanisms involved in the production of endocan and its clearance from the circulation via the kidney in RT patients.

The limitations of the present study include the small number of patients recruited, its cross-sectional design, and the single rather than multiple measurements of the serum endocan concentrations. In conclusion, pediatric RT patients with both HT and a loss of renal function have elevated endocan levels. The presence of correlations between the endocan levels and the SBP, the PP, and the eGFR strengthens the hypothesis that endocan is an important marker of cardiorenal risk. Although the pathological implications are not completely understood, the data from this study may help to explain the kidney damage and the increased risks of HT and other cardiovascular diseases that occur in pediatric RT patients. Further studies are necessary to clarify the importance of these correlations and to elucidate the clinical significance of endocan.

Acknowledgments

This research was supported by a Project Grant from the *FAPESP* (Fundação de Amparo à Pesquisa do Estado de São Paulo, Brazil) (Project no. 2013/03139-0) and *CNPq* (Conselho Nacional de Desenvolvimento Científico e Tecnológico) (Project no. 443248/2014-1).

References

[1] B. A. Warady, D. Hébert, E. K. Sullivan, and S. R. Alexander, "Renal transplantation, chronic dialysis and chronic renal insufficiency in children and adolescents. The 1995 annual report of the North American Pediatric Renal Transplant Cooperative study," *Pediatric Nephrology*, vol. 11, pp. 49–64, 1997.

[2] B. J. van der Heijden, P. C. W. van Dijk, K. Verrier-Jones, K. J. Jager, and J. D. Briggs, "Renal replacement therapy in children: data from 12 registries in Europe," *Pediatric Nephrology*, vol. 19, no. 2, pp. 213–221, 2004.

[3] S. P. McDonald and J. C. Craig, "Long-term survival of children with end-stage renal disease," *The New England Journal of Medicine*, vol. 350, no. 26, pp. 2654–2662, 2004.

[4] A. Mehrabi, A. Kashfi, B. Tönshoff et al., "Long-term results of paediatric kidney transplantation at the University of Heidelberg: a 35 year single-centre experience," *Nephrology Dialysis Transplantation*, vol. 19, S4, pp. iv69–iv74, 2004.

[5] M. Wigger, E. Drückler, J. Muscheites, and H. J. Stolpe, "Course of glomerular filtration rate after renal transplantation and the influence of hypertension," *Clinical Nephrology*, vol. 56, no. 6, pp. S30–S34, 2001.

[6] R. Büscher, U. Vester, A.-M. Wingen, and P. F. Hoyer, "Pathomechanisms and the diagnosis of arterial hypertension in pediatric renal allograft recipients," *Pediatric Nephrology*, vol. 19, no. 11, pp. 1202–1211, 2004.

[7] T. Seeman, "Hypertension after renal transplantation," *Pediatric Nephrology*, vol. 24, no. 5, pp. 959–972, 2009.

[8] G. Opelz, T. Wujciak, and E. Ritz, "Association of chronic kidney graft failure with recipient blood pressure," *Kidney International*, vol. 53, no. 1, pp. 217–222, 1998.

[9] A. Moudgil, K. Martz, D. M. Stablein, and D. P. Puliyanda, "Variables affecting estimated glomerular filtration rate after renal transplantation in children: a NAPRTCS data analysis," *Pediatric Transplantation*, vol. 14, no. 2, pp. 288–294, 2010.

[10] M. M. Mitsnefes, P. R. Khoury, and P. T. McEnery, "Early posttransplantation hypertension and poor long-term renal allograft survival in pediatric patients," *Journal of Pediatrics*, vol. 143, no. 1, pp. 98–103, 2003.

[11] J. W. Groothoff, K. Cransberg, M. Offringa et al., "Long-term follow-up of renal transplantation in children: a Dutch cohort study," *Transplantation*, vol. 78, no. 3, pp. 453–460, 2004.

[12] B. Afsar, M. Takir, O. Kostek, A. Covic, and M. Kanbay, "Endocan: a new molecule playing a role in the development of hypertension and chronic kidney disease?" *Journal of Clinical Hypertension*, vol. 16, no. 12, pp. 914–916, 2014.

[13] M. I. Yilmaz, D. Siriopol, M. Saglam et al., "Plasma endocan levels associate with inflammation, vascular abnormalities, cardiovascular events, and survival in chronic kidney disease," *Kidney International*, vol. 86, no. 6, pp. 1213–1220, 2014.

[14] H. G. Lee, H. Y. Choi, and J. Bae, "Endocan as a potential diagnostic or prognostic biomarker for chronic kidney disease," *Kidney International*, vol. 86, no. 6, pp. 1079–1081, 2014.

[15] D. Béchard, T. Gentina, M. Delehedde et al., "Endocan is a novel chondroitin sulfate/dermatan sulfate proteoglycan that promotes hepatocyte growth factor/scatter factor mitogenic activity," *The Journal of Biological Chemistry*, vol. 276, no. 51, pp. 48341–48349, 2001.

[16] S. M. Zhang, L. Zuo, Q. Zhou et al., "Expression and distribution of endocan in human tissues," *Biotechnic and Histochemistry*, vol. 87, no. 3, pp. 172–178, 2012.

[17] P. Lassalle, S. Molet, A. Janin et al., "ESM-1 is a novel human endothelial cell-specific molecule expressed in lung and regulated by cytokines," *The Journal of Biological Chemistry*, vol. 271, no. 34, pp. 20458–20464, 1996.

[18] S. Balta, D. P. Mikhailidis, S. Demirkol, C. Ozturk, T. Celik, and A. Iyisoy, "Endocan: a novel inflammatory indicator in cardiovascular disease?" *Atherosclerosis*, vol. 243, no. 1, pp. 339–343, 2015.

[19] S. Balta, D. P. Mikhailidis, S. Demirkol et al., "Endocan-a novel inflammatory indicator in newly diagnosed patients with hypertension: a pilot study," *Angiology*, vol. 65, no. 9, pp. 773–777, 2014.

[20] National High Blood Pressure Education Program Working Group on High Blood Pressure in Children and Adolescents, "The fourth report on the diagnosis, evaluation, and treatment of high blood pressure in children and adolescents," *Pediatrics*, vol. 114, supplement 2, pp. 1–22, 2004.

[21] G. J. Schwartz and D. F. Work, "Measurement and estimation of GFR in children and adolescents," *Clinical Journal of the American Society of Nephrology*, vol. 4, no. 11, pp. 1832–1843, 2009.

[22] A. S. Levey, J. Coresh, E. Balk et al., "National Kidney Foundation practice guidelines for chronic kidney disease: evaluation, classification, and stratification," *Annals of Internal Medicine*, vol. 139, no. 2, pp. 137–147, 2003.

[23] M. A. Cikrikcioglu, Z. Erturk, E. Kilic et al., "Endocan and albuminuria in type 2 diabetes mellitus," *Renal Failure*, pp. 1–7, 2016.

[24] S. Li, L. Wang, C. Wang et al., "Detection on dynamic changes of endothelial cell specific molecule-1 in acute rejection after renal transplantation," *Urology*, vol. 80, no. 3, pp. 738.e1–738.e8, 2012.

[25] Y.-H. Su, K.-H. Shu, C.-P. Hu et al., "Serum endocan correlated with stage of chronic kidney disease and deterioration in renal transplant recipients," *Transplantation Proceedings*, vol. 46, no. 2, pp. 323–327, 2014.

[26] C. A. Peralta, D. R. Jacobs Jr., R. Katz et al., "Association of pulse pressure, arterial elasticity, and endothelial function with kidney function decline among adults with estimated GFR >60 mL/min/1.73 m^2: the multi-ethnic study of atherosclerosis (MESA)," *American Journal of Kidney Diseases*, vol. 59, no. 1, pp. 41–49, 2012.

[27] L. M. Carrillo, E. Arciniegas, H. Rojas, and R. Ramírez, "Immunolocalization of endocan during the endothelial-mesenchymal transition process," *European Journal of Histochemistry*, vol. 55, article e13, 2011.

[28] M. Delehedde, L. Devenyns, C.-A. Maurage, and R. R. Vivès, "Endocan in cancers: a lesson from a circulating dermatan sulfate proteoglycan," *International Journal of Cell Biology*, vol. 2013, Article ID 705027, 11 pages, 2013.

[29] A. Icli, E. Cure, M. C. Cure et al., "Endocan levels and subclinical atherosclerosis in patients with systemic lupus erythematosus," *Angiology*, vol. 67, no. 8, pp. 749–755, 2016.

[30] N. Altintas, L. C. Mutlu, D. C. Akkoyun et al., "Effect of CPAP on new endothelial dysfunction marker, endocan, in people with obstructive sleep apnea," *Angiology*, vol. 67, no. 4, pp. 364–374, 2016.

[31] Y. H. Lee, J. S. Kim, S. Kim et al., "Plasma endocan level and prognosis of immunoglobulin A nephropathy," *Kidney Research and Clinical Practice*, vol. 35, no. 3, pp. 152–159, 2016.

[32] T. Celik, S. Balta, M. Karaman et al., "Endocan, a novel marker of endothelial dysfunction in patients with essential hypertension: comparative effects of amlodipine and valsartan," *Blood Pressure*, vol. 24, no. 1, pp. 55–60, 2015.

[33] P. Menon, O. N. Kocher, and W. C. Aird, "Endothelial cell specific molecule-1 (ESM-1), a novel secreted proteoglycan stimulates vascular smooth muscle cell proliferation and migration," *Circulation*, vol. 124, Article ID A15455, 2011.

6

High Steroid Sensitivity among Children with Nephrotic Syndrome in Southwestern Nigeria

Taiwo Augustina Ladapo,[1,2] **Christopher Imokhuede Esezobor,**[1,2] **and Foluso Ebun Lesi**[1,2]

[1] *Department of Paediatrics, College of Medicine, University of Lagos, PMB 12003, Lagos, Nigeria*
[2] *Department of Paediatrics, Lagos University Teaching Hospital, Idi-Araba, PMB 12003, Lagos, Nigeria*

Correspondence should be addressed to Taiwo Augustina Ladapo; drteeladapo@yahoo.com

Academic Editor: Tibor Nadasdy

Recent reports from both Caucasian and black populations suggest changes in steroid responsiveness of childhood nephrotic syndrome. This study was therefore undertaken to determine the features and steroid sensitivity pattern of a cohort of black children with nephrotic syndrome. Records of children managed for nephrotic syndrome from January 2008 to April 2013 were reviewed. Details including age, response to treatment, and renal histology were analysed. There were 108 children (median age: 5.9 years, peak: 1-2 years), 90.2% of whom had idiopathic nephrotic syndrome. Steroid sensitivity was 82.8% among children with idiopathic nephrotic syndrome but 75.9% overall. Median time to remission was 7 days. Median age was significantly lower in steroid sensitive compared with resistant patients. The predominant histologic finding in resistant cases was focal segmental glomerulosclerosis (53.3%). No cases of quartan malaria nephropathy or hepatitis B virus nephropathy were diagnosed. Overall mortality was 6.5%. In conclusion, unusually high steroid sensitivity is reported among a cohort of black children. This is likely attributable to the lower age structure of our cohort as well as possible changing epidemiology of some other childhood diseases. Surveillance of the epidemiology of childhood nephrotic syndrome and corresponding modifications in practice are therefore recommended.

1. Introduction

Childhood nephrotic syndrome (NS) is the commonest glomerular lesion encountered in childhood [1, 2]. Although various histological features have been described, the most important determinant of outcome of this condition is steroid responsiveness which is, however, not uniformly distributed globally. High steroid responsiveness has traditionally been demonstrated in temperate regions of the world and, conversely, high steroid resistance in tropical regions of the world like Nigeria [3–10]. Consequently, the black race is often considered an indication for kidney biopsy in children with NS.

Recent reports however suggest changes in steroid responsiveness of nephrotic syndrome, with steroid resistance being increasingly reported in non-blacks while some regions have experienced increasing steroid sensitivity [11–15]. Previous reports from Nigeria demonstrated high steroid resistance ranging between 35% and 92% [6–9, 15–18]. Cursory observations of the cohort of children receiving care in our centre suggested high steroid sensitivity, hence the need for this report. This study therefore evaluates the pattern of steroid sensitivity among a cohort of black children with childhood nephrotic syndrome.

2. Materials and Methods

The study was conducted at the Paediatric Nephrology Unit of the Lagos University Teaching Hospital, a 760-bed tertiary hospital in Southwest Nigeria. The hospital is one of the two referral centres in the state providing renal care to children in Lagos State and its environs. It therefore caters for children across all socioeconomic strata. The records of all children managed for nephrotic syndrome between January 2008 and April 2013 were reviewed. Nephrotic syndrome was diagnosed based on the following: 24-hour urine protein > 40 mg/m^2/hr or spot urine protein: creatinine ratio > 200 mg/mmol, hypoalbuminemia (serum albumin < 25 g/L), generalized oedema, and hypercholesterolemia (serum cholesterol > 5.2 mmol/L) [1, 2].

The following results were retrieved: blood pressure, urine microscopy and culture, serum electrolytes, calcium, phosphate, urea and creatinine, blood film for malaria parasite, haemoglobin genotype, renal ultrasound scan and screening for hepatitis B, hepatitis C, and human immunodeficiency virus, antinuclear antibodies, ANCA, and Complement levels. Microscopic haematuria was defined as >5 red blood cells (RBCs) per high field of a centrifuged urine specimen and glomerular filtration rate (eGFR) was estimated using the modified Schwartz formula. Chronic disease was defined according to the Kidney Disease Outcomes Qualitative Initiative (KDOQI) guidelines [19]. Hypertension was defined as blood pressure > 95th centile for age, gender, and height on three consecutive occasions [20]. Urinary tract infection was diagnosed in the presence of supportive urinalysis findings and significant growth of uropathogenic organism in an appropriately collected urine specimen [2]. Systemic lupus erythematosus (SLE) was diagnosed using the revised American College of Rheumatology criteria [21]. Socioeconomic classification was done using the classification by Oyedeji [22] which employs the educational status and occupation of parents.

3. Treatment Regimen

At first presentation, patients receive oral prednisolone at $60 \, \text{mg/m}^2$ daily for 4–6 weeks. Since 2012, following KDIGO (Kidney Disease Improving Global Outcomes) recommendations, we have extended treatment to 8 weeks to define steroid resistance [23]. Following remission, the dose is reduced to $40 \, \text{mg/m}^2$ on alternate days for 4 weeks and gradually tapered over 3–5 months. Steroid dependence (SD) was treated with the addition of levamisole (2.5 mg/kg/day) on alternate days or cyclophosphamide (oral or intravenous). Steroid resistance was treated with oral (2 mg/kg/day for 8weeks) or intravenous ($500 \, \text{mg/m}^2$/month for 6 months) cyclophosphamide, angiotensin converting enzyme (ACE) inhibitors, or cyclosporine. Since 2012, cyclosporine rather than cyclophosphamide has become the preferred drug for the management of steroid resistance [23]. Renal biopsies were performed by the paediatric nephrologists for steroid resistant or secondary cases of NS. Tissue was considered adequate for reporting if at least 5 glomeruli were present.

4. Definition of Terms [1, 2]

Terms are defined as follows: remission: nil or trace proteinuria < 30 mg/dL for 3 consecutive days after commencing treatment; steroid resistant nephrotic syndrome (SRNS): failure to achieve remission after 6–8 weeks of daily prednisolone; relapse: recurrence of 100 mg/dL (≥2+) proteinuria for ≥3 consecutive days after having been in remission; steroid dependent nephrotic syndrome (SDNS): two consecutive relapses during alternate day steroid therapy or within 14 days after cessation of steroids; frequently relapsing nephrotic syndrome (FRNS): two or more relapses within 6 months of initial response or ≥4 relapses in any 12-month period.

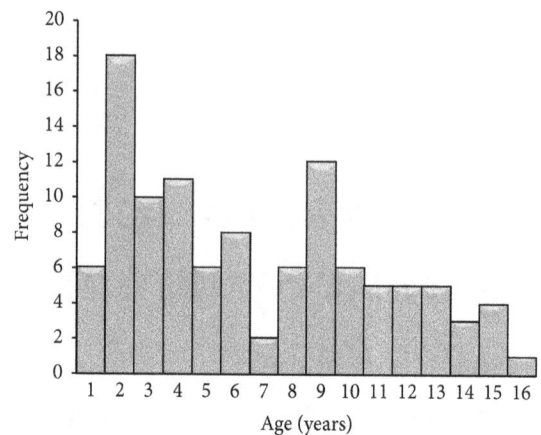

FIGURE 1: Age distribution of 108 patients with nephrotic syndrome.

5. Statistical Analysis

Data was analysed using the Statistical Package for Social Sciences software version 20. Continuous data were represented as mean or median while categorical data were presented as percentages. Significance between steroid sensitivity and some variables was determined using chi-square test while comparison of means was done with Student's t-test. A P value of <0.05 was considered statistically significant.

6. Results

We managed 108 children, 68 males and 40 females (m : f = 1.7 : 1). Age range was 8 months to 15.4 years (median 5.9 years). Their age distribution is shown in Figure 1, reflecting a bimodal distribution with a peak at 1 to 2 years and a slightly lesser one at about 9-10 years. About half, 53 (49.1%), were aged less than ≤5 years. Of 88 children with complete data on socioeconomic status, majority, 38 (45.2%), were from the lower socioeconomic class while 31 (36.9%) and 15 (17.9%) were from the middle and upper socioeconomic classes, respectively. Mean serum albumin was 2.05 g/L ± 0.82 with mean serum cholesterol of 10.4 ± 4.4 mmol/L. Most of the children, 94 (87%), had normal creatinine levels at presentation. Haematuria was present in (48) 44%, hypertension in (46) 43%, while (27) 25% had urinary tract infection.

6.1. Aetiology and Steroid Response. Records on aetiology were available for 102 patients. Of these, the majority (92; 90.2%) were idiopathic. A secondary cause was found in 10 children as follows: systemic lupus erythematosus (3), sickle cell disease (3), chronic glomerulonephritis (2), infantile NS (1) and Down's syndrome with cyanotic glomerulopathy (1). Steroid sensitivity pattern was available for 95 children (Figure 2). Five died before steroid sensitivity could be determined while others were unavailable due to loss to follow-up. Steroid sensitivity among children with INS was 82.8% (72/87) but 75.9% (72/95) overall. Twelve (16.7%) of those with SSNS were either steroid dependent or frequently

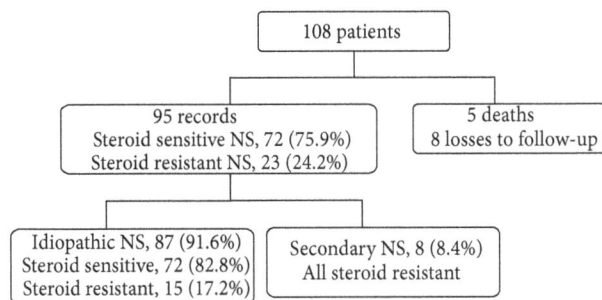

FIGURE 2: Flow chart of steroid sensitivity of patients with nephrotic syndrome.

relapsing, and 23 children (24.2%) were steroid resistant. Time to remission in steroid sensitive patients ranged from 3 to 38 days (median 7 days).

Fifteen children were biopsied: 14 with SRNS of whom 8 had idiopathic SRNS and an 11-year-old male at presentation on account of age, macroscopic haematuria, and hypertension. Biopsy was not done in the others due to refusal to consent, transfer to another facility, or death. Histological findings were as follows: focal segmental glomerulosclerosis (FSGS) in 8 (53.3%), minimal change disease (MCNS) in 3 (20%) and 1 (6.7%) each of membranous nephropathy, membranoproliferative glomerulonephritis (MPGN), diffuse proliferative glomerulonephritis, and class 3 lupus nephritis. Histologic patterns among the 8 with idiopathic SRNS were FSGS in 5 (62.5%), MCNS in 2 (25%), and MPGN in 1 (12.5%).

Table 1 shows a comparison of variables between the steroid resistant and responsive groups. Lower serum albumin, higher serum cholesterol, older age, haematuria, and raised serum creatinine were all associated with steroid resistance. Only association with albumin and UTI did not reach statistical significance.

6.2. Outcome. Seven children (6.5%), all with SRNS, developed chronic kidney disease (CKD) of whom 5 progressed to end-stage kidney disease (ESKD) during the review period. One was with haemoglobin SS disease (HBSS) presented in CKD while the others (SLE: 2; FSGS: 2; idiopathic: 2) developed CKD within 2 years of diagnosis. There were 7 deaths as follows: complications of ESKD in 3 (lupus nephritis: 1, FSGS: 1, and INS: 1); AKI in 2 patients, one of whom had lupus nephritis, and 2 newly diagnosed patients with undetermined steroid sensitivity one of whom died from a cerebrovascular accident. Overall mortality was therefore 6.5% but 21.8% in those with SRNS.

7. Discussion

Our study revealed high prevalence of steroid sensitivity among a cohort of black children with NS. In summary about 76% of the whole cohort and approximately 83% of the cohort with idiopathic childhood nephrotic syndrome achieved remission following treatment with steroids. The high proportion of steroid sensitivity in this study is remarkable because such high sensitivity has rarely been described

in a large sample of black children and ranks similar to that described among children of other races [2–4]. Various studies describe NS in children of African descent as being predominantly steroid resistant and nonminimal change on histology. In Nigeria, steroid resistance ranges between 35% and 92% among different geographical locations [6–9, 15–17] Table 2, higher than the 23% in the current study. Doe et al. in Ghana [24] reported steroid resistance of 50% amongst their cohort while Bhimma's group in South Africa [25] reported about 86% steroid resistance among black children. In the latter study, steroid sensitivity among Indian children in the same cohort was over 65% again highlighting racial differences in steroid sensitivity. This has led to the recommendation of a kidney biopsy as part of the initial evaluation of black children with NS.

The reasons for this striking observation of high steroid sensitivity likely include the younger age structure of our cohort. The statistically significant lower median age of the steroid sensitive compared with steroid resistant patients supports this. A small study from southern Nigeria [14] that reported 80% steroid sensitivity had a young population with a mean age of 5.8 years. Asinobi's group [13] also from Nigeria reported higher steroid sensitivity but their cohort comprised only children aged ≤ 5 years. This age pattern is similar to that reported among Caucasians and Asian children where high steroid sensitivity has been reported [1–4]. For instance, in a report from the United Kingdom [3], median age of children with SSNS was 4.5 years compared with 6 years in those with SRNS. We therefore argue that age and race should be considered together as strong predictors of response to steroid rather than the sole reliance on race.

Another plausible explanation for the increased sensitivity observed in our cohort is the absence of certain previously prominent secondary aetiologies of NS in our environment resulting in a relatively higher idiopathic pool, the majority of whom were steroid sensitive. This is a likely consequence of intensified efforts by the Government to reduce the burden of some childhood conditions in the region. For instance, we did not diagnose any case of quartan malaria nephropathy (QMN), which was previously reported to be a leading cause of steroid resistant nephrotic syndrome in our environment [26]. Previous Nigerian authors [8, 27] have similarly alluded to the reduced incidence of QMN in the region. Malaria control programs have resulted in improved access to antimalarial drugs over the last two decades and this is likely to have contributed to the decline in associated nephropathy. Doe's group in Ghana [2] also found no evidence of a tropical form of nephrotic syndrome in their patients. In the same vein, in contrast with reports from South Africa [5] and Ghana [24], we did not diagnose infections such as hepatitis and schistosomiasis, which we attribute to improved vaccination rates and access to portable water, respectively. These diseases have seemingly been replaced by others like SLE and sickle cell anaemia, as also observed by Olowu et al. [27]. Recent availability of diagnostic facilities for the former and improved survival beyond early childhood for the latter could account for this observation.

Contrariwise, on the global scene, the incidence of steroid resistant NS in various parts of the world such as the

TABLE 1: Comparison of variables between steroid responsive and nonresponsive groups.

	SSNS	SRNS	P
Mean age (years)	5.8 ± 3.9 (median 5)	8.8 ± 4.8 (median 10.1)	0.004
Age group (years/number)			0.01
0–5 (48)	41 (85.4%)	7 (14.6%)	
6–10 (27)	20 (74.1%)	7 (25.9%)	
>10 (20)	10 (50%)	10 (50%)	
Serum albumin	2.1 ± 0.8	1.9 ± 0.8	0.57
Serum cholesterol	9.8 ± 4.0	12.6 ± 5.0	0.03
Hypertension* (89)	21/62 (33.9%)	16/23 (69.6%)	0.006
Haematuria* (95)	25/72 (36.2%)	12/23 (60%)	<0.001
UTI* (89)	15 (22.7%)	7 (35.0%)	0.32
Raised creatinine	2/72 (2.7%)	11/23 (47.8%)	<0.001

UTI: urinary tract infection. *Indicates number available for review for variable; percentages are of the total within the group.

TABLE 2: Steroid responsiveness of nephrotic syndrome across Nigeria.

Authors/year of publication	Region of Nigeria	Total No (mean/median age) years	SSNS, N (%)
F. U. Eke and N. N. Eke (1994) [6]	Port-Harcourt, south-south	102 (—)	23 (22.5)
Ibadin and Abiodun (1998) [7]	Benin, south-south	58 (8.2 ± 0.5)	30 (51.7)
Asinobi et al. (1999) [8]	Ibadan, south-west	41 (—)	3 (8.0)
Okoro and Okafor (1999) [9]	Enugu, south-east	346 (5–7)	104 (30)
*Adedoyin et al. (2001) [16]	Ilorin, north-central	17 (8.8)	3 (17.6)
Ibadin and Ofovwe (2003) [18]	Benin, south-south	51 (5)	35 (68.6)
Asinobi et al. (2005) [15]	Ibadan, south-west	20 (4.0)	12 (60)
XAnochie et al. (2006) [14]	Port-Harcourt, south-south	20 (5.8 ± 3.8)	16 (80)
XOlowu et al. (2010) [17]	Ile-Ife, south-west	42 (9.95 ± 3.15)	19 (45.2)
Current study	Lagos, south-west	108 (6.6 ± 4.2/5.9)	72 (75.9) X72 (82.8)

Note: *8 defaulted, Xidiopathic nephrotic syndrome only, (—) data not given.

USA [11, 28], Poland [12], India [13], and Canada [29] is reportedly on increase which has been linked to increasing FSGS among these populations. Although Kim's group [11] and Bonilla-Felix et al. [28] attributed their findings to the large proportion of the African-Africans in their cohort, similar observations in homogenous or near homogenous Caucasian populations [12, 28] suggest the role of other factors. The reasons for these changes however remain of continued research interest [30].

Socioeconomic class is thought to play a role in NS although the exact associations are not very clear. The majority of our patients were from the lower socioeconomic class similar to a report from India [31] where 84% of study participants were from the lower socioeconomic class. While this may suggest a role for infections which are more prevalent in this socioeconomic class of children, we did not find a high prevalence of infection associated NS in this study. We however also reported a significant proportion of children from the middle socioeconomic class suggesting the role of other factors which are not apparent from this study. The aetiology of INS remains of continued research interest globally with extensive research into genetic mechanisms howbeit largely in the developed world.

FSGS was also our predominant histologic finding, a finding consistent with other African studies [16, 24, 25], especially since the era when kidney biopsy was reserved commonly for those with clinical and treatment features not in keeping with minimal change disease. Since minimal change NS is predominantly steroid sensitive, it is safe to assume that if all the children in the present study were to undergo kidney biopsies, it would have been the most predominant histological pattern. Higher cholesterol levels, hypertension, and haematuria were associated with increased steroid resistance, consistent with published data [32]. Our findings also support the reportedly high frequency of UTI in NS, particularly SRNS [33], and emphasize the need for screening for this infection in affected children.

As expected, progression to CKD and mortality were predominantly a function of with steroid resistance [1, 4, 7]; hence, our lower overall mortality of 6.5%, compared with 6.6–14.3% in other African reports [7, 16, 24], is not surprising. Mortality was particularly high among those with steroid resistant nephrotic syndrome who progressed to ESKD. This is largely a consequence of a combination of factors which include high cost of care, inadequate facilities for long-term dialysis, and lack of transplant facilities. Late presentation, hence advanced disease in two patients one of whom presented with a cerebrovascular accident, also contributed to the high mortality reported.

In conclusion, our study reports high steroid sensitivity in a large group of black children. Although its retrospective nature resulted in incomplete data in some cases, this was compensated for by its large sample size. This study and few others in the region [14, 15] suggest a changing pattern of steroid sensitivity of childhood NS which may reflect an adaptation to the changing epidemiology of some childhood diseases as alluded to by previous authors. Surveillance of the epidemiology of childhood NS and corresponding modifications in practice guidelines over time are therefore recommended.

Acknowledgment

The authors thank the International Paediatric Nephrology Association for sponsorship of Fellowship Training in Paediatric Nephrology for Taiwo Augustina Ladapo and Christopher Imokhuede Esezobor.

References

[1] International study of kidney disease in children, "Nephrotic syndrome in children: prediction of histopathology from clinical and laboratory characteristics at the time of diagnosis," *Kidney International*, vol. 13, pp. 159–165, 1978.

[2] P. Niaudet and O. Boyer, "Idiopathic nephrotic syndrome in childhood: clinical aspects," in *Pediatric Nephrology*, E. D. Avner, W. E. Harmon, and N. Yoshikawa, Eds., pp. 667–692, Springer, Berlin, Germany, 6th edition, 2009.

[3] P. A. McKinney, R. G. Feltbower, J. T. Brocklebank, and M. M. Fitzpatrick, "Time trends and ethnic patterns of childhood nephrotic syndrome in Yorkshire, UK," *Pediatric Nephrology*, vol. 16, no. 12, pp. 1040–1044, 2001.

[4] W. Wong, "Idiopathic nephrotic syndrome in New Zealand children, demographic, clinical features, initial management and outcome after twelve-month follow-up: results of a three-year national surveillance study," *Journal of Paediatrics and Child Health*, vol. 43, no. 5, pp. 337–341, 2007.

[5] M. Adhikari, H. M. Coovadia, V. Chrystal, and L. Morel-Maroger, "Absence of "tru" minimal change nephrotic syndrome in African children in South Africa," *Journal of Tropical Medicine and Hygiene*, vol. 86, no. 6, pp. 223–228, 1983.

[6] F. U. Eke and N. N. Eke, "Renal disorders in children: a Nigerian study," *Pediatric Nephrology*, vol. 8, no. 3, pp. 383–386, 1994.

[7] M. O. Ibadin and P. O. Abiodun, "Epidemiology and clinico-pathologic characteristics of childhood nephrotic syndrome in Berlin-City, Nigeria," *Journal of the Pakistan Medical Association*, vol. 48, no. 8, pp. 235–238, 1998.

[8] A. O. Asinobi, R. A. Gbadegesin, A. A. Adeyemo et al., "The predominance of membranoproliferative glomerulonephritis in childhood nephrotic syndrome in Ibadan, Nigeria," *West African Journal of Medicine*, vol. 18, no. 3, pp. 203–206, 1999.

[9] B. A. Okoro and H. U. Okafor, "Pattern of childhood renal disorders in Enugu," *Nigerian Journal of Paediatrics*, vol. 26, pp. 14–18, 1999.

[10] E. Ingulli and A. Tejani, "Racial differences in the incidence and renal outcome of idiopathic focal segmental glomerulosclerosis in children," *Pediatric Nephrology*, vol. 5, no. 4, pp. 393–397, 1991.

[11] S. K. Jung, C. A. Bellew, D. M. Silverstein, D. H. Aviles, F. G. Boineau, and V. M. Vehaskari, "High incidence of initial and late steroid resistance in childhood nephrotic syndrome," *Kidney International*, vol. 68, no. 3, pp. 1275–1281, 2005.

[12] B. Banaszak and P. Banaszak, "The increasing incidence of initial steroid resistance in childhood nephrotic syndrome," *Pediatric Nephrology*, vol. 27, no. 6, pp. 927–932, 2012.

[13] S. Gulati, A. P. Sharma, R. K. Sharma, and A. Gupta, "Changing trends of histopathology in childhood nephrotic syndrome," *American Journal of Kidney Diseases*, vol. 34, no. 4, pp. 646–650, 1999.

[14] I. Anochie, F. Eke, and A. Okpere, "Childhood nephrotic syndrome: change in pattern and response to steroids," *Journal of the National Medical Association*, vol. 98, no. 12, pp. 1977–1981, 2006.

[15] A. O. Asinobi, R. A. Gbadegesin, and O. O. Ogunkunle, "Increased steroid responsiveness of young children with nephrotic syndrome in Nigeria," *Annals of Tropical Paediatrics*, vol. 25, no. 3, pp. 199–203, 2005.

[16] O. T. Adedoyin, H. O. D. Gbele, and A. Adeniyi, "Childhood nephrotic syndrome in Ilorin," *Nigerian Journal of Paediatrics*, vol. 28, pp. 68–72, 2001.

[17] W. A. Olowu, K. A. Adelusola, and O. Adefehinti, "Childhood idiopathic steroid resistant nephrotic syndrome in Southwestern Nigeria," *Saudi Journal of Kidney Diseases and Transplantation*, vol. 21, no. 5, pp. 979–990, 2010.

[18] M. O. Ibadin and G. E. Ofovwe, "Pattern of renal diseases in children in mid-western zone of Nigeria," *Saudi Journal of Kidney Diseases and Transplantation*, vol. 14, pp. 539–544, 2003.

[19] National Kidney Foundation, "Kidney disease outcome quality initiative clinical guidelines for chronic disease: evaluation, classification and stratification—part 4: definition and classification of stages of chronic kidney disease," *American Journal of Kidney Diseases*, vol. 39, pp. S46–S75, 2002.

[20] National High Blood Pressure Education Program Working Group on High Blood Pressure in Children and Adolescents, "The fourth report on the diagnosis, evaluation, and treatment of high blood pressure in children and adolescents," *Pediatrics*, vol. 114, supplement 2, pp. 555–576, 2004.

[21] M. C. Hochberg, "Updating the American College of Rheumatology revised criteria for the classification of systemic lupus erythematosus," *Arthritis and Rheumatism*, vol. 40, no. 9, article 1725, 1997.

[22] E. A. Oyedeji, "Socioeconomic and cultural background of hospitalised children in Ilesha," *Nigerian Journal of Paediatrics*, vol. 12, pp. 111–117, 1985.

[23] Kidney Disease: Improving Global Outcomes (KDIGO) Glomerulonephritis Work Group, "KDIGO clinical practice guideline for glomerulonephritis," *Kidney International Supplements*, vol. 2, pp. 139–274, 2012.

[24] J. Yao Doe, M. Funk, M. Mengel, E. Doehring, and J. H. H. Ehrich, "Nephrotic syndrome in African children: lack of evidence for "tropical nephrotic syndrome"?" *Nephrology Dialysis Transplantation*, vol. 21, no. 3, pp. 672–676, 2006.

[25] R. Bhimma, H. M. Coovadia, and M. Adhikari, "Nephrotic syndrome in South African children: changing perspectives over 20 years," *Pediatric Nephrology*, vol. 11, no. 4, pp. 429–434, 1997.

[26] M. B. Abdurrahman, B. M. Greenwood, P. Narayana, F. A. Babaoye, and G. M. Edington, "Immunological aspects of nephrotic syndrome in northern Nigeria," *Archives of Disease in Childhood*, vol. 56, no. 3, pp. 199–202, 1981.

[27] W. A. Olowu, K. A. Adelusola, O. Adefehinti, and T. G. Oyetunji, "Quartan malaria-associated childhood nephrotic syndrome: now a rare clinical entity in malaria endemic Nigeria," *Nephrology Dialysis Transplantation*, vol. 25, no. 3, pp. 794–801, 2010.

[28] M. Bonilla-Felix, C. Parra, T. Dajani et al., "Changing patterns in the histopathology of idiopathic nephrotic syndrome in children," *Kidney International*, vol. 55, no. 5, pp. 1885–1890, 1999.

[29] G. Filler, E. Young, P. Geier, B. Carpenter, A. Drukker, and J. Feber, "Is there really an increase in non-minimal change nephrotic syndrome in children?" *The American Journal of Kidney Diseases*, vol. 42, no. 6, pp. 1107–1113, 2003, Review.

[30] E. Machuca, G. Benoit, and C. Antignac, "Genetics of nephrotic syndrome: connecting molecular genetics to podocyte physiology," *Human Molecular Genetics*, vol. 18, no. 2, pp. R185–R194, 2009.

[31] P. Guha, A. De, and M. Ghosal, "Behavior profile of children with nephrotic syndrome," *Indian Journal of Psychiatry*, vol. 51, no. 2, pp. 122–126, 2009.

[32] F. Mortazavi and Y. S. Khiavi, "Steroid response pattern and outcome of pediatric idiopathic nephrotic syndrome: a single-center experience in Northwest Iran," *Therapeutics and Clinical Risk Management*, vol. 7, pp. 167–171, 2011.

[33] S. Gulati, V. Kher, P. Arora, S. Gupta, and S. Kale, "Urinary tract infection in nephrotic syndrome," *Pediatric Infectious Disease Journal*, vol. 15, no. 3, pp. 237–240, 1996.

7

Comparative Performance of Creatinine-Based Estimated Glomerular Filtration Rate Equations in the Malays: A Pilot Study in Tertiary Hospital in Malaysia

Maisarah Jalalonmuhali, Ng Kok Peng, and Lim Soo Kun

University Malaya Medical Centre, 59100 Kuala Lumpur, Malaysia

Correspondence should be addressed to Maisarah Jalalonmuhali; mai_jalal@yahoo.com

Academic Editor: Suresh C. Tiwari

Aim. To validate the accuracy of estimated glomerular filtration rate (eGFR) equations in Malay population attending our hospital in comparison with radiolabeled measured GFR. *Methods*. A cross-sectional study recruiting volunteered patients in the outpatient setting. Chromium EDTA (51Cr-EDTA) was used as measured GFR. The predictive capabilities of Cockcroft-Gault equation corrected for body surface area (CGBSA), four-variable Modification of Diet in Renal Disease (4-MDRD), and Chronic Kidney Disease Epidemiology Collaboration (CKD-EPI) equations were calculated. *Results*. A total of 51 subjects were recruited with mean measured GFR 42.04 (17.70–111.10) ml/min/1.73 m^2. Estimated GFR based on CGBSA, 4-MDRD, and CKD-EPI were 40.47 (16.52–115.52), 35.90 (14.00–98.00), and 37.24 (14.00–121.00), respectively. Higher accuracy was noted in 4-MDRD equations throughout all GFR groups except for subgroup of GFR $\geq$ 60 ml/min/1.73 m^2 where CGBSA was better. *Conclusions*. The 4-MDRD equation seems to perform better in estimating GFR in Malay CKD patients generally and specifically in the subgroup of GFR < 60 ml/min/1.73 m^2 and both BMI subgroups.

1. Introduction

According to the 21st Malaysian Dialysis and Transplant Registry report, in the year 2013, a total of 31,637 patients received dialysis, an increase from a mere 11,842 in 2004. A staggering 61% of end-stage renal disease (ESRD) in Malaysia was reported to be caused by diabetes mellitus [1]. Chronic kidney disease (CKD) can lead to various complications and is well known to be an independent risk factor for cardiovascular disease [2]. A reduced glomerular filtration rate (GFR) to <60 ml/min/1.73 m^2 alone is sufficient to diagnose CKD [3]. Direct assessment of GFR is measured from urinary or plasma clearance of an ideal filtration marker such as inulin or other alternative exogenous markers such as iothalamate, chromium 51 ethylenediaminetetraacetic acid (^{51}Cr-EDTA), technetium-99 m diethylenetriaminepentaacetic acid (^{99m}TC-DTPA), and iohexol. ^{51}Cr-EDTA and ^{99m}TC-DTPA are radioactive tracers that were reported in radiological studies used to obtain accurate measurement of

GFR [4, 5]. However, measuring clearance with exogenous markers is complex, expensive, and difficult to do in routine clinical practice. Therefore, an accurate, convenient, and precise method to estimate GFR is important to overcome this problem.

Traditionally, serum creatinine has been used as a marker to assess kidney function. It is now an established fact that serum creatinine alone is not an accurate marker of GFR as it is dependent on muscle mass [6]. Apart from that, serum creatinine usually does not increase until GFR has decreased by 50% or more and thus many patients with normal serum creatinine may have lower GFR [7]. Therefore, a calculated GFR from creatinine-based method is recommended. In Malaysia, Cockcroft-Gault (CG) formula for estimating kidney function is still widely used. Unfortunately it has been reported to overestimate true GFR. The Modification of Diet in Renal Disease (MDRD) formula derived from MDRD study was proposed to overcome this limitation [8]. Based on the study, four-variable MDRD (4-MDRD) that consists of serum creatinine, gender, age, and ethnicity was derived and became commonly used in clinical practice and research. The 4-MDRD formula provides good GFR estimation particularly in the group of GFR <60 mL/min/1.73 m^2 White Americans [9]. This subsequently leads to the new equation proposed for Caucasian and African-American CKD populations, known as Chronic Kidney Disease Epidemiological Collaboration (CKD-EPI) equation [10]. The development of this equation is mainly to overcome some of the limitations from MDRD equation, particularly in estimating GFR of >60 ml/min/1.73 m^2.

Among Asian population, namely, in Chinese, Japanese, and Thais, racial coefficient has been identified and incorporated in eGFR formulas [11–14]. To date, studies comparing different methods of kidney function assessment in our unique multiethnic population are very scarce. Evaluation of these methods in the Malays as the dominant ethnic group of this country is very interesting. A good eGFR formula needs to have lower bias and limits of agreement, in addition to excellent precision and accuracy. The objective of this study is to evaluate the accuracy of creatinine-based eGFR formulas compared to the measured GFR in Malay population.

2. Materials and Methods

This is a cross-sectional study conducted in University Malaya Medical Centre (UMMC), Kuala Lumpur, Malaysia, and approved by UMMC ethic committee. We used power and sample size software version 3 to calculate sample size. Single mean formula was used. Under a significance level of 0.05 and power of 0.90, the estimated sample size is 46 ± 10% patients. Our study cohort involved patients presented to UMMC nephrology clinic for their regular follow-up. Volunteered participants were recruited in continuous manner. All patients older than 18 years old with stable renal function for at least 3 months prior to recruitment were eligible to participate. Patients with acute deterioration of renal function, bedridden patients, patients with malnutrition, limb amputees, patients who are less than 18 years old, and pregnant women were excluded.

2.1. ^{51}Cr-EDTA Measurement.
Measured GFR is determined by collecting blood sample from different arm 2, 2.5, 3, and 4 hours later following ^{51}Cr-EDTA single injection technique. Plasma clearance of ^{51}Cr-EDTA from 4 samples was obtained based on the interval above. Patient's height and weight were measured for body surface area (BSA) calculation. GFR was calculated using the slope-intercept method and normalized to BSA, which was calculated using du Bois formula. The result was then corrected using Brochner-Mortensen equation.

Volume distribution (Vd) is calculated by

$$Vd = \frac{\text{Standard activity (cpm)} \times \text{weight of dose} \times 100\,ml}{\text{Po (cpm)} \times \text{weight of standard}}. \tag{1}$$

(i) Standard activity is calculated using computer generated chromium result.

(ii) Weight of dose is calculated from weight of syringe and dose before injection − after injection.

(iii) Po (zero time plasma activity) is corrected by extrapolating the curve to zero time.

Slope clearance (C-slope) is calculated by

$$\frac{\text{C-slope}}{\text{slope intercept}} = \frac{0.693}{T\,(1/2)} \times Vd. \tag{2}$$

Normalized GFR is calculated by

$$\text{Normalized GFR} = \frac{\text{C-slope}}{\text{Patient's BSA}} \times 1.73. \tag{3}$$

2.2. Calibration for the Serum Creatinine Assay.
Serum creatinine was measured on a Dimension Vista system clinical chemistry analyzer (Siemens) with an assay using a modification of the kinetic Jaffe reaction (alkaline picrate reaction). This modified technique was reported to be less susceptible than conventional methods to interference from noncreatinine Jaffe positive compounds [15]. The creatinine assay was adjusted for calibration with the isotope dilution mass spectrometry (IDMS).

2.3. Estimated GFR Calculations.
The eGFR values were calculated by using CG, 4-MDRD, and CKD-EPI equations. 4-MDRD and CKD-EPI derived eGFR are expressed as ml/min/1.73 m^2. Meanwhile CG equation was converted from ml/min to ml/min/1.73 m^2 by multiplying the calculated values by 1.73 and dividing by BSA (Table 1).

2.4. Statistical Analysis.
SPSS version 20.0 was used to calculate baseline characteristics frequency, mean, median, range, and standard deviation. Mean GFR were given with a 95% confidence interval (CI) unless indicated otherwise. p values < 0.05 were considered significant. Pearson's correlation coefficients (r) were calculated between ^{51}Cr-EDTA clearance and estimated GFR by a linear correlation analysis. Pairwise comparison of the mean was performed using paired t-test.

Bias, precision, and accuracy within 10% and 30% of the measured GFR were determined. Bias is defined as mean difference between estimated GFR and the measured GFR (^{51}Cr-EDTA). The precision of the estimates was determined as SD of the mean difference between measured GFR and eGFR. Accuracy was determined by integrating precision and bias and was calculated as the percentage of GFR estimates within 10 and 30% of the measured GFR. Moreover, a graphical analysis was carried out according to Bland and Altman plots. This was used to assess the limits of agreement between the eGFR and the measured GFR.

In our study, accuracy is the most important determinants for a good estimated GFR and it is best if further supported by lower bias, greater precision, and lower limits of agreement. However, as we understand that bias, precision and limits of agreement may be affected by the overall means and outliers; therefore the individual parameter may not reflect the best estimated GFR.

TABLE 1: Different eGFR formula according to gender.

eGFR methods	Gender	Equations
Cockcroft-Gault	Male	$\dfrac{(140\text{-Age}) \times \text{mass (kg)} \times 1.23}{\text{Serum Creatinine (umol/L)}}$
	Female	$\dfrac{(140\text{-Age}) \times \text{mass (kg)} \times 1.04}{\text{Serum Creatinine (umol/L)}}$
4-MDRD	Male	$32788 \times \text{Serum Creatinine}^{-1.154} \times \text{Age}^{-0.203} \times \{1.212 \text{ if Black}\}$
	Female	$32788 \times \text{Serum Creatinine}^{-1.154} \times \text{Age}^{-0.203} \times \{1.212 \text{ if Black}\} \times 0.742$
		(Serum creatinine in umol/L)
CKD-EPI	Male	$141 \times \min(\text{SCr}/0.9, 1)^{-0.411} \times \max(\text{SCr}/0.9, 1)^{-1.209} \times 0.993^{\text{Age}} \times \{1.159 \text{ if Black}\}$
	Female	$141 \times \min(\text{SCr}/0.7, 1)^{-0.329} \times \max(\text{SCr}/0.7, 1)^{-1.209} \times 0.993^{\text{Age}} \times \{1.159 \text{ if Black}\} \times 1.018$
Cockcroft-Gault BSA		$\dfrac{\text{Calculated Cockcroft-Gault} \times 1.73}{\text{BSA}}$

3. Results

A total of 51 patients were recruited with mean age of 58.7 years, where the youngest was 26 years old and the eldest was 78 years old. Majority of our patients are males representing 90.2%. The mean height and weight in our patient were 164.5 cm and 71.9 kg, respectively, with mean BMI of 26.5 kg/m^2. Vast majority of our study patients had diabetic nephropathy (35.3%) and hypertension (19.6%) as the main cause of their CKD. Summary of patient's baseline characteristics is tabulated in Table 2.

From our cohort, mean measured GFR was 42.04 (17.70–111.10) ml/min/1.73 m^2, while the estimated GFR based on CGBSA, 4-MDRD, and CKD-EPI formula were 40.47 (16.52–115.52), 35.90 (14.00–98.00), and 37.24 (14.00–121.00), respectively. The calculated GFR of the 4-MDRD and CKD-EPI differed significantly from measured GFR with p value = 0.001 and 0.005. The correlation between estimated and measured GFR is illustrated in Table 3.

Bias of CGBSA (1.573 ml/min/1.73 m^2) was smaller than 4-MDRD (6.137 ml/min/1.73 m^2) and CKD-EPI (4.804 ml/min/1.73 m^2), while the precisions of the estimated GFR showed that CGBSA is more precise followed by CKD-EPI and 4-MDRD formula. However, from our cohort we found that 4-MDRD is the most accurate formula with the accuracy of 13.7 and 54.9% within 10 and 30% of measured GFR, respectively. Nevertheless, we noted that 4-MDRD formula underestimated GFR by 6.137 ml/min/1.73 m^2; this was likely because of the outliers in this study cohort.

The differences between estimated and measured GFR were illustrated using a graphical technique according to Bland and Altman plot (Figures 1(a)–1(c)). These figures display the span between +2SD and −2SD of the mean difference (limits of agreement between 2 methods), which represent 95% CI. From the chart below it showed that smaller limits of agreement were found for the CGBSA (43.21 ml/min/1.73 m^2), followed by CKD-EPI (46.78 ml/min/1.73 m^2) and 4-MDRD (48.23 ml/min/1.73 m^2) formula.

TABLE 2: Baseline characteristics of patients.

Characteristic ($n = 51$)	Mean ± SD (median) or n (%)
Male	46 (90.2)
Age (year)	58.7 ± 12.6 (61.0)
BMI (kg/m^2)	26.5 ± 4.6 (25.5)
Plasma creatinine (umol/l)	192.5 ± 66.7 (190.0)
Plasma urea nitrogen (mmol/l)	9.8 ± 3.5 (9.4)
Plasma albumin (g/l)	37.9 ± 3.0 (38.0)
Measured GFR (ml/min/1.73m^2)	42.04 ± 22.5 (35.1)
Causes of CKD	
Diabetic nephropathy	18 (35.3)
Hypertension	10 (19.6)
Nondiabetic glomerulopathy	4 (7.8)
Renal calculi/nephrocalcinosis	4 (7.8)
Other causes	10 (19.7)
Unknown	5 (9.8)
CKD stages	
1	2 (3.9)
2	8 (15.7)
3	26 (51.0)
4	15 (29.4)
Medical history	
Diabetes mellitus	33 (64.7)
Hypertension	46 (90.2)
Medications	
Diuretics	14 (27.5)
Antihypertensive	48 (94.1)
OHA/insulin	32 (62.7)
Statin	41 (80.4)
Smoking status	
Current smoker	6 (11.8)
Ex-smoker	21 (41.2)
Nonsmoker	24 (47.1)

TABLE 3: Correlation coefficient (r), mean, bias, precision, and accuracy for CGBSA, 4-MDRD, and CKD-EPI formula.

	Correlation coefficient (r)	Mean GFR	Range (IQR)		p value	Mean difference (bias)	SD of mean bias (precision)	Accuracy within	
			Lower	Upper				10%	30%
Measured GFR		42.039	17.70	111.10					
CGBSA	0.877*	40.467	16.52	115.52	0.303	−1.573	10.802	9.8	47.1
4-MDRD	0.848*	35.902	14.00	98.00	0.001	−6.137	12.058	13.7	54.9
CKD-EPI	0.854*	37.235	14.00	121.00	0.005	−4.804	11.697	13.7	49.0

*Significantly correlating with $p < 0.001$.

(Bias: mean difference of estimated GFR and measured GFR; accuracy: n percentage of GFR estimates within n% of measured GFR; IQR: interquartile range).

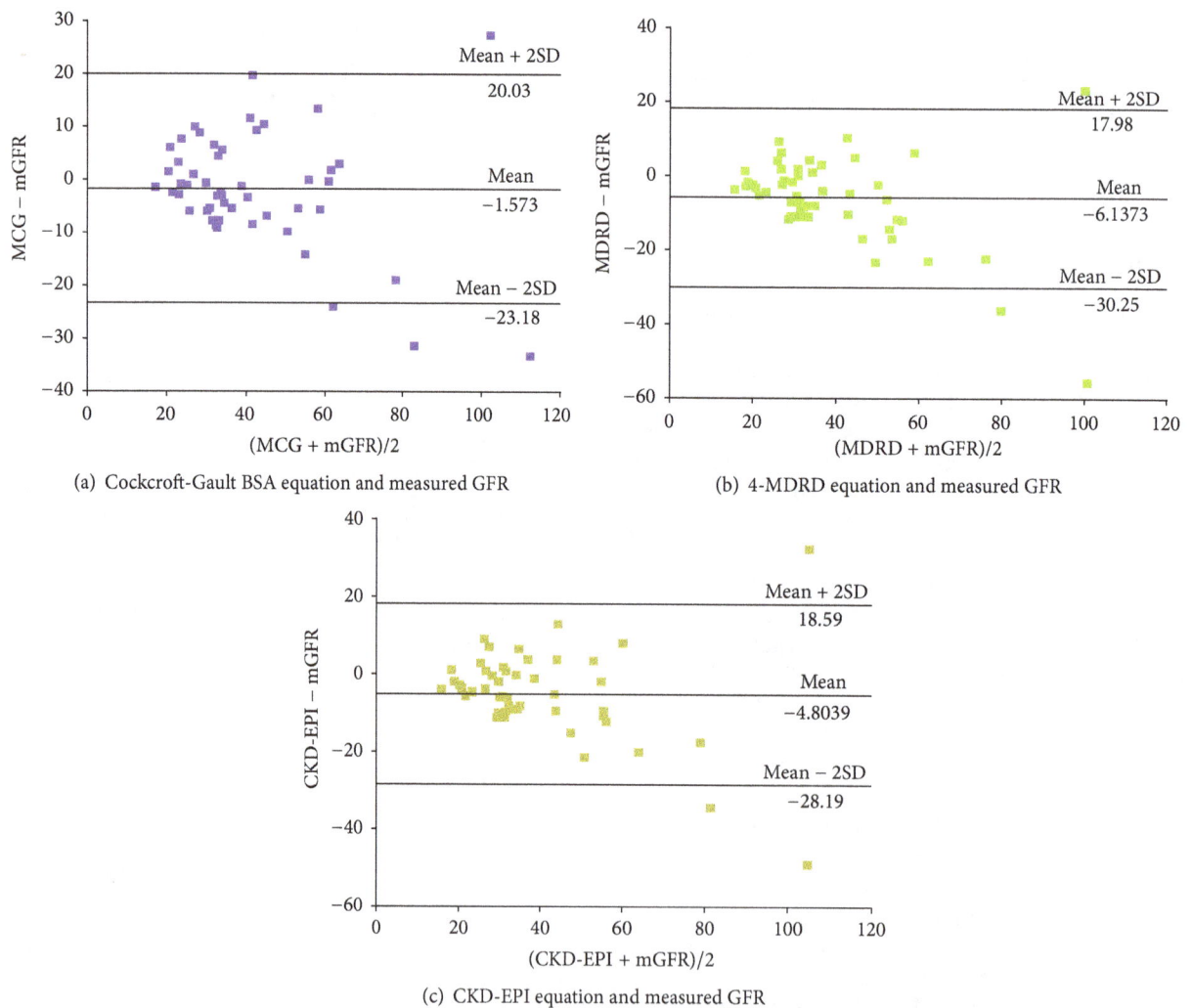

(a) Cockcroft-Gault BSA equation and measured GFR

(b) 4-MDRD equation and measured GFR

(c) CKD-EPI equation and measured GFR

FIGURE 1: (a–c) Bland and Altman analysis of GFR estimates. In this analysis, the differences between estimated and measured GFR are plotted against the average of the estimated and measured GFR for each individual patient.

Even though limits of agreement in 4-MDRD formula are wider, Figure 1(b) illustrated that each patient distribution is closer from one another and these wider limits of agreement can be explained by the extreme outliers (underestimated by almost 60 mls/min/1.73 m^2) that present in this group. Thus, this make 4-MDRD formula the most accurate estimated GFR in comparison with ^{51}Cr-EDTA throughout all ranges of GFR in our study cohort.

Patients were further divided into two groups according to the measured GFR: GFR < 60 ml/min/1.73 m^2 or GFR ≥ 60 ml/min/1.73 m^2. In subgroup GFR < 60 ml/min/1.73 m^2, lower bias was found for CGBSA formula (0.34 ml/min/1.73 m^2) followed by CKD-EPI (2.24 ml/min/1.73 m^2) and 4-MDRD (2.95 ml/min/1.73 m^2). However, better accuracy within 10% of measured GFR was found in 4-MDRD and CKD-EPI formula. In subgroup GFR ≥ 60 ml/min/1.73 m^2, a

TABLE 4: Mean, bias, precision, and accuracy of GFR estimates within two GFR subgroups.

Variable	GFR < 60 ml/min/1.73 m^2 ($n = 41$)	GFR ≥ 60 ml/min/1.73 m^2 ($n = 10$)
GFR (ml/min/1.73 m^2)		
Measured	33.19 ± 10.39	78.32 ± 22.61
CGBSA	33.53 ± 10.79*	68.92 ± 21.10**
4-MDRD	30.24 ± 10.27*	59.10 ± 21.35**
CKD-EPI	30.95 ± 11.14*	63.00 ± 23.49**
Median bias		
CGBSA	−0.99 (−9.6, 19.81)	−9.80 (−33.00, 27.35)
4-MDRD	−2.60 (−17.10, 10.20)	−19.70 (−55.80, 23.60)
CKD-EPI	−1.80 (−15.10, 13.20)	−14.70 (−48.80, 32.60)
Mean difference		
CGBSA	0.34 ± 7.04	−9.40 ± 18.53
4-MDRD	−2.95 ± 6.13	19.22 ± 20.11
CKD-EPI	−2.24 ± 6.22	−15.32 ± 20.86
Accuracy within 10%		
CGBSA	24.4	40.0
4-MDRD	31.7	20.0
CKD-EPI	31.7	10.0
Accuracy within 30%		
CGBSA	63.4	70.0
4-MDRD	65.9	80.0
CKD-EPI	65.9	80.0

*Mean CGBSA GFR versus measured GFR $p = 0.761$, mean 4-MDRD GFR versus measured GFR $p = 0.004$, and mean CKD-EPI GFR versus measured GFR $p = 0.026$.
**Mean CGBSA GFR versus measured GFR $p = 0.143$, mean 4-MDRD GFR versus measured GFR $p = 0.014$, and mean CKD-EPI GFR versus measured GFR $p = 0.045$.

different pattern of bias and accuracy was noted. In this subgroup, CGBSA formula was found to be better in terms of bias (9.40 ml/min/1.73 m^2) and accuracy within 10% of measured GFR (40%), while 4-MDRD and CKD-EPI formula were noted to have higher bias, 19.22 and 15.32 ml/min/1.73 m^2, respectively, and lower accuracy within 10% of measured GFR. Precisions of all the equations were significantly lower in the patients with GFR <60 ml/min/1.73 m^2 (Table 4).

Assessment of eGFR formula in patients with BMI < 23 kg/m^2 and BMI ≥ 23 kg/m^2 was performed. In both subgroups, better accuracy within 10 and 30% of measured GFR was found in 4-MDRD formula, which was 14.3 and 50% in BMI < 23 kg/m^2 while in subgroup BMI ≥ 23 kg/m^2 was 16.2 and 54.0% (Table 5).

4. Discussions

This study investigated the performance of different creatinine-based eGFR formula in Malay population in a tertiary hospital in Malaysia. An accurate eGFR measurement is extremely important as a tool for CKD diagnosis, drug dosage preparations, and procedural preparation and subsequently to determine the efficacy of novel treatments to delay CKD progression in clinical practice. Performing labor-intensive

radio-labelled GFR measurement is not practical and economical particularly in developing country like Malaysia.

It is known that racial coefficient is an important factor to determine accurate GFR [11–14, 16, 17]. In our cohort, the eGFR obtained from each formula showed significant correlation with measured GFR (^{51}Cr-EDTA). However, the eGFR by 4-MDRD formula in general was found to be more accurate than the other eGFR equations in estimating GFR in our small cohort.

In the subgroup analysis of measured GFR < 60 mls/min/1.73 m^2, our data showed that CKD-EPI and 4-MDRD formulas showed better performance pertaining to the accuracy in comparison with other estimates GFR. The results corresponded with MDRD study that was performed in White American patients, which revealed that MDRD equation showed a reliable performance in estimating GFR in CKD patients with GFR < 60 mls/min/1.73 m^2. However, in Singaporean multiethnic study, it revealed that CKD-EPI was more accurate than the 4-MDRD in GFR < 60 ml/min/1.73 m^2 and overestimated reference GFR when the reference GFR was ≥ 60 ml/min/1.73 m^2 [18].

Estimating GFR in overweight and obese populations is another interesting factor to look into as weight and body size may influence the level of creatinine. In subgroup analysis

TABLE 5: Mean, bias, precision, and accuracy of GFR estimates within two BMI subgroups.

Variable	BMI < 23 kg/m² (n = 14)	BMI ≥ 23 kg/m² (n = 37)
GFR (ml/min/1.73 m²)		
Measured	43.19 ± 19.44	41.61 ± 23.78
CGBSA	41.80 ± 23.96*	39.94 ± 17.67**
4-MDRD	43.14 ± 23.28*	33.16 ± 13.90**
CKD-EPI	44.57 ± 25.73*	34.46 ± 15.40**
Median bias		
CGBSA	−1.34 (−23.8, 27.35)	−1.66 (−33.07, 19.81)
4-MDRD	0.04 (−22.8, 23.6)	−8.44 (−55.80, 6.10)
CKD-EPI	1.39 (−19.8, 32.6)	−7.15 (−48.80, 7.10)
Mean difference		
CGBSA	−1.34 ± 11.54	−1.66 ± 10.68
4-MDRD	−0.04 ± 11.06	8.44 ± 11.74
CKD-EPI	1.39 ± 12.31	−7.15 ± 10.71
Accuracy within 10%		
CGBSA	7.0	8.1
4-MDRD	14.3	16.2
CKD-EPI	14.3	10.8
Accuracy within 30%		
CGBSA	50.0	48.6
4-MDRD	50.0	54
CKD-EPI	42.9	54.1

*Mean CGBSA GFR versus measured GFR $p = 0.672$, mean 4-MDRD GFR versus measured GFR $p = 0.989$, and mean CKD-EPI GFR versus measured GFR $p = 0.680$.
**Mean CGBSA GFR versus measured GFR $p = 0.350$, mean 4-MDRD GFR versus measured GFR $p < 0.001$, and mean CKD-EPI GFR versus measured GFR $p < 0.001$.

of BMI ≥ 23 kg/m², greater accuracy was noted in 4-MDRD formula. Similar result was noted in another local study done by National University of Malaysia (UKM) that revealed MDRD equation showed greater accuracy and precision in obese individuals [19]. Interestingly, in BMI < 23 kg/m², 4-MDRD fared better as well unlike in lean population in African that showed that CG was better than MDRD and CKD-EPI formula with regard to the narrow limits of agreement [16].

5. Limitations of the Study

This is a small single-centre cohort of CKD patients, who are predominantly male and mainly consisted of CKD stages 3 and 4. Due to the continuous sampling method used in this study, we are unable to ensure equal distribution of patients in different arms of subgroup analysis. Thus, to further validate the more recent CKD-EPI formula, more inclusion of other stages of CKD is needed. Although this study has the above-mentioned limitations, this is the first study to be conducted in Malaysia using ^{51}Cr-EDTA as reference GFR.

6. Conclusion

We found that 4-MDRD equation seems to be more accurate in estimating GFR in our small cohort of Malay CKD patients

except in subgroup of GFR ≥ 60 mls/min/m², where CGBSA was found to be better. We would like to propose further studies to look into the need for racial correction factor to improve the performance of the original 4-MDRD formula in Malay population.

Acknowledgments

Special thanks are due to the dedicated staffs of Nuclear Medicine Unit of Department of Biomedical Imaging, University Malaya Medical Centre, for their contribution in performing the GFR measurement for the subjects.

References

[1] B. L. Goh, L. M. Ong, and Y. N. Lim, "21st Report of the Malaysian Dialysis and Transplant Registry 2013," Tech. Rep., 2014.

[2] J. F. E. Mann, H. C. Gerstein, J. Poque, J. Bosch, and S. Yusuf, "Renal insufficiency as a predictor of cardiovascular outcomes and the impact of ramipril: the HOPE randomized trial," *Annals of Internal Medicine*, vol. 134, no. 8, pp. 629–636, 2001.

[3] L. A. Inker, B. C. Astor, C. H. Fox et al., "KDOQI US commentary on the 2012 KDIGO clinical practice guideline for

the evaluation and management of CKD," *The American Journal of Kidney Diseases*, vol. 63, no. 5, pp. 713–735, 2014.

[4] A. J. Hilson, R. D. Mistry, and M. N. Maisey, "Tc-99m-DTPA for the measurement of glomerular filtration rate," *The British Journal of Radiology*, vol. 49, no. 585, pp. 794–796, 1976.

[5] J. S. Fleming, J. Wilkinson, R. M. Oliver, D. M. Ackery, G. M. Blake, and D. G. Waller, "Comparison of radionuclide estimation of glomerular filtration rate using technetium 99m diethylenetriaminepentaacetic acid and chromium 51 ethylene-diaminetetraacetic acid," *European Journal of Nuclear Medicine*, vol. 18, no. 6, pp. 391–395, 1991.

[6] G. Manjunath, M. J. Sarnak, and A. S. Levey, "Prediction equations to estimate glomerular filtration rate: An update," *Current Opinion in Nephrology and Hypertension*, vol. 10, no. 6, pp. 785–792, 2001.

[7] R. D. Perrone, N. E. Madias, and A. S. Levey, "Serum creatinine as an index of renal function: new insights into old concepts," *Clinical Chemistry*, vol. 38, no. 10, pp. 1933–1953, 1992.

[8] A. S. Levey, J. P. Bosch, J. B. Lewis, T. Greene, N. Rogers, and D. Roth, "A more accurate method to estimate glomerular filtration rate from serum creatinine: a new prediction equation. Modification of Diet in Renal Disease Study Group," *Annals of Internal Medicine*, vol. 130, no. 6, pp. 461–470, 1999.

[9] E. D. Poggio, X. Wang, T. Greene, F. Van Lente, and P. M. Hall, "Performance of the modification of diet in renal disease and Cockcroft-Gault equations in the estimation of GFR in health and in chronic kidney disease," *Journal of the American Society of Nephrology*, vol. 16, no. 2, pp. 459–466, 2005.

[10] A. S. Levey, L. A. Stevens, C. H. Schmid et al., "A new equation to estimate glomerular filtration rate," *Annals of Internal Medicine*, vol. 150, no. 9, pp. 604–612, 2009.

[11] Y. Ma, L. Zuo, J. Chen et al., "Modified glomerular filtration rate estimating equation for Chinese patients with chronic kidney disease," *Journal of the American Society of Nephrology*, vol. 17, no. 10, pp. 2937–2944, 2006.

[12] E. Imai, M. Horio, K. Nitta et al., "Estimation of glomerular filtration rate by the MDRD study equation modified for Japanese patients with chronic kidney disease," *Clinical and Experimental Nephrology*, vol. 11, no. 1, pp. 41–50, 2007.

[13] S. Matsuo, E. Imai, M. Horio et al., "Revised equations for estimated GFR from serum creatinine in Japan," *The American Journal of Kidney Diseases*, vol. 53, no. 6, pp. 982–992, 2009.

[14] K. Praditpornsilpa, N. Townamchai, T. Chaiwatanarat et al., "The need for robust validation for MDRD-based glomerular filtration rate estimation in various CKD populations," *Nephrology Dialysis Transplantation*, vol. 26, no. 9, pp. 2780–2785, 2011.

[15] C. A. Burtis and E. R. Ashwood, *Tietz Fundamentals of Clinical Chemistry*, W.B. Saunders, Philadelphia, Pa, USA, 5th edition, 2001.

[16] J. B. Eastwood, S. M. Kerry, J. Plange-Rhule et al., "Assessment of GFR by four methods in adults in Ashanti, Ghana: the need for an eGFR equation for lean African populations," *Nephrology Dialysis Transplantation*, vol. 25, no. 7, pp. 2178–2187, 2010.

[17] S. Srinivas, R. A. Annigeri, M. K. Mani, B. S. Rao, P. C. Kowdle, and R. Seshadri, "Estimation of glomerular filtration rate in South Asian healthy adult kidney donors," *Nephrology*, vol. 13, no. 5, pp. 440–446, 2008.

[18] B. W. Teo, H. Xu, D. Wang et al., "GFR estimating equations in a multiethnic Asian population," *The American Journal of Kidney Diseases*, vol. 58, no. 1, pp. 56–63, 2011.

[19] N. H. Shaharudin, A. H. A. Gafor, S. Zainudin, N. C. T. Kong, A. A. Aziz, and S. A. Shah, "Estimating glomerular filtration rate in overweight and obese malaysian subjects," *Nephro-Urology Monthly*, vol. 3, no. 1, pp. 15–22, 2011.

8

Morphological Retrospective Study of Peritoneal Biopsies from Patients with Encapsulating Peritoneal Sclerosis: Underestimated Role of Adipocytes as New Fibroblasts Lineage?

Monika Tooulou,[1] **Pieter Demetter,**[2] **Anwar Hamade,**[3] **Caroline Keyzer,**[4]
Joëlle L. Nortier,[1,3] **and Agnieszka A. Pozdzik**[1,3]

[1]*Laboratory of Experimental Nephrology, Department of Biochemistry, Faculty of Medicine,*
Université Libre de Bruxelles (ULB), 1070 Brussels, Belgium
[2]*Department of Pathology, Cliniques Universitaires de Bruxelles (CUB), Erasme Hospital,*
Université Libre de Bruxelles (ULB), 1070 Brussels, Belgium
[3]*Department of Nephrology, Cliniques Universitaires de Bruxelles (CUB), Erasme Hospital,*
Université Libre de Bruxelles (ULB), 1070 Brussels, Belgium
[4]*Department of Radiology, Cliniques Universitaires de Bruxelles (CUB), Erasme Hospital,*
Université Libre de Bruxelles (ULB), 1070 Brussels, Belgium

Correspondence should be addressed to Agnieszka A. Pozdzik; agnieszka.pozdzik@erasme.ulb.ac.be

Academic Editor: Jaime Uribarri

Background. Encapsulating peritoneal sclerosis (EPS) is a rare but serious complication of peritoneal dialysis (PD). Besides the endothelial-to-mesenchymal transition (EMT), recently peritoneal adipocytes emerged as a potential source of fibrosis. We performed immunohistochemistry to approach EMT and to localize peritoneal adipocytes in peritoneal biopsies from PD-related EPS patients. *Material and Methods.* We investigated tissue expression of podoplanin, cytokeratin AE1/AE3 (mesothelium), calretinin (adipocytes), alpha-smooth muscle actin [α-SMA] (mesenchymal cells), interstitial mononuclear cell inflammation, and neoangiogenesis (CD3, CD4, CD8, CD20, CD68, and CD31 immunostainings, resp.). *Results.* Three patients (1 man/2 women; 17, 64, and 39 years old, resp.) developed EPS after 21, 90, and 164 months of PD therapy. In patients with EPS, we observed (1) loss of AE1/AE3 cytokeratin+ mesothelial cells without any evidence of migration into the interstitium, (2) disappearance of adipose tissue, (3) diffuse infiltration of calretinin+ cells in the areas of submesothelial fibrosis with a huge number of α-SMA and calretinin+ fusiform cells, and (4) increased vascular density. *Conclusion.* We report that the involvement of EMT in peritoneal fibrosis is difficult to demonstrate and that the calretinin+ adipocytes might be an underestimated component and a new source of myofibroblasts in peritoneal remodeling during PD-related EPS.

1. Introduction

Peritoneal dialysis (PD) is a first choice and successful home-based dialysis modality for patients with end-stage kidney disease (ESKD), with great advantages for their quality of life: preservation of residual renal function, no vascular access requirement, and possibility of continuing scholar or professional activities [1, 2]. Moreover, the International Society of Nephrology and International Society of Peritoneal Dialysis strongly advise PD therapy for acute kidney injury, especially in a pediatric population [3]. Despite the above-mentioned benefits, PD therapy deserves some particular attention. Indeed, long-term PD may prompt the remodeling of peritoneal membrane and loss of mesothelial cells mono-layer, increase in vascular density with diabetes-like vascular abnormalities (typical PD-associated venular subendothelial hyalinosis), vascular calcifications, and interstitial fibrosis [4]. These pathological structural changes of the peritoneal membrane are most frequently followed by functional consequences resulting in progressive loss of peritoneal membrane ultrafiltration capacity leading to discontinuation of PD therapy [5, 6].

Encapsulating peritoneal sclerosis (EPS) is still worrying and is an uncommon life-threatening complication of peritoneal dialysis with an incidence of 0.5 to 2.5% and a high mortality rate (25% to 55%) [7]. Following the International Society of Peritoneal Dialysis guidelines, diagnosis criteria of EPS include the association of clinical symptoms, radiological and histological findings [8]. The main pathological feature of EPS consists in a marked peritoneal fibrosis; however it lacks specificity as various degrees of submesothelial thickening have been reported in patients with chronic kidney disease [9, 10]. The pathophysiology of EPS is still unknown [11]. Nowadays, it appears that peritoneal fibrosis cannot be entirely explained on the basis of the simple model of wound healing (a three-phase model including injury of mesothelial cells, inflammation, and repair) [7, 12, 13]. This epithelial to mesenchymal transdifferentiation (EMT) process, first described in kidney fibrosis, states that the mesothelial cells change into a mesenchymal phenotype, migrate to submesothelial areas, and differentiate into "activated myofibroblasts," the cells responsible for fibrosis. The EMT was proposed to be involved mainly in the early stage of peritoneal fibrosis [14]. Recent data demonstrate that the resident peritoneal interstitial cells are early activated following the aggression of mesothelial cells (or epithelium), the inflammatory infiltrate, and profibrosing cytokine microenvironment. Currently, new data suggest that peritoneal adipocytes could also contribute to this pathological process [15].

In our study, we approached the EMT process and adipocytes involvement in peritoneal fibrosis in a morphohistological retrospective analysis of 6 peritoneal tissue biopsies (3 cases with PD-related EPS, 2 cases with normal peritoneal tissue, and 1 case with acute peritonitis, for a histological study during an acute inflammatory process). Our presented data show that the resident peritoneal adipocytes represent an underestimated source of peritoneal myofibroblasts in PD-induced EPS.

2. Material and Methods

The study was evaluated and approved by the Local Ethic Committee (Erasme Hospital number P2014/184). We included peritoneal biopsies samples of the 3 patients with EPS diagnosed between 1995 and 2013 in our center. We selected the 2 control patients with normal peritoneum (randomly selected in our database of patients who had abdominal surgery in our center and with normal renal function). We also analyzed 1 case with acute peritonitis, with normal renal function (so without any ESKD or peritoneal fibrosis), in order to evaluate the hypothesis of early crosstalk between inflammatory cells, mesothelial cells, and adipocytes. For EPS diagnosis, we applied the clinical and biological criteria adapted from Nakamoto [16]: (i) stage 1

(pre-EPS), characterized by loss of ultrafiltration, high transport status, hypoproteinaemia, bloody dialysate, ascites, and peritoneal calcifications; (ii) stage 2 (inflammatory), increase in C-reactive protein level and white blood cell count, fever, weight, and appetite loss; (iii) stage 3 (encapsulating or progressive), disappearance of signs of inflammation and appearance of signs of ileus (nausea, vomiting, abdominal pain, and constipation), abdominal mass with ascites, and (iv) stage 4 (obstructive or cocooning). We used the formalin-fixed peritoneal tissue embedded in paraffin blocks available in the files of the pathology department of our hospital. Medical records analysis of included cases provided epidemiological data (age, gender), PD characteristics (dialysis modality, type of solution, and PD duration), clinical, radiological, and laboratory parameters at EPS diagnosis, time between renal transplantation and the onset of EPS symptoms, and prescribed immunosuppressive agents. Treatment modalities and outcomes of EPS were also recorded and included.

2.1. Standard Stainings and Immunohistochemistry. Standard stainings (Masson's trichrome and haematoxylin-eosin (HE)) were used to illustrate peritoneal fibrosis, mesothelial cells, and inflammatory infiltrate. The entire sample of each peritoneal tissue specimen was analyzed by optical microscopy using low (×40 and ×100), medium (×200), and high (×400) magnifications (Carl Zeiss, Oberkochen, Germany).

The study of tissue expression of podoplanin, AE1/AE3 cytokeratin (mesothelial phenotype), calretinin (expressed by mesothelial cells and adipocytes), vimentin (mesenchymal phenotype), α-SMA (myofibroblasts), CD4, CD8, CD20, CD68 (immunophenotyping of inflammatory cells), and CD31 (endothelial cells marker) was performed on sections of $4\,\mu m$ thickness using an immunohistochemistry analysis technique (Ventana XT-Discovery, Tucson, USA). Immunoperoxidase procedures counterstained with hematoxylin were applied. We chose the following human tissues as positive controls for immunohistochemistry of used antibodies: tonsil for immunostaining of anti-CD4, anti-CD8, anti-CD20, and anti-CD68 antibodies (3-membrane and 1-membrane-cytoplasm patterns, resp.); colon for anti-AE1/AE3 cytokeratin antibodies (cytoplasm pattern); vessels for anti-α-SMA and anti-CD31 antibodies (cytoplasm pattern); sarcoma for anti-vimentin antibodies (cytoplasm pattern); and adipose tissue for anti-calretinin antibodies (nuclear and cytoplasm pattern). The negative controls were performed in the absence of primary antibodies and showed no staining (Table 1).

2.2. Quantification of Immunostainings. The semiquantitative score for cytokeratin AE1/AE3, calretinin, vimentin, and α-SMA expression was applied as follows: strong expression (+++), moderate expression (++), low expression (+), or no expression (0).

The quantitative analysis of CD4 expression (subpopulation of T helper cells and infiltration macrophages), CD8 expression (subpopulation of cytotoxic/suppressor T cells), CD20 (B cells population), and CD68 (circulating monocyte and macrophages) was performed by calculating the number of positive cells per field (high magnification, ×400).

TABLE 1: Details of immunohistochemistry studies performed on peritoneal tissue biopsies (primary antibodies and corresponding cells specificity, retrieval processes, dilution, and type of secondary antibodies).

Antigen	Specificity	Retrieval (time in minutes)	Dilution	Manufacturer
Secondary antibody: monoclonal				
Podoplanin	Mesothelium, lymphatics endothelium	H1 (20)	1/50	Covance, Princeton, New Jersey, USA
Secondary antibody: polyclonal				
AE1/AE3	Mesothelium	H1 (20)	1/800	Dako, Glostrup, Denmark
Calretinin	Mesothelium	H1 (20)	1/150	Menarini, Zaventem, Belgium
CD8	Cytotoxic/suppressor T cells subpopulation	H1 (20)	1/800	Dako, Glostrup, Denmark
CD20	B cells	H1 (30)	1/3000	Dako, Glostrup, Denmark
CD68	Monocytes/macrophages	H1 (30)	1/100	Menarini, Zaventem, Belgium
Secondary antibody: peroxidase				
CD4	Helper T cells subpopulation	H2 (20)	1/50	Klinipath, Duiven, Netherlands
CD31	Endothelium	H2 (30)	1/1000	Menarini, Zaventem, Belgium
Vimentin	Mesenchymal cells	/	1/100	Klinipath, Duiven, Netherlands
α-SMA	Myofibroblasts	/	1/100	Menarini, Zaventem, Belgium

H1: citrate buffer, pH 6.0; H2: EDTA buffer, pH 8.0.

For quantitative analysis of CD31 expression (vascular density), we counted CD31 positive vessels per field (medium magnification, ×200).

We analyzed 20 fields at random in each case using an optical microscope (Carl Zeiss, Oberkochen, Germany).

3. Results

3.1. Clinical, Biological, and Radiological Characteristics of Studied Patients.
The clinical and biological characteristics at diagnosis of EPS are summarized in Table 2. We identified a 17-year-old man (case 1) and two women aged 64 years (case 2) and 39 years (case 3) treated with PD (for 21, 90, and 164 months, resp.), who developed EPS after shift to hemodialysis (case 1) and after first (case 2) and second kidney transplantation (case 3).

In all cases, the diagnosis was suspected because of digestive symptoms, systemic inflammation, and normocytic anemia. Furthermore, cases 2 and 3 had hemorrhagic ascites. Their abdominal CT scan showed, in addition to abundant ascites, diffuse peritoneal calcifications, with parietal and visceral involvement (Figure 1). Positron emission tomography with [18F] fluorodeoxyglucose (FDG-PET) was available only in one case (case 3) and demonstrated significant FDG uptake by the parietal peritoneal membrane (Figure 1).

3.2. Histological and Immunohistochemical Findings.
Compared with the normal peritoneal tissue biopsies (controls), massive submesothelial thickening corresponding to fibrosis was associated with the disappearance of the mesothelium in all EPS cases (Figure 2). In controls, we observed a distinct monolayer of cubic mesothelial cells closely attached to one another and affixed to the thin basement membrane, which was in direct contact with a waste area of adipose tissue. In the control 3 biopsy (acute peritonitis), mesothelium was well preserved but we found a marked hyperplasia of mesothelial cells attached to the basement membrane and the apposition

of inflammatory connective tissue containing predominantly polymorphonuclear neutrophils infiltrate (Figure 2).

3.3. The Mesothelial Cells in Controls, Acute Peritonitis, and EPS Biopsies.
In all 3 control peritoneal biopsies, the thin layer of mesothelial cells strongly expressed podoplanin, cytokeratin AE1/AE3, and calretinin (mesothelial markers) (Figure 3, Table 3); these data are consistent with literature [17].

Podoplanin expression was also found in the endothelial cells of lymphatic vessels and mesothelium (Figures 3(a)–3(d)). In case with acute peritonitis, mesothelial cells did not express podoplanin. Only in case 1 of EPS, hyperplastic podoplanin positive mesothelial cells were clearly identified in the interstitium, which had a completely remodeled architecture. In this case, an acute inflammatory component was present at the time of peritoneal biopsy. Interestingly, in case 3 of EPS, we objectified increased podoplanin expression by deep vascular structures. This may suggest an increase in lymphatic vessels density.

High expression of cytokeratin AE1/AE3 by mesothelial cells was observed in the 3 controls but was lacking in all cases of EPS (Figures 3(e)–3(h), Table 3). In the acute peritonitis case, mesothelial cells did not express cytokeratin AE1/AE3. Despite basement membrane rupture, we did not find AE1/AE3+ cells migrating to interstitial areas. Only in case 1 of EPS, hyperplastic cytokeratin AE1/AE3+ mesothelial cells were clearly identified in the remodeled interstitium. These cells did not present typical for myofibroblasts fusiform morphology.

Expression of calretinin in mesothelium was similar to AE1/AE3. Interestingly, expression of calretinin by adipocytes, although in low intensity (+), was constant in all of our 3 controls and acute peritonitis. Nevertheless, we clearly objectified an interstitial accumulation of calretinin positive spindle cells in the 3 EPS cases (Figures 3(i)–3(l), Table 3).

TABLE 2: Patients with encapsulating peritoneal sclerosis: epidemiological characteristics, diagnostic criteria, risk factors, treatment, and outcomes.

	Case EPS 1	Case EPS 2	Case EPS 3
Sex/age at diagnosis (years)	M/19	F/64	F/39
Primitive nephropathy	CAKUT	Diabetes	MPGN
Status at EPS diagnosis	HD	KTx	KTx
Time from peritoneal dialysis arrest to EPS diagnosis (months)	5	18	55
Peritoneal dialysis modality	CAPD	CAPD	CAPD
Time on peritoneal dialysis (months)	21	90	164
Peritonitis episodes (n)	3	ND	8
Microorganisms	S. aureus (3)	ND	E. coli (3) S. aureus (3) P. aeruginosa (2)
Glucose overexposure	Yes	No	Yes
Chlorhexidine use	No	No	No
Ciclosporin	No	No	Yes
Everolimus	No	No	Yes
Clinical and radiological diagnostic criteria of EPS			
Clinical symptoms/hemoperitoneum	Yes/no	Yes/yes	Yes/yes
Abdominal CT findings	Intestinal subocclusion Adherence	Loculated ascites Peritoneal thickening and calcifications	Loculated severe ascites Peritoneal thickening and calcifications
Treatment of EPS			
Azathioprine (mg/day)	50	75	50
Tamoxifen (mg/day)	/	20	10
Dexamethasone (mg/day)	/	32	8
Current state	HD	Died (septicemia)	KTx
Follow-up (months)	237	ND	57
Outcome	Nausea Abdominal pain	ND	Recurrent ascites, bacterial peritonitis (2)

EPS: encapsulating peritoneal sclerosis; M: man; W: woman; CAKUT: congenital abnormality of kidney and urinary tract; MPGN: membranoproliferative glomerulonephritis; HD: haemodialysis; KTx: kidney transplantation CAPD: continuous ambulatory peritoneal dialysis; ND: no data available.

3.4. Interstitial Infiltration by Polymorphonuclear Cells in Acute Peritonitis and by Mononuclear Cells in EPS Biopsies. In comparison with controls, we found diffuse mononuclear cells infiltration containing macrophages, T cells, and few B cells in all EPS cases. We observed a marked heterogeneity between the EPS cases, with a highly variable degree of mononuclear cell infiltration, containing mainly CD68+ and CD8+ cells. Those cells were absent in the interstitium from patient with acute peritonitis that contained several polymorphonuclear cells (Figure 4, Table 3).

3.5. The Mesenchymal Cells in Controls, Acute Peritonitis, and EPS Biopsies. The constitutional expression of α-SMA was mainly found in the vessels and in some rare interstitial cells. In all cases, many spindle cells expressed vimentin and α-SMA and corresponded to mesenchymal cells and myofibroblasts accumulation (Figure 5). A significant increase in vascular density (CD31 positive endothelial cells) was observed in all EPS cases, as compared with controls (Figure 6, Table 3).

4. Discussion

The main finding of our study was the discovery of fusiform calretinin positive cells in areas of severe submesothelial fibrosis in all EPS patients. In normal peritoneal tissue biopsy, weak calretinin staining was found in adipocytes and more enhanced in mesothelial cells according to literature [18]. Calretinin (29 kDa calbindin) is a vitamin D-dependent calcium-binding protein coded by the *CALB2* gene and emerges as a multifunctional protein associated with cells development, proliferation, differentiation, and cell death [19].

Our EPS cases were recognized after discontinuation of PD, suggesting the need for vigilance of the nephrologists taking care about transplanted or on hemodialysis patients previously treated by PD [7]. As the incidence of EPS increases with time after renal transplantation [11], the immunosuppressive regimen involvement in the pathogenesis of posttransplant EPS remains an unresolved question.

Several other risk factors have been identified such as high glucose concentration dialysate, long duration of PD,

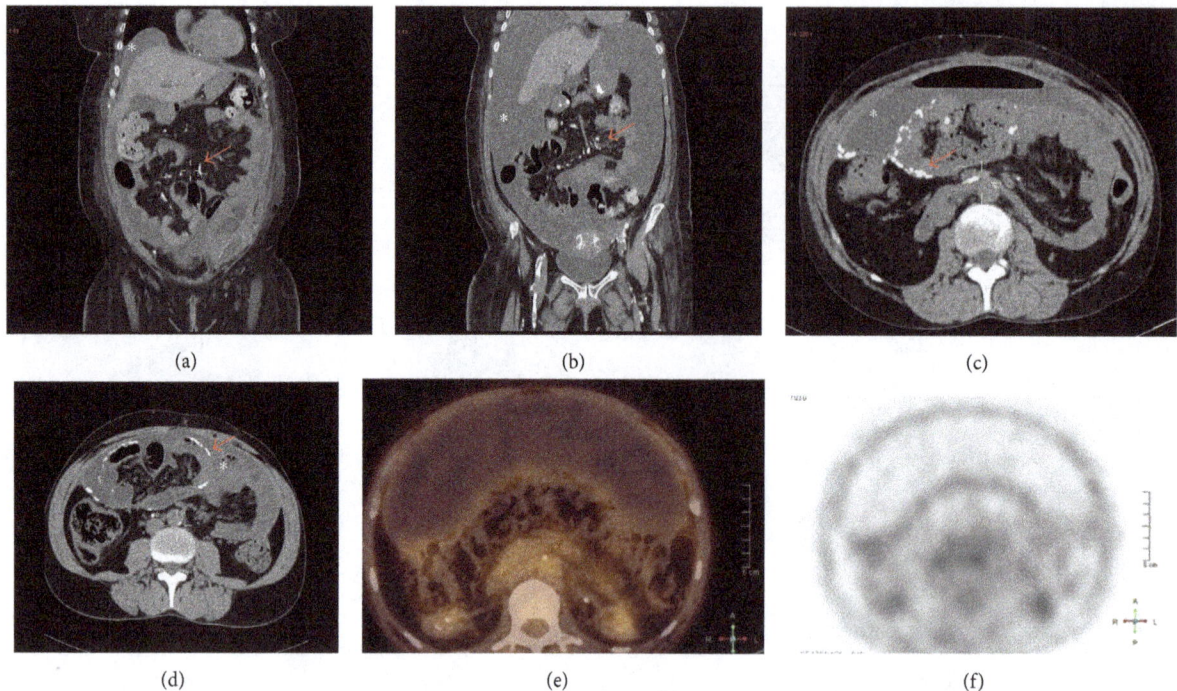

(a)   (b)   (c)

(d)   (e)   (f)

FIGURE 1: Radiological findings suggesting encapsulating peritoneal sclerosis (EPS). (a, c and b, d correspond to cases EPS 2 and EPS 3, resp.) Abdominal computed tomography without contrast agent showed massive nonloculated fluid and bowel loops drowned into the center of the abdominal cavity suggestive of bowel adhesions. As compared with EPS case 2, EPS case 3 presented more abundant abdominal ascites, marked narrowing of bowel lumen and thickening of visceral and parietal peritoneum, absence of dilated bowel loop, air-fluid levels or entrapped fluid collections, and several calcifications in both parietal and visceral peritoneum. (e and f, case EPS 3) Fluorodeoxyglucose[18] positron emission tomography (F^{18} PET) scan showed a mild increase in the tracer uptake in the peritoneal areas.

TABLE 3: Results of immunohistochemical quantifications of mesothelio-mesenchymal transdifferentiation process, evaluation of interstitial inflammation, and vasculature in peritoneal biopsies samples from controls, case of acute peritonitis, and patients with encapsulating peritoneal sclerosis.

	Control 1	Control 2	Case of acute peritonitis	Case EPS 1	Case EPS 2	Case EPS 3
Markers of mesothelial cells phenotype						
AE1/AE3						
Mesothelium	(+++)	(+++)	(+++)	0	(0)	0
Interstitium	0	0	0	(+++)	(+++)	(+++)
Calretinin						
Mesothelium	(+++)	(+++)	(+++)	0	0	0
Interstitium	0	0	(+/−)	(++)	(+)	(+)
Immunohistochemical phenotyping of inflammatory infiltrating cells						
CD4*	19.6	11.5	8.85	1.05	10.8	ND
CD8*	1.15	0	1.05	0.9	2.25	130
CD68*	0.9	1.25	4.7	2.75	1.66	18.8
CD20*	3	0	0	3	10	1
Markers of endothelial cells phenotype						
CD31#	0.95	0.8	4.2	6.5	0.5	ND
Markers of mesenchymal cells phenotype						
Vimentin						
Mesothelium	0	0	(+)	(+++)	(+++)	(+)
Interstitium	0	0	(+)	(+++)	(+++)	(+++)
Markers of myofibroblasts						
Alpha SMA	0	0	(+)	(+++)	(+++)	(+++)

EPS: encapsulating peritoneal sclerosis; SMA: alpha-smooth muscle actin. ND: no data available (insufficiency of biopsy material). Semiquantitative score analysis: expression; high: (+++), moderate: (++), low: (+), and absent: 0. Score of quantitative evaluations: (*) mean number of cells or (#) vessels per field (details of all immunostaining analysis are described in Material and Methods).

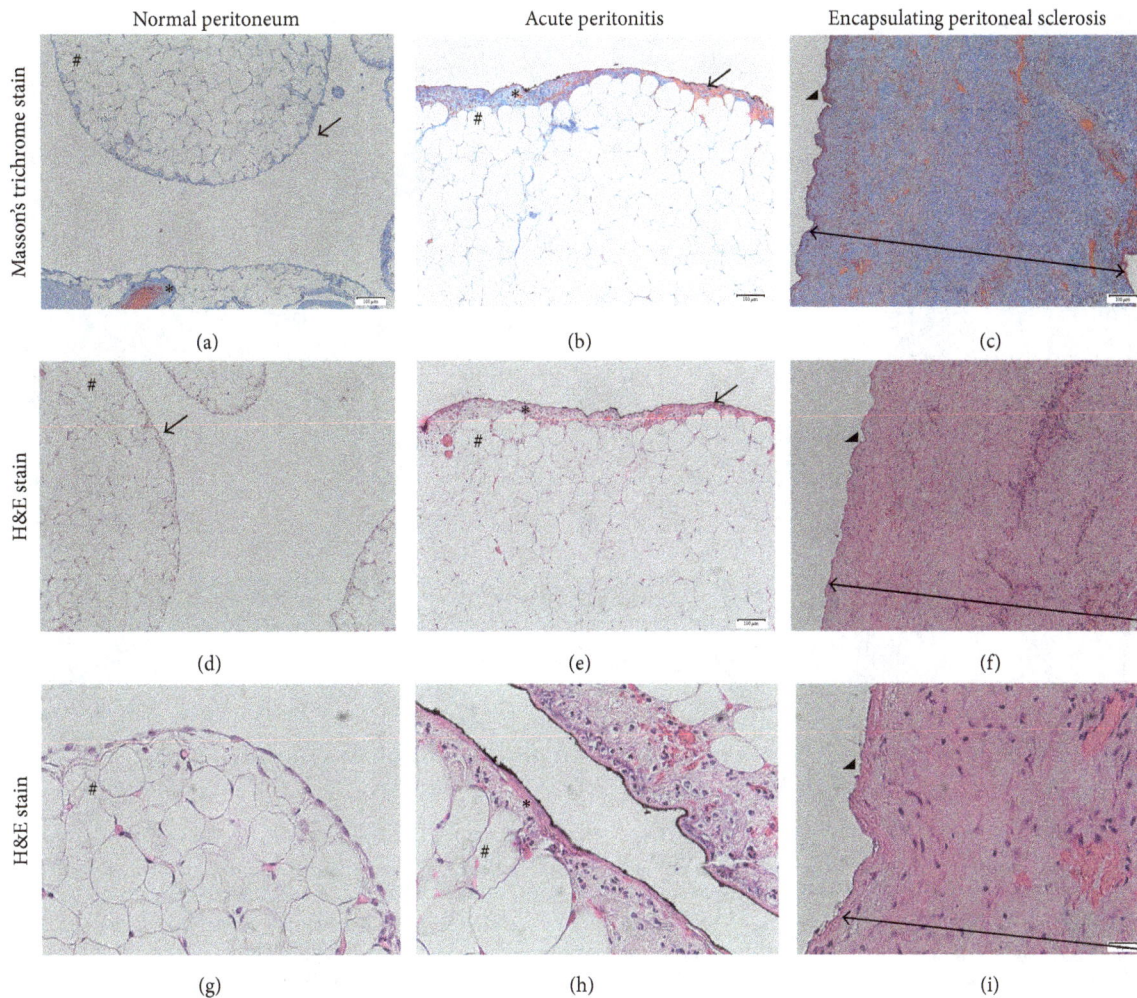

FIGURE 2: Peritoneal biopsies representative photomicrographs of haematoxylin-eosin and Masson's trichrome stainings in studied cases (a, d, and g). Mesothelium (→) and adipocytes (#) in the submesothelial area in normal peritoneal membrane (b, e, and h). Well preserved mesothelium with hyperplasic mesothelial cells and increase in conjunctive tissue (∗) associated with interstitial submesothelial infiltrate mainly polymorphonuclear neutrophils (++) in acute peritonitis case. *Superficial black lining related to the surgery technique (use of Indian ink).* (c, f, and i) Disappearance of mesothelium (arrowhead), major submesothelial fibrosis containing mainly mononuclear cells, and sever fibrosis (← →) in case of EPS. Original magnifications: (a–f) ×10, (g–i) ×40.

young age, and the use of beta-blockers or cyclosporine and peritonitis [7, 11, 16]. One constant in these factors is the duration of PD, confirmed recently by two independent groups [20, 21]. Indeed, more severe fibrosis is observed in transplanted patient with longest PD vintage and who had a high glucose exposure.

Besides the duration of PD therapy, the number of peritonitis episodes is still a significant risk factor [20, 21]. For this reason, in our morphohistological study we included a case of acute peritonitis not related to PD or ESKD, in order to evaluate the hypothesis of early crosstalk between inflammatory cells and resident peritoneal membrane cells (adipocytes and mesothelial cells). These interactions could be an early link between the PD-related peritonitis (acute inflammation) and peritoneal fibrosis [22]. Interestingly, we found some morphological similarities between mesothelial cells hyperplasia observed in acute peritonitis and in EPS

cases, which is in accordance with the findings by others [17]. The reason for mesothelial cells hyperplasia is unknown; however it may be postulated that the cells are activated secondarily by cytokines (released by inflammatory cells) or by hypertonic solutions.

Peritoneal thickening and lowering in the lumen/vessels diameter ratio related to uremia have been reported in patients with chronic kidney diseases [10]. The EMT process has been proposed as a chief pathway of peritoneal fibrosis, mainly in its early stage [23], so early before beginning PD [10]. Despite extensive studies on EMT [14, 23, 24], many aspects of peritoneal membrane remodeling and EPS remain poorly understood [25, 26] suggesting that additional novel mechanisms and pathways need to be explored [13]. Interpretation of our data is unfortunately limited by the small number of studied biopsies as well as the fact that they were obtained at advanced stages of EPS. Indeed, agreeing

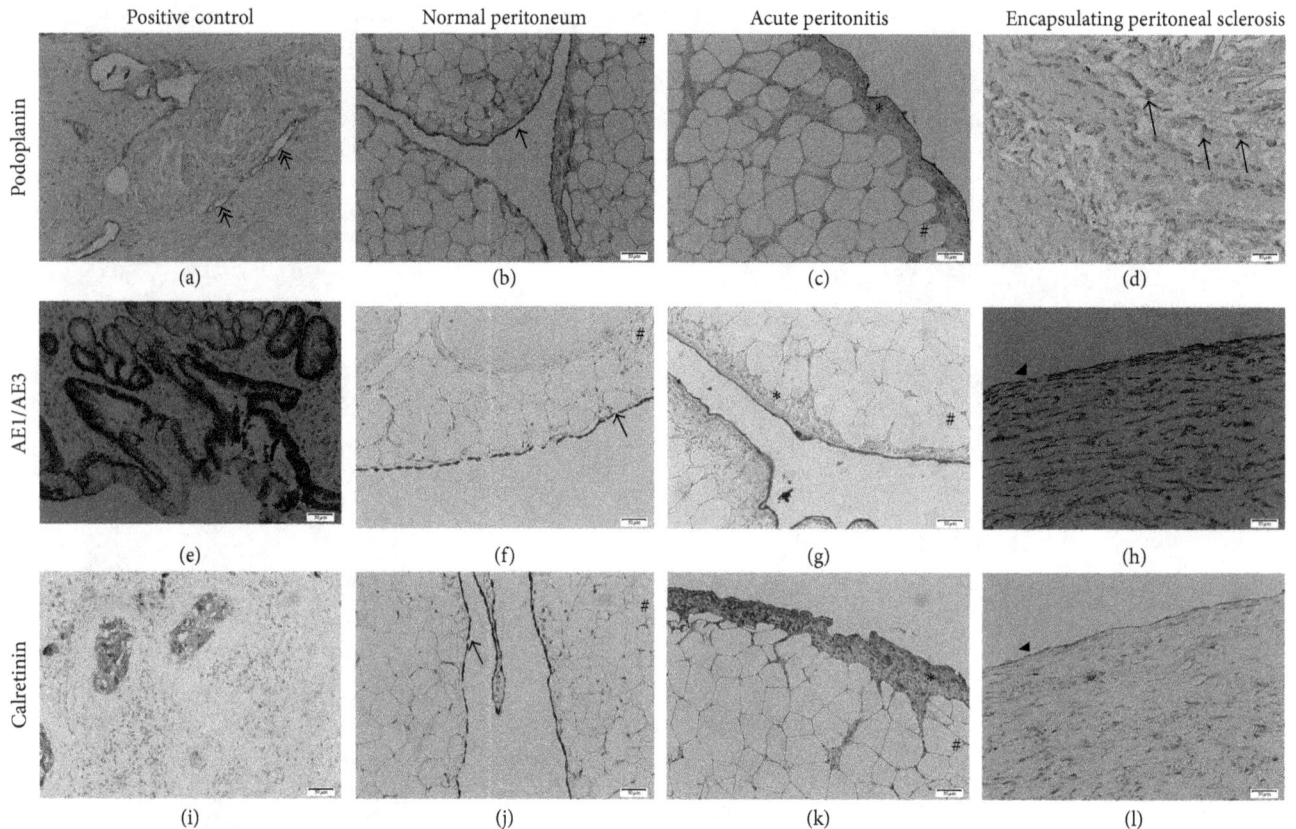

| Positive control | Normal peritoneum | Acute peritonitis | Encapsulating peritoneal sclerosis |

Podoplanin: (a), (b), (c), (d)

AE1/AE3: (e), (f), (g), (h)

Calretinin: (i), (j), (k), (l)

FIGURE 3: Peritoneal biopsy representative photomicrographs of mesothelial phenotype markers expression: podoplanin (a–d), cytokeratin AE1/AE3 (e–h), and calretinin (i–l). Positive control of immunostainings for used antibodies (internal controls) (a, e, and i), control case: normal peritoneum (b, f, and j), case of acute peritonitis (control 3, c, g, and k), and case 1 of encapsulating peritoneal sclerosis (EPS) (d, h, and l). Physiologic expression of podoplanin (cytoplasm of endothelium in lymphatics (→)), AE1/AE3 cytoplasm in epithelial cells of stomach and calretinin (cytoplasm in epithelial cells) (a, e, and i, resp.). (b, f, and j) Intact peritoneal membrane biopsy in controls; mesothelial cells (→) with obvious expression of adipocytes (#). (c, g, and k) Acute peritonitis case: hyperplasia of mesothelial cells. *Superficial black lining related to the surgery technique (use of Indian ink).* (d, h, and l) EPS case: loss of mesothelial cells (arrowheads) as attested by absence of podoplanin, AE1/AE3, and calretinin expressions. Note hyperplasia of mesothelial cells expressed all mesothelial markers podoplanin, cytokeratin AE1/AE3, and calretinin located in interstitial areas. The architecture of interstitium is strongly modified and contains several calretinin+ fusiform (fibroblasts-like) cells (arrow). Immunoperoxidase staining counterstained with haematoxylin. Original magnification: (a–l) ×20.

to Nakamoto [16], cases 1, 2, and 3 corresponded to pre-EPS and inflammatory and progressive or encapsulating EPS, respectively. Moreover, we observed a highly variable degree of interstitial inflammation. Similar to previous report [17], we did not find a transmembrane migration of mesothelial cells into the interstitium, a pivotal phase of EMT. Our results did not confirm that peritoneal interstitial fibroblasts derive from EMT.

The role of EMT in peritoneal fibrosis has been adapted from mechanisms reported in kidney fibrosis (KF). However today, this model begins to be questioned [27–30]. In fact, resident cells (fibroblasts) are considered as the main source as only 5% of myofibroblasts derived from EMT in experimental models of KF [31]. As in the renal fibrosis, already present resident peritoneal cells should be considered as a potential source for myofibroblasts generation. Indeed, peritoneal adipocytes are pluripotent cells and they are active players in fibrosis [32–34]. Therefore, peritoneal calretinin positive adipocytes might be a new

and actually underestimated source of myofibroblasts. As compared with controls, the submesothelial adipose tissue containing several calretinin positive adipocytes completely disappeared; nonetheless numerous fusiform calretinin positive cells were observed in the areas of peritoneal fibrosis in EPS biopsies. Intriguingly, in case of acute peritonitis, we found that a submesothelial layer of inflammatory cells closely bordered adipocytes. Unfortunately because of insufficient quantity of peritoneal tissue biopsies, the expression of adipose cells mRNA was not performed. Besides dialysate, several cytokines and growth factors such as transforming growth factor-beta (TGF-β) a pivotal profibrotic cytokine secreted by injured mesothelial cells and/or inflammatory cells could be involved in adipocytes differentiation into the peritoneal fibroblasts [35]. In fact, strong evidence suggests a possible crosstalk between the PD solutions, adipose tissue, and peritoneal fibrosis [15, 32]. Moreover, adipocytes mediate numerous physiological processes, secreted adipokines (leptin, adiponectin), cytokines (TNFα, IL-6), and growth

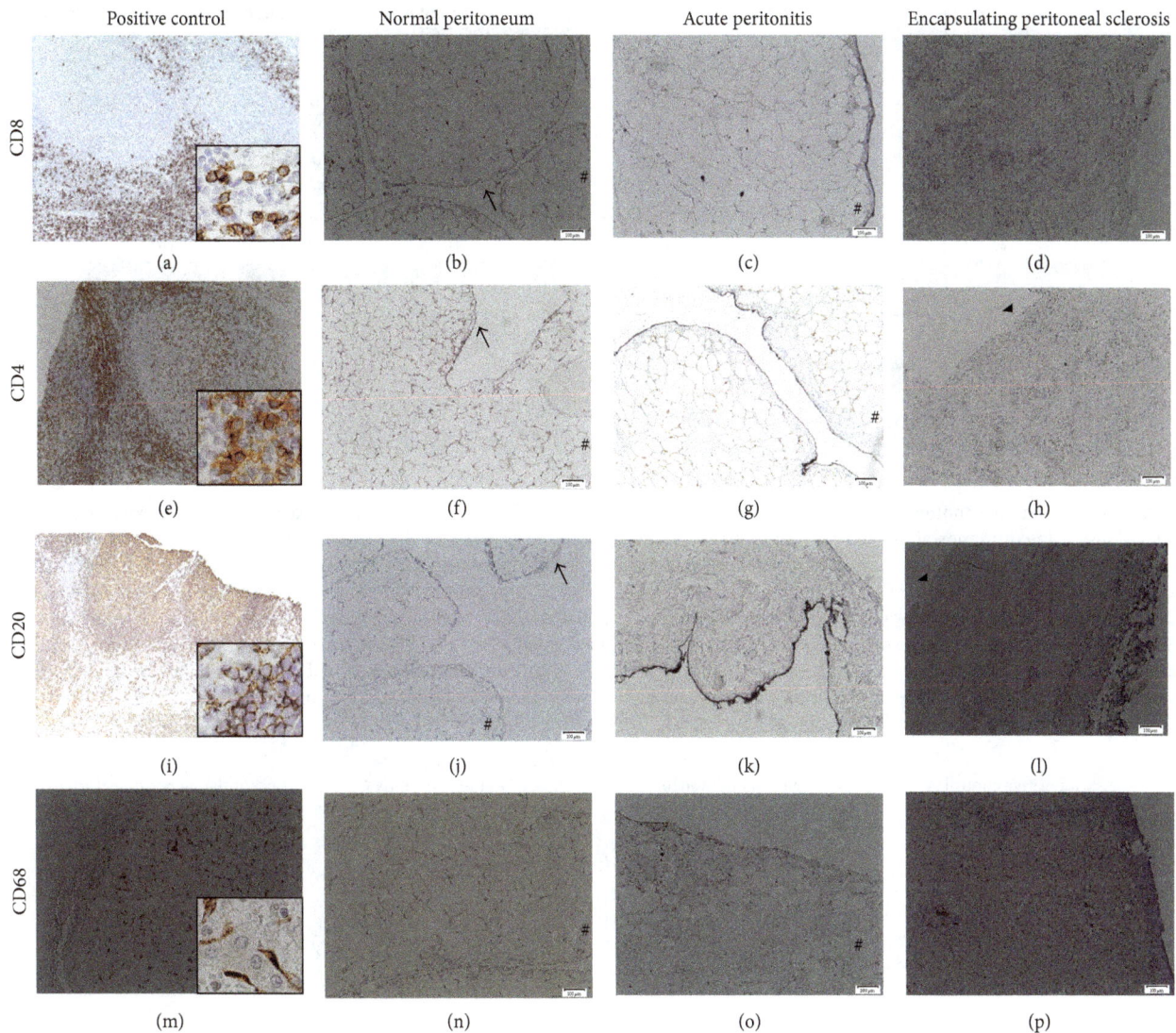

FIGURE 4: Representative photomicrographs demonstrating histopathological data of interstitial inflammatory cells infiltration in parietal peritoneal tissues biopsy using immunostaining of CD8 (a–d), CD4 (e–h), CD20 (i–l), and CD68 (m–p). Positive control of immunostainings for used antibodies (internal controls) (a, e, i, and m), control: normal peritoneum (b, f, j, and n), case of acute peritonitis (control 3; c, g, k, and o), and case 1 of encapsulating peritoneal sclerosis (EPS) (d, h, l, and p). Absence of mononuclear cells in normal peritoneum. Weak expression of all CD8, CD4, CD20, and CD68 in conjunctive tissue areas adjacent to mesothelium in case with acute peritonitis characterized mainly by polymorphonuclear cells infiltration. Marked interstitial inflammatory cells identified (d) several CD8+ cells (T lymphocytes), (h) few CD4+ cells (T lymphocytes), and (l) CD20+ (B cells), which were accompanied by several (f) CD68+ cells (macrophages) diffusely infiltrating fibrotic areas. Immunoperoxidase staining counterstained with hematoxylin. Original magnification: (a–p) ×20. Small pictures (a, e, i, and m): ×40.

factors including transforming growth factor-beta (TGF-β) [32]. Leptin stimulates lipolysis and inhibits lipogenesis [32]. In human peritoneal mesothelial cells, it has been reported that glucose increased the leptin mRNA expression and its synthesis. Concomitantly, the leptin receptor was upregulated in mesothelial cells and leptin induced the release of TGF-β by mesothelial cells. Interestingly, glucose markedly amplified this process [36]. It must be taken into account that adipocytes could be potentially in direct contact with the glucose contained in PD solution after disruption of mesothelium integrity. Indeed shedding of mesothelial cells into the peritoneal cavity by alteration of cell junctions and basement membrane denudation are induced by recurrent mechanical stress related to the daily variations in intra-abdominal pressure and to turbulences of in- and outflow of PD solutions (volume, number of cycles) [1, 7]. Above data could be a plausible way to explain the observed loss of adipose tissue as our cases were exposed to high glucose concentration PD solutions during a long time.

In conclusion, we report that the involvement of EMT in peritoneal fibrosis is difficult to demonstrate. The calretinin positive cells accumulate in the submesothelial fibrosis so

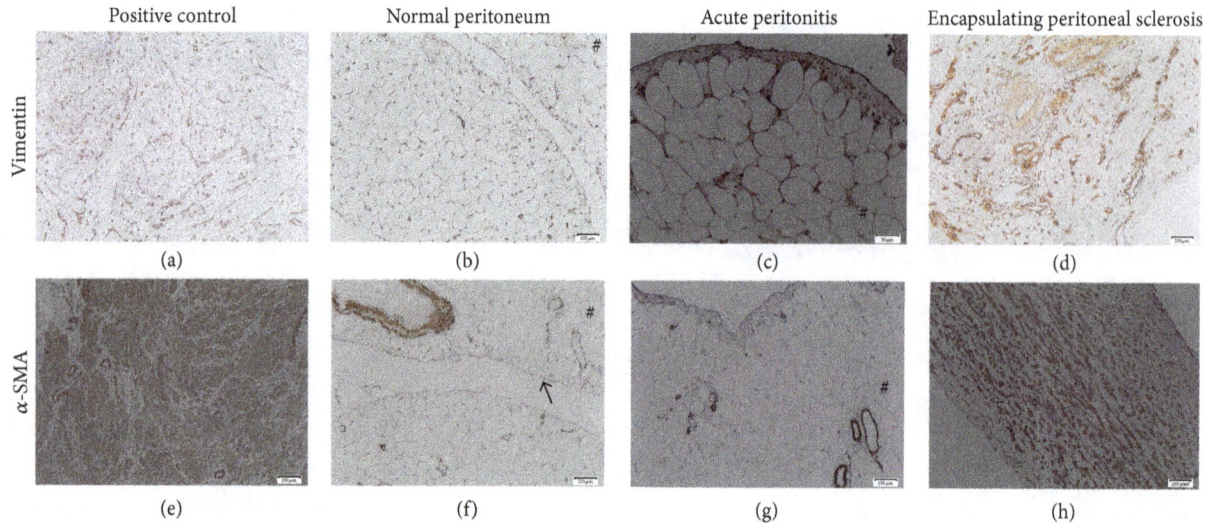

FIGURE 5: Representative photomicrographs demonstrating histopathological data of mesenchymal markers expression in parietal peritoneal tissues biopsy using immunostaining of vimentin (a–d) and alpha-smooth muscle actin (α-SMA) (e–h). Positive control of immunostainings for used antibodies (internal controls) (a, e), control: normal peritoneum (b, f), case of acute peritonitis (control 3; c and g), and case 1 of encapsulating peritoneal sclerosis (EPS) (d and h). (a, e) Normal peritoneum, expression of vimentin ($\rightarrow$) limited to few interstitial cells and of α-SMA expression to vascular walls. (c, g) Acute peritonitis: interstitial vimentin+ cells, lack of expression of vimentin in mesothelial cell layer; α-SMA found only in the vessels. (d, h) Case of encapsulating peritoneal sclerosis (EPS): absence of expression of both markers in the mesothelial cell layer. Note diffuse accumulation of vimentin+ cells identifying interstitial mesenchymal cells and α-SMA immunostaining of numerous interstitial cells entrapped in the fibrotic areas reflecting the presence of myofibroblasts. Immunoperoxidase staining counterstained with haematoxylin. Original magnification: (a–g) ×20. (h) ×4.

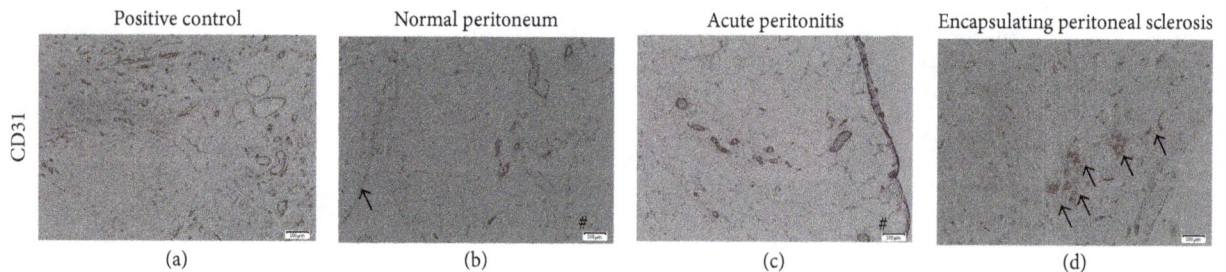

FIGURE 6: Representative photomicrographs demonstrating histopathological data of endothelial cells marker expression in parietal peritoneal tissues biopsy using immunostaining of CD31 (a). Positive control of immunostainings for used antibodies (internal controls) (a), control: normal peritoneum (b), case of acute peritonitis (control 3; c), and case 1 of encapsulating peritoneal sclerosis (EPS) (d). As compared with normal and acute peritonitis cases, increases in endothelial CD31 expression identifying nonlymphatic vascular network were localized in the deep areas of peritoneum and reflected increased vessels density. Immunoperoxidase staining counterstained with hematoxylin. Original magnification: (a–d) ×20.

that adipocytes might be an underestimated component and a new source of myofibroblasts in peritoneal remodeling during EPS related to PD.

Disclosure

Parts of this work have been presented at the Annual Scientific Meeting of the Belgian Society of Nephrology (October 2014, Brussels, Belgium) and at the 47th Annual Meeting of the American Society of Nephrology (November 2014, Philadelphia, USA).

References

[1] S. J. Davies, "Peritoneal dialysis—current status and future challenges," *Nature Reviews Nephrology*, vol. 9, no. 7, pp. 399–408, 2013.

[2] J. M. Bargman, "Peritoneal dialysis should be the first choice for renal replacement therapy in the elderly," *Seminars in Dialysis*, vol. 25, no. 6, pp. 668–670, 2012.

[3] B. Cullis, M. Abdelraheem, G. Abrahams et al., "Peritoneal dialysis for acute kidney injury," *Peritoneal Dialysis International*, vol. 34, no. 5, pp. 494–517, 2014.

[4] R. T. Krediet and D. G. Struijk, "Peritoneal changes in patients on long-term peritoneal dialysis," *Nature Reviews Nephrology*, vol. 9, no. 7, pp. 419–429, 2013.

[5] E. A. Brown, W. Van Biesen, F. O. Finkelstein et al., "Length of time on peritoneal dialysis and encapsulating peritoneal

sclerosis: position paper for ISPD," *Peritoneal Dialysis International*, vol. 29, no. 6, pp. 595–600, 2009.

[6] O. Devuyst, P. J. Margetts, and N. Topley, "The pathophysiology of the peritoneal membrane," *Journal of the American Society of Nephrology*, vol. 21, no. 7, pp. 1077–1085, 2010.

[7] C. Goodlad and E. A. Brown, "Encapsulating peritoneal sclerosis: what have we learned?" *Seminars in Nephrology*, vol. 31, no. 2, pp. 183–198, 2011.

[8] Y. Kawaguchi, A. Saito, H. Kawanishi et al., "Recommendations on the management of encapsulating peritoneal sclerosis in Japan, 2005: diagnosis, predictive markers, treatment, and preventive measures," *Peritoneal Dialysis International*, vol. 25, supplement 4, pp. S83–S95, 2005.

[9] K. Honda and H. Oda, "Pathology of encapsulating peritoneal sclerosis," *Peritoneal Dialysis International*, vol. 25, supplement 4, pp. S19–S29, 2005.

[10] K. Honda, C. Hamada, M. Nakayama et al., "Impact of uremia, diabetes, and peritoneal dialysis itself on the pathogenesis of peritoneal sclerosis: a quantitative study of peritoneal membrane morphology," *Clinical Journal of the American Society of Nephrology*, vol. 3, no. 3, pp. 720–728, 2008.

[11] M. R. Korte, D. E. Sampimon, M. G. H. Betjes, and R. T. Krediet, "Encapsulating peritoneal sclerosis: the state of affairs," *Nature Reviews Nephrology*, vol. 7, no. 9, pp. 528–538, 2011.

[12] T. A. Wynn, "Cellular and molecular mechanisms of fibrosis," *Journal of Pathology*, vol. 214, no. 2, pp. 199–210, 2008.

[13] J. S. Duffield, M. Lupher, V. J. Thannickal, and T. A. Wynn, "Host responses in tissue repair and fibrosis," *Annual Review of Pathology: Mechanisms of Disease*, vol. 8, pp. 241–276, 2013.

[14] L. S. Aroeira, A. Aguilera, J. A. Sánchez-Tomero et al., "Epithelial to mesenchymal transition and peritoneal membrane failure in peritoneal dialysis patients: pathologic significance and potential therapeutic interventions," *Journal of the American Society of Nephrology*, vol. 18, no. 7, pp. 2004–2013, 2007.

[15] S. Aoki, K. Udo, H. Morimoto et al., "Adipose tissue behavior is distinctly regulated by neighboring cells and fluid flow stress: a possible role of adipose tissue in peritoneal fibrosis," *Journal of Artificial Organs*, vol. 16, no. 3, pp. 322–331, 2013.

[16] H. Nakamoto, "Encapsulating peritoneal sclerosis—a clinician's approach to diagnosis and medical treatment," *Peritoneal Dialysis International*, vol. 25, supplement 4, pp. S30–S38, 2005.

[17] N. Braun, D. M. Alscher, P. Fritz et al., "Podoplanin-positive cells are a hallmark of encapsulating peritoneal sclerosis," *Nephrology Dialysis Transplantation*, vol. 26, no. 3, pp. 1033–1041, 2011.

[18] J. M. M. Cates, B. N. Coffing, B. T. Harris, and C. C. Black, "Calretinin expression in tumors of adipose tissue," *Human Pathology*, vol. 37, no. 3, pp. 312–321, 2006.

[19] B. Schwaller, "Calretinin: from a 'simple' Ca²⁺ buffer to a multifunctional protein implicated in many biological processes," *Frontiers in Neuroanatomy*, vol. 8, article 3, 2014.

[20] E. De Sousa-Amorim, G. Del Peso, M. A. Bajo et al., "Can EPS development be avoided with early interventions? The potential role of tamoxifen—a single-center study," *Peritoneal Dialysis International*, vol. 34, no. 6, pp. 582–593, 2014.

[21] C. Goodlad, F. W. K. Tam, S. Ahmad, G. Bhangal, B. V. North, and E. A. Brown, "Dialysate cytokine levels do not predict encapsulating peritoneal sclerosis," *Peritoneal Dialysis International*, vol. 34, no. 6, pp. 594–604, 2014.

[22] M. N. Schilte, J. W. A. M. Celie, P. M. Ter Wee, R. H. J. Beelen, and J. van den Born, "Factors contributing to peritoneal tissue remodeling in peritoneal dialysis," *Peritoneal Dialysis International*, vol. 29, no. 6, pp. 605–617, 2009.

[23] G. Del Peso, J. A. Jiménez-Heffernan, M. A. Bajo et al., "Epithelial-to-mesenchymal transition of mesothelial cells is an early event during peritoneal dialysis and is associated with high peritoneal transport," *Kidney International*, vol. 73, no. 108, pp. S26–S33, 2008.

[24] R. Selgas, A. Bajo, J. A. Jiménez-Heffernan et al., "Epithelial-to-mesenchymal transition of the mesothelial cell—its role in the response of the peritoneum to dialysis," *Nephrology Dialysis Transplantation*, vol. 21, supplement 2, 2006.

[25] Y. Kawaguchi and A. Tranaeus, "A historical review of encapsulating peritoneal sclerosis," *Peritoneal Dialysis International*, vol. 25, supplement 4, pp. S7–S13, 2005.

[26] J. M. Bargman, "Advances in peritoneal dialysis: a review," *Seminars in Dialysis*, vol. 25, no. 5, pp. 545–549, 2012.

[27] V. S. Lebleu, G. Taduri, J. O'Connell et al., "Origin and function of myofibroblasts in kidney fibrosis," *Nature Medicine*, vol. 19, no. 8, pp. 1047–1053, 2013.

[28] B. D. Humphreys, S.-L. Lin, A. Kobayashi et al., "Fate tracing reveals the pericyte and not epithelial origin of myofibroblasts in kidney fibrosis," *American Journal of Pathology*, vol. 176, no. 1, pp. 85–97, 2010.

[29] J. S. Duffield and B. D. Humphreys, "Origin of new cells in the adult kidney: results from genetic labeling techniques," *Kidney International*, vol. 79, no. 5, pp. 494–501, 2011.

[30] A. A. Eddy, "Overview of the cellular and molecular basis of kidney fibrosis," *Kidney International Supplements*, vol. 4, pp. 2–8, 2014.

[31] L. L. Falke, S. Gholizadeh, R. Goldschmeding, R. J. Kok, and T. Q. Nguyen, "Diverse origins of the myofibroblast—implications for kidney fibrosis," *Nature Reviews Nephrology*, vol. 11, pp. 233–244, 2015.

[32] K. Sun, J. Tordjman, K. Clément, and P. E. Scherer, "Fibrosis and adipose tissue dysfunction," *Cell Metabolism*, vol. 18, no. 4, pp. 470–477, 2013.

[33] L. Yin, W. Cai, J. Sheng, and Y. Sun, "Hypoxia induced changes of SePP1 expression in rat preadipocytes and its impact on vascular fibroblasts," *International Journal of Clinical and Experimental Medicine*, vol. 7, no. 1, pp. 41–50, 2014.

[34] R. R. Driskell, B. M. Lichtenberger, E. Hoste et al., "Distinct fibroblast lineages determine dermal architecture in skin development and repair," *Nature*, vol. 504, no. 7479, pp. 277–281, 2013.

[35] Y. Cho, C. M. Hawley, and D. W. Johnson, "Clinical causes of inflammation in peritoneal dialysis patients," *International Journal of Nephrology*, vol. 2014, Article ID 909373, 9 pages, 2014.

[36] J. C. K. Leung, L. Y. Y. Chan, S. C. W. Tang, K. M. Chu, and K. N. Lai, "Leptin induces TGF-β synthesis through functional leptin receptor expressed by human peritoneal mesothelial cell," *Kidney International*, vol. 69, no. 11, pp. 2078–2086, 2006.

Management Practice, and Adherence and its Contributing Factors among Patients with Chronic Kidney Disease at Tikur Anbessa Specialized Hospital: A Hospital Based Cross-Sectional Study

Belayneh Kefale [iD],[1] **Yewondwossen Tadesse**,[2]
Minyahil Alebachew [iD],[3] and **Ephrem Engidawork**[3]

[1]*Department of Pharmacy, College of Medicine and Health Science, Ambo University, P.O. Box 19, Ambo, Ethiopia*
[2]*Department of Internal Medicine, School of Medicine, College of Health Sciences, Addis Ababa University, Addis Ababa, Ethiopia*
[3]*Department of Pharmacology and Clinical Pharmacy, School of Pharmacy, College of Health Sciences, Addis Ababa University, Addis Ababa, Ethiopia*

Correspondence should be addressed to Belayneh Kefale; belayneh.kefale@yahoo.com

Academic Editor: Franca Anglani

The objective of this study was to assess the management practice, medication adherence, and factors affecting medication adherence in CKD patients at Tikur Anbessa Specialized Hospital (TASH). *Methods.* A cross-sectional study was conducted at the nephrology clinic of TASH. A total of 256 CKD (stages 1 and 2=50, stage 3=88, stage 4=55, and stage 5=63) patients were recruited through systematic random sampling. Data were collected from medical records and interviewing patients. The rate of adherence was determined using 8-item Morisky medication adherence scale. The data were analyzed using SPSS version 20.0 statistical software. Univariate and multivariate binary logistic regression were used to investigate the potential predictors of medication nonadherence. *Results.* About 57.3% of diabetes mellitus with hypertension were treated with combination of insulin and ACEI based regimens. Other cardiovascular comorbidities were predominantly treated with Acetyl Salicylic Acid in combination with β-blocker. Only 61.3% (stages 1 and 2=70%, stage 3=73.9%, stage 4=54.5%, and stage 5=43%) of the study population were adherent to their treatment regimens. Forgetfulness (79.8%) was the major reason for medication nonadherence. Patients who had an average and high monthly income were 4.14 (AOR=4.14, 95% CI: 1.45-11.84, p=0.008) and 6.17 times (AOR=6.17, 95% CI: 1.02-37.46, p=0.048) more likely to adhere as compared to those who had very low income. Patients who were prescribed with ≥5 drugs were 0.46 times (AOR= 0.54, 95% CI: 0.27-1.10, p=0.049) less likely to adhere compared to their counterpart. Patients who were students, drivers, or teachers working in private school were about 7.46 times (AOR=7.46, 95% CI: 1.49-37.26, p=0.014) more likely to adhere compared with patients who were farmers. *Conclusion.* Insulin and ACEIs based regimens were the most frequently used regimens in the treatment of diabetes mellitus and hypertension comorbidities. Very low income, increased number of prescribed medications, and being a farmer were the predictors of medication nonadherence.

1. Introduction

Chronic kidney disease (CKD) is defined as abnormal kidney structure or function persisting greater than 3 months [1]. It is a progressive, irreversible deterioration in renal function in which the body's ability to sustain metabolic and fluid and electrolyte balance fails, resulting in uremia or azotemia [2]. Increasing prevalence of declining renal function, diabetes, hypertension, primary renal disorders, and obesity [3, 4] has contributed to CKD becoming one of the most common chronic diseases [5].

CKD has a complicated interrelationship with other diseases, most commonly diabetes and hypertension [6]. It is a global public health problem due to the rapid rise of common risk factors such that diabetes and hypertension will result in more profound burden that developing

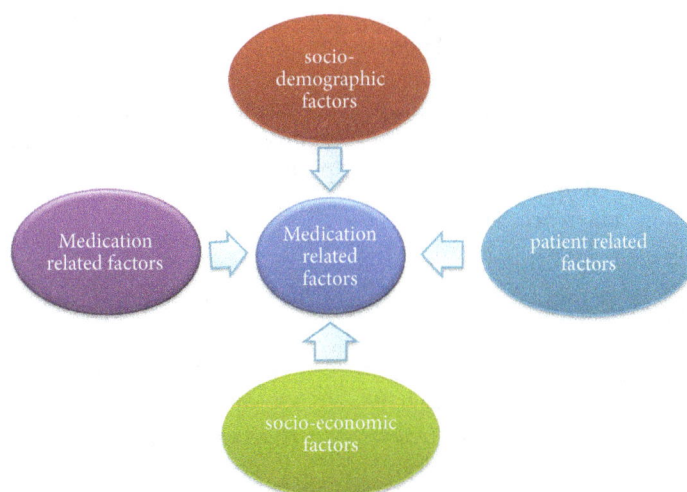

FIGURE 1: Structural framework for factors affecting medication adherence.

nations are not equipped to handle [7]. It is associated with serious consequences, including increased risk of mortality, accelerated CVD, and increased risk of acute kidney injury [1]. Mortality from CVD is estimated to be at least 8- to 10-fold higher in CKD patients as compared to non-CKD patients [7]. Recent studies have reported that CKD is an independent and major risk factor for cardiovascular disease (CVD) [1, 8]. Attention to cardiovascular risk factors remains the cornerstone of management to delay progression of CKD and prevent cardiovascular events. The direct management of CKD focuses on renin angiotensin aldosterone system, blood pressure, and glycemic control. Optimal management of common comorbid conditions and addressing cardiovascular risk factors are important to slow down its progression and reduce the risk of developing CVD for as long as possible [9].

Globally, 10% of the population is affected by CKD, and millions die each year due to high economic cost treatment [1]. It affects 10–15% (western countries) [10], 17.2% (India) [11], and 14.82% (China) [12] of the adult population, many of whom require costly treatments. With increasing of aging population, elderly people are the highest risk group for CKD. Studies in US and China population showed prevalence of CKD (US & China) as follows: stage 1 (1.8% & 3.33%), stage 2 (3.2% & 2.49%), stage 3 (7.7% & 7.07%), and stages 4 and 5 (0.35 % & 0.97%) [12, 13].

Incidence of the disease increases at an annual rate of 8% and consumes up to 2% of the total global health expenditure [14]. The treatment of CKD in developing countries is expensive, unaffordable, and unavailable [15]. Suboptimal management of comorbid conditions and nonadherence to prescribed medication schedule have been the major problems in CKD patients and their occurrence can adversely impact the course of the disease [16, 17]. Poor adherence to medication regimens is common, contributing to substantial worsening of disease, death, and increased healthcare costs. According to World Health Organization, it is estimated that only 50% of people with chronic diseases take their medications consistently as prescribed because they consider them ineffective or experience untoward side effects [18]. The

pill burden in CKD patients is high, having to take on average around 8–10 tablets/day, due to comorbidities and dominant risk factors of CKD [19]. Hence, CKD patients belong to the group of subjects with one of the highest burdens of daily pill intake depending on severity of their disease [20]. This imposes high personal and economic burden on patients and their families [5, 17, 21].

Though nonadherence to treatment is an increasing problem for patients with CKD, it has not been extensively studied in patients with CKD [22]. Previous studies have reported that 24.8% [23], 26–28% [16], 46.1% [24], 22% [25], 18.4% [26], and 23.8% [27] of CKD patients were nonadherent in California, Brazil, the Netherlands, India, Germany, and southern Ethiopia, respectively.

The incidence of CKD in Ethiopia is rising because of increased risk factors [27]. Evidence-based research that evaluates management practice and medication adherence among patients with CKD in developing countries is scanty [28]. Thus, there should be a continuing need to routinely assess management practice and factors affecting adherence among patients with CKD in clinical practice [23, 29]. This is especially important in resource-limited countries like Ethiopia, as the preponderance of economic instability, low literacy level, and restricted access to healthcare facilities, pill burden, side effects of medication, inadequate follow-up, and comorbidities might have led to the increased incidence of medication nonadherence (Figure 1) [30, 31].

Evaluating the management practice, adherence, and identification of the factors leading to nonadherence to a prescribed treatment through a continued research can assist in planning interventions to overcome the barriers. Hence, this study was carried out to

(i) give information on CKD management practice, and nonadherence and its contributing factors that may help in the healthcare system for whom it concerns;

(ii) design an interventional method that can solve problems related to management practice and nonadherence;

(iii) give recommendations on how to manage problems associated with inappropriate management and non-adherence in CKD patients;

(iv) help as a baseline for further study on management and adherence of renal patients.

Hence, the present study was carried out to assess the management practice, medication adherence, and factors affecting adherence in CKD patients at TASH.

2. Methods and Materials

2.1. Study Settings. The study was conducted in the renal ambulatory clinics of Tikur Anbessa Specialized Hospital (TASH), which is located in Addis Ababa, Ethiopia. TASH is the largest general public hospital, where tertiary care is being provided in Ethiopia, with over 800 beds. TASH serves about 500,000 patients per year in its outpatient department, 40,000 in the inpatient and same number in the emergency department, and about >600 CKD patients. The renal clinic has nephrologists, nurses, and pharmacists. It provides treatment to different types of renal disease and its complications.

2.2. Study Design and Period. A cross-sectional study was conducted in two phases. The first was a patient interview phase, while the second was a retrospective patient chart review. The two phases were done for the same patient from May 1st – September 30th 2017 to assess management practice and adherence.

2.3. Sample Size and Sampling Methods. The sample size was calculated using single population proportion formula [32] as follows:

$$n = \frac{Z_{\alpha/2^2} p\,(1-p)}{d^2} \quad (1)$$

where

n is desired sample size for population >10,000;

Z is standard normal distribution usually set as 1.96 (which corresponds to 95% confidence level);

P means that we use positive prevalence estimated, to maximize sample size; negative prevalence = 1 − 0.5 = 0.5;

d is the degree of accuracy desired (marginal error is 0.05); then the sample size is

$$n = \frac{1.96^2 0.5\,(1-0.5)}{(0.05)^2} = 384.16 = \sim 384 \quad (2)$$

The expected number of source population in the study period (N), based on the average number of patients coming to the clinic three days in a week with a total of 20 weeks, was 600 (20∗6+20∗12+20∗12). The corrected sample size, using the following correction formula, was 233.1 ~ 233:

$$\text{Corrected sample size} = \frac{n \times N}{n + N} \quad (3)$$

Then 10% contingency was added on 233:

$$233 \times 10\% = 23$$

$$233 + \text{contingency} = \text{Nf} = \underline{\textbf{256}}$$

$$(4)$$

A systematic random sampling method was used to recruit samples for the study in each day of the data collection process.

2.4. Inclusion and Exclusion Criteria

2.4.1. Inclusion Criteria

(i) All CKD ambulatory patients and on medications for more than 6 months

(ii) ≥18 years of age

2.4.2. Exclusion Criteria

(i) Patients who refused to participate in the study

(ii) Patients with cognitive impairment

2.5. Data Collection and Analysis

2.5.1. Instruments. Data were collected using structured questionnaire and data abstraction format to extract information from the patients and medical records, respectively. The questionnaire for the interview contained sociodemographic characteristics, 8-item Morisky medication adherence scale, and reasons for nonadherence to medications. In addition, data abstraction format was prepared to extract information such as management practices and clinical data.

2.5.2. Data Collectors Recruitment and Training. Three nurses were recruited as data collectors. Training was given to them regarding appropriate use of the data collection instruments focusing on uniform interpretation of questions, strict use of study criterion, explanation of study objectives and getting verbal consent from study participants, implementation of sampling technique, and confidentiality of the collected data.

2.5.3. Data Quality Control. The data collection instrument which consisted of the questionnaire and the data abstraction format was assessed by an expert physician in the field of nephrology for clarity and comprehensiveness of its contents. Pretesting was done on 5% of the study participants before the start of the actual study. All the necessary modifications and adjustments were done before implementing in the main study.

2.5.4. Data Analysis and Interpretation. Data were sorted, cleaned, coded, and entered into SPSS version-20.0 statistical software for management and analysis. Descriptive statistics including frequency, mean, and standard deviation were used to summarize patients' baseline sociodemographic data and evaluate distribution of responses. Bivariate analysis was conducted to see the existence of association between adherence and independent variables. All variables with p<0.2 in the bivariate analysis were included in the multivariate binary logistic regression, which was performed to determine the potential predictors of nonadherence. Adjusted Odds Ratio (AOR) with its p value and confidence interval (95%) was reported in each logistic regression analysis. P value < 0.05 was considered as statistically significant.

2.6. Ethical Consideration. Ethical clearance and approval of the study protocols were obtained from the Ethical Review Board of School of Pharmacy, Addis Ababa University. In addition, permission was sought from the respective heads of Department of Internal Medicine and renal clinic to conduct the study in the clinic. Prior to data collection, individuals were informed about the study and verbal consent was obtained from the study participants. Each patient was informed about the objective of the study, procedures of selection, and assurance of confidentiality and their right to refuse was maintained. No identifiers were used to minimize social desirability bias and enhance anonymity.

3. Results

3.1. Sociodemographic Characteristics. Males comprised 58% of the sex category. Majority of the participants were in the age group of less than 61 years, which accounted for 54.3%. Mean age of the study population was 52.5 (SD=16.8) years (range 18 to 90 years). Married participants accounted for 69.9% and being retired (25.4%) and government employee (23.4%) accounted for the highest percentage of occupation. Education-wise, 34.4% and 27.7% attended primary and higher education, respectively. Majority of the participants were non-health professionals (97.3%). A significant proportion of the study participants (29.7%) had low level of monthly family income. Stage 3 and 5 CKD patients accounted for the highest percentage of the study participants (Table 1).

3.2. Disease Related Characteristics. Overall, patients had been diagnosed with CKD for an average of 4.7 (SD=3.5) years, ranging from under five years (158, 61.7 %) through 5-10 years (75, 29.3%) to above ten years (23, 9%) (Figure 2).

Regarding clinical and laboratory parameters, ≥3 comorbidities (31.7%) and complications (6.9%) were commonly found in stage 5 CKD patients. Fasting blood sugar, serum creatinine, and blood urea nitrogen increased, while hemoglobin decreased across the stages (Table 2).

About two-thirds (64.4%) of the study participants did not have long term complications. Cardiovascular disease and anemia accounted for the highest percentage among patients that had at least one long term CKD complications. Almost all (96.5%) patients had at least one comorbid condition, hypertension being the major type of comorbidity (91.1%) (Table 3).

3.3. Nonpharmacological Management Approaches. The present study revealed that diet restriction, exercise, and no-smoking were the most commonly used nonpharmacological approaches. Agreed dietary plan was found to be present in most (68.8%) of the patients (Table 4).

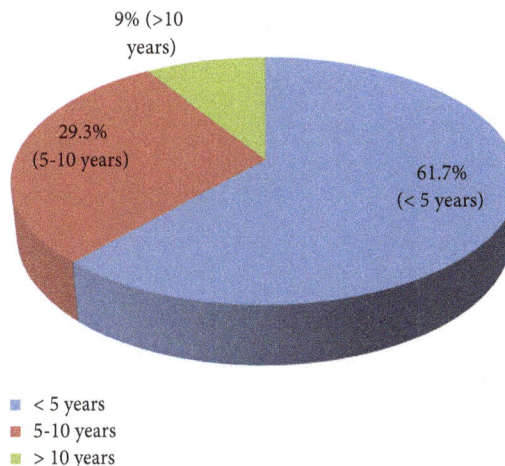

FIGURE 2: Duration of chronic kidney disease among patients attending the renal clinic of Tikur Anbessa Specialized Hospital.

3.4. Profile of Prescribed Medications. Table 5 presents medication profile of patients based on CKD stages. It revealed that enalapril (133, 52%) was the most commonly prescribed drug followed by furosemide (128, 50%) and amlodipine (124, 48.4%). Insulin and ASA (Acetyl Salicylic Acid) were found to be the major type of antidiabetic and cardiovascular medications which were prescribed for 69 (27%) and 70 (27.3%) patients, respectively. The average number of prescribed drugs per patient was 3.9 (SD=2.2) with a range of 0-12 drugs (Table 5).

3.5. Management Practice for Comorbidities and Complications. Respondents were placed on different medications for treatment of CKD comorbidities or complications. Hypertension was managed by combination of drugs, non-ACEI based (55%) being the most commonly used combination followed by ACEI based (45%). Insulin and metformin were the most commonly prescribed drugs in the management of diabetes mellitus alone. In diabetes mellitus and hypertension comorbidities, insulin and ACEI based combinations (57.3%) and ACEI based combinations (19.8%) were the two most commonly used combinations (Table 6).

3.6. Types of Regimens Used in the Management of Complications of Chronic Kidney Disease. ACEIs alone (18%) or in combination (52%) were the most commonly prescribed agent for treating CVD related complications. About three-fourth of anemia and osteodystrophy were treated with iron preparation and calcium-based formulations, respectively. Likewise, 92.3% of fluid buildup, 40% of hyperkalemia, and 88.9% of peripheral neuropathy were treated with furosemide, calcium gluconate, and amitriptylin, respectively (Figure 3).

3.7. Rate of Adherence and Reasons for Nonadherence. Assessment of patients' responses to the 8-item Morisky medication adherence scale showed that 157 (61.3%), 51 (19.9%), and 48 (18.8%) patients exhibited high, medium, and poor adherence to the prescribed regimens, respectively (Figure 4).

TABLE 1: Sociodemographic characteristic of chronic kidney disease patients attending the renal clinic of Tikur Anbessa Specialized Hospital.

Variables	Stage of CKD				
	1 & 2 (n=50)	3 (n = 88)	4 (n = 55)	5 (n = 63)	Total (n= 256)
Sex					
Male	25 (50)	60 (68.2)	31 (56.4)	33 (52.4)	149 (58)
Female	25 (50)	28 (31.2)	24 (43.6)	30 (47.6)	107 (42)
Age (years)					
≤60	38 (76)	41 (46.6)	28(50.9)	32(50.8)	139 (54.3)
>60	12(24)	47 (53.4)	27(49.1)	31(49.2)	117 (45.7)
Marital status					
Single✝	14(28)	23(26.1)	20(36.4)	20(31.7)	77 (30.1)
Married	36(72)	65(73.9)	35(63.6)	43(68.3)	179 (69.9)
Occupation					
Farmer	6(12)	8(9.1)	4(7.3)	6(9.5)	24 (9.4)
Gov't employee	18(36)	19(25.6)	11(20)	12(19.1)	60 (23.4)
Merchant/trade	7(14)	5(5.7)	5(9.1)	6(9.5)	23 (9)
Daily laborer	2(4)	6(6.8)	4(7.3)	7(11.1)	19 (7.4)
House wife	7(14)	11(12.5)	8(14.5)	11(17.5)	37 (14.5)
Retired	6(12)	27(30.7)	18(32.7)	14(22.2)	65 (25.4)
Others∗	4(8)	12(13.6)	5(9.1)	7(11.1)	28 (10.9)
Profession					
Health professional	3(6)	1(1.1)	2(3.6)	1(1.6)	7 (2.7)
Non-health professional	47(94)	87(98.9)	53(96.4)	62(98.4)	249 (97.3)
Educational status					
Cannot read and write	5(10)	11(12.5)	7(12.7)	7(11.1)	30 (11.7)
Primary	13(26)	31(35.23)	20(36.4)	24(38.1)	88 (34.4)
Secondary	10(20)	23(26.1)	19(34.5)	15(23.8)	67 (26.2)
Higher Education	22(44)	23(26.1)	9(16.4)	17(27)	71 (27.7)
Monthly family income (ETB)∗∗					
Very low (≤860)	4(8)	10(11.4)	11(20)	15(23.8)	40 (15.6)
Low (861-1500)	13(26)	21(23.9)	17(30.9)	21(33.3)	72 (28.1)
Average (1501-3000)	10(20)	33(37.5)	18(32.7)	15(23.8)	76 (29.7)
Above average (3001-5000)	17(34)	20(22.7)	6(10.9)	8(12.7)	51 (19.9)
High (≥5001)	6(12)	4(4.5)	3(5.5)	4(6.4)	17 (6.7)

✝Single, divorced, and widowed; ∗students, driver, garage (mechanic), guard, or teacher working in private school; ∗∗ based on the Ethiopian Civil Service monthly salary scale for civil servants.

Up on evaluation of the reasons for CKD medication nonadherence, it was identified that forgetfulness (79.8%) was the main reason for their nonadherence. Furthermore, side effects of the medications and high cost of medications accounted for 49.5% and 38.4% of medication nonadherence, respectively. Feeling well without treatment and physicians mode of approach were, however, the least common reasons for nonadherence (Figure 5).

3.8. Factors Associated with Medication Adherence. Based on the results of univariate binary logistic regression analysis, variables such as sex, age, occupation, educational status, family income, CKD stage, number of medications, and comorbidities were included in the multivariate logistic regression analysis. After controlling different demographic, economical, and other factors through the use of multivariate logistic regression analysis, this study showed that only family income, total number of prescribed drugs, and occupation had significant association with CKD medication adherence. Accordingly, patients who had an average and high family monthly income were about four (AOR=4.14, 95% CI: 1.45-11.84, p=0.008) and six (AOR=6.17, 95% CI: 1.02-37.46, p=0.048) times, respectively, more likely to adhere as compared to those who had very low income. During a multivariate logistic regression analysis, it was also found that patients with other groups (students, driver, and teacher working in private school) of occupation had a significant association with their adherence condition and were about seven (AOR=7.46, 95% CI: 1.49-37.26, p=0.014) times more likely to adhere compared with patients who were farmers. On the other hand, patients who were prescribed with five and above drugs were 0.46 (AOR= 0.54, 95% CI: 0.27-1.10, p=0.049) times less likely to adhere compared to those prescribed with less than five drugs (Table 7).

TABLE 2: Clinical and laboratory parameters according to the stage of chronic kidney disease patients attending the renal clinic of Tikur Anbessa Specialized Hospital.

Clinical/laboratory parameters	Stage of CKD				
	1 & 2 (n = 50)	3 (n = 88)	4 (n = 55)	5 (n = 63)	Total (n=256)
Number of comorbidities					
≤ 2	43 (91.5)	77 (90.6)	46 (83.6)	41 (68.3)	207 (83.8)
3 or more	4 (8.5)	8 (9.4)	9 (16.4)	19 (31.7)	40 (15.6)
Number of complications					
≤ 2	9 (100)	29 (100)	23 (95.8)	27 (93.1)	88 (96.7)
3 or more	0	0	1 (4.2)	2 (6.9)	3 (3.3)
FBS	125 ± 46	140 ± 46	149 ± 69	155 ± 57	141 ± 56
Scr	1.6 ± 0.8	2.0 ± 0.8	3.5 ± 1.6	7.6 ± 3.1	3.6 ± 3
BUN	41 ± 20	56 ± 34	93 ± 46	136 ± 66	80 ± 57
Hgb	16.0 ± 18.9	13.6 ± 14.1	10.5 ± 2.6	10.3 ± 2.8	12.6 ± 12.0
MAP	104.9 ± 12.2	101.7 ± 9.6	104.3 ± 14.3	103.6 ± 14.3	103.4 ± 12.4
GFR	74.7 ± 15.4	43.3 ± 8.4	23 ± 4.8	10.4 ± 2.9	37 ± 24.2

FBS = fast blood sugar, Scr = serum creatinine, BUN = blood urea nitrogen, Hgb = hemoglobin, MAP = mean arterial pressure, and GFR = glomerular filtration rate.

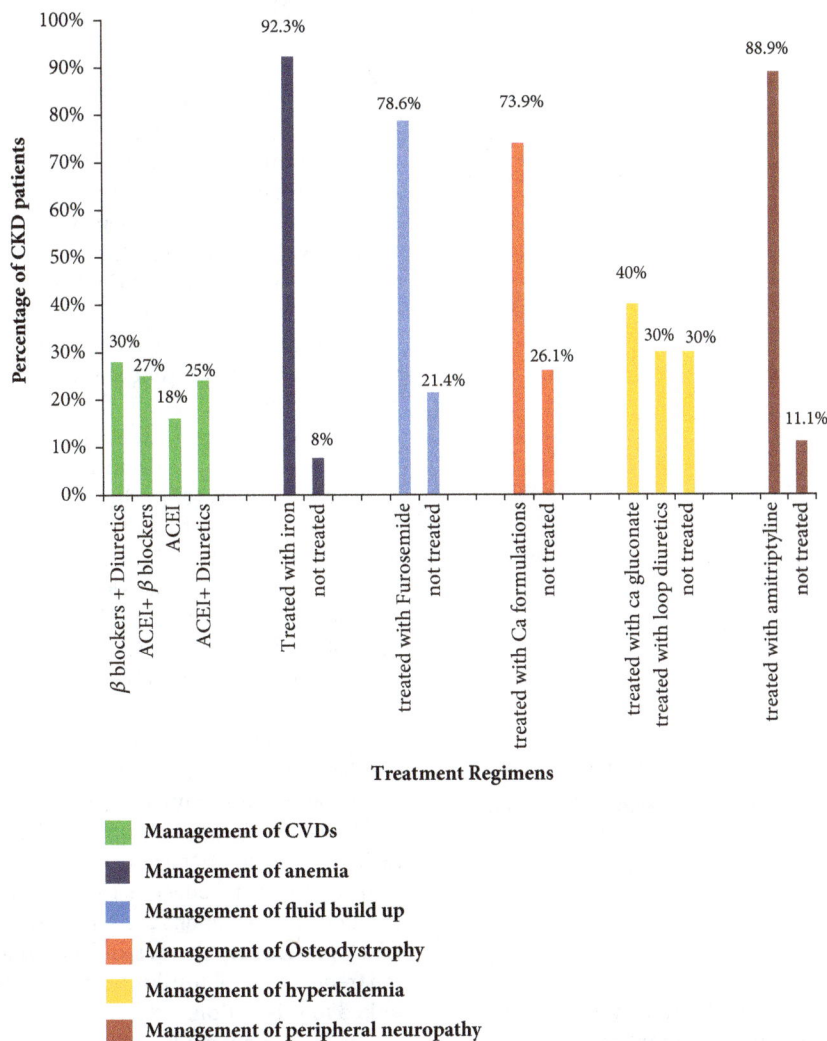

FIGURE 3: Management practice of complications among chronic kidney disease patients attending the renal clinic of Tikur Anbessa Specialized Hospital. ACEI: angiotensin converting enzyme inhibitor.

TABLE 3: Presence of comorbidities and complications among chronic kidney disease patients attending the renal clinic of Tikur Anbessa Specialized Hospital.

Variables	Frequency	Percent
Comorbidities		
Absent	9	3.5
Present	247	96.5
Specific Comorbidities (n=247)		
Hypertension	225	91.1
Diabetes mellitus	114	46.2
Ischemic Heart Disease	33	13.4
Dyslipidemia	31	12.6
Stroke	10	4.1
Others*	22	13
Complications		
Absent	165	64.4
Present	91	35.6
Specific complications (n=91)		
Cardiovascular disease	29	31.9
Anemia	28	30.8
Osteodystrophy	23	25.2
Fluid build up	14	15.3
Hyperkalemia	10	11
Peripheral neuropathy	9	9.9

*Gouty arthritis, asthma, Parkinson, nephritic syndrome, and pyelonephritis.

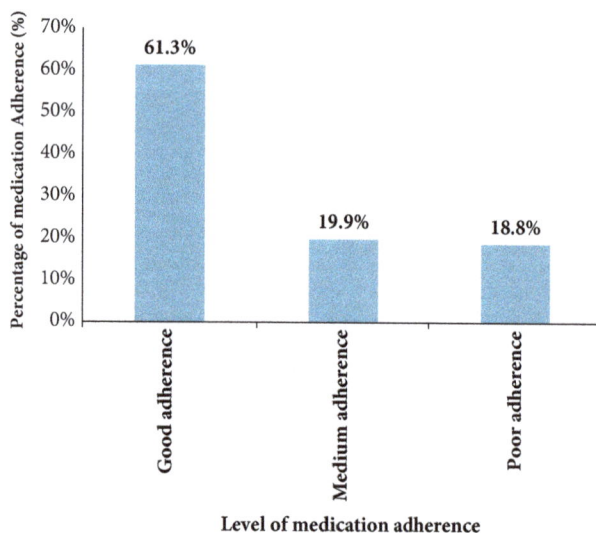

FIGURE 4: Rate of adherence to medications among chronic kidney disease patients in renal clinic of Tikur Anbessa Specialized Hospital.

4. Discussion

In the present study, different medications were used in the management of comorbidities and complications of CKD. Enalapril and hydrochlorothiazide were prescribed in 50.8% and 32.7% of CKD stage 4 and 5 patients, although little robust evidence exists on the use of ACEIs in advanced CKD. ACEIs/ARBs increase potassium and decrease GFR [33, 34] and withdrawal of ACEIs/ARBs increase eGFR and hence delay the onset of renal replacement therapy [35]. Hydrochlorothiazide was used inappropriately in advanced CKD patients, since thiazide diuretics are deemed ineffective [36]. Based on comorbidity status, non-ACEI based combinations were the most commonly used treatment regimens in the management of hypertension alone. Contrastingly, various clinical guidelines done by Stevens and Levin [37] and Bilo et al. [38] stated that ARBs or ACEIs are considered as the first-line agents in both diabetic and nondiabetic patients with CKD. ARBs or ACEIs are used not only to decrease BP but also slow down the progression of CKD by reducing proteinuria [39, 40]. The probable reason for this variation in TASH may be due to the absence of local standard treatment guideline for the management of CKD patients and lack of awareness of physicians practicing in the renal clinic. Besides, it might be due to difficulty in communication between physicians, shortage of multidisciplinary care team, and heavy workload on nephrologists. Coordinated multidisciplinary care team could improve management and outcomes of patients with CKD and essential for the appropriate management of CKD due to associated comorbidities and complex regimens. Indeed, a systematic review showed that lack of awareness of evidence-based guidelines for CKD results in large variability in the treatment of CKD comorbidities and complications [41]. A deficiency in the nephrology workforce especially nephrologists for the provision of appropriate management is a critical problem in developing countries [15]. Hence, targeted training for physicians to raise awareness about the management of CKD and development of clinical guidelines should be emphasized.

Regarding the management of diabetes mellitus and hypertension, the present study revealed that combinations of insulin and ACEI based combinations were the most commonly used treatment regimens. This is in agreement with studies done by Levin et al. [42], Tomson and Baily [43], and Bilo et al. [38], which stated that ACEIs based combinations were the first-line regimens in the management of diabetes mellitus and hypertension comorbidities in CKD patients. Previous studies demonstrated that if ACEIs were not effective in controlling BP, then CCB might be added but not used alone since CCBs may lead to albuminuria and greater hyperfiltration [42].

Insulin was the most widely used treatment agent in the management of diabetes alone comorbidity with CKD at TASH accounting for 44.4%. The finding of this study is comparable with similar studies by Albers et al. [44] and Dasari et al. [45], which indicated that renal patients with diabetes suitably managed with insulin. Though metformin is inexpensive and effective for type 2 diabetes mellitus, there is much concern about the safety of metformin in advanced CKD, particularly the risk of lactic acidosis [45, 46]. Hence, the frequent use of insulin as first-line agent may probably be linked to this notion.

In the present study, statins were predominantly used for the treatment of dyslipidemia and reduction of the relative risk of cardiovascular events in CKD patients. Likewise, studies [45] and practice guidelines [47] have shown that

Table 4: Nonpharmacological management approaches used among chronic kidney disease patients attending the renal clinic of Tikur Anbessa Specialized Hospital.

Variables	Frequency	Percent
Dietary Approach		
Presence of agreed dietary plan with physician		
Yes	175	68.4
No	81	31.6
Salt restriction (n = 175)		
Yes	167	95.4
No	8	4.6
Cut off sweet carbohydrate meals (n=114)	114	100
Exercise		
Presence of agreed exercise plan with physicians		
Yes	130	50.8
No	126	49.2
Exercising according to plan (n=130)		
Yes	120	92.3
No	10	7.7
Days per week doing moderate intense exercise		
< 3 Days	7	5.4
≥3 Days	123	94.6
Duration of moderate intense exercise per week in minutes		
< 140 Minutes	64	49.2
≥140 Minutes	66	50.8
Cigarette		
Ever smoked		
Yes	28	10.9
No	228	89.1
Smoking now (n = 28)		
Yes	4	14.3
No	24	85.7

statins are routinely used in the treatment of dyslipidemia and reduction of cardiovascular risk. This frequent usage might be due to the superior pharmacological effects of statins to reduce cardiovascular complications as compared to other lipid lowering agents. In addition, statins may have a role in preventing progression of kidney disease and reducing albuminuria [48]. Thus, statins are the standard treatment of choice in the prevention of cardiovascular risks in patients with and without CKD [49]. Furthermore, ASA and β-blocker combinations were predominantly used treatment regimens in ischemic heart disease. This finding is in agreement with a study [45] and practice guideline [47] that reported β-blockers should be initiated for the relief of symptoms and ASA in the primary prevention of cardiovascular events.

Regarding the management of CKD complications, ACEI based combinations were the most commonly used treatment regimens in cardiovascular complications. This finding is in line with a systematic review that reported ACEIs or ARBs appeared to be the most commonly used regimens to treat heart failure in renal patients [50]. The present study also revealed that iron preparations were predominantly used in the treatment of anemia in CKD patients. Contrastingly,

various studies reported that the use of erythropoietin stimulating agents with iron preparations was routinely used in the treatment of anemia in renal patients [51]. Hence, the lesser usage of erythropoietin stimulating agent could probably be due to the financial constraints and limited availability of this agent at TASH. Although Malluche et al. [52] and Miller [53] demonstrated that the use of calcium-based phosphate binders has been associated with the development of low bone turnover, bone loss, and worsening of vascular calcifications, calcium containing phosphate binders were the most commonly used agents in the management of osteodystrophy at TASH. This could probably be due to the inaccessibility of new nonaluminum, noncalcium (sevelamer hydrochloride and lanthanum carbonate) phosphate binders in this setting, which have lower risk of vascular calcification [54].

Adherence to CKD medications was observed in 61.3% of the study participants. This finding is similar with previous studies conducted in Netherland [24], India [55], and Spain [56] and different from other studies conducted in Saudi Arabia [20], India [25], German [26], southern Ethiopia [27], Italy [57], United States [58], and Australia [59]. This variation could be attributed to differences in the definition of

TABLE 5: Profile of prescribed medications for chronic kidney disease patients attending the renal clinic of Tikur Anbessa Specialized Hospital.

Variables	Stage of CKD				
	1 & 2 (n = 50)	3 (n = 88)	4 (n = 55)	5 (n = 63)	Total (n=256)
ACEI					
Enalapril	41 (82)	47 (53.4)	32(58.2)	28(44.4)	148 (57.8)
CCB					
Amlodipine	21(42)	41(46.6)	25(45.5)	37(58.7)	124 (48.4)
Nifedipine	8(16)	13(14.8)	17(30.9)	13(20.6)	51 (19.9)
Diuretics					
Furosemide	14(28)	38(43.2)	30(54.5)	46(73)	128 (50)
Hydrochlorothiazide	10(20)	23(26.1)	14(24.5)	22(34.9)	69 (27)
Spironolactone	4(8)	12(13.6)	4(7.3)	10(15.9)	30 (11.7)
β-blocker					
Atenolol	6(12)	13(14.8)	10(18.2)	20(31.7)	49 (19.1)
Metoprolol	4(8)	5(5.7)	3(5.5)	1(1.6)	13 (5.1)
Carvedilol	0(0)	4(4.5)	1(1.8)	2(3.2)	7 (2.74)
ARB					
Losartan	1(2)	2(2.3)	2(3.6)	0(0)	5(2)
Antidiabetic Medications					
Insulin	14(28)	14(15.9)	20(36.4)	21(33.3)	69 (27)
Metformin	9(18)	8(9.1)	4(7.3)	5(7.9)	26 (10.2)
Glibenclamide	1(2)	5(5.7)	2(3.6)	0(0)	8 (3.1)
Other medications					
ASA	8(16)	23(26.1)	20(36.4)	19(30.2)	70 (27.3)
Statins	9(18)	18(20.5)	8(14.5)	15(23.8)	50 (19.5)
Calcium supplement	1(2)	3(3.4)	6(10.9)	15(23.8)	25 (9.8)
Iron	0(0)	4(4.5)	9(16.4)	15(23.8)	28 (10.9)
Antibiotics	1(2)	5(5.7)	5(9.1)	5(7.9)	16 (6.3)
Others*	15(30)	23(26.1)	13(23.6)	17(27)	68 (26.6)
Number of medications	3.2 ± 1.6	3.5 ± 1.7	4.3 ± 2	4.9 ± 2.9	3.9 ± 2.2

* Phenobarbitone, warfarin, prednisolone, antiretroviral therapy, carbamazepine, and chlorpromazine; ACEI = angiotensin converting enzyme inhibitor; CCB = calcium channel blocker; ARB = angiotensin receptor blocker; ASA = Acetyl Salicylic Acid.

nonadherence between studies. In addition, methodologies may differ between studies, contributing to variation in the data. For example, direct monitoring methods include drug concentration assays, use of pill markers, and direct observation of pill taking; indirect methods include patient self-reports, structured interview, compliance ratings by nurses, prescription refills, and pill counts [60].

Prevalence of adherence in the present study was below the recommended level in the literature to attain optimum outcomes [61]. In the light of poor management of CKD comorbidities and alleged failure of therapeutic regimen, healthcare providers are urged to measure CKD patients' treatment adherence. Efforts are needed to increase the medication adherence of these patients so that they could realize the full benefits of prescribed therapies. When accurate and clear information on the importance of medication adherence is provided, patients are encouraged towards self-care and adherence to drug therapy. Healthcare professionals should be more vigilant towards identifying these concerns to address adherence issues. Nonadherence to drug therapy is detrimental and costly in renal patients [62], as these patients have increased burden of coexisting illness and are

prescribed with multiple complex regimens to treat various comorbidities [63–65]. Different studies demonstrated that medication nonadherence has been associated with presence of comorbidity [66], increased risk of hospitalization, medication and hospitalization-related costs, and death [67].

In this study, multivariate logistic regression analysis showed that total number of prescribed drugs, occupation, and family income were found to be significantly associated with CKD medication adherence. As the number of prescribed drugs increased from <5 medications to ≥5 medications, the odds of being adherent were about 0.46 times less and this implies that patients with ≥5 medications were found to be less likely to adhere to their medications. Numerous literatures support this finding, as pill burden negatively affects patient adherence to treatment. A study done in USA and Italy demonstrated that patients with high pill burden were more likely to be nonadherent [57, 58]. Similar studies also reported that the number of prescribed medications had a significant inverse association with CKD medication adherence [25, 62, 68]. Moreover, occupation had significant association with CKD medication adherence. Patients who were students, drivers, and teachers working

TABLE 6: Types of regimens used in the management of chronic kidney disease comorbidities patients attending the renal clinic of Tikur Anbessa Specialized Hospital.

Comorbidities	Frequency	Percent (%)
Hypertension (n=129)		
ACEI based regimens	58	45
Non-ACEI based regimens	71	55
DM + HTN (n=96)		
Insulin + ACEI based regimens	55	57.3
ACEI based regimens	19	19.8
Metformin + ACEI based regimens	13	13.5
Insulin + Non-ACEI based regimens	5	5.2
Metformin + Non-ACEI based regimens	4	4.2
DM (n=18)		
Insulin	8	44.4
Metformin	6	33.3
Glibenclamide	3	16.7
Insulin + Glibenclamide	1	5.6
IHD (n=33)		
ASA + β-Blocker	33	100
Dyslipidemia (n=31)		
Statins	31	100
Stroke (n=10)		
ASA	10	100
Others* (n=12)		
ASA + others[†]	7	58.3
Statins + others[†]	5	41.7

DM = diabetes mellitus; HTN = hypertension; IHD = ischemic heart disease; ACEI = angiotensin converting enzyme inhibitor or an angiotensin receptor blocker; ASA = Acetyl Salicylic Acid; *asthma, HIV/AIDS, gout, and nephritic syndrome; [†]phenobarbitone, antibiotics, prednisolone, antiretroviral therapy, and carbamazepine.

in private school were more likely to engage in adherence compared to those who were farmers. This could probably be due to the fact that farmers might be less aware of their disease and the importance of medication adherence when compared with students, driver, and teacher working in private school and thus more likely to be more nonadherent.

On the other hand, monthly family income was significantly associated with medication adherence as the family income increased, and patients were found to be more likely to adhere to their medications. This finding is in line with previous study, which reported that socioeconomic status had a significant association with medication adherence [69]. A qualitative study done in Australia to explore factors associated with medication adherence in ESRD patients indicated that financial constraints had contributed to medication nonadherence [59]. Income status has been implicated in nonadherence in several studies of renal patients. In addition, low socioeconomic status has been significantly associated for medication nonadherence among CKD patients [16]. Most CKD patients in developing countries have no access to health insurance and this makes care for CKD unaffordable and consequently affects their adherence rates to the prescribed treatment regimen. According to World Kidney Day [70], the majority of patients commencing dialysis in low income countries die or stop treatment within three months

of initiating dialysis due to cost constraints. Limited economic resources of patients in developing countries result in reduced frequency of dialysis and eventually discontinuation of therapy [71].

In this study, patients with poor adherence reported several reasons for not adhering to their medications. The most common reasons were found to be forgetfulness, experiencing side effects, cost, and complex regimen. Most of the patients missed their CKD medications due to forgetfulness which is similar with other studies [25, 59]. A qualitative study by Lindberg and Lindberg [72] revealed that forgetfulness and complex regimen due to polypharmacy were identified as the main obstacle for medication adherence.

Adherence to therapies is a primary determinant of treatment success. Failure to adherence is a serious problem, which affects not only the patient but also the healthcare system. Medication nonadherence in patients leads to substantial worsening of disease, death, and increased healthcare costs. Varieties of factors are likely to affect adherence. This could be classified as patient centered, therapy related, social and economic, disease, and healthcare system factors, with interactions among them. Identifying specific barriers for each patient and adopting suitable techniques to overcome them will be necessary to improve medication adherence. Healthcare professionals such as physicians, pharmacists, and

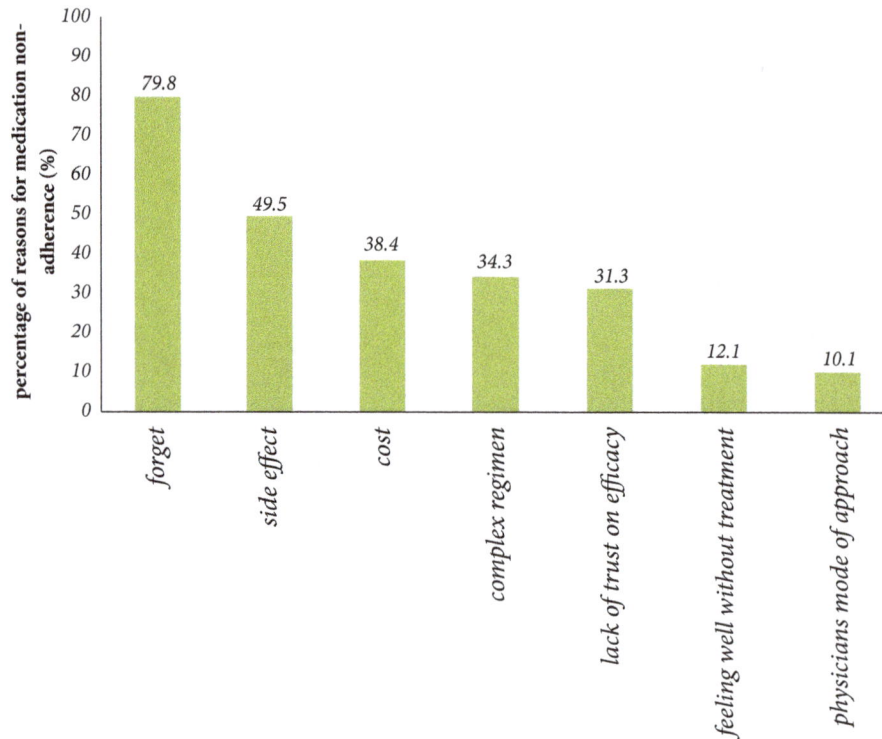

FIGURE 5: Reasons for medication nonadherence among chronic kidney disease patients attending the renal clinic of Tikur Anbessa Specialized Hospital.

nurses have significant role in their daily practice to improve patient medication adherence [73]. Even though a number of sociodemographic (age, sex, and educational status) and clinical factors (number of comorbidities and complications, severity of the disease, and laboratory parameters) were found to be significantly associated with nonadherence in various studies [73], in this study they were not statistically significant associated. The probable reason for this variation could be due to the sample size and methodological difference. Hence, prospective studies with multiple methods of adherence assessment may be required to identify different factors which affect medication adherence.

5. Conclusions

In summary, the present study showed that 55% of hypertensive patients were treated with non-ACEI based regimens, which are inappropriate. Insulin and ACEIs based regimens were the most frequently used regimen in the management of diabetes mellitus and hypertension with diabetes comorbidities. Calcium containing phosphate binders were used inappropriately in the management of osteodystrophy CKD complications. In addition, medication adherence in CKD patients at TASH was found to be suboptimal (61.3%). Forgetfulness was the most important reason preventing optimal adherence to prescribed medications. Socioeconomic status and pill burden had an important role in determining adherence rate to medications. Very low family income, increased number of prescribed drugs, and being a farmer were significant predictor of medication nonadherence.

Abbreviations

ACEI: Angiotensin converting enzyme inhibitor
AOR: Adjusted odds ratio
ARB: Angiotensin receptor blocker
CCB: Calcium channel blocker
CI: Confidence interval
CKD: Chronic kidney disease
COR: Crude odds ratio
CVD: Cardiovascular disease
GFR: Glomerular filtration rate
MMAS-8: 8-item Morisky medication adherence scale
RAAS: Renin Angiotensin Aldosterone System
SPSS: Statistical Package for Social Sciences
TASH: Tikur Anbessa Specialized Hospital
USA: United States of America.

Ethical Approval

Approval and permission were sought from Ethical Review Board of School of Pharmacy and Department of Internal Medicine of Addis Ababa University.

TABLE 7: Univariate and multivariate binary logistic regression analysis of predictors of medication nonadherence.

Variables	Adherence		COR, 95 % CI	AOR, 95% CI
	Low to moderate adherence	High adherence		
Sex				
Female	51	56	1.00	1.00
Male	48	101	1.92(1.15, 3.20)*	1.56(0.76, 3.2)
Age in years				
≤60	43	96	1.00	1.00
> 60	56	61	0.49(0.29, 0.81) *	0.64 (0.29, 1.42)
Occupation				
Farmer	13	11	1.00	1.00
Gov't Employee	20	40	2.36(0.90, 6.21)	1.14(0.30, 4.34)
Merchant/Trade	6	17	3.35(0.98, 11.45)	2.99(0.67, 13.36)
Daily Laborer	7	12	2.03(0.59, 6.93)	2.03(0.43, 9.52)
House wife	21	16	0.90(0.32, 2.53)	1.41(0.34, 5.88)
Retired	27	38	1.66(0.65, 4.27)	2.52(0.63, 10.13)
Others*	5	23	5.44(1.55, 19.11)*	7.46(1.49, 37.26)*
Educational status				
Cannot read & write	16	14	1.00	1.00
Primary	43	45	1.2(0.52, 2.74)	0.49(0.14, 1.68)
Secondary	24	43	2.05 (0.85, 4.91)	0.69(0.18, 2.69)
Higher Education	16	55	3.93(1.59, 9.74)*	1.14 (0.24, 5.38)
Family income category				
Very Low	25	15	1.00	1.00
Low	39	33	1.41(0.64, 3.1)	1.37(0.49, 3.85)
Average	19	57	5.0(2.19, 11.4)**	4.14(1.45, 11.84)*
Above Average	13	38	4.88(1.99, 11.96)**	3.39(0.91, 12.66)
High	3	14	7.78(1.92, 31.59)*	6.17(1.02, 37.46)*
CKD stage				
1 & 2	15	35	1.00	1.00
3	23	65	1.21(0.56, 2.61)	1.42(0.58, 3.47)
4	25	30	0.51 (0.23, 1.15)	0.68(0.27, 1.71)
5	36	27	0.32 (0.15, 0.70)*	0.45(0.18, 1.13)
Number of medications				
<5	57	120	1.00	1.00
≥ 5	42	37	0.42 (0.24, 0.72)*	0.54 (0.27, 1.10)*
Number of comorbidities				
0-2	75	141	1.00	1.00
≥ 3	24	16	0.36(0.18, 0.71)*	0.85(0.35, 2.11)

COR = crude odd ratio; AOR = adjusted odd ratio; *statistically significant at P≤0.05 and **statistically significant at p ≤ 0.001; *students, driver, garage (mechanic), guard, or teacher working in private school.

Authors' Contributions

Belayneh Kefale conducted the actual study and the statistical analysis. Belayneh Kefale, Yewondwossen Tadesse, Minyahil Alebachew, Ephrem Engidawork were involved in developing the idea, designing of the study, and the write up of the manuscript. All authors approved the submitted version of the manuscript.

Acknowledgments

The authors would like to acknowledge Addis Ababa University for financial support towards this project.

References

[1] N. R. Hill, S. T. Fatoba, J. L. Oke et al., "Global prevalence of chronic kidney disease - A systematic review and meta-analysis," *PLoS ONE*, vol. 11, no. 7, Article ID e0158765, 2016.

[2] "KDIGO clinical practice guideline for the diagnosis, evaluation, prevention, and treatment of Chronic Kidney

Disease-Mineral and Bone Disorder (CKD-MBD)," *Kidney International Supplements*, vol. 13, pp. S1–130, 2009.

[3] K. Eckardt, J. Coresh, O. Devuyst et al., "Evolving importance of kidney disease: from subspecialty to global health burden," *The Lancet*, vol. 382, no. 9887, pp. 158–169, 2013.

[4] D. W. Johnson, E. Atai, M. Chan et al., "KHA-CARI guideline: early chronic kidney disease: detection, prevention and management," *Nephrology*, vol. 18, no. 5, pp. 340–350, 2013.

[5] L. Osterberg and T. Blaschke, "Adherence to medication," *The New England Journal of Medicine*, vol. 353, no. 5, pp. 487–497, 2005.

[6] C. S. Snively and C. Gutierrez, "Chronic kidney disease: Prevention and treatment of common complications," *American Family Physician*, vol. 70, no. 10, pp. 1921–1930, 2004.

[7] V. Jha, A. Y. Wang, and H. Wang, "The impact of CKD identification in large countries: the burden of illness," *Nephrology Dialysis Transplantation* , vol. 27, supplement 3, pp. iii32–iii38, 2012.

[8] J. F. E. Mann, H. C. Gerstein, J. Poque, J. Bosch, and S. Yusuf, "Renal insufficiency as a predictor of cardiovascular outcomes and the impact of ramipril: the HOPE randomized trial," *Annals of Internal Medicine*, vol. 134, no. 8, pp. 629–636, 2001.

[9] M. J. Sarnak, A. S. Levey, A. C. Schoolwerth et al., "Kidney disease as a risk factor for development of cardiovascular disease: a statement from the American Heart Association Councils on Kidney in Cardiovascular Disease, High Blood Pressure Research, Clinical Cardiology, and Epidemiology and Prevention," *Circulation*, vol. 108, no. 17, pp. 2154–2169, 2003.

[10] A. S. Levey, L. A. Stevens, C. H. Schmid et al., "A new equation to estimate glomerular filtration rate," *Annals of Internal Medicine*, vol. 150, no. 9, pp. 604–612, 2009.

[11] A. K. Singh, Y. M. K. Farag, B. V. Mittal et al., "Epidemiology and risk factors of chronic kidney disease in India—results from the SEEK (Screening and Early Evaluation of Kidney Disease) study," *BMC Nephrology*, vol. 14, no. 1, article 114, 2013.

[12] B.-C. Liu, X.-C. Wu, Y.-L. Wang et al., "Investigation of the prevalence of CKD in 13,383 Chinese hospitalized adult patients," *Clinica Chimica Acta*, vol. 387, no. 1-2, pp. 128–132, 2008.

[13] C.-Y. Hsu, E. Vittinghoff, F. Li, and M. G. Shlipak, "The incidence of end-stage renal disease is increasing faster than the prevalence of chronic renal insufficiency," *Annals of Internal Medicine*, vol. 141, no. 2, pp. 95–101, 2004.

[14] J. M. López-Novoa, C. Martínez-Salgado, A. B. Rodríguez-Peña, and F. J. Hernández, "Common pathophysiological mechanisms of chronic kidney disease: therapeutic perspectives," *Pharmacology & Therapeutics*, vol. 128, no. 1, pp. 61–81, 2010.

[15] I. G. Okpechi, A. K. Bello, O. I. Ameh, and C. R. Swanepoel, "Integration of Care in Management of CKD in Resource-Limited Settings," *Seminars in Nephrology*, vol. 37, no. 3, pp. 260–272, 2017.

[16] E. J. C. Magacho, L. C. Ribeiro, A. Chaoubah, and M. G. Bastos, "Adherence to drug therapy in kidney disease," *Brazilian Journal of Medical and Biological Research*, vol. 44, no. 3, pp. 258–262, 2011.

[17] M. C. Cruz, C. Andrade, M. Urrutia, S. Draibe, L. A. Nogueira-Martins, and R. D. C. C. Sesso, "Quality of life in patients with chronic kidney disease," *Clinics*, vol. 66, no. 6, pp. 991–995, 2011.

[18] P. V. Burkhart and E. Sabaté, "Adherence to long-term therapies: evidence for action," *Journal of Nursing Scholarship*, vol. 35, no. 3, p. 207, 2003.

[19] H. J. Manley, C. G. Garvin, D. K. Drayer et al., "Medication prescribing patterns in ambulatory haemodialysis patients: Comparisons of USRDS to a large not-for-profit dialysis provider," *Nephrology Dialysis Transplantation* , vol. 19, no. 7, pp. 1842–1848, 2004.

[20] M. Burnier, M. Pruijm, G. Wuerzner, and V. Santschi, "Drug adherence in chronic kidney diseases and dialysis," *Nephrology Dialysis Transplantation* , vol. 30, no. 1, pp. 39–44, 2015.

[21] H. P. McDonald, A. X. Garg, and R. B. Haynes, "Interventions to enhance patient adherence to medication prescriptions: Scientific review," *Journal of the American Medical Association*, vol. 288, no. 22, pp. 2868–2879, 2002.

[22] A. Victoria, "Family Support, Social and Demographic Correlations of Non-Adherence among Haemodialysis Patients," *American Journal of Nursing Science*, vol. 4, no. 2, p. 60, 2015.

[23] M. R. DiMatteo, "Variations in patients' adherence to medical recommendations: A quantitative review of 50 years of research," *Medical Care*, vol. 42, no. 3, pp. 200–209, 2004.

[24] A. C. Drenth-Van Maanen, R. J. Van Marum, P. A. F. Jansen, J. E. F. Zwart, W. W. Van Solinge, and T. C. G. Egberts, "Adherence with dosing guideline in patients with impaired renal function at hospital discharge," *PLoS ONE*, vol. 10, no. 6, Article ID e0128237, 2015.

[25] R. Ahlawat and P. Tiwari, "Prevalence and Predictors of Medication Non-Adherence in Patients of Chronic Kidney Disease: Evidence from A Cross Sectional Study," *Journal of Pharmaceutical Care & Health Systems*, vol. 03, no. 01, 2016.

[26] C. Kugler, I. Maeding, and C. L. Russell, "Non-adherence in patients on chronic hemodialysis: An international comparison study," *Journal of Nephrology*, vol. 24, no. 3, pp. 366–375, 2011.

[27] T. Fiseha, "Prevalence of Chronic Kidney Disease and Associated Risk Factors among Diabetic Patients in Southern Ethiopia," *American Journal of Health Research*, vol. 2, no. 4, p. 216, 2014.

[28] K. T. Awuah, S. H. Finkelstein, and F. O. Finkelstein, "Quality of life of chronic kidney disease patients in developing countries," *Kidney International Supplements*, vol. 3, no. 2, pp. 227–229, 2013.

[29] P. MahboobLessan and R. Zohreh, "Contributing factors in health-related quality of life assessment of ESRD patients: a single center study," *International Urology and Nephrology*, vol. 1, no. 2, pp. 129–136, 2009.

[30] P. Tuso, "SERVE Ethiopia," *The Permanente Journal*, vol. 13, no. 3, 2009.

[31] C. A. Johnson, A. S. Levey, J. Coresh, A. Levin, J. Lau, and G. Eknoyan, "Clinical practice guidelines for chronic kidney disease in adults: Part I. Definition, disease stages, evaluation, treatment, and risk factors," *American Family Physician*, vol. 70, no. 5, pp. 869–876, 2004.

[32] M. A. Pourhoseingholi, M. Vahedi, and M. Rahimzadeh, "Sample size calculation in medical studies," *Gastroenterology and Hepatology from Bed to Bench*, vol. 6, no. 1, pp. 14–17, 2013.

[33] F. H. Fan, X. Zhang, H. Z. Guo et al., "Efficacy and safety of benazepril for advanced chronic renal insufficiency," *The New England Journal of Medicine*, vol. 354, no. 2, pp. 131–140, 2006.

[34] M. Z. Molnar, K. Kalantar-Zadeh, E. H. Lott et al., "Angiotensin-converting enzyme inhibitor, angiotensin receptor blocker use, and mortality in patients with chronic kidney disease," *Journal of the American College of Cardiology*, vol. 63, no. 7, pp. 650–658, 2014.

[35] A. K. Ahmed, N. S. Kamath, M. El Kossi, and A. M. El Nahas, "The impact of stopping inhibitors of the renin-angiotensin system in patients with advanced chronic kidney disease," *Nephrology Dialysis Transplantation* , vol. 25, no. 12, pp. 3977–3982, 2010.

[36] R. Agarwal and A. D. Sinha, "Thiazide diuretics in advanced chronic kidney disease," *Journal of the American Society of Hypertension*, vol. 6, no. 5, pp. 299–308, 2012.

[37] P. E. Stevens and A. Levin, "Evaluation and management of chronic kidney disease: synopsis of the kidney disease: improving global outcomes 2012 clinical practice guideline," *Annals of Internal Medicine*, vol. 158, no. 11, pp. 825–830, 2013.

[38] H. Bilo, L. Coentrão, C. Couchoud, A. Covic, J. De Sutter, and C. Drechsler, "Clinical Practice Guideline on management of patients with diabetes and chronic kidney disease stage 3b or higher (eGFR< 45 mL/min)," *Nephrology Dialysis Transplantation*, vol. 30, supplement 2, pp. iii–ii142, 2015.

[39] R. D. Toto, "Treatment of hypertension in chronic kidney disease," *Seminars in Nephrology*, vol. 25, no. 6, pp. 435–439, 2005.

[40] L. A. Inker, B. C. Astor, C. H. Fox et al., "KDOQI US commentary on the 2012 KDIGO clinical practice guideline for the evaluation and management of CKD," *American Journal of Kidney Diseases*, vol. 63, no. 5, pp. 713–735, 2014.

[41] C. M. Junaid Nazar, T. B. Kindratt, S. M. Ahmad, M. Ahmed, and J. Anderson, "Barriers to the successful practice of chronic kidney diseases at the primary health care level; A systematic review," *Journal of Renal Injury Prevention*, vol. 3, no. 3, pp. 61–67, 2014.

[42] A. Levin, B. Hemmelgarn, B. Culleton et al., "Guidelines for the management of chronic kidney disease," *Canadian Medical Association Journal*, vol. 179, no. 11, pp. 1154–1162, 2008.

[43] C. Tomson and P. Bailey, "Management of chronic kidney disease," *Medicine*, vol. 39, no. 7, pp. 407–413, 2011.

[44] J. W. Albers, W. H. Herman, R. Pop-Busui et al., "Effect of prior intensive insulin treatment during the Diabetes Control and Complications Trial (DCCT) on peripheral neuropathy in type 1 diabetes during the Epidemiology of Diabetes Interventions and Complications (EDIC) study," *Diabetes Care*, vol. 33, no. 5, pp. 1090–1096, 2010.

[45] P. Dasari, K. Venkateshwarlu, and R. Venisetty, "Management of comorbidities in chronic kidney disease: a prospective observational study," *International Journal of Pharmacy and Pharmaceutical Sciences*, vol. 6, no. 2, pp. 363–367, 2014.

[46] C. E. Koro, B. H. Lee, and S. J. Bowlin, "Antidiabetic medication use and prevalence of chronic kidney disease among patients with type 2 diabetes mellitus in the United States," *Clinical Therapeutics*, vol. 31, no. 11, pp. 2608–2617, 2009.

[47] G. Eknoyan, N. Lameire, K. Eckardt, B. Kasiske, D. Wheeler, and A. Levin, "KDIGO 2012 clinical practice guideline for the evaluation and management of chronic kidney disease," *Kidney International*, vol. 3, pp. 5–14, 2013.

[48] S. D. S. Fraser, P. J. Roderick, C. R. May et al., "The burden of Comorbidity in people with chronic kidney disease stage 3: A cohort study," *BMC Nephrology*, vol. 16, no. 1, Article ID 0189-z, 2015.

[49] J. A. Rivera, A. M. O'Hare, and G. Michael Harper, "Update on the management of chronic kidney disease," *American Family Physician*, vol. 86, no. 8, pp. 749–754, 2012.

[50] J. A. Vassalotti, R. Centor, B. J. Turner, R. C. Greer, M. Choi, and T. D. Sequist, "Practical Approach to Detection and Management of Chronic Kidney Disease for the Primary Care Clinician," *American Journal of Medicine*, vol. 129, no. 2, pp. 153–162.e7, 2016.

[51] S. Padhi, J. Glen, B. A. J. Pordes, and M. E. Thomas, "Management of anaemia in chronic kidney disease: Summary of updated NICE guidance," *BMJ*, vol. 350, 2015.

[52] H. H. Malluche, H. Mawad, and M.-C. Monier-Faugere, "Effects of treatment of renal osteodystrophy on bone histology.," *Clinical journal of the American Society of Nephrology : CJASN*, vol. 3, pp. S157–163, 2008.

[53] P. D. Miller, "Chronic kidney disease and osteoporosis: evaluation and management," *BoneKEy Reports*, vol. 3, 2014.

[54] S. Mathew, R. J. Lund, F. Strebeck, K. S. Tustison, T. Geurs, and K. A. Hruska, "Reversal of the adynamic bone disorder and decreased vascular calcification in chronic kidney disease by sevelamer carbonate therapy," *Journal of the American Society of Nephrology*, vol. 18, no. 1, pp. 122–130, 2007.

[55] S. Sontakke, R. Budania, C. Bajait, K. Jaiswal, and S. Pimpalkhute, "Evaluation of adherence to therapy in patients of chronic kidney disease," *Indian Journal of Pharmacology*, vol. 47, no. 6, pp. 668–671, 2015.

[56] M. D. Arenas, T. Malek, M. T. Gil, A. Moledous, F. Alvarez-Ude, and A. Reig-Ferrer, "Challenge of phosphorus control in hemodialysis patients: A problem of adherence?" *Journal of Nephrology*, vol. 23, no. 5, pp. 525–534, 2010.

[57] L. Neri, A. Martini, V. E. Andreucci, M. Gallieni, L. A. Rocca Rey, and D. Brancaccio, "Regimen complexity and prescription adherence in dialysis patients," *American Journal of Nephrology*, vol. 34, no. 1, pp. 71–76, 2011.

[58] Y.-W. Chiu, I. Teitelbaum, M. Misra, E. M. de Leon, T. Adzize, and R. Mehrotra, "Pill burden, adherence, hyperphosphatemia, and quality of life in maintenance dialysis patients," *Clinical Journal of the American Society of Nephrology*, vol. 4, no. 6, pp. 1089–1096, 2009.

[59] S. Ghimire, R. L. Castelino, M. D. Jose, and S. T. R. Zaidi, "Medication adherence perspectives in haemodialysis patients: a qualitative study," *BMC Nephrology*, vol. 18, no. 1, 2017.

[60] H. Schmid, B. Hartmann, and H. Schiffl, "Adherence to prescribed oral medication in adult patients undergoing chronic hemodialysis: A critical review of the literature," *European Journal of Medical Research*, vol. 14, no. 5, pp. 185–190, 2009.

[61] L. Roy, B. White-Guay, M. Dorais, A. Dragomir, M. Lessard, and S. Perreault, "Adherence to antihypertensive agents improves risk reduction of end-stage renal disease," *Kidney International*, vol. 84, no. 3, pp. 570–577, 2013.

[62] S. Ghimire, R. L. Castelino, N. M. Lioufas, G. M. Peterson, and S. T. R. Zaidi, "Nonadherence to medication therapy in haemodialysis patients: A systematic review," *PLoS ONE*, vol. 10, no. 12, Article ID 0144119, 2015.

[63] N. A. Mason, "Polypharmacy and medication-related complications in the chronic kidney disease patient," *Current Opinion in Nephrology and Hypertension*, vol. 20, no. 5, pp. 492–497, 2011.

[64] K. L. Hsu, J. C. Fink, J. S. Ginsberg et al., "Self-reported medication adherence and adverse patient safety events in CKD," *American Journal of Kidney Diseases*, vol. 66, no. 4, pp. 621–629, 2015.

[65] D. E. Rifkin, M. B. Laws, M. Rao, V. S. Balakrishnan, M. J. Sarnak, and I. B. Wilson, "Medication adherence behavior and priorities among older adults with CKD: A semistructured interview study," *American Journal of Kidney Diseases*, vol. 56, no. 3, pp. 439–446, 2010.

[66] P. Muntner, S. E. Judd, M. Krousel-Wood, W. M. McClellan, and M. M. Safford, "Low medication adherence and hypertension control among adults with CKD: Data from the REGARDS (Reasons for Geographic and Racial Differences in Stroke) Study," *American Journal of Kidney Diseases*, vol. 56, no. 3, pp. 447–457, 2010.

[67] C. B. Raymond, L. D. Wazny, and A. R. Sood, "Medication adherence in patients with chronic kidney disease.," *CANNT journal = Journal ACITN*, vol. 21, no. 2, pp. 47–52, 2011.

[68] A. Covic and A. Rastogi, "Hyperphosphatemia in patients with ESRD: assessing the current evidence linking outcomes with treatment adherence," *BMC Nephrology*, vol. 14, article 153, 2013.

[69] A. Salini and C. Sajeeth, "Prevalence, risk factors, adherence and non adherence in patient with chronic kidney disease: A prospective study," *IJRPC*, vol. 3, pp. 2231–2781, 2013.

[70] G. G. Garcia, P. N. Harden, and J. R. Chapman, "The global role of kidney transplantation," *Kidney International*, vol. 81, no. 5, pp. 425–427, 2012.

[71] A. Schieppati, N. Perico, and G. Remuzzi, "Preventing end-stage renal disease: The potential impact of screening and intervention in developing countries," *Kidney International*, vol. 63, no. 5, pp. 1948–1950, 2003.

[72] M. Lindberg and P. Lindberg, "Overcoming obstacles for adherence to phosphate binding medication in dialysis patients: A qualitative study," *Pharmacy world and science*, vol. 30, no. 5, pp. 571–576, 2008.

[73] B. Jimmy and J. Jose, "Patient medication adherence: measures in daily practice," *Oman Medical Journal*, vol. 26, no. 3, pp. 155–159, 2011.

The Clinical Efficacy and Safety of Ertapenem for the Treatment of Complicated Urinary Tract Infections Caused by ESBL-Producing Bacteria in Children

Ayse Karaaslan, Eda Kepenekli Kadayifci, Serkan Atici, Gulsen Akkoc, Nurhayat Yakut, Sevliya Öcal Demir, Ahmet Soysal, and Mustafa Bakir

Department of Pediatric Infectious Diseases, Marmara University School of Medicine, 34890 Istanbul, Turkey

Correspondence should be addressed to Ahmet Soysal; asoysal@marmara.edu.tr

Academic Editor: Danuta Zwolinska

Background. Urinary tract infections (UTIs) are common and important clinical problem in childhood, and extended-spectrum-beta-lactamase- (ESBL-) producing organisms are the leading cause of healthcare-related UTIs. In this study, we aimed to evaluate the clinical efficacy and safety of ertapenem therapy in children with complicated UTIs caused by ESBL-producing organisms. *Methods.* Seventy-seven children with complicated UTIs caused by ESBL-producing organisms were included in this retrospective study, and all had been treated with ertapenem between January 2013 and June 2014. *Results.* Sixty-one (79%) females and sixteen (21%) males with a mean ± standard deviation (SD) age of 76.6 ± 52 months (range 3–204, median 72 months) were enrolled in this study. *Escherichia coli* (*E. coli*) ($n = 67$; 87%) was the most common bacterial cause of the UTIs followed by *Klebsiella pneumoniae* (*K. pneumoniae*) ($n = 9$; 11.7%) and *Enterobacter cloacae* (*E. cloacae*) ($n = 1$; 1.3%). The mean duration of the ertapenem therapy was 8.9 ± 1.6 days (range 4–11). No serious drug-related clinical or laboratory adverse effects were observed, and the ertapenem therapy was found to be safe and well tolerated in the children in our study. *Conclusion.* Ertapenem is a newer carbapenem with the advantage of once-daily dosing and is highly effective for treating UTIs caused by ESBL-producing microorganisms.

1. Introduction

Urinary tract infections (UTIs) are common bacterial infections in infants and children and have high prevalence and morbidity rates. Urinary tract infections are simply classified as acute pyelonephritis/upper urinary tract infection and cystitis/lower urinary tract infection. In a community with low antimicrobial resistance rates, UTIs in children older than 3 months can be treated with oral antibiotics for 7–10 days, for example, with cephalosporins or co-amoxiclav [1]. In conditions that oral antibiotics therapy is not possible (poor feeding, lethargy, toxic appearance, immunosuppression, etc.) intravenous (IV) antibiotics such as cefotaxime and ceftriaxone are appropriate therapeutic regimens for inpatient care. Parenteral antibiotic therapy may be stopped at 2nd–4th days and followed by oral antibiotics [1]. However, cephalosporins are mostly not effective for UTIs caused by ESBL-producing

microorganisms, with the management of these infections being complicated by the increasing prevalence of these microorganisms in both healthcare-related and community-acquired UTIs. In our country, the data showed that prevalence of ESBL-producing bacteria in children is increasing, ranging from 20% to 54% [2, 3]. Kizilca et al. [4] reported that, in community-acquired UTIs caused by *E. coli* and *Klebsiella* species, ESBL productions were 41% and 53%, respectively.

Carbapenems, such as meropenem, imipenem, ertapenem, and doripenem, are one of the best antimicrobial therapy choices for infections caused by ESBL-producing microorganisms. Ertapenem is newer and has a narrower spectrum of activity than the others. It is effective against most Enterobacteriaceae and anaerobes, which are common causes of intra-abdominal infections, but it is less effective than the other carbapenems for *P. aeruginosa*, *Acinetobacter*, and Gram-positive bacteria [5]. The major benefit of ertapenem is that it has long half-life and it can be administered in a once-daily dose in contrast to three-four times daily for the other carbapenems.

Ertapenem is a beta-lactam antimicrobial agent that was licensed in the United States in November 2001 and in Europe in 2002. In addition, since 2005, it has been approved for use in children who are more than three months old with complicated skin and soft tissue infections, complex intra-abdominal infections, community-acquired pneumonia, UTIs, and acute pelvic infections [6].

In this study, we aimed to evaluate the clinical efficacy and safety of ertapenem in 77 children with complicated UTIs caused by ESBL-producing microorganisms.

2. Methods

Seventy-seven children aged three months to 18 years with UTIs caused by ESBL-producing organisms were included in this study. All had been treated with ertapenem between January 2013 and June 2014 in a tertiary care hospital. In this facility, the use of carbapenem for children is feasible after gaining the approval of the pediatric infectious diseases department.

In this retrospective study, the study participants were identified through the department's patient files archive, and their demographic information (age and gender), underlying diseases, clinical manifestations, and laboratory and radiological test results were evaluated.

Complicated UTI was identified by the presence all of the followings: (i) pyuria (a urinary white blood cell (WBC) count of >five bacteria per high-power field (HPF) for centrifuged urine); (ii) a positive dipstick for leukocyte esterase and/or nitrate; (iii) the presence of a recognized uropathogen at $\geq 10^5$ colony-forming units (CFU)/mL for midstream urine, $\geq 10^4$ CFU/mL for catheter urine, or >0 CFU/mL for suprapubic puncture urine; and (iv) the presence of two or more UTI symptoms such as fever, hypothermia, suprapubic tenderness, dysuria, urgency, or frequency [7]. The patients with UTIs who did not match these criteria were excluded from the study.

We used the Vitek 2 automated system (bioMèrieux) to identify the microorganisms and assess their susceptibility, and the antimicrobial susceptibility results and ESBL production were determined according to the guidelines of the Clinical and Laboratory Standards Institute (CLSI) [8]. In addition, all isolates were evaluated for ESBL production via the double-disk synergy test (DDST) using Mueller-Hinton agar.

When the patients were hospitalized, empirical antibiotic therapy was started depending on community or nosocomial urinary tract infection that was diagnosed. Cephalosporins were started for community-acquired complicated UTIs and meropenem was started for nosocomial UTIs, empirically. On the third day of empirical antibiotic therapy urine culture and antibiogram results were achieved and then changed to appropriate antibiotic. In this study, we focused on only patients treated with ertapenem. We administered ertapenem 30 mg/kg/day by dividing it into two intravenous doses.

TABLE 1: Predisposing factors for urinary tract infection, n (%).

Neurological (myelomeningocele with a neurogenic bladder) abnormality	14 (18.2)
Vesicoureteral reflux (VUR)	10 (13)
Anatomic anomaly (e.g., obstructive uropathy, bladder exstrophy, or a neurogenic bladder)	10 (13)
Bladder dysfunction representing with enuresis	6 (7.8)
Patients had undergone chronic hemodialysis	4 (5.2)
Urolithiasis	3 (3.8)
Others (malignancy, etc.)	4 (5.2)

TABLE 2: Distribution of the bacterial isolates, n (%).

E. coli	67 (87)
K. pneumoniae	9 (11.7)
E. cloacae	1 (1.3)

3. Results

There were 61 (79%) females and 16 (21%) males with a mean age of 76.6 ± 52 months (range 3–204, median 72 months). We determined that 51 (66%) patients had an underlying predisposing factor for a UTI. Fourteen (18.2%) had a neurological (myelomeningocele with a neurogenic bladder) abnormality, 10 (13%) had vesicoureteral reflux (VUR), 10 (13%) had an anatomic anomaly (e.g., obstructive uropathy, bladder exstrophy, or a neurogenic bladder), six (7.8%) had bladder dysfunction representing with enuresis, four (5.2%) had undergone chronic hemodialysis, three (3.8%) had urolithiasis, and four (5.2%) had other anomalies, including two with cerebral palsy (CP), one with a malignancy, and one with congenital myasthenia gravis (Table 1). We accepted patients who had undergone chronic hemodialysis as secondary immunocompromised patients. The patients with underlying risk factors for UTIs were receiving prophylaxis including trimethoprim-sulfamethoxazole, nitrofurantoin, or amoxicillin. Ertapenem was initiated in all of the patients after the results of the microbiological cultures became available, and we determined that Escherichia coli (E. coli) ($n = 67$; 87%) was the most common bacterial cause of the UTIs. Klebsiella pneumonia (K. pneumonia) was identified as the source in nine patients (11.7%), whereas Enterobacter cloacae (E. cloacae) was the culprit in another patient (1.3%) (Table 2). All of the isolates were susceptible to the carbapenems including ertapenem, meropenem, and imipenem, but the ESBL-producing Enterobacteriaceae isolates were most frequently resistant to ampicillin ($n = 75$; 97.4%) and ceftriaxone ($n = 75$; 97.4%) followed by trimethoprim-sulfamethoxazole ($n = 46$; 59.7%), piperacillin-tazobactam ($n = 42$; 54.5%), gentamicin ($n = 23$; 29.9%), and nitrofurantoin ($n = 16$; 20.8%) (Table 3). The ESBL-producing E. coli was most often resistant to ampicillin ($n = 65$, 97%) and ceftriaxone ($n = 65$, 97%), but it was also resistant to trimethoprim-sulfamethoxazole ($n = 39$; 58.2%), piperacillin-tazobactam ($n = 37$; 55.2%),

TABLE 3: Resistance rates of Enterobacteriaceae strains against antimicrobial agents, n (%).

Ampicillin	75 (97.4)
Ceftriaxone	75 (97.4)
Trimethoprim-sulfamethoxazole	46 (59.7)
Piperacillin-tazobactam	42 (54.5)
Gentamicin	23 (29.9)
Nitrofurantoin	16 (20.8)
Carbapenems (ertapenem, meropenem, and imipenem)	—

gentamicin (n = 22; 32.8%), and nitrofurantoin (n = 9; 13.4%). On the third day of ertapenem therapy, we obtained control urine cultures, and all resulted to be sterile. Clinical cure was accepted as the resolution of infection-related signs and symptoms after 48-hour onset of ertapenem therapy. And clinical cure was achieved in all patients. The blood culture results were available for all patients and all cultures resulted to be negative. None of the patients were bacteremic. The mean duration of ertapenem therapy was 8.9 ± 1.6 days (range 4–11), and we observed two drug-related adverse events (AEs), with one patient having a mildly elevated level of alanine aminotransferase and another patient developing a short-term maculopapular rash.

4. Discussion

Urinary tract infections caused by community-acquired and healthcare-related ESBL-producing *E. coli* and other Gram-negative bacilli have become widespread around the world since community-acquired ESBL-producing microorganisms were first discovered in 1998 in Ireland [9–12]. Carbapenems, such as meropenem, imipenem, ertapenem, and doripenem, are the most common antimicrobial agents used for treating several infections caused by ESBL-producing microorganisms because ESBLs are the enzymes which confer resistance to most beta-lactam antibiotics, including penicillins, cephalosporins, and aztreonam. Aminoglycosides can be used even after documentation of in vitro activity; however, the potential for emergence of resistance on treatment often limits their use. Furthermore, genes responsible for ESBLs are in close relation with resistance determinants to other antimicrobials (aminoglycosides, fluoroquinolones, and trimethoprim-sulfamethoxazole) [13, 14].

There are few reports regarding the clinical efficacy of the use of carbapenems for UTIs in children caused by ESBL-producing microorganisms. Ertapenem may be preferred over imipenem or meropenem because of its lower cost, feasibility for outpatient intramuscular therapy, and potential value for reducing carbapenem resistance in *Acinetobacter baumannii* (*A. baumannii*) and *Pseudomonas aeruginosa* (*P. aeruginosa*). In addition, there is also scarcity of reports concerning the clinical efficacy of ertapenem in the treatment of UTIs in children caused by ESBL-producing microorganisms. However, we believe that this particular carbapenem

may be suitable for the first-line treatment of UTIs caused by these microorganisms in children.

The safety and efficacy of the use of ertapenem in children between the ages of three months and 17 years are based on evidence from well-controlled adult studies, pediatric pharmacokinetic data, and additional data from comparator-controlled studies that focused on pediatric patients [12, 15]. All of the patients in our study were at least three months old.

The duration of UTI therapy usually lasts from seven to 10 days; however, we suggest a longer course of therapy for children with an underlying predisposing factor for this type of infection. Unfortunately, the extended therapy necessitates longer hospital stays, exposure to more hospital-related infections, and higher treatment costs. Ertapenem can be given once a day intravenously in the hospital or intramuscularly as an outpatient, with the latter shortening the length of hospital stays. In turn, this decreases the costs and risks associated with the longer treatment.

Having an anomaly in the urinary tract increases the risk of UTIs [16], and predisposing obstructive abnormalities, for example, posterior urethral valves and ureteropelvic junction obstruction, as well as neurological abnormalities, such as myelomeningocele with a neurogenic bladder, and functional abnormalities, for instance, bladder dysfunction, may be anatomical in nature. In previous studies, VUR was the most common urological anomaly and the most common predisposing factor for UTIs in children [17, 18]. However, in our study, myelomeningocele with a neurogenic bladder was the most common underlying predisposing factor while VUR with the source was present in only 10 (13%) patients.

Ertapenem is primarily metabolized by the kidneys with minimal hepatic metabolism, which results in high antibiotic levels in the urine. The most common ertapenem-related AEs in previous studies were elevated hepatic transaminase levels (8.8%), diarrhea (5.0%), thrombophlebitis (4.5%), nausea (2.5%), and seizures (0.2%) [19], whereas the only two drug-related AEs that we observed were a mild elevation in alanine aminotransferase levels and a short-term maculopapular rash, both of which were reversible without having to discontinue the ertapenem therapy. Hence, ertapenem was well-tolerated in all our patients without any serious AEs.

Repeating the urine culture during the treatment of UTIs is no longer recommended [20], but, in our hospital, after the beginning of the therapy control urine cultures are obtained in clinical practice, especially in patients with underlying urinary anomalies. In this study, we obtained control urine cultures on the third day of the therapy, and all of the cultures resulted to be sterile with ertapenem therapy.

In addition, 66% of the patients in our study had underlying abnormalities that required at least ten days of treatment with hospitalization, but since the urine cultures were sterile on the third day of ertapenem treatment, the patients were then discharged and only needed single-dose intramuscular ertapenem maintenance therapy as outpatients for the next seven days.

Limitations of this study were as follows. (1) The data for episodes of UTIs was not given because of multicenter follow-up of patients. The patients' files in other hospitals were not available. For this reason, we did not give the episode data because of its unreliability. (2) We did not compare ertapenem with any other therapeutic agents in this study because of the retrospective study design. (3) We did not perform cost analysis of different antibiotic therapy regimens and their comparison with ertapenem therapy.

5. Conclusion

Ertapenem appears to be a good choice for first-line therapy for UTIs caused by ESBL-producing microorganisms in children. Not only did we find that it was an effective treatment option in this study, but also it was well tolerated by the patients. Furthermore, ertapenem has the advantage of shorter hospital stays and lower healthcare costs.

Authors' Contribution

All authors have participated in drafting of the paper and/or critical revision of the paper for important intellectual content. All authors read and approved the final paper.

References

[1] NICE (National Institute for Health and Care Excellence), "Urinary tract infection in children: diagnosis, treatment and long-term management," Clinical Guideline 54, NICE, 2007.

[2] S. Çelebi, N. Yüce, D. Çakır, M. Hacımustafaoğlu, and G. Öakaya, "Çocuklarda genişlemiş spektrumlu β-laktamaz üreten E. coli enfeksiyonlarında risk faktörleri ve klinik sonuçları, beş yıllık çalışma," Çocuk Enfeksiyon Hastalıkları Derneği, vol. 3, pp. 5–10, 2009.

[3] N. Demir, S. Gençer, S. Özer, and M. Doğan, "Genişlemiş spektrumlu β-laktamaz üreten gram negatif bakteri infeksiyonları için çeşitli risk faktörlerinin araştırılması," Flora, vol. 13, pp. 179–188, 2008.

[4] O. Kizilca, R. Siraneci, A. Yilmaz et al., "Risk factors for community-acquired urinary tract infection caused by ESBL-producing bacteria in children," Pediatrics International, vol. 54, no. 6, pp. 858–862, 2012.

[5] UpToDate Database, http://www.uptodate.com/contents/combination-beta-lactamase-inhibitors-inhibitors-carbapenems-andmonobactams?source=machineLearning&search=ertapenem&selectedTitle=5~36&sectionRank=1&anchor=H3#H3.

[6] G. M. Keating and C. M. Perry, "Ertapenem: a review of its use in the treatment of bacterial infections," Drugs, vol. 65, no. 15, pp. 2151–2178, 2005.

[7] J. S. Elder, "Urinary tract infections," in Nelson Textbook of Pediatrics, R. M. Kliegman, R. Behrman, H. Jenson, and B. Stanton, Eds., chapter 538, pp. 2223–2228, Saunders Elsevier, Philadelphia, Pa, USA, 18th edition, 2007.

[8] National Committee for Clinical Laboratory Standards, Methods for Dilution Antimicrobial Susceptibility Tests for Bacteria That Grow Aerobically, Approved Standard M7-A5 and Informational Supplement M100-S10, National Committee for Clinical Laboratory Standards, Wayne, Pa, USA, 2000.

[9] M. D. Zilberberg and A. F. Shorr, "Secular trends in gram-negative resistance among urinary tract infection hospitalizations in the United States, 2000–2009," Infection Control and Hospital Epidemiology, vol. 34, no. 9, pp. 940–946, 2013.

[10] D. L. Paterson and R. A. Bonomo, "Extended-spectrum β-lactamases: a clinical update," Clinical Microbiology Reviews, vol. 18, no. 4, pp. 657–686, 2005.

[11] R. Ben-Ami, J. Rodríguez-Baño, H. Arslan et al., "A multinational survey of risk factors for infection with extended-spectrum beta-lactamase-producing enterobacteriaceae in nonhospitalizd patients," Clinical Infectious Diseases, vol. 49, no. 5, pp. 682–690, 2009.

[12] N. Dalgic, M. Sancar, B. Bayraktar, E. Dincer, and S. Pelit, "Ertapenem for the treatment of urinary tract infections caused by extended-spectrum β-lactamase-producing bacteria in children," Scandinavian Journal of Infectious Diseases, vol. 43, no. 5, pp. 339–343, 2011.

[13] M. Fernández-Reyes, D. Vicente, M. Gomariz et al., "High rate of fecal carriage of extended-spectrum-β-lactamase-producing Escherichia coli in healthy children in Gipuzkoa, northern Spain," Antimicrobial Agents and Chemotherapy, vol. 58, no. 3, pp. 1822–1824, 2014.

[14] T. M. Coque, F. Baquero, and R. Canton, "Increasing prevalence of ESBL-producing Enterobacteriaceae in Europe," Eurosurveillance, vol. 13, no. 47, article 4, 2008.

[15] A. Parakh, S. Krishnamurthy, and M. Bhattacharya, "Ertapenem," Kathmandu University Medical Journal, vol. 7, no. 28, pp. 454–460, 2009.

[16] A. L. Freedman, "Urinary tract infections in children," in Urologic Diseases in America. U.S. Department of Health and Human Services, Public Health Service, National Institutes of Health, National Institute of Diabetes and Digestive and Kidney Diseases, M. S. Litwin and C. S. Saigal, Eds., NIH Publication 07-5512, pp. 439–458, U.S. Government Printing Office, Washington, DC, USA, 2007.

[17] S. Hansson, I. Bollgren, E. Esbjörner, B. Jakobsson, and S. Mårild, "Urinary tract infections in children below two years of age: a quality assurance project in Sweden," Acta Paediatrica, vol. 88, no. 3, pp. 270–274, 1999.

[18] E. Stokland, M. Hellström, B. Jacobsson, U. Jodal, and R. Sixt, "Evaluation of DMSA scintigraphy and urography in assessing both acute and permanent renal damage in children," Acta Radiologica, vol. 39, no. 4, pp. 447–452, 1998.

[19] H. Teppler, R. M. Gesser, I. R. Friedland et al., "Safety and tolerability of ertapenem," Journal of Antimicrobial Chemotherapy, vol. 53, supplement 2, pp. 75–81, 2004.

[20] M. L. Currie, L. Mitz, C. S. Raasch, and L. A. Greenbaum, "Follow-up urine cultures and fever in children with urinary tract infection," Archives of Pediatrics and Adolescent Medicine, vol. 157, no. 12, pp. 1237–1240, 2003.

11

Mortality in Patients on Renal Replacement Therapy and Permanent Cardiac Pacemakers

Gabriel Vanerio,[1,2] **Cristina García,**[1] **Carlota González,**[1,3] **and Alejandro Ferreiro**[1,3,4]

[1] *CASMU Arrhythmia Service, 8 de Octubre 3310, 11600 Montevideo, Uruguay*
[2] *British Hospital, Avenida Italia 2420, 11600 Montevideo, Uruguay*
[3] *Uruguayan Registry of Dialysis, Uruguay*
[4] *Nephrology Clinic, Hospital de Clinicas, Faculty of Medicine, The University of the Republic, Avenida Italia s/n, 11600 Montevideo, Uruguay*

Correspondence should be addressed to Gabriel Vanerio; gabvaner@gmail.com

Academic Editor: David B. Kershaw

End stage renal disease is a relatively frequent disease with high mortality due to cardiac causes. Permanent pacemaker (PM) implantation rates are also very common; thus combination of both conditions is not unusual. We hypothesized that patients with chronic kidney disease with a PM would have significantly higher mortality rates compared with end stage renal disease patients without PM. Our objectives were to analyze mortality of patients on renal replacement therapy with PM. 2778 patients were on renal replacement therapy (RRT) and 110 had a PM implanted during the study period. To reduce the confounding effects of covariates, a propensity-matched score was performed. 52 PM patients and 208 non-PM matched patients were compared. 41% of the PM were implanted before entering the RRT program and 59% while on RRT. Mortality was higher in the PM group. Cardiovascular disease and infections were the most frequent causes of death. Propensity analysis showed no differences in long-term mortality between groups. We concluded that in patients on RRT and PM mortality rates are higher. Survival curves did not differ from a RRT propensity-matched group. We concluded that the presence of a PM is not an independent mortality risk factor in RRT patients.

1. Background

Permanent cardiac pacing (PM) is the treatment of choice in severe and symptomatic bradycardia. Several independent factors such as age, gender, comorbidities, presence of structural heart disease, stimulation modalities, index arrhythmia, and initial symptoms are associated with mortality [1–4].

End-stage renal disease is a relatively common condition associated with high mortality due to cardiovascular causes. Most deaths in patients on renal replacement therapy (RRT) are attributed to sudden cardiac death, which accounts for approximately one-quarter of all deaths [5–9]. Therefore, as chronic kidney disease is an increasingly prevalent condition and an independent risk factor for cardiovascular mortality, the presence of a permanent pacemaker is likely to increase mortality.

To our knowledge, no data is available regarding mortality in patients on RRT with permanent pacemakers (PM) [10–12]. These groups of patients are not included in the current

guidelines [13, 14]. Mortality rates are likely to be higher due to the advanced age, the high incidence of stroke, and comorbidities. Estimation of outcomes after PM placement in long-term dialysis patients is needed to evaluate the risks and benefits of permanent cardiac stimulation [5, 6, 15–21].

Our objectives were

(1) to analyze mortality in RRT patients with and without a PM;

(2) to compare survival and describe baseline characteristics of patients with PM on a RRT program.

2. Methods

We performed a longitudinal retrospective study from January 2003 to December 2008. Data was obtained from the Uruguayan National Resource Fund (FNR) database (which includes 99% of PM implants and all dialysis units in Uruguay) [22]. The FNR is a nongovernmental public organization that provides financial coverage of medical procedures for the entire Uruguayan population. The FNR ensures financing and evaluates the quality of care provided to patients, controlling the processes and outcomes of the funded procedures.

Demographic data, comorbidities, time on RRT, clinical conditions, and the functional status evaluated by Karnofsky modified score (4 categories) were registered to perform comparisons between groups [23]. Data on comorbid conditions at the beginning of the study and the evolution were prospectively recorded using a standardized data collection tool (Basic Data and Evolution Questionnaire). We restricted the analysis to the first device implanted. Participants were followed up from PM implant date until March 30, 2010, or death.

2.1. Baseline Covariates. For each patient, we obtained demographic data and cause of renal failure from the FNR database. Variables included risk factors for mortality, such as history of myocardial infarction, coronary heart disease, ischemic stroke or transient ischemic attack, congestive heart failure, cardiac arrest, atrial fibrillation, chronic obstructive lung disease, cancer, and diabetes.

2.2. Outcomes. Outcomes of interest were all-cause mortality. Mortality date and cause of death were extracted from the FNR database.

2.3. Statistical Analysis. Categorical and continuous data are presented as absolute numbers and percentages or mean values and standard deviations, respectively. Variables were compared by the χ^2 test, Fisher's exact test or Student's *t*-test, Wilcoxon test, and binary logistic regression when appropriate. Survival curves were constructed by the Kaplan-Meier method. Pooled-over strata log rank test or Breslow test was used for comparing the equality of survival distributions for the different levels of the factors. The log-rank test was used to compare curves. Due to the important imbalance of mortality-associated comorbidities between groups, patients who received a PM device while on RRT were propensity-matched accordingly with a logistic regression derived probability of death, adjusted to the confounding effects of covariates (age, sex, comorbidities, Karnofsky-based functional status, and previous time on dialysis). All variables significant at the $P < 0.2$ level were entered into the multivariate model (forward stepwise binary logistic regression analysis) provided they were present in at least 2% of the sample. Variables were entered into the model separately, beginning with the variable having the highest statistically significant score. Variables that significantly improved the fit of the model were retained and forced into subsequent models. Stability of the model was assessed every time a variable was entered. The final step was to search for first-degree interaction. Criteria to include an interaction term were: (1) significant at $P < 0.05$, (2) 1% of the sample had to exhibit the same combination factors, and (3) the combination should be clinically relevant. All patients were propensity-matched accordingly with the derived probability of death,

on a 1 PM × 4 non-PM number of patients basis (1 : 4 ratio). 52/65 (80%) PM patients (all on RRT before the device was implanted) and 208 non-PM matched subjects were suitable for comparison. A two-sided alpha level of 0.05 was considered statistically significant.

3. Results

From 2003 to 2008, 7129 new PMs were implanted in Uruguay (1188 per year); during this period, 1432 (20%) PM patients died.

During the same time period, 2778 patients were on RRT, with an unadjusted annual mortality rate of 13.4%. Chronic kidney diseases determinant of the loss of renal function were primary glomerulopathies (12.6%), diabetic nephropathy (21.5%), vascular nephropathy (24.4%), obstructive nephropathy (8.2%), tubule-interstitial nephropathy (2.8%), other causes (28.5%), and unknown cause (2%). Mortality was secondary to cardiovascular diseases in 39.7% (95% CI 34–44), infectious diseases in 19.25% (15–23), discontinuation of treatment in 7.9 (2–12), cancer in 8 (6–9), and other causes in 26% (22–28).

110 of the 2778 (3.9%) RRT patients were recipients of a PM, 41% (45/110) before entering the RRT program, and 59% (65/110) while on RRT.

The PM population on RRT corresponded to 1.9% of all PM implants in Uruguay in the observation period.

3.1. RRT Population. Mean followup was 93.6 ± 63 months. Patients in the PM group were older and predominantly male. (Figure 1) Comorbidities were extremely common. Table 1 shows baseline characteristics and comparison between groups; PM patients were older, with a significant male predominance; Kaplan-Meier survival time was significantly shorter. Within the PM group, there was a slightly higher prevalence of diabetes, and the functional status was significantly lower. A significantly higher incidence of stroke and neoplasic disease was observed. Those who received a PM while on RRT had the highest burden of comorbidities (Table 1).

3.2. Study Outcomes. Crude all-cause mortality was higher in the pacemaker group (60% versus 54% $P = 0.2$) with a different mean survival time (29.7 ± 2 months versus 96.2 ± 6 months, resp.; $P < 0.05$). The mortality rate was 24.3 versus 14.9 per 100 patient-years, respectively, $P < 0.05$ (Figure 2).

Variables associated with long-term mortality were: odds ratio (95% CI); age 1.053 (1.043–1.062); age > 70 years; 1.5 (1.1–2.0) coronary heart disease; 1.8 (1.4–2.3) diabetes; 2.1 (1.5–2.8) COPD; 2.9 (1.9–4) Karnofsky modified score 1; 1.9 (1.5–2.3) Karnofsky modified score 2; 4.3 (3.09–6) Karnofsky modified score 3; 7.4 (3.3–16) peripheral vascular disease; 3 (2.1–4.3).

3.3. Propensity Matched Adjusted Groups. After propensity adjustment, no differences were observed in long-term mortality between both groups (Table 3 and Figure 3).

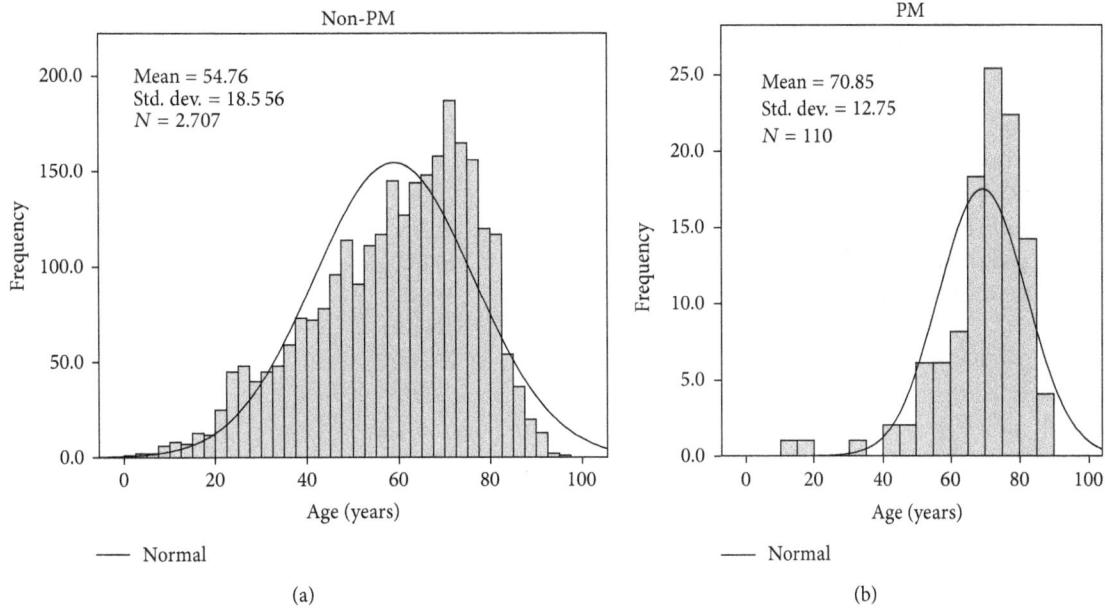

FIGURE 1: Age histograms from both groups without pacemaker (a) and with pacemaker (b).

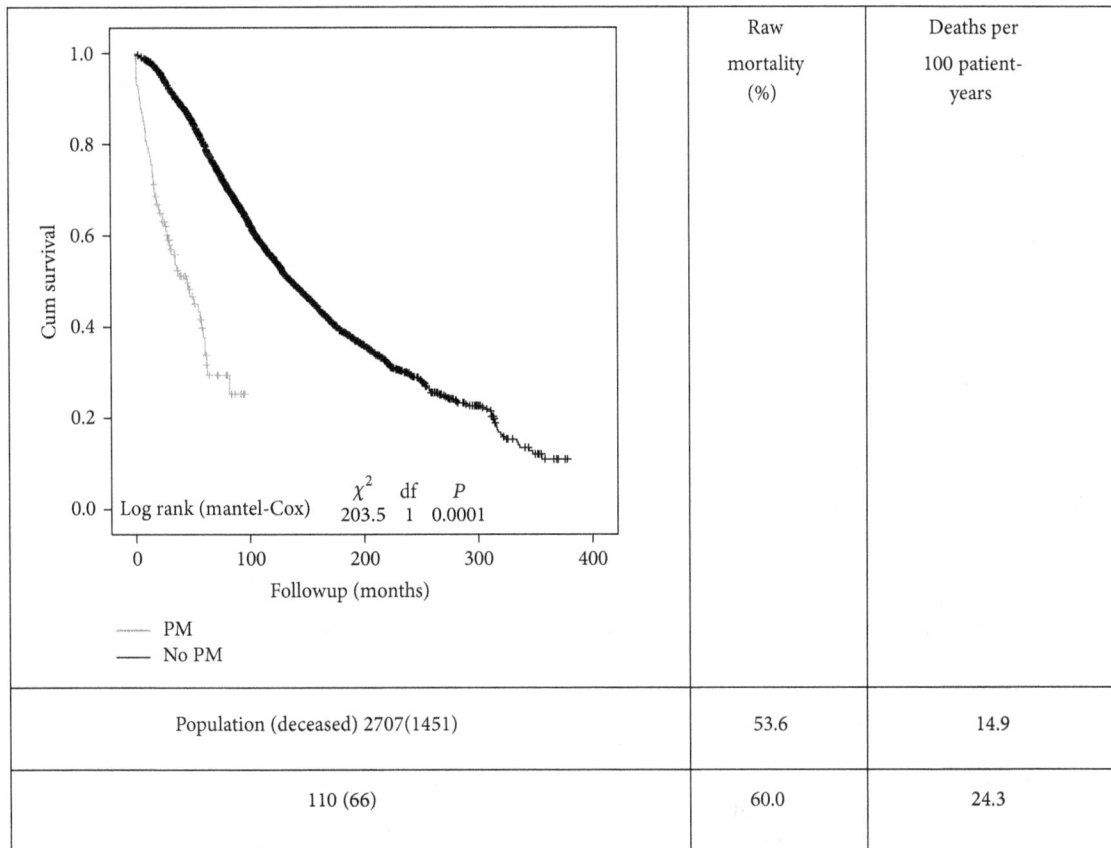

FIGURE 2: Kaplan-Meier survival curves comparing both groups (PM-pacemaker grey line and non-PM black line). Curves are quite different and show a high mortality in both groups, particularly in the PM group. Mortality (raw and adjusted) rates are shown on the right side of the figure.

TABLE 1: Patient demographics.

	No PM	PM	PM after RRT (group A + C); see text
n (%)	2668 (96)	110 (4)	83 (2.9)
Age (years)	59.0 ± 1	70.8 ± 1[*]	69.5 ± 14.5[**]
Female gender n (%)	1140 (42)	29 (26)[TT]	27 (32.1)[T]
Mean survival time (months)	96.2 ± 62	29.7 ± 22[*]	24 ± 19[**]
Previous time in RRT (years)	5.2 ± 4.6	NA	4.8 ± 4.6
Arterial hypertension n (%)	1272 (47)	61 (55)	50 (60)
SBP > 140 mmHg predialysis n (%)	983 (37)	44 (40)	34 (41)
Antihypertensive treatment n (%)	1042 (38)	53 (48)	45 (54)
Hb ≥ 10 g% n (%)	609 (22)	8/29 (25)	5/25 (20)
Coronary artery disease n (%)	569 (22)	35 (32)	42 (51.5)[**]
Atrial fibrillation n (%)	16[§]	35 (32)	20 (35)
Valvular heart disease n (%)	NA	13 (11.8)	8 (9)
Diabetes n (%)	575 (21)	26 (23)	23 (27.9)[*]
(a) Karnofsky 1 n (%)	1425 (53)	25 (22)[TT]	25 (30.9)[**]
(a) Karnofsky 2 n (%)	749 (28)	61 (55)[*]	31 (38.2)[*]
(a) Karnofsky 3 n (%)	392 (15)	24 (22)	19 (23.5)[*]
(a) Karnofsky 4 n (%)	100 (3.7)	8 (5.4)	6 (7.4)[*]
Previous stroke n (%)	216 (8.3)	24 (22)[T]	29 (35.3)[**]
Smoker n (%)	347 (13)	18 (16)	21 (27.3)[**]
Neoplastic disease n (%)	202 (7)	19 (17)[TT]	22 (27.5)[TT]
Peripheral vascular disease n (%)	417 (15)	19 (17)	22 (27.5)[**]
COPD n (%)	212 (7.9)	12 (11)	6 (7.5)
Mortality n (mortality/rate 100 patient-years)	1451 (14.9)	66 (24.3)[*]	29 (35.2)[TT]

All comparisons versus the non-PM group; [*]$P < 0.05$, [**]$P < 0.01$, [T]$P < 0.001$, and [TT]$P < 0.0001$.
[§]Data estimated from the international dialysis outcomes and practice patterns study (DOPPS).
NA: not available.
(a) 1: Able to carry on normal activity and to work; no special care needed. 2: Normal activity with effort; some signs or symptoms of disease; unable to work; able to live at home and care for most personal needs; varying amount of assistance needed. 3: Cares for self; unable to carry on normal activity or to do active work; requires occasional assistance but is able to care for most of his personal needs. 4: Unable to care for self; requires equivalent of institutional or hospital care; disease may be progressing rapidly.

Survival curves were not different in the RRT propensity-matched group. Coronary artery disease, age, and the Karnofsky modified score were the only independent variables associated with mortality in the propensity population, without differences between groups.

3.4. *PM Population.* The PM population could be divided into three groups: 64 (58%) patients who received the PM while on RRT (group A), mean time of 68 ± 56 months on RRT before PM implantation. Group B: 27 (24%) patients received the pacemaker before entering the RRT program (mean time −26 ± 21 months) and Group C: 19 (17%) patients received the device within 3 months before or after entering the RRT program (1 ± 1.35 months). Group A had a significantly higher mortality (65% versus 52% $P = 0.05$, versus group B) and a shorter mean survival time (24 ± 19 versus 36 ± 25 months), with a different age at implantation (68 ± 15 versus 74 ± 7 years, $P < 0.05$) (Figure 4). In these subgroups, the presence of atrial fibrillation was associated with a significantly higher mortality, group A versus group B plus group C, 21% versus 9% ($P < 0.006$). VVI pacing was also associated with higher mortality rates, particularly in group A, 38% ($P < 0.003$) versus 15% in groups B and C together.

TABLE 2: Cause of death in the PM group.

	$N = 66$ (%)
Cardiovascular	17 (20.9)
Cardiac arrest	8 (21.1)
End-stage dilated cardiomyopathy	2 (3)
Myocardial infarction	3 (4.5)
Stroke, including intracranial hemorrhage	3 (4.5)
Pulmonary edema due to exogenous fluid	1 (1.5)
Infection	12 (18.1)
Neoplasic disease	1 (1.5)
Unknown	36 (54.5)

Most deaths were cardiovascular (20.9%), and approximately 10% were attributed to cardiac arrest or ventricular arrhythmias (Table 2). Deaths due to infections were common and observed in 18% of the patients, most of them not related to PM infections.

Survival within the PM group was longer in males than females (32 ± 23 versus 23 ± 16 months, $P < 0.05$) despite an older but non-significant age at implantation (male 71.7 ± 11

TABLE 3: Characteristics of the propensity-matched adjusted groups.

Variable	No PM ($n = 208$)	PM ($n = 52$)[a]	P
Predicted probability	0.64 ± 0.26	0.64 ± 0.25	NS
Age (years)	65.2 ± 13.4	66.9 ± 13.6	NS
Female gender (%)	41.8	42.6	NS
Diabetes (%)	20.1	25	NS
Previous time on RRT (years)	5.06 ± 4.4	5.8 ± 4.6	NS
Coronary heart disease (%)	46.2	49.8	NS
Previous stroke (%)	16.3	23.5	NS
Smoker (%)	11.5	17.3	NS
Neoplastic disease (%)	7.7	15.4	NS
Peripheral vascular disease (%)	21.5	28.8	NS
COPD (%)	6.2	9.6	NS
Functional status			
Karnofsky* 1 (%)	35.9	30.8	NS
Karnofsky* 2 (%)	36.8	40.4	NS
Karnofsky* 3 (%)	21.2	22	NS
Karnofsky* 4 (%)	7.7	5.3	NS

* As in Table 1.
[a] All patients in this group had the PM implanted while on RRT.

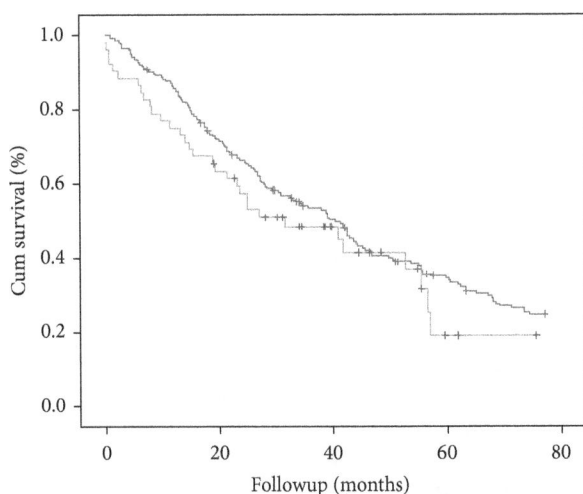

FIGURE 3: KM survival curve after propensity-matched adjustment. The darker grey line corresponds to the non-PM group and the lighter grey to PM group. There are no differences regarding survival between both groups (P = NS).

TABLE 4: Characteristics of the PM patients by survival outcome.

	Alive	Dead	P
n (%)	44 (40)	66 (60)	
Age (mean $\pm$ SD)	69.7 ± 11	71.6 ± 13	0.3 NS
Female gender n (%)	11 (25)	18 (27)	0.8 NS
Followup (months) (mean $\pm$ SD)	43 ± 21	21 ± 18	0.05
Arterial hypertension n (%)	29 (66)	32 (48)	0.08 NS
Diabetes n (%)	4 (9)	10 (15)	0.4 NS
Atrial fibrillation n (%)	17 (38)	18 (27)	0.2 NS
Coronary artery disease n (%)	6 (13)	13 (19)	0.4 NS
Dilated cardiomyopathy n (%)	2 (4)	7 (10)	0.3 NS
LVEF % (mean $\pm$ SD)	52.8 ± 2	50.8 ± 1	0.4 NS
Valvular heart disease n (%)	3 (7)	10 (15)	0.2 NS
AV block n (%)	23 (52)	42 (63)	0.24 NS
Sick sinus syndrome n (%)	18 (41)	23 (34)	0.5 NS
VVI PM n (%)	8 (18)	32 (48)	0.0013

NS: not significant.

4. Discussion

Although PM implant is routinely performed in patients on RRT, there is no relevant data available in this group of patients. Patients on RRT have increased morbidity and mortality and are at increased risk of developing cardiac device-related infections. Interestingly, there is much more information of implantable cardioverter defibrillators (ICDs) and RRT [10, 24–40].

In our study, we found that crude mortality rates were higher in the PM group, averaging 24.3 deaths per 100 patient-years versus 14.9 deaths per 100 patient-years in the RRT population without PM. This finding is probably related to older age and associated comorbidities. However, after propensity adjustment, mortality was similar between groups.

Global mortality rates in patients on RRT and patients without PM were lower when compared to other countries, 18.6 deaths per 100 patient-years of unselected dialysis patients reported in 2008 in the US [5, 41].

Cardiovascular disease and particularly malignant arrhythmias remain the predominant cause of death in RRT patients; however, infections were a very frequent cause of death [31, 32].

Patients with ICDs have much higher mortality rates, with 45 deaths/100 patient-years of followup. Cardiovascular mortality accounts for two-thirds of all deaths, and more than half those deaths were due to arrhythmia despite the type of the implanted device [28, 41, 42].

The high rate of deaths from arrhythmia after ICD-defibrillator or PM placement is consistent with studies showing higher defibrillation thresholds in dialysis patients than in individuals with preserved kidney function [33, 42]. The uremic milieu, the major shifts in potassium and calcium concentrations during hemodialysis [41–44], may increase the likelihood of a sudden increase of capture thresholds, resulting in defibrillation-resistant arrhythmias, bradycardia,

years versus female 68 ± 14 years). The type of arrhythmia leading to the PM implant had no influence on survival. Patients with a VVI PM had a higher mortality compared to those with dual chamber PMs, with a significantly shorter mean survival time, 16 ± 15 months versus 47 ± 23 months, $P < 0.05$ (Table 4 and Figure 4).

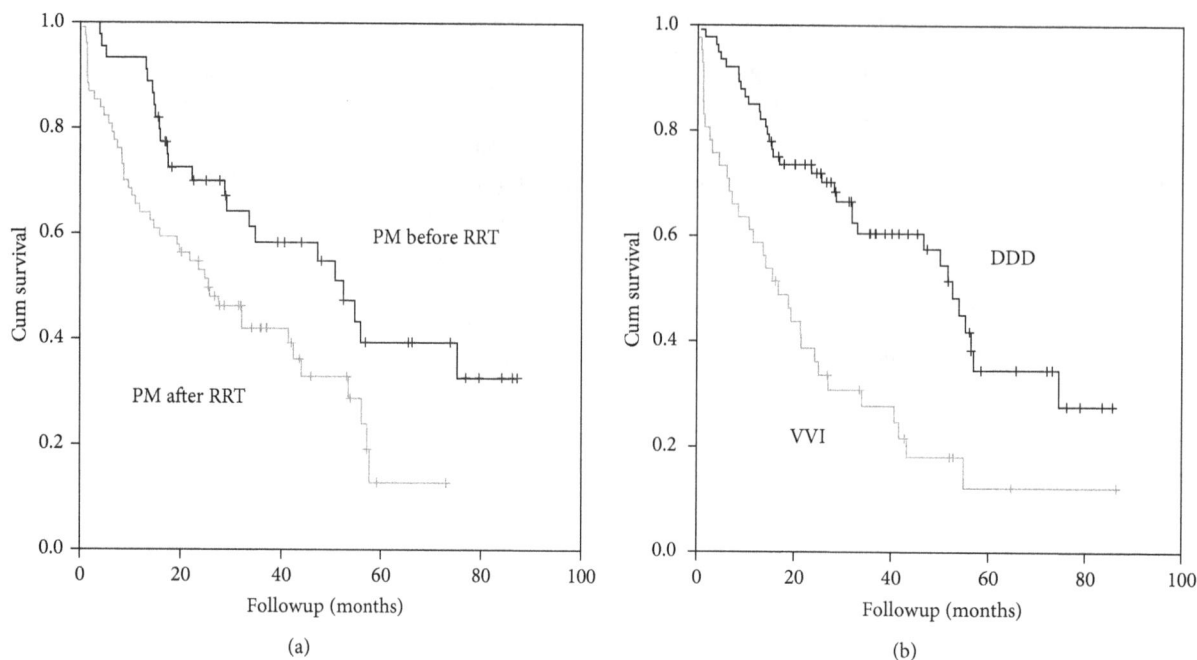

FIGURE 4: KM survival curves. (a) Mortality related to RRT; the grey lines correspond to the group of PM patients who received the device while on RRT and the black line corresponds to those who received the PM before entering the RRT program. Log rank (mantel-Cox); Chi-Square 6,2 df 1; $P = 0.012$. (b) Mortality regarding PM mode, DDD versus VVI pacing. The grey line corresponds to the VVI PMs and the black line to the DDD devices. Log rank (mantel-Cox) Chi-Square 11,31 df 1; $P = 0.001$.

heart block, and primary pulseless electrical activity in RRT patients [19, 35].

Although not important in our population as a significant mortality cause, clinicians considering PM therapy should carefully evaluate a history of infections before device placement, an assessment that may be particularly important in patients with catheters or grafts. RRT patients are at great risk of infection due to the repeated exposure during intravenous access creating a permanent potential menace of infection long after PM implantation. Reduction of device-related infections continues to be a clinical challenge. Irrigation of the pocket with antibiotics, antibacterial meshs coated with antibiotics, and/or use of prophylactic antibiotics had been shown to reduce infection rates [45].

Cost-effectiveness analyses should be implemented to assess mortality risk factors in order to clearly define the optimal PM indications in the RRT population, particularly the need for cardiac resynchronization therapy with or without an ICD. Those with depressed left ventricular function and atrial fibrillation have a significantly higher mortality rate.

In the near future, this population will definitively benefit form leadless PM to overcome infections.

4.1. Study Limitations. There are several limitations to our study. It was a retrospective observational study and the information contains administrative data rather than clinical records, but the data was prospectively recorded using a standardized data collection instrument, allowing for the best

quality of data acquisition in these types of observational studies. The number of patients suitable for the propensity analysis in the PM group was quite small. However, 80% of patients that received a PM while on RRT were included in the propensity risk-adjusted analysis.

Cardiovascular outcomes were not adjudicated independently, and important conditions, device-related complications, potassium level, and medication, were unavailable for analysis.

5. Conclusions

Patients on RRT with an implanted PM had significantly higher mortality rates; however, this observation is related to the burden of comorbidity. The presence of a PM is not an independent risk factor for mortality.

Patients on RRT that receive a PM have a worse prognosis than those that had the PM implanted before entering RRT.

Single chamber pacemakers had a significantly higher mortality and should be avoided if possible.

Acknowledgment

The authors are thankful to the National Resource Fund of Uruguay.

References

[1] S. S. Raza, J.-M. Li, R. John et al., "Long-term mortality and pacing outcomes of patients with permanent pacemaker implantation after cardiac surgery," *Pacing and Clinical Electrophysiology*, vol. 34, no. 3, pp. 331–338, 2011.

[2] M. Brunner, M. Olschewski, A. Geibeli, C. Bode, and M. Zehender, "Long-term survival after pacemaker implantation: prognostic importance of gender and baseline patient characteristics," *European Heart Journal*, vol. 25, no. 1, pp. 88–95, 2004.

[3] B. Schmidt, M. Brunner, M. Olschewski et al., "Pacemaker therapy in very elderly patients: long-term survival and prognostic parameters," *American Heart Journal*, vol. 146, no. 5, pp. 908–913, 2003.

[4] J. R. Pyatt, J. D. Somauroo, M. Jackson et al., "Long-term survival after permanent pacemaker implantation: analysis of predictors for increased mortality," *Europace*, vol. 4, no. 2, pp. 113–119, 2002.

[5] US Renal Data System, *USRDS, 2008 Annual Data Report: Atlas of End-Stage Renal Disease in the United States*, National Institutes of Health, National Institute of Diabetes and Digestive and Kidney Diseases, Bethesda, Md, USA, 2008.

[6] B. Kestenbaum, K. D. Rudser, M. G. Shlipak et al., "Kidney function, electrocardiographic findings, and cardiovascular events among older adults," *Clinical Journal of the American Society of Nephrology*, vol. 2, no. 3, pp. 501–508, 2007.

[7] Y. Ishikawa, "Arrhythmia and conduction abnormalities in hemodialysis patients," *Nippon Rinsho*, vol. 62, pp. 237–245, 2004.

[8] C. A. Herzog, "Can we prevent sudden cardiac death in dialysis patients?" *Clinical Journal of the American Society of Nephrology*, vol. 2, no. 3, pp. 410–412, 2007.

[9] A. A. Alsheikh-Ali, T. A. Trikalinos, R. Ruthazer et al., "Risk of arrhythmic and nonarrhythmic death in patients with heart failure and chronic kidney disease," *American Heart Journal*, vol. 161, no. 1, pp. 204.e1–209.e1, 2011.

[10] C. Arsenescu, G. I. Georgescu, A. Covic, and L. Briotă, "Permanent cardiac pacing for chronic symptomatic atrioventricular block in uremic hemodialysed patients. A prospective study," *Revista Medico-Chirurgicala a Societatii de Medici si Naturalisti din Iasi*, vol. 106, no. 1, pp. 112–121, 2002.

[11] H. Kohno, M. Hisahara, M. Umesue et al., "Permanent cardiac pacing in patients on chronic dialysis," *Nihon Kyobu Geka Gakkai Zasshi*, vol. 39, no. 7, pp. 992–995, 1991.

[12] R. B. Leman, J. M. Kratz, and P. C. Gazes, "Permanent cardiac pacing in patients on chronic renal dialysis," *American Heart Journal*, vol. 110, no. 6, pp. 1242–1244, 1985.

[13] A. E. Epstein, J. P. DiMarco, K. A. Ellenbogen et al., "ACC/AHA/HRS 2008 Guidelines for Device-Based Therapy of Cardiac Rhythm Abnormalities. A Report of the American College of Cardiology/American Heart Association Task Force on Practice Guidelines (Writing Committee to Revise the ACC/AHA/NASPE 2002 Guideline Update for Implantation of Cardiac Pacemakers and Antiarrhythmia Devices)," *Journal of the American College of Cardiology*, vol. 51, no. 21, pp. e1–e62, 2008.

[14] P. E. Vardas, A. Auricchio, J.-J. Blanc et al., "Guidelines for cardiac pacing and cardiac resynchronization therapy. The Task Force for Cardiac Pacing and Cardiac Resynchronization Therapy of the European Society of Cardiology. Developed in collaboration with the European Heart Rhythm Association," *Europace*, vol. 9, no. 10, pp. 959–998, 2007.

[15] D. A. Drew, K. B. Meyer, and D. E. Weiner, "Transvenous cardiac device wires and vascular access in hemodialysis patients," *American Journal of Kidney Diseases*, vol. 58, no. 3, pp. 494–496, 2011.

[16] A. Asif, L. H. Salman, G. G. Lopera, and R. G. Carrillo, "The dilemma of transvenous cardiac rhythm devices in hemodialysis patients: time to consider the epicardial approach," *Kidney International*, vol. 79, no. 12, pp. 1267–1269, 2011.

[17] H. Bloom, B. Heeke, A. Leon et al., "Renal insufficiency and the risk of infection from pacemaker or defibrillator surgery," *Pacing and Clinical Electrophysiology*, vol. 29, no. 2, pp. 142–145, 2006.

[18] C.-F. Chang, B. I.-T. Kuo, T.-L. Chen, W.-C. Yang, S.-D. Lee, and C.-C. Lin, "Infective endocarditis in maintenance hemodialysis patients: fifteen years' experience in one medical center," *Journal of Nephrology*, vol. 17, no. 2, pp. 228–235, 2004.

[19] K. Mischke, T. Schimpf, C. Knackstedt, and P. Schauerte, "Pacemaker with 2:1 hyperkalemic ventricular exit block," *International Journal of Cardiology*, vol. 116, no. 1, pp. 117–119, 2007.

[20] T. H. Teruya, A. M. Abou-Zamzam Jr., W. Limm, L. Wong, and L. Wong, "Symptomatic subclavian vein stenosis and occlusion in hemodialysis patients with transvenous pacemakers," *Annals of Vascular Surgery*, vol. 17, no. 5, pp. 526–529, 2003.

[21] F. Cavatorta, S. Campisi, and A. Zollo, "Subclavian vein stenosis: a potentially serious complication in chronic hemodialysis patients with permanent cardiac pacemakers," *International Journal of Artificial Organs*, vol. 20, no. 6, pp. 316–318, 1997.

[22] N. Mazzuchi, E. Schwedt, L. Solá, C. González, and A. Ferreiro, "Risk factors and prevention of end stage renal disease in Uruguay," *Renal Failure*, vol. 28, no. 8, pp. 617–625, 2006.

[23] N. Mazzuchi, E. Schwedt, C. Gonzalez et al., "Uruguayan registry committee of dialysis: evaluation of the dialysis program for the treatment of chronic kidney disease in Uruguay," *Archives of Internal Medicine Uruguay*, vol. 22, pp. 1–71, 2000.

[24] E. S. Williams, S. H. Shah, J. P. Piccini et al., "Predictors of mortality in patients with chronic kidney disease and an implantable defibrillator: an EPGEN substudy," *Europace*, vol. 13, no. 12, pp. 1717–1722, 2011.

[25] C. Tompkins, R. McLean, A. Cheng et al., "End-stage renal disease predicts complications in pacemaker and ICD implants," *Journal of Cardiovascular Electrophysiology*, vol. 22, no. 10, pp. 1099–1104, 2011.

[26] I. Ahmed, E. Gertner, W. B. Nelson, C. M. House, and D. W. X. Zhu, "Chronic kidney disease is an independent predictor of pocket hematoma after pacemaker and defibrillator implantation," *Journal of Interventional Cardiac Electrophysiology*, vol. 29, no. 3, pp. 203–207, 2010.

[27] C. S. Hager, S. Jain, J. Blackwell, B. Culp, J. Song, and C. D. Chiles, "Effect of renal function on survival after implantable cardioverter defibrillator placement," *American Journal of Cardiology*, vol. 106, no. 9, pp. 1297–1300, 2010.

[28] D. M. Charytan, A. R. Patrick, J. Liu et al., "Trends in the use and outcomes of implantable cardioverter-defibrillators in patients undergoing dialysis in the united states," *American Journal of Kidney Diseases*, vol. 58, no. 3, pp. 409–417, 2011.

[29] S. Hiremath, S. R. Punnam, S. S. Brar et al., "Implantable defibrillators improve survival in end-stage renal disease: results from a multi-center registry," *American Journal of Nephrology*, vol. 32, no. 4, pp. 305–310, 2010.

[30] R. Sakhuja, M. Keebler, T.-S. Lai, C. McLaughlin Gavin, R. Thakur, and D. L. Bhatt, "Meta-analysis of mortality in dialysis patients with an implantable cardioverter defibrillator," *American Journal of Cardiology*, vol. 103, no. 5, pp. 735–741, 2009.

[31] J. Robin, K. Weinberg, J. Tiongson et al., "Renal dialysis as a risk factor for appropriate therapies and mortality in implantable cardioverter-defibrillator recipients," *Heart Rhythm*, vol. 3, no. 10, pp. 1196–1201, 2006.

[32] D. S. Lee, J. V. Tu, P. C. Austin et al., "Effect of cardiac and noncardiac conditions on survival after defibrillator implantation," *Journal of the American College of Cardiology*, vol. 49, no. 25, pp. 2408–2415, 2007.

[33] A. Wase, A. Basit, R. Nazir et al., "Impact of chronic kidney disease upon survival among implantable cardioverter-defibrillator recipients," *Journal of Interventional Cardiac Electrophysiology*, vol. 11, no. 3, pp. 199–204, 2004.

[34] J. I. Koontz, D. Haithcock, V. Cumbea et al., "Rationale and design of the Duke Electrophysiology Genetic and Genomic Studies (EPGEN) biorepository," *American Heart Journal*, vol. 158, no. 5, pp. 719–725, 2009.

[35] A. Dasgupta, J. Montalvo, S. Medendorp et al., "Increased complication rates of cardiac rhythm management devices in ESRD patients," *American Journal of Kidney Diseases*, vol. 49, no. 5, pp. 656–663, 2007.

[36] T. Kusaba, S. Tanda, H. Kameyama et al., "Efficacy of biventricular pacing for dialysis-related hypotension due to idiopathic dilated cardiomyopathy," *Clinical and Experimental Nephrology*, vol. 9, no. 3, pp. 255–259, 2005.

[37] F. G. Hage, W. AlJaroudi, H. Aggarwal et al., "Outcomes of patients with chronic kidney disease and implantable cardiac defibrillator: primary versus secondary prevention," *International Journal of Cardiology*, vol. 165, no. 1, pp. 113–116, 2013.

[38] N. Lam, P. Leong-Sit, and A. X. Garg, "The role of implantable cardioverter-defibrillators in long-term dialysis patients," *American Journal of Kidney Diseases*, vol. 58, no. 3, pp. 338–339, 2011.

[39] L. A. Cannizzaro, J. P. Piccini, U. D. Patel, and A. F. Hernandez, "Device therapy in heart failure patients with chronic kidney disease," *Journal of the American College of Cardiology*, vol. 58, no. 9, pp. 889–896, 2011.

[40] O. A. Ajijola, E. A. MacKlin, S. A. Moore et al., "Inpatient vs. elective outpatient cardiac resynchronization therapy device implantation and long-term clinical outcome," *Europace*, vol. 12, no. 12, pp. 1745–1749, 2010.

[41] J.-W. Chae, C. S. Song, H. Kim, K.-B. Lee, B.-S. Seo, and D.-I. Kim, "Prediction of mortality in patients undergoing maintenance hemodialysis by Charlson Comorbidity Index using ICD-10 database," *Nephron: Clinical Practice*, vol. 117, no. 4, pp. c379–c384, 2011.

[42] US Renal Data System, *USRDS 2010 Annual Data Report: Atlas of Chronic Kidney Disease and End-Stage Renal Disease in the United States*, National Institutes of Health, National Institute of Diabetes and Digestive and Kidney Diseases, Bethesda, Md, USA, 2010.

[43] A. J. Bleyer, G. B. Russell, and S. G. Satko, "Sudden and cardiac death rates in hemodialysis patients," *Kidney International*, vol. 55, no. 4, pp. 1553–1559, 1999.

[44] A. J. Bleyer, J. Hartman, P. C. Brannon, A. Reeves-Daniel, S. G. Satko, and G. Russell, "Characteristics of sudden death in hemodialysis patients," *Kidney International*, vol. 69, no. 12, pp. 2268–2273, 2006.

[45] J. C. de Oliveira, M. Martinelli, S. A. Nishioka et al., "Efficacy of antibiotic prophylaxis before the implantation of pacemakers and cardioverter-defibrillators: Results of a large, prospective, randomized, double-blinded, placebo-controlled trial," *Circulation: Arrhythmia and Electrophysiology*, vol. 2, pp. 29–34, 2009.

12

Factors Predicting Renal Function Outcome after Augmentation Cystoplasty

Shahbaz Mehmood,[1] **Raouf Seyam,**[1] **Sadia Firdous,**[2] **and Waleed Mohammad Altaweel**[1]

[1]*Department of Urology, King Faisal Specialist Hospital & Research Centre, P.O. Box 3354, Riyadh 11211, Saudi Arabia*
[2]*Fatima Jinnah Medical University, Lahore, Pakistan*

Correspondence should be addressed to Shahbaz Mehmood; shahbazmalik49@gmail.com
and Waleed Mohammad Altaweel; drwt1@hotmail.com

Academic Editor: Anil K. Agarwal

We determined the cause of renal deterioration after augmentation cystoplasty (AC). Twenty-nine adult patients with refractory bladder dysfunction and who underwent ileocystoplasty from 2004 to 2015 were studied. Patients with a decline in glomerular filtration rate (GFR) after augmentation were reviewed. The primary outcome was to determine the factors that might lead to deterioration of estimated GFR. Median follow-up was 7.0 ± 2.6 years. Significant bladder capacity, end filling pressure, and bladder compliance were achieved from median 114 ± 53.6 to 342.1 ± 68.3 ml ($p = .0001$), 68.5 ± 19.9 to 28.2 ± 6.9 cm H_2O ($p = .0001$), and 3.0 ± 2.1 to 12.8 ± 3.9 ($p = .0001$), respectively. Renal function remained stable and improved in 22 (76%) patients from median eGFR 135 ± 81.98 to 142.82 ± 94.4 ml/min/1.73 m^2 ($p = .160$). Significant deterioration was found in 7 (24%) patients from median eGFR 68.25 ± 42 to 36.57 ± 35.33 ($p = .001$). The causes of renal deterioration were noncompliance to self-catheterization (2 patients), posterior urethral valve/dysplastic kidneys (2 patients), and reflux/infection (2 patients). On multivariate analysis, recurrent pyelonephritis (OR 3.87, $p = 0.0155$) and noncompliance (OR 30.78, $p = 0.0156$) were significant. We concluded that AC is not the cause of progression to end-stage renal disease in patients with renal insufficiency.

1. Introduction

Augmentation cystoplasty (AC) has traditionally been used in the management of small capacity, poorly compliant, or refractory overactive bladder. Severe bladder dysfunction has deleterious effects on the upper renal tract in terms of renal function deterioration in both native and transplanted kidneys [1]. High storage pressure because of bladder dysfunction can cause vesicoureteric reflux and subsequently impair renal function [2]. It has been estimated that almost 15% of end-stage renal disease (ESRD) cases were caused by lower urinary tract dysfunction.

Various congenital anomalies may result in small capacity, poor compliance, and high intravesical pressure, which threaten upper tract function. When these bladder conditions are refractory to conservative therapy, augmentation cystoplasty is required to preserve renal function. These diverse groups of conditions include posterior urethral valve (PUV), bladder and cloacal exstrophy, and epispadias and myelomeningocele [3–5].

In properly selected patients, augmentation cystoplasty is an excellent procedure that provides a safe and effective way of improving urinary storage. It provides long-term therapy in patients with refractory neurogenic bladder, but stomal problems continue to be a source of complication in the continent outflow channel [6]. Bladder emptying is almost universally impaired, and the patient must be prepared to perform lifelong intermittent catheterization. The patient and physician must recognize the need for surveillance to identify potential problems. Stones, metabolic and nutritional abnormalities, renal insufficiency, and malignancy are best treated through early recognition and prompt therapy [7].

Augmentation cystoplasty is used in an attempt to preserve and improve renal function. In spite of this, deterioration in renal function has been observed in 0 to 15% of patients after augmentation cystoplasty [8]. A few authors proposed that this is because of baseline renal function status. Some authors argued that augmentation cystoplasty may hasten the ESRD, proposing chronic renal insufficiency to be a relative contraindication for augmentation cystoplasty [9]. Others are of the opinion that augmentation cystoplasty does not appear to cause renal function deterioration in patients with chronic renal insufficiency [10]. In another large retrospective cohort study, it was found that that deterioration of renal function after augmentation cystoplasty was strongly associated with preoperative diagnosis of lower urinary tract dysfunction. It was further concluded that impairment of renal function is likely related to primary pathology rather than augmentation cystoplasty [11].

In view of the above controversy, we need to know the exact etiopathogenesis of renal deterioration after augmentation cystoplasty. The primary objective of our study was to determine factors that might predict the progression rate of renal insufficiency in patients with severe lower urinary tract dysfunction treated with AC.

2. Material and Method

After approval from the Office of Research Administration, adult patients with refractory bladder dysfunction who underwent augmentation ileocystoplasty by a single surgeon from 2004 to 2015 were retrospectively reviewed. All patients had refractory bladder dysfunction because of neurogenic and nonneurogenic etiology exhausted from all conservative and minimally invasive treatment.

2.1. Inclusion and Exclusion Criteria. Our inclusion criteria considered all adult patients over the age of 18 years who presented with bladder dysfunction. All patients with small capacity, noncompliant bladder with high or normal intravesical pressures proven by urodynamic testing were included in the study. Patients who failed maximum conservative therapy with strict (CIC), anticholinergic medication, and minimally invasive therapy in the form of intravesical botulinum toxin therapy were chosen for the study. We excluded patients with ESRD already on renal replacement therapy or those who underwent staged pretransplant augmentation cystoplasty because renal deterioration cannot be determined in these patients. We also excluded those patients who underwent ureterocystoplasty or augmentation done in another hospital. Patients in which only continent reconstruction were done, such as creation of Mitrofanoff, Monte, and bladder neck reconstruction without AC, were also excluded.

Patient demographics, diagnosis, surgical details, pre and postoperative urodynamic parameters, renal function, and postoperative complications were abstracted from patient medical records at our institution. Renal function was determined by calculating eGFR at baseline and last clinical follow-up using and age appropriate MDRD formula, such as GFR (ml/min/1.73 m^2) = 186 × (Serum creatinine)$^{-1.154}$ × (age)$^{-0.203}$ × 0.742 (if female) × 1.212 (if black).

Patients were categorized according to the National Kidney Foundation criteria for Chronic Kidney Disease (CKD) on the basis of eGFR value in which stage 1 CKD is described as normal kidney function with eGFR > 90 ml/min/1.73 m^2,

stage 2 as kidney damage with a mildly decreased eGFR (60 to 89), stage 3 as moderately decreased eGFR (30 to 59), stage 4 as severely decreased eGFR (15 to 29), and stage 5 as kidney failure < 15 ml/min/1.73 m^2 or requiring dialysis. All patients had some form of renal insult due to vesicoureteral reflux (VUR), pyelonephritis, scarring, or dysplastic kidneys fulfilling the CKD criteria.

The primary outcome of this study was to see renal deterioration from baseline and determine factors that might lead to renal insufficiency. Secondary outcome is to determine overall complication rates after augmentation.

2.2. Statistical Analysis. Data were analyzed by using Statistical Analysis Software (SAS) V. 9.3. Renal function and urodynamic parameters were presented as median ± standard deviation. Statistical analysis was performed using paired Student's t-test and Fisher's exact test. Univariate logistic regression analysis was performed to identify independent predictors of renal function deterioration after AC. Variables attaining $p < .05$ on univariate analysis or considered clinically relevant were included in the multivariate analysis. p value < .05 was considered significant.

3. Results

Of the 41 patients who had undergone lower tract reconstruction, 29 patients, 16 males (55%) and 13 females (45%), met inclusion and exclusion criteria. Median age at ileocystoplasty was 26 ± 08 (range 17–55) years. Patients were followed up for a median of 7.0 ± 2.6 (range 1–10) years after lower urinary tract reconstruction. Primary diagnosis for lower urinary tract dysfunction was neurogenic in 62% of patients (myelomeningocele: 10; spinal cord injury: 3; sacral agenesis: 3; postspinal surgery: 2) and nonneurogenic in 38% of patients (PUV: 2; bladder exstrophy: 6; nonneurogenic bladder: 2; schistosomiasis: 1). Preoperative urodynamic parameter revealed that 24 out of 29 patients had small capacity, low compliance, and high intravesical pressure. Five patients had small capacity, low compliance, and normal intravesical pressure. Baseline renal function was normal (eGFR > 90 ml/min/1.73 m^2) in 18 of 29 patients (62%), 5 patients (17.24%) had CKD stage 2, 5 patients (17.24%) had CKD stage 3, and one patient had CKD stage 4. Bladder augmentation was done with ileum in all patients. Concomitant procedures included creation of continent outflow like Mitrofanoff in 14 patients, Monti neourethra in 2 patients, bilateral ureteric reimplantation in 2 patients, cecostomy button in 4 patients, bladder neck reconstruction in 4 patients, and pubovaginal sling in 3 patients. Two patients had nephrectomy for nonfunctioning kidney along with AC. The characteristics of study population are shown in Table 1.

Of the 18 patients with baseline normal renal function, 16 patients remained stable and improved their eGFR, except for 2 patients who progressed to CKD stage 2. One was having persistent vesicoureteral reflux and recurrent pyelonephritis confirmed on urine culture, voiding cystourethrogram (VCUG), and DMSA renal scan. The other patient was noncompliant to CIC and having high residual and recurrent urinary tract infection (UTI). Both patients remained stable

TABLE 1: Demographic data.

Total number of patients	29
Gender	
Male	16
Female	13
Median age (years)	26 ± 08 (17–55)
Median follow-up (years)	7.0 ± 2.6 (range 1–10)
Pre-op renal function	
Normal eGFR	18
CKD stage 2	05
CKD stage 3	05
CKD stage 4	01
Pre-op diagnosis	
(1) Neurogenic	18
MMC	10
SCI	03
SA	03
Postspinal surgery	02
(2) Nonneurogenic	11
PUV	02
BE	06
NNB	02
Schistosomiasis	01
Urodynamic findings	
Small capacity, low compliance, and high pressure	24
Small capacity, low compliance, and normal pressure	05
Additional procedures	
Mitrofanoff	14
Monti	02
Pubovaginal sling	03
B/L ureteric reimplantation	02
Bladder neck reconstruction	04
Cecostomy button	04

PUV = posterior urethral valve; MMC = myelomeningocele; BE = bladder exstrophy; SA = sacral agenesis; SCI = spinal cord injury; NNG = nonneurogenic neurogenic bladder.

TABLE 2: Categorization of patients on the basis of eGFR.

Groups	Preoperative eGFR	Postoperative eGFR	p value
eGFR > 90 ml/min/1.73 m^2 ($n = 18$)	160.4 ± 73.3	164.4 ± 91	.567
CKD 2 ($n = 05$)	70.4 ± 10.8	56.6 ± 28.2	.636
CKD 3 ($n = 5$)	40.2 ± 7.9	29.0 ± 21.4	.148
CKD 4 ($n = 01$)	19.0	10.0	n/a

augmentation. This patient experienced the complication of recurrent bladder and renal stones treated with PCNL, ESWL, and cystolithotripsy before progressing to ESRD.

Of the 5 patients with stage 3 CKD, one improved to stage 2, 2 remained stable at stage 3, and 2 deteriorated to ESRD and began hemodialysis. One of the 2 had a primary diagnosis of myelomeningocele and experienced persistent high intravesical pressure with recurrent symptomatic UTI. Another patient with posterior urethral valve fulgurated at childhood had dysplastic kidneys and renal scarring confirmed on renal ultrasound and DMSA renal scan. One patient had stage 4 CKD with fulgurated PUV and bilateral VUR as the primary diagnosis at the time of bladder augmentation and progressed to ESRD on follow-up. Overall, 22 patients (76%) remained stable and improved renal function ($p = .160$), and 07 patients (24%) deteriorated significantly from baseline ($p = .0001$) as shown in (Table 3).

We investigated certain factors (Table 4) in these progressive renal insufficiency patients after AC. Noncompliance to CIC, baseline creatinine, and preaugmentation renal insult, such as dysplastic kidneys, especially in patients with PUV, are some of the factors that might predict renal function deterioration after AC. Similarly persistent high intravesical pressure with VUR, recurrent symptomatic UTI, and metabolic disturbances are also factors that predict renal insufficiency on long-term follow-up after AC.

On univariate logistic regression analysis, factors like persistent vesicoureteral reflux (OR 13.333, 95% CI 1.65, 107.42, p value = .0150), recurrent pyelonephritis (OR = 125.97 95% CI 6.81, 999.99, p value = .0012), and noncompliance to CIC (OR = 52.500 95% CI 3.935, 700.52, p value = .0027) were found to be independent risks for renal function deterioration with respect to binary status, such as stable versus deteriorated renal function. When these significant factors were compared to each other on multivariate regression analysis, it was found that noncompliance to CIC was more significant (OR = 30.78, 95% CI = 1.913, 495.191, p value = .0156) than persistent vesicoureteral reflux (OR = 3.356, 95% CI = 0.193, 58.4, p value = .4064), and recurrent pyelonephritis was more significant (OR = 3.87, 95% CI = 2.089, 999.99, p value = .0155) than noncompliance to CIC (OR = 10.16, 95% CI = 0.314, 328.91, p value = .191). Although two patients had posterior urethral valves and both deteriorated, it was not found significant on univariate logistic regression analysis as shown in Table 5.

Regarding urodynamic study, patients achieved significant increase in bladder capacity with mean 342.1 ± 68.3 ml

after successful therapy on further follow-up. Categorization on the basis of eGFR is shown in Table 2.

Of the 5 patients with stage 2 CKD, 3 patients remained stable at stage 2. One patient progressed to stage 3, and the other progressed to ESRD. Both patients had a solitary functioning kidney, with contralateral nephrectomy done for nonfunctioning status along with bladder augmentation. Stage 3 patient had grade 5 reflux in the remaining kidney managed with ureteric reimplantation and strict CIC.

Renal function remained stable at stage 3 on further follow-up. One patient was incontinent and underwent bladder neck closure with Mitrofanoff created along with bladder

TABLE 3: Overall stabilized and deteriorated renal function patients.

Category	Number of patients	Preoperative eGFR (ml/min/1.73 m²)	Postoperative eGFR (ml/min/1.73 m²)	p value
Stabilized/improved renal function	22 (76%)	135.50 ± 81.98	142.82 ± 94.45	.160
Deteriorated renal function	07 (24%)	68.29 ± 42.01	36.57 ± 35.33	.001

TABLE 4: Factors predicting renal deterioration.

S. number	Diagnosis	Pre-op Cr.	Post-op Cr.	Pre-op eGFR	Post-op eGFR	Probable cause of renal deterioration
1	MMC	73	98	120	85 (CKD 2)	Persistent VUR & recurrent UTI
2	BE	56	79	122	82 (CKD 2)	Noncompliance to CIC, recurrent pyelonephritis
3	MMC	102	157	83 (CKD 2)	50 (CKD 3)	Solitary left kidney with grade 4 reflux treated with ureteric reimplant, stabilized at CKD 3
4	MMC	120	612	66 (CKD 2)	10 (CKD 5)	Solitary kidneys with bladder neck closure and Mitrofanoff created having bladder & kidneys stone, noncompliant to CIC
5	MMC	250	426	30 (CKD 3)	6 (CKD 5)	Persistent high intravesical pressure, recurrent pyelonephritis, incontinent
6	PUV	200	510	38 (CKD 3)	13 (CKD 5)	Dysplastic & scarred kidneys
7	PUV(B/L VUR)	280	504	19 (CKD 4)	10 (CKD 5)	Dysplastic & scarred kidneys

(p = .0001), decrease in end filling pressure 28.1 ± 6.9 cm H_2O (p = .0001), and significant increase in bladder compliance 12.8 ± 3.9 ml/cm H_2O (p = .0001) measured with formula: bladder compliance = $\Delta v/\Delta p$. This represents a 300% increase in bladder capacity (Table 6).

Regarding early complications, 2 patients who failed conservative management developed gross hematuria and underwent cystoscopy and coagulation of bleeding sites from augmented ileovesical junction. Three patients developed vesicocutaneous fistula; 2 were managed by keeping suprapubic and urethral catheter for one extra week. One patient was diverted with nephrostomy tubes and urethral and suprapubic catheter. Wound infection was found in 3 patients who were treated with IV antibiotics according to swab culture. Three patients were incontinent and two developed ileus managed conservatively (Table 7).

Three patients sustained bladder perforation. Although this is a dreadful complication, especially in neurogenic patients, we successfully managed all these cases by performing laparotomy and closure of the perforation. Perforation was found at ileovesical junction in all three cases. Mucus retention was also detected in all of the cases, which was primarily due to noncompliance of manual bladder irrigation and CIC. Two patients developed kidneys stones, and 5 patients got bladder stones, which were treated with ESWL, URS laser lithotripsy, and cystolitholapaxy, respectively. Out

of 5 patients who complained of persistence of incontinence, 3 patients were managed with bladder neck reconstruction, with macroplastique injection at bladder neck, and 2 patients were managed successfully with anticholinergic medications. We did not find a single patient with bladder malignancy in our series.

Asymptomatic bacteriuria was found in most of the patients as >90% of our patients were doing CIC. Asymptomatic bacteriuria was found in 57% (15/29) of patients, and febrile UTI was found in 17% (05/29) of patients which were managed with oral or intravenous antibiotics according to culture and sensitivity and hemodynamic status of the patients.

4. Discussion

The primary objective of our study was to assess long-term renal function and to determine factors that might lead to deterioration of renal function after AC at our institution. The therapeutic goal of AC is to create low-pressure storage, large capacity, and a continent urinary reservoir. Decreased compliance and high pressure storage put the upper tract at risk for renal deterioration. Wang et al. [12] presented the deleterious effect of high detrusor leak point pressure on the upper urinary tract by calculating urodynamic risk score including a detrusor leak point pressure (DLPP) >40 cm

TABLE 5: Predictive factors for renal function deterioration on univariate logistic and multivariate regression analysis.

Serial number	Predictive factors	Univariate analysis		Multivariate analysis	
		OR (95% CI)	p value	OR (95% CI)	p value
1	Persistent vesicoureteral reflux	13.333 (1.65, 107.42)	.0150	3.356 (0.193, 58.4)	.4064
2	Recurrent pyelonephritis	125.97 (6.81, 999.99)	.0012	3.87 (2.089, 999.99)	.0155
3	Solitary kidney with reflux	999.99 (0.001, 999.99)	.963		
4	Noncompliance to CIC	52.500 (3.935, 700.52)	.0027	30.78 (1.913, 495.191)	.0156
5	High pressure reservoir	13.556 (0.001, 999.99)	.963	—	—
6	Posterior urethral valves (PUV) with scarring and dysplasia	13.55 (0.001, 999.99)	.963	—	—
7	Renal/bladder stone/recurrent pyelonephritis	0.567 (0.055, 5.88)	.634	—	—
8	Solitary kidney without reflux	0.001 (.001)	.9831	—	—

TABLE 6: Pre- and postoperative urodynamic parameters.

Variables	Preoperative mean $\pm$ SD (range)	Preoperative mean $\pm$ SD (range)	p value
Mean capacity (ml)	114 ± 53.6 (40–270)	342.1 ± 68.3 (220–520)	.0001
Mean end filling pressure (cm H_2O)	68.5 ± 19.9 (34–98)	28.2 ± 6.9 (18–45)	.0001
Compliance (ml/cm H_2O)	3.0 ± 2.1 (.3 to 9.2)	12.8 ± 3.9 (7.1–21.6)	.0001

TABLE 7: Early and late complications.

	Number
Early complications	
Gross hematuria	2
Vesicocutaneous fistula	3
Incontinence	3
Ileus	2
Wound infection	3
Late complications	
Bladder perforation	03
Mucus retention	03
Bladder & kidney stones	05
Incontinence	05
Renal deterioration	07
Febrile UTI	07
Malignancy	Nil

H_2O, bladder compliance of <9 mL/cm H_2O, and evidence of an acontractile detrusor, in children with neurogenic lower urinary tract dysfunction. They found these three factors to be the main risk factors for upper tract dilatation and subsequent renal damage. None of them had reflux when DLPP was <40 cm H_2O.

There is some controversy among authors on the role of AC in the preservation of renal function. A few studies have addressed this important issue [13, 14]. All of these showed good preservation of renal function after AC. Significant renal insufficiency is a more controversial relative contraindication. Few studies have addressed this issue in detail. Küss et al. [15] found that augmentation of patients with a creatinine clearance of >15 mL/min/1.73 m^2 was associated with a 44% deterioration of renal function in one series while only 4.1% of renal deterioration was found when clearance was >40 ml/min/1.73 m^2 [16]. They attested that this renal

impairment may result in an inability to cope with the metabolic complication of AC.

In our series, AC stabilized and improved renal function in (n = 22) 76% of the patients, and 24% of the patients deteriorated to various stages. We found certain factors that can stabilize deteriorated renal function when corrected promptly. Fontaine et al. [17] achieved similar results. They observed that results of 10 years of follow-up study of AC in 53 patients showed that 19% of the patients experienced renal function deterioration expressed by a decrease in GFR of more than 20%. The most common reason for renal deterioration in these patients was chronic retention or infection because of inadequate catheterization due to poor compliance.

In younger age groups, the persistence of VUR after AC and its associated febrile UTI can impair renal function by recurrent pyelonephritis and renal scarring. Two of the patients in our series were having persistent VUR in their solitary functioning kidney. One of them stabilized after ureteric reimplantation. Soygur et al. found the necessity of ureteric reimplant after AC and observed that renal scarring and febrile UTI caused by VUR can impair renal function [18]. AC increases bladder compliance, by lowering intravesical pressure during the urinary storage phase; so in most cases, reflux improves after AC, making reimplantation unnecessary [19]. In our series asymptomatic bacteriuria was 57% (n = 15/29) and febrile UTI were found in 17% of our patients. Febrile UTI patients were treated with either IV or oral antibiotics according to sensitivity and patient's hemodynamic status. Greenwell et al. [20] found the same frequency of asymptomatic bacteriuria of 75% and troublesome febrile UTI of 20% in patients on CIC with AC.

More than 90% of our patients were on CIC. Three of our deteriorated patients were noncompliant to CIC associated with high residual and recurrent febrile UTI and pyelonephritis. One progressed to CKD 2 from normal eGFR > 90 ml/min/1.73 m^2 and was stabilized at CKD 2 when CIC was enforced, and the other two progressed to ESRD from CKD 2 and CKD 3. These last two patients had other risk factors, such as solitary kidney complicated with bladder and renal stones, along with noncompliance to CIC. Noncompliance or inability to perform CIC is a relative contraindication to AC. Intermittent self-catheterization is simple, safe, and effective but underused procedure mandatory in neuropathic bladder, postoperative retention, and following bladder reconstruction like AC [21]. Intermittent catheterization preserves the upper urinary tract by eliminating residual urine, decreasing intravesical pressure, and reducing urinary infection. CIC is excellent in the preservation of the upper urinary tract. Noncompliance to CIC deteriorates renal function with reported range of 0 to 14% in various series [22]. Dik et al. stated that early start of therapy in the form of CIC and anticholinergic medications preserve renal function in patients with neuropathic bladder dysfunction and deteriorate in patients who were noncompliant to CIC [23].

We failed to achieve low intravesical pressure and higher compliance bladder and were unable to relieve lower urinary tract symptoms in one patient (3.44%) with myelomeningocele in our series. Unfortunately, that patient progressed to ESRD and required revision AC surgery before proceeding to renal transplantation. Failure of AC to relieve lower urinary tract symptoms and urodynamic parameter required to preserve upper tract has been reported in 5 to 42% of the patients in various studies [24, 25]. The success rate is lower in idiopathic detrusor overactivity patients (53–58%) [26] when compared to the higher success rate (almost 92%) reported in neuropathic patients [27].

A primary diagnosis of PUV is a nonmodifiable factor that has the worst prognosis in terms of renal function deterioration. PUV can lead to deleterious effects on bladder and renal function in long-term follow-up [28]. Renal function in PUV patients depends upon various well-known factors like age at presentation, GFR, renal dysplasia, VUR, renal scarring, extent of bladder dysfunction, and UTI. As many as 25 to 60% of PUV patients may have significant renal function impairment despite efforts made to treat these patients in long-term follow-up [29].

Two patients with primary diagnosis of PUV, one with CKD stage 3 and other with stage 4, progressed to ESRD after AC. Both patients had renal dysplasia and scarring on USG and DMSA scans. In contrast, congenital renal deterioration is rare in exstrophy patients before surgical reconstruction. Therefore, renal dysplasia, scarring, or intrauterine nephropathy can be ruled out as a cause of subsequent renal function deterioration [30]. One out of 6 bladder exstrophy patients deteriorated from normal renal function to CKD 2 due to noncompliance to CIC and recurrent UTI. We managed this patient with antibiotics, reeducated and reenforced to do CIC. This patient stabilized at CKD 2 on further follow-up.

These data show that overall AC stabilized and improved renal function in 76% of patients, and 24% deteriorated from baseline. We found certain remedial and nonmodifiable factors that lead to deterioration of renal function. Out of 7 deteriorated patients, 2 had primary PUV diagnosis and had

inherent disease that lead to ESRD. All other factors like noncompliance to CIC, persistent VUR, recurrent pyelonephritis, and high pressure reservoir are modifiable when corrected lead to stabilization of kidney functions. Our data showed that close follow-up is essential in deteriorated patients to search for early modifiable factors. Although baseline renal function and primary diagnosis are significant, we need to correct modifiable factors to stabilize and at least prolong the time to develop ESRD after AC.

The strengths of our study are its long-term follow-up and detailed renal function analysis using eGFR. We admit methodologic constraints of retrospective analysis and low number of patients as main limitation of this study. The result of this study might not be generalized because of small sample size and heterogeneous group of the patients. Missing data and selection bias are inherent limitation of any retrospective study. Furthermore, our investigation is not without limitation. Serum creatinine was used to calculate eGFR which is only reliable in individuals in a steady state. The most important factors affecting serum creatinine are hydration status, exposure to contrast dye, variation in diet, muscle mass, and urinary tract infection. We did not control any of these factors in our retrospective analysis. However, the widespread clinical use of creatinine measurement makes it frequently available for analysis.

5. Conclusion

There is no evidence that AC causes renal damage. Close follow-up is necessary in patients with deteriorated renal function to search for remedial and modifiable factors that lead to renal function deterioration.

Disclosure

Proposal of this study was accepted by Office of Research Assistance (ORA) committee in our hospital.

References

[1] C. A. Sheldon, R. Gonzalez, M. W. Burns, A. Gilbert, H. Buson, and M. E. Mitchell, "Renal transplantation into the dysfunctional bladder: the role of adjunctive bladder reconstruction," *Journal of Urology*, vol. 152, no. 3, pp. 972–975, 1994.

[2] U. Sillén, P. Brandström, U. Jodal et al., "The swedish reflux trial in children: V. bladder dysfunction," *Journal of Urology*, vol. 184, no. 1, pp. 298–304, 2010.

[3] V. Bhatnagar, S. Dave, S. Agarwala, and D. K. Mitra, "Augmentation colocystoplasty in bladder exstrophy," *Pediatric Surgery International*, vol. 18, no. 1, pp. 43–49, 2002.

[4] J. C. Austin, "Long-term risks of bladder augmentation in pediatric patients," *Current Opinion in Urology*, vol. 18, no. 4, pp. 408–412, 2008.

[5] M. Youssif, H. Badawy, A. Saad, A. Hanno, and I. Mokhless, "Augmentation ureterocystoplasty in boys with valve bladder syndrome," *Journal of Pediatric Urology*, vol. 3, no. 6, pp. 433–437, 2007.

[6] J. G. Blaivas, J. P. Weiss, P. Desai, A. J. Flisser, D. S. Stember, and P. J. Stahl, "Long-term followup of augmentation enterocystoplasty and continent diversion in patients with benign disease," *Journal of Urology*, vol. 173, no. 5, pp. 1631–1634, 2005.

[7] P. M. S. Gurung, K. H. Attar, A. Abdul-Rahman, T. Morris, R. Hamid, and P. J. R. Shah, "Long-term outcomes of augmentation ileocystoplasty in patients with spinal cord injury: a minimum 10-year follow-up," *BJU International*, 2011.

[8] D. A. Husmann, "Long-term complications following bladder augmentations in patients with spina bifida: bladder calculi, perforation of the augmented bladder and upper tract deterioration," *Translational Andrology and Urology*, vol. 5, no. 1, pp. 3–11, 2016.

[9] E. J. Alfrey, O. Salvatierra Jr., D. C. Tanney et al., "Bladder augmentation can be problematic with renal failure and transplantation," *Pediatric Nephrology*, vol. 11, no. 6, pp. 672–675, 1997.

[10] V. Ivančić, W. DeFoor, E. Jackson et al., "Progression of renal insufficiency in children and adolescents with neuropathic bladder is not accelerated by lower urinary tract reconstruction," *Journal of Urology*, vol. 184, no. 4, pp. 1768–1774, 2010.

[11] B. J. Schlomer and H. L. Copp, "Cumulative incidence of outcomes and urologic procedures after augmentation cystoplasty," *Journal of Pediatric Urology*, vol. 10, no. 6, pp. 1043–1049, 2014.

[12] Q. W. Wang, J. G. Wen, D. K. Song et al., "Is it possible to use urodynamic variables to predict upper urinary tract dilatation in children with neurogenic bladder-sphincter dysfunction?" *BJU International*, vol. 98, no. 6, pp. 1295–1300, 2006.

[13] A. Kristjansson and W. Mansson, "Renal function in the setting of urinary diversion," *World Journal of Urology*, vol. 22, no. 3, pp. 172–177, 2004.

[14] G. Abd-el-Gawad, K. Abrahamsson, E. Hanson et al., "Kock urinary reservoir maturation in children and adolescents: consequences for kidney and upper urinary tract," *European Urology*, vol. 36, no. 5, pp. 443–449, 1999.

[15] R. Küss, M. Bitker, M. Camey, C. Chatelain, and J. P. Lassau, "Indications and early and late results of intestino-cystoplasty: a review of 185 cases," *Journal of Urology*, vol. 103, no. 1, pp. 53–63, 1970.

[16] R. M. Decter, S. B. Bauer, J. Mandell, A. H. Colodny, and A. B. Retik, "Small bowel augmentation in children with neurogenic bladder: an initial report of urodynamic findings," *Journal of Urology*, vol. 138, no. 4, pp. 1014–1016, 1987.

[17] E. Fontaine, R. Leaver, and C. R. J. Woodhouse, "The effect of intestinal urinary reservoirs on renal function: a 10-year follow-up," *BJU International*, vol. 86, no. 3, pp. 195–198, 2000.

[18] T. Soygur, B. Burgu, A. Zümrütbas, and E. Süer, "The need for ureteric re-implantation during augmentation cystoplasty: video-urodynamic evaluation," *BJU International*, vol. 105, no. 4, pp. 530–532, 2010.

[19] Y. Soylet, H. Emir, Z. Ilce, E. Yesildag, S. N. C. Buyukunal, and N. Danismend, "Quo vadis? Ureteric reimplantation or ignoring reflux during augmentation cystoplasty," *BJU International*, vol. 94, no. 3, pp. 379–380, 2004.

[20] T. J. Greenwell, S. N. Venn, and A. R. Mundy, "Augmentation cystoplasty," *BJU International*, vol. 88, no. 6, pp. 511–525, 2001.

[21] J. J. Wyndaele, "Complications of intermittent catheterization: their prevention and treatment," *Spinal Cord*, vol. 40, no. 10, pp. 536–541, 2002.

[22] G. Holmdahl, U. Sillén, A.-L. Hellström et al., "Does treatment with clean intermittent catheterization in boys with posterior urethral valves affect bladder and renal function?" *Journal of Urology*, vol. 170, no. 4, pp. 1681–1685, 2003.

[23] P. Dik, A. J. Klijn, J. D. van Gool, C. C. E. de Jong-de Vos van Steenwijk, and T. P. V. M. de Jong, "Early start to therapy preserves kidney function in spina bifida patients," *European Urology*, vol. 49, no. 5, pp. 908–913, 2006.

[24] C. Edlund, R. Peeker, and M. Fall, "Clam ileocystoplasty: successful treatment of severe bladder overactivity," *Scandinavian Journal of Urology and Nephrology*, vol. 35, no. 3, pp. 190–195, 2001.

[25] B. Shekarriz, J. Upadhyay, S. Demirbilek, J. Spencer Barthold, and R. González, "Surgical complications of bladder augmentation: comparison between various enterocystoplasties in 133 patients," *Urology*, vol. 55, no. 1, pp. 123–128, 2000.

[26] P. Reyblat and D. A. Ginsberg, "Augmentation cystoplasty: what are the indications?" *Current Urology Reports*, vol. 9, no. 6, pp. 452–458, 2008.

[27] F. Obermayr, P. Szavay, J. Schaefer, and J. Fuchs, "Outcome of augmentation cystoplasty and bladder substitution in a pediatric age group," *European Journal of Pediatric Surgery*, vol. 21, no. 2, pp. 116–119, 2011.

[28] P. Caione and S. G. Nappo, "Posterior urethral valves: long-term outcome," *Pediatric Surgery International*, vol. 27, no. 10, pp. 1027–1035, 2011.

[29] P. Lopez Pereira, L. Espinosa, M. J. Martinez Urrutina, R. Lobato, M. Navarro, and E. Jaureguizar, "Posterior urethral valves: prognostic factors," *BJU International*, vol. 91, no. 7, pp. 687–690, 2003.

[30] P. C. Gargollo, J. G. Borer, D. A. Diamond et al., "Prospective followup in patients after complete primary repair of bladder exstrophy," *Journal of Urology*, vol. 180, no. 4, pp. 1665–1670, 2008.

13

Arterial Stiffness and Renal Replacement Therapy: A Controversial Topic

Edmundo Cabrera Fischer,[1,2] Yanina Zócalo,[3] Cintia Galli,[1,2] Sandra Wray,[1] and Daniel Bia[3]

[1]*Favaloro University (AIDUF-CONICET), Solís 453, C1078AAI Buenos Aires, Argentina*
[2]*Technological National University, C1179AAQ Buenos Aires, Argentina*
[3]*Physiology Department, School of Medicine, CUiiDARTE, Republic University, 11800 Montevideo, Uruguay*

Correspondence should be addressed to Daniel Bia; dbia@fmed.edu.uy

Academic Editor: Francesca Mallamaci

The increase of arterial stiffness has been to have a significant impact on predicting mortality in end-stage renal disease patients. Pulse wave velocity (PWV) is a noninvasive, reliable parameter of regional arterial stiffness that integrates the vascular geometry and arterial wall intrinsic elasticity and is capable of predicting cardiovascular mortality in this patient population. Nevertheless, reports on PWV in dialyzed patients are contradictory and sometimes inconsistent: some reports claim the arterial wall stiffness increases (i.e., PWV increase), others claim that it is reduced, and some even state that it augments in the aorta while it simultaneously decreases in the brachial artery pathway. The purpose of this study was to analyze the literature in which longitudinal or transversal studies were performed in hemodialysis and/or peritoneal dialysis patients, in order to characterize arterial stiffness and the responsiveness to renal replacement therapy.

1. Introduction

Hemodialyzed and peritoneal dialysis patients are currently evaluated in order to detect structural and functional alterations in the arterial tree. Since it has been demonstrated that renal function replacement therapy significantly improves survival rates of end-stage renal disease (ESRD) patients, the improvement of biochemical and hemodynamic parameters is desirable aims. Nevertheless, the underlying mechanism by which these improvements occur is not entirely understood, and not all cardiovascular parameters tend to reach their normal values. Pulse wave velocity (PWV) is a well-known independent predictor of cardiovascular disease that is currently obtained by using a simple, noninvasive technique. This method to quantify arterial stiffness has been used during the last decades, and a good number of analyses have been reported, including longitudinal studies. Furthermore, cross-sectional studies were performed, including the comparative analysis between hemodialysis and peritoneal dialysis patients. Nevertheless, the relationship between renal replacement therapy and arterial stiffness remains unclear, since the research results are controversial; sometimes they are inconsistent and other times it is not possible to compare them.

The purpose of this work was to analyze the literature in which longitudinal or transversal studies were performed in hemodialysis and/or peritoneal dialysis patients and (1) to summarize the effects of the dialysis modality on arterial stiffness and (2) to comment on the relationship of arterial stiffness impairment with the etiological factors mentioned in the revised literature. For practical reasons, the text was organized taking into account the dialysis modality and the nature of the research: whether it is a transversal or a longitudinal study. When comparisons among the reported researches were feasible, the results were included in tables.

2. Arterial Stiffness and End-Stage Renal Diseases

In recent years, great emphasis has been placed on the role of arterial stiffness in the development of cardiovascular diseases. Aortic stiffness, which results in increased pulse pressure (PP), cardiac overload, and left ventricular hypertrophy, is an established predictor for cardiovascular morbidity and mortality in several disease (i.e., chronic kidney disease, CKD). Indeed, the assessment of arterial stiffness is increasingly used in the clinical assessment of patients.

Basically, arterial stiffness can be measured "systemically" (the cardiovascular system as a whole), "regionally" (large arterial segments or pathways), or locally (arterial rings or short arterial segments) [1, 2]. In contrast to systemic arterial stiffness, which can only be estimated from models of the circulation (i.e., Windkessel model), regional and local arterial stiffness can be measured directly and noninvasively, at various sites along the arterial tree. A major advantage of the regional and local evaluations of arterial stiffness is that they are based on direct measurements of parameters strongly linked to wall stiffness [1, 2]. Local arterial stiffness is directly determined, from the change in pressure driving the change in arterial diameter (distension or volume). However, because it requires a high degree of technical expertise and different techniques (i.e., pressure measurement using applanation tonometry and diameter measurement using ultrasound) and takes longer than measuring "regional stiffness", local measurement of arterial stiffness is only really indicated for mechanistic analyses in pathophysiology, pharmacology, and therapeutics, rather than for epidemiological or clinical studies [1, 2].

In contrast, the measurement of arterial pulse wave velocity (PWV: a regional stiffness marker) is generally accepted as the most simple, noninvasive, robust, and reproducible method to determine arterial regional stiffness. Measured along the aortic and aortoiliac pathway, it is the most clinically relevant, since the aorta and its first branches are what the left ventricle "sees" and are thus responsible for most of the pathophysiological effects of arterial stiffness. Carotid-femoral PWV has been used in the epidemiological studies demonstrating the predictive value of aortic stiffness for cardiovascular events. In contrast, PWV measured outside the aortic pathway (i.e., at the upper or lower limb) allows determining the arterial stiffness in those regions but has no predictive value. The Moens-Korteweg equation states that PWV is proportional to the square root of the incremental elastic modulus (E_{inc}) of the vessel wall given constant ratio of wall thickness, h, to vessel radius, r, and blood density, ρ, assuming that that the artery wall is isotropic and experiences isovolumetric change with pulse pressure [1, 2]:

$$\text{PWV} = \sqrt{\frac{E_{inc} \cdot h}{2r\rho}}. \tag{1}$$

Epidemiological studies in almost all populations have clearly shown that aging is the most determinant risk factor for cardiovascular diseases. This age-associated risk for the development of cardiovascular complications is associated with numerous normal or physiological deleterious changes in the structure and function of the arterial system (i.e., increase in aortic PWV) [3]. Among the most characteristic changes associated with aging are central arteries stiffening and remodeling (i.e., intima and/or media layers thickness increase, increased length, and tortuousness) of large arteries.

The degeneration of elastic (elastine) fibers is associated with an increase in collagen fibers and ground substance and depositions of calcium. In this context, in end-stage renal disease (ESRD) patients the arterial structural and functional changes are characterized by an accelerated influence of aging [4]. Premature or early vascular aging (EVA syndrome) are observed with progression of CKD and in ESRD. This accelerated aging is associated with outward remodeling of large and medium arteries, characterized by an increased arterial diameter not totally compensated for by artery wall thickness increase. In addition, despite the fact that deposition of calcium salts in the walls of human arteries is a "normal or physiologically" inevitable consequence of aging, the extent of calcifications is more pronounced in ESRD [4]. As will be discussed, arterial stiffening in CKD and ESRD patients is of multifactorial origin.

3. Hemodialysis and Arterial Stiffness

3.1. Transversal Studies. As was mentioned, the role of vascular calcifications has been pointed out as a determinant factor associated to arterial aging. In 2013, London et al. reported that the incremental elastic modulus (E_{inc}, i.e., the arterial wall stiffness) of the carotid artery was increased in hemodialyzed patients [4]. This research included 155 hemodialyzed patients whose age (abscissa) versus arterial stiffness (ordinate) relationship (x/y graph) was higher (a significantly steeper slope) than that obtained in 105 healthy control subjects. Curiously, in the same cohort of hemodialyzed patients, the age versus arterial stiffness relationship of patients without arterial calcifications was lower than that obtained in healthy subjects. This finding is coincident with those reported (by our group) in an animal model of arterial calcinosis [5]. On the contrary, hemodialyzed patients with carotid calcification showed the highest age versus arterial stiffness relationship. Since the age versus arterial stiffness relationship of the noncalcified hemodialyzed patients is lower than that obtained in the healthy cohort, the beneficial role of renal replacement therapy could be ensured. Calcinosis of the media in hemodialysis patients has been linked to increases of arterial stiffness by several authors [6, 7].

On the other hand, an interesting research by Shinohara and coworkers, published a decade ago, demonstrated that hemodialysis has no adverse effects on renal replacement therapy when compared to uremic predialysis patients [8]. The authors emphasized on the active role of the control of metabolic alterations patients have in ESRD (Table 1). The probably most important finding of this research was that hemodialysis patients ($n = 144$) showed significantly lower PWV values ($p < 0.05$) than predialysis patients ($n = 71$).

3.2. Longitudinal Studies. In 2001, Guerin and coworkers reported a follow-up (51 ± 38 months) of 150 hemodialyzed patients in which the decrease of PWV values in response to blood pressure declined was associated with a significant improvement of survival rates, which was attributed to the use of ACE inhibitors [9]. The authors divided the patients into blood pressure responders and nonresponders and

TABLE 1: Arterial (Aortic) stiffness in hemodialyzed patients.

	cfPWV in HD	Longitudinal study	Transversal study
Shinohara et al., 2004 [8]	Decrease (1)		X
Charitaki and Davenport, 2013 [13]	Increase (1)	X	
London et al., 2001* [14]	Decrease (2)	X	
London et al., 2001** [14]	Increase (2)	X	
Utescu et al., 2013 [11]	Increase (3)	X	

Pulse wave velocity in the carotid-femoral pathway (cfPWV) was measured in hemodialyzed patients (HD).
*Responders: patients having a decrease of left ventricular mass by >10% after follow-up.
**Nonresponders: patients having an increase of left ventricular mass or decrease <10% after follow-up.
(1) With respect to predialysis values obtained in uremic patients.
(2) With respect to patients receiving hemodialysis for at least 3 months.
(3) With respect to baseline values obtained in hemodialyzed patients (mean = 2.3 years).

emphasized on the fact that normalization of mean arterial pressure *per se* was unable to determine a decrease in mortality.

In 2005, Takenaka and Suzuki demonstrated that patients in hemodialysis ($n = 15$) showed a significant increase of PWV in a short period of six months (from 11.82 ± 0.54 m/sec to 14.56 ± 1.20 m/sec; $p < 0.05$). Following the mentioned impairment of the arterial stiffness, the same cohort of patients significantly decreased their PWV values after six months of administration of Sevelamer (13.34 ± 0.90 m/sec). In this small cohort, patients with marked hyperparathyroidism and/or receiving Vitamin D pulse therapy were excluded [10].

An interesting study was carried out by a Canadian group in hemodialyzed patients after a follow-up of 1.2 years [11]. Surprisingly, in this cohort the aortic (carotid-femoral) PWV increased (from 13.27 m/s to 14.26 m/s; $p < 0.001$) (Table 1) and the carotid-radial PWV decreased (from 8.80 m/s to 8.05 m/s; $p < 0.001$) although no convincing argument was provided about this rather strange finding.

A 36-month follow-up of hemodialyzed patients ($n = 80$) and general population patients ($n = 60$) concluded that arterial stiffening was accelerated in hemodialyzed patients. Furthermore, the authors mentioned that cholesterol and uremia-related factors were determinants of the increased arterial stiffness in hemodialyzed patients [12].

Recently, a group from London (United Kingdom) analyzed the relationship of dialysate calcium concentrations on aortic PWV in 289 hemodialysis patients [13]. Arterial stiffness was measured in four subgroups of patients at the beginning of the research and after six months, during which four different calcium concentrations were used. The authors concluded that PWV increased in the whole population ($p < 0.001$), with no changes in the augmentation index (a wave reflection parameter) nor in central (aortic) blood pressure. No significant changes in PWV were found at the start or end of the study in the four subgroups. It was observed that PWV increased in the subgroup of hemodialyzed patients using the lowest dialysate calcium over the six months study. The authors concluded that factors other than the calcium concentration used during hemodialysis are involved in arterial stiffening.

The effects of hemodialysison aortic stiffness have been reported in an old paper by London and coworkers, whose purpose was to study the left ventricular hypertrophy and survival of 153 hemodialyzed patients [14]. The follow-up period was 54 ± 37 months and baseline value of PWV was 11.15 ± 2.70 m/s versus 11.03 ± 3.18 m/s at the end of follow-up, showing a nonsignificant decrease. According to the response in terms of left ventricular hypertrophy, this cohort was divided into responders (decreased by > 10%) and nonresponders (increased or decreased by < 10%); interestingly the responders significantly decreased PWV at the end of the follow-up period (from a baseline value of 11.37 ± 2.80 m/s to 10.18 ± 2.57 m/s; $p < 0.001$). See Table 1.

This distinct response to hemodialysis was not observed in a five-year follow-up of 25 hemodialyzed patients carried out by our group (Argentina and Uruguay), in which a significant decrease of carotid-femoral pulse wave velocity was demonstrated [15].

4. Peritoneal Dialysis and Arterial Stiffness

4.1. Transversal Studies. Brachial-ankle PWV (a parameter influenced for the aortic and lower-limb arterial stiffness levels) has been used to analyze the correlation between arterial stiffness and several different parameters in a sample of peritoneal dialysis patients in Macao, China [16]. The patients included in the study ($n = 96$) were divided into two groups: (a) low brachial-ankle PWV group including those patients with values below the mean value of the entire population and (b) high brachial-ankle PWV group including those patients with values higher than the mean value of the entire population. The latter were significantly older than the former and included a high proportion of females ($p < 0.004$). The whole population of peritoneal dialysis patients showed that brachial-ankle PWV is independently correlated with age, serum albumin level C-reactive protein, and residual renal creatinine clearance.

4.2. Longitudinal Studies. Szeto and coworkers affirmed, in a very simple way, that peritoneal dialysis patients significantly increased carotid-femoral PWV in 24 months [17]. This increase was also observed in carotid-radial PWV. In contrast, Tang and coworkers showed that a PWV improvement found in peritoneal dialysis patients is associated with modifiable risk factors [18]. The authors found that 23% of patients undergo a decrease of carotid-femoral PWV values after a six-month follow-up, compared to the baseline data (Table 2). The outcomes in PWV obtained in these peritoneal dialysis patients were divided into "progressors" (increases higher than 1 m/s or 15% between baselines to 6-month follow-up) and "regressors" (decreases lower than 1 m/s or 15% between baselines to 6-month follow-up).

TABLE 2: Arterial (aortic) stiffness in peritoneal dialysis patients.

	cfPWV in PD	Longitudinal study	Transversal study
Demirci et al., 2012* [19]	Increase (1)		X
Demirci et al., 2012** [19]	Decrease (1)		X
Szeto et al., 2012 [17]	Increase (2)		X
Tang et al., 2012* [18]	Increase (3)		X
Tang et al., 2012** [18]	Decrease (1)		X

Pulse wave velocity in the carotid-femoral pathway (cfPWV) was measured in peritoneal dialysis (PD) patients.
*Progressors: patients having an increase of cfPWV after follow-up.
**Regressors: patients having a decrease of cfPWV after follow-up.
(1) With respect to baseline values obtained in peritoneal dialysis patients for at least 6 months.
(2) With respect to baseline values obtained in peritoneal dialysis patients for at least 6 months.
(3) With respect to baseline values obtained in the first week of PD training.

Coincidentally with the above-mentioned publication of Tang et al., another study in which the cohort outcome of peritoneal dialysis patients was divided was reported by Demirci and coworkers [19]. They analyzed carotid-femoral PWV in 89 peritoneal dialysis patients at baseline and after a nine-month follow-up. Patients with an aortic PWV variation higher than 5% were considered progressors, and, on the contrary, patients with equal or lower values than 5% of variation were considered nonprogressors (Table 2). Patients included in the nonprogressor group showed a significant decrease of carotid-femoral PWV (from 8.56 ± 2.73 m/s in baseline to 7.30 ± 2.02 m/s after 9 months; $p < 0.0001$).

5. Hemodialysis versus Peritoneal Dialysis: Arterial Stiffness

5.1. Transversal Studies. A polish group reported an interesting research in which peritoneal dialysis and hemodialyzed patients were compared. No statistically significant differences between groups were found [20]. The carotid-femoral PWV of 35 ambulatory patients receiving peritoneal dialysis was 9.9 ± 1.2 m/s, while aortic PWV of hemodialyzed patients was 10.0 ± 1.4 m/s. The authors concluded that both hemodialysis and peritoneal dialysis increase aortic stiffness. The comparison between PWV of nondiabetic and that of diabetic patients showed significant differences ($p < 0.01$) in both peritoneal dialysis and hemodialyzed patients (Table 3).

On the contrary, hemodialysis and peritoneal dialysis have been shown to improve arterial stiffness comparatively with predialysis subjects [21]. This study included ambulatory peritoneal dialysis patients ($n = 62$), hemodialyzed subjects ($n = 56$), a cohort of uremic patients ($n = 128$), and a control group ($n = 40$) of healthy subjects. The comparative analysis included control, peritoneal dialysis, hemodialysis, and nondialyzed patients in ESRD. The authors concluded that dialysis improved arterial stiffness evaluated through PWV and augmentation index (Table 3).

It has been pointed out that the dialysis modality (peritoneal or hemodialysis) may impact arterial stiffness in different ways. In an interesting in vivo and in vitro work of Chung and coworkers, it has been reported that the duration of renal replacement therapy did not correlate with arterial stiffness [22]. The study was performed in patients undergoing living-donor renal transplantation. The most important finding of this work perhaps is the difference between the in vivo and in vitro (measured in the) determination of arterial PWV. No differences in noninvasive PWV were found among nondialysis, peritoneal dialysis, and hemodialysis patients (Table 3). On the contrary, the in vitro determination of PWV showed that peritoneal dialysis and hemodialysis patients exhibit higher values than nondialyzed patients ($p < 0.01$).

5.2. Longitudinal Studies. PWV has been found to be higher in hemodialyzed patients than in those on continuous ambulatory peritoneal dialysis after 12 months of renal replacement therapy [23] (Table 3). Curiously, the cohort of patients on peritoneal dialysis exhibit higher serum cholesterol levels.

6. The Nature of the Arterial Stiffening

Aortic stiffening has been demonstrated in early stages of kidney disease and, as mentioned above, is increased in both hemodialyzed and peritoneal dialysis patients. Furthermore, it has been pointed out that continuous peritoneal dialysis could contribute to determine the most important increases of arterial stiffness.

Peritoneal-dialysis and hemodialyzed patients with abnormal increases of aortic stiffness showed a direct correlation between PWV and blood pressure (systolic, diastolic, and mean) values [8, 17, 19]. Nevertheless, the lowering of blood pressure levels is not always followed by decreases of aortic stiffness evaluated through PWV measurements [9]. This fact obviously shows the multifactorial nature of the arterial stiffening observed in uremic patients.

In 2010, Gao and coworkers reported a follow-up in 107 peritoneal dialyzed patients in which carotid-femoral and carotid-radial PWV were measured and the fluid overload was determined [24]. The authors pointed out that the resulting mean values of carotid-femoral PWV were lower than those obtained in a similar population in which salt intake was higher.

Recently, a report by Sipahioglu et al. showed that the aortic stiffness index (β; a local marker of the ascending aorta stiffness) measured in a cohort of peritoneal dialysis patients showed higher values than that obtained in healthy subjects [25]. Moreover, in this 2-year longitudinal follow-up, 156 patients showed a significant correlation of the β index with age ($p < 0.001$) and Kt/V ($p < 0.023$).

In patients with ESRD there is an increase of degenerative processes that affect the structural integrity of the arterial wall, which involve the deposit of abnormal product derived from proteins or lipids [26]. Several reports mentioned that the reduction of AGEs (Advanced Glycation End Products) improves arterial stiffening [6].

TABLE 3: Arterial (aortic) stiffness and modality of dialysis.

	cfPWV in PD	cfPWV in HD	Longitudinal study	Transversal study
Mimura et al., 2005 [23]	Decrease (1)	Increase (1)	X	
Yang et al., 2011 [21]	Decrease (2)	Decrease (2)		X
Strózecki et al., 2012 [20]	Increase (3)	Increase (3)		X
Chung et al., 2010 [22]	Increase (4)	pNS		X

Pulse wave velocity in the carotid-femoral pathway (cfPWV) was measured in peritoneal dialysis (PD) and hemodialyzed patients (HD).
(1) With respect to baseline values obtained in dialyzed patients between 3 and 5 months.
(2) With respect to predialysis values obtained in uremic patients.
(3) With respect to the theoretical value according to Blacher equation.
(4) With respect to nondialysis uremic patients (in vitro studies in humans).

TABLE 4: Arterial (upper-limb or carotid-radial) stiffness in dialyzed patients.

	PD	HD	Longitudinal study	Transversal study
Utescu et al., 2013 [11]		X (PWV)	Decrease (1)	
Szeto et al., 2012 [17]	X (PWV)		Increase (2)	
Mourad et al., 1997 [34]		X (E_{inc})		Increase (3)

Pulse wave velocity (PWV) in the carotid-radial pathway or incremental elastic modulus (E_{inc}) was measured in peritoneal dialysis (PD) or hemodialyzed patients (HD). X indicates the used dialysis modality.
(1) With respect to baseline values obtained in hemodialyzed patients (mean = 2.3 years).
(2) With respect to baseline values obtained in peritoneal dialysis patients for at least 6 months ($p < 0.0001$).
(3) With respect to values obtained in normal normotensive and hypertensive patients ($p < 0.05$).

Alteration of calcium and phosphate metabolism has been found to be associated with structural and functional changes of the arterial wall. Particularly, the development of mediacalcinosis has been linked to increases of elastic arterial stiffening [7]. This pathological process which involves the extracellular matrix is accompanied by cellular changes of the arterial wall. As previously reported, uremic toxins resulted in the transformation of vascular smooth muscle cells in osteoblast-like cell [27]; considering this fact together with the increase of arterial stiffness in patients in which the dialysate calcium was high [28], the association between vascular calcification and arterial stiffening is clear. Furthermore, carotid-radial PWV was found to be significantly associated with vascular calcification in a study that included three groups: chronic kidney disease in stage 5, hemodialyzed, and peritoneal dialysis patients [29].

Carotid-femoral PWV was found to inversely correlate with serum albumin levels, obtained in a cohort of peritoneal dialysis patients [30]. Additionally, increases in brachial-ankle PWV have been associated with proteinuria and low creatinine clearance in nondialyzed patients participating in a health-check Japanese program [31]. Phosphate levels have been found to be significantly correlated with arterial wall stiffness in uremic patients [22].

Endothelial dysfunction has been observed in uremic patients and their reversibility was reported in hemodialyzed patients [32]. Hemodialysis has no acute effects on endothelial function and aortic PWV in patients who are on continuous renal replacement function therapy [33].

Arterial stiffness has demonstrated to be correlated with C-reactive protein serum levels [4, 12, 16]. Very few authors performed carotid-radial PWV measurements in patients under renal replacement therapy (Table 4). The reported findings are sometimes inconsistent. For instance, Utescu

and coworkers concluded that after a 1.2-year follow-up hemodialysis determined a significant decrease of PWV in upper limbs (arterial stiffness reduction) simultaneous to aortic stiffness significant increases [11]. On the other hand, Szeto and coworkers demonstrated significant increases of carotid-radial PWV after a 2-year follow-up of peritoneal dialysis patients (from 10.05 ± 1.44 m/s to 10.80 ± 1.90 m/s) [17]. Mourad and coworkers concluded that radial arteries showed an increase of arterial stiffness (evaluated through E_{inc}) in hemodialyzed patients, compared to hypertensive and normotensive control subjects [34]. See Table 4. According to a previous research reported by our group in hemodialysis patients, a significative reduction in the carotid-brachial PWV was demonstrated in the arm where the arteriovenous fistula was confectioned [35]. Moreover, this reduction was greater in patients with the arteriovenous fistula performed in the upper arm than in those with the shunt in the forearm [36].

7. Final Comments

The outcome examination of the reports in which a follow-up of arterial stiffness in hemodialyzed patients was performed shows differences, perhaps determined by the lack of a unique data collection methodology. So, the effects of renal replacement therapy on arterial stiffness are a controversial topic. The nature of the differences in terms of arterial stiffness outcomes observed among the above-mentioned reports could be attributed to

(a) differences among pharmacological drug resources used to control comorbidities and metabolic alterations secondary to renal failure in the analyzed population,

(b) the use of higher dialysate calcium, which would result in impairment of aortic stiffness,

(c) the presence or absence of calcinosis of the arterial wall, which was found to be associated with changes in vascular stiffness,

(d) differences in data collection and type of analysis (transversal and or longitudinal studies).

The list of the factors involved in the source of arterial stiffness alterations at present seems to be incomplete. Nevertheless, the therapeutically connotations of the commented findings are very important, since the stiffening process evidences a high risk for both peritoneal dialysis and hemodialyzed patients.

Finally, it is important to mention that several authors demonstrated a positive relationship between PWV and body volume overload parameters [37, 38]. Furthermore, the arterial stiffness changes could be originated in variations in the exchangeable sodium pool involving the arterial wall, as suggested by Hogas and coworkers [39]. Consequently, it is hypothetically possible that the origin of the observed discrepancies among the analyzed reports in this review could be explained by tissue hydration changes.

8. Conclusions

(1) The renal replacement therapy effects on arterial stiffness remain controversial.

(2) The origin of the arterial wall stiffening found in hemodialyzed and peritoneal dialysis patients is multifactorial.

(3) Arterial stiffness increases and decreases seem to be part of a generalized process that involves territories different from the aortic territory, such as the carotid-radial pathway.

(4) Contradictory results in arterial stiffness should be analyzed considering all of the variables involved in the determinants of the vascular dynamic behavior, both in elastic and in muscular arteries.

(5) Arterial stiffening of elastic and muscular arteries should be evaluated in order to check preventive and therapeutic options that were capable of stopping the impairment of the arterial wall stiffness in hemodialyzed and peritoneal dialysis patients.

Acknowledgments

This work was supported by the René Favaloro University Foundation and funds of "PICT 2008 OC AR 0340" (Argentina) and Espacio Interdisciplinario and Agencia Nacional de Investigación e Innovación (Uruguay).

References

[1] S. Laurent, J. Cockcroft, L. Van Bortel et al., "Expert consensus document on arterial stiffness: methodological issues and clinical applications," *European Heart Journal*, vol. 27, no. 21, pp. 2588–2605, 2006.

[2] D. Bia and Y. Zócalo, "Rigidez arterial: evaluación no invasiva en la práctica clínica. Importancia clínica y análisis de las bases metodológicas de los equipos disponibles para su evaluación," *Revista Uruguaya de Cardiología*, vol. 29, no. 1, pp. 39–59, 2014.

[3] W. Nichols and M. F. O'Rourke, Eds., *McDonald's Blood Flow in Arteries: Theoretical, Experimental and Clinical Principles*, Hodder Arnold, London, UK, 5th edition, 2005.

[4] G. M. London, B. Pannier, and S. J. Marchais, "Vascular calcifications, arterial aging and arterial remodeling in ESRD," *Blood Purification*, vol. 35, no. 1–3, pp. 16–21, 2013.

[5] E. I. Cabrera-Fischer, R. L. Armentano, J. Levenson et al., "Paradoxically decreased aortic wall stiffness in response to vitamin D3-induced calcinosis. A biphasic analysis of segmental elastic properties in conscious dogs," *Circulation Research*, vol. 68, no. 6, pp. 1549–1559, 1991.

[6] A. Covic, P. Gusbeth-Tatomir, and D. J. A. Goldsmith, "Arterial stiffness in renal patients: an update," *American Journal of Kidney Diseases*, vol. 45, no. 6, pp. 965–977, 2005.

[7] B. Pannier, A. P. Guérin, S. J. Marchais, F. Métivier, and G. M. London, "Arterial structure and function in end-stage renal disease," *Artery Research*, vol. 1, no. 2, pp. 79–88, 2007.

[8] K. Shinohara, T. Shoji, Y. Tsujimoto et al., "Arterial stiffness in predialysis patients with uremia," *Kidney International*, vol. 65, no. 3, pp. 936–943, 2004.

[9] A. P. Guerin, J. Blacher, B. Pannier, S. J. Marchais, M. E. Safar, and G. M. London, "Impact of aortic stiffness attenuation on survival of patients in end-stage renal failure," *Circulation*, vol. 103, no. 7, pp. 987–992, 2001.

[10] T. Takenaka and H. Suzuki, "New strategy to attenuate pulse wave velocity in haemodialysis patients," *Nephrology Dialysis Transplantation*, vol. 20, no. 4, pp. 811–816, 2005.

[11] M. S. Utescu, V. Couture, F. Mac-Way et al., "Determinants of progression of aortic stiffness in hemodialysis patients: a prospective longitudinal study," *Hypertension*, vol. 62, no. 1, pp. 154–160, 2013.

[12] P. Avramovski, P. Janakievska, K. Sotiroski, and A. Sikole, "Accelerated progression of arterial stiffness in dialysis patients compared with the general population," *Korean Journal of Internal Medicine*, vol. 28, no. 4, pp. 464–474, 2013.

[13] E. Charitaki and A. Davenport, "Do higher dialysate calcium concentrations increase vascular stiffness in haemodialysis patients as measured by aortic pulse wave velocity?" *BMC Nephrology*, vol. 14, no. 1, article 189, 2013.

[14] G. M. London, B. Pannier, A. P. Guerin et al., "Alterations of left ventricular hypertrophy in and survival of patients receiving hemodialysis: follow-up of an interventional study," *Journal of the American Society of Nephrology*, vol. 12, no. 12, pp. 2759–2767, 2001.

[15] E. I. Cabrera Fischer, D. Bia, C. N. Galli et al., "Hemodialysis decreases carotid-brachial and carotid-femoral pulse wave velocities: a 5-year follow-up study," *Hemodialysis International*, 2015.

[16] D.-W. Kuang, C.-L. Li, U.-I. Kuok, K. Cheung, W.-I. Lio, and J. Xin, "Risk factors associated with brachial-ankle pulse wave velocity among peritoneal dialysis patients in Macao," *BMC Nephrology*, vol. 13, no. 1, article 143, 2012.

[17] C.-C. Szeto, B. C.-H. Kwan, K.-M. Chow, C.-B. Leung, M.-C. Law, and P. K.-T. Li, "Prognostic value of arterial pulse wave velocity in peritoneal dialysis patients," *American Journal of Nephrology*, vol. 35, no. 2, pp. 127–133, 2012.

[18] M. Tang, A. Romann, G. Chiarelli et al., "Vascular stiffness in incident peritoneal dialysis patients over time," *Clinical Nephrology*, vol. 78, no. 4, pp. 254–262, 2012.

[19] M. S. Demirci, O. Gungor, F. Kircelli et al., "Impact of mean arterial pressure on progression of arterial stiffness in peritoneal dialysis patients under strict volume control strategy," *Clinical Nephrology*, vol. 77, no. 2, pp. 105–113, 2012.

[20] P. Strózecki, R. Donderski, A. Kardymowicz, and J. Manitius, "Comparison of arterial stiffness in end-stage renal disease patients treated with peritoneal dialysis or hemodialysis," *Polskie Archiwum Medycyny Wewnetrznej*, vol. 122, no. 1-2, pp. 33–39, 2012.

[21] L. Yang, Y. Lin, C. Ye et al., "Effects of peritoneal dialysis and hemodialysis on arterial stiffness compared with predialysis patients," *Clinical Nephrology*, vol. 75, no. 3, pp. 188–194, 2011.

[22] A. W. Y. Chung, H. H. C. Yang, J. M. Kim et al., "Arterial stiffness and functional properties in chronic kidney disease patients on different dialysis modalities: an exploratory study," *Nephrology Dialysis Transplantation*, vol. 25, no. 12, pp. 4031–4041, 2010.

[23] T. Mimura, T. Takenaka, Y. Kanno, H. Aoki, J. Ohshima, and H. Suzuki, "Comparison of changes in pulse wave velocity in patients on continuous ambulatory peritoneal dialysis and hemodialysis one year after introduction of dialysis therapy," *Advances in Peritoneal Dialysis*, vol. 21, pp. 139–145, 2005.

[24] N. Gao, B. C.-H. Kwan, K.-M. Chow et al., "Arterial pulse wave velocity and peritoneal transport characteristics independently predict hospitalization in Chinese peritoneal dialysis patients," *Peritoneal Dialysis International*, vol. 30, no. 1, pp. 80–85, 2010.

[25] M. H. Sipahioglu, H. Kucuk, A. Unal et al., "Impact of arterial stiffness on adverse cardiovascular outcomes and mortality in peritoneal dialysis patients," *Peritoneal Dialysis International*, vol. 32, no. 1, pp. 73–80, 2012.

[26] A. Goldin, J. A. Beckman, A. M. Schmidt, and M. A. Creager, "Advanced glycation end products: sparking the development of diabetic vascular injury," *Circulation*, vol. 114, no. 6, pp. 597–605, 2006.

[27] S. M. Moe, D. Duan, B. P. Doehle, K. D. O'Neill, and N. X. Chen, "Uremia induces the osteoblast differentiation factor Cbfa1 in human blood vessels," *Kidney International*, vol. 63, no. 3, pp. 1003–1011, 2003.

[28] A. Leboeuf, F. Mac-Way, M. S. Utescu et al., "Impact of dialysate calcium concentration on the progression of aortic stiffness in patients on haemodialysis," *Nephrology Dialysis Transplantation*, vol. 26, no. 11, pp. 3695–3701, 2011.

[29] M. Sigrist, P. Bungay, M. W. Taal, and C. W. McIntyre, "Vascular calcification and cardiovascular function in chronic kidney disease," *Nephrology Dialysis Transplantation*, vol. 21, no. 3, pp. 707–714, 2006.

[30] L.-T. Cheng, L.-J. Tang, H.-M. Chen, W. Tang, and T. Wang, "Relationship between serum albumin and pulse wave velocity in patients on continuous ambulatory peritoneal dialysis," *Vascular Health and Risk Management*, vol. 4, no. 4, pp. 871–876, 2008.

[31] Y. Ohya, K. Iseki, C. Iseki, T. Miyagi, K. Kinjo, and S. Takishita, "Increased pulse wave velocity is associated with low creatinine clearance and proteinuria in a screened cohort," *American Journal of Kidney Diseases*, vol. 47, no. 5, pp. 790–797, 2006.

[32] J. M. Cross, A. Donald, P. J. Vallance, J. E. Deanfield, R. G. Woolfson, and R. J. MacAllister, "Dialysis improves endothelial function in humans," *Nephrology Dialysis Transplantation*, vol. 16, no. 9, pp. 1823–1829, 2001.

[33] M. Kosch, A. Levers, M. Barenbrock et al., "Acute effects of haemodialysis on endothelial function and large artery elasticity," *Nephrology Dialysis Transplantation*, vol. 16, no. 8, pp. 1663–1668, 2001.

[34] J.-J. Mourad, X. Girerd, P. Boutouyrie, S. Laurent, M. Safar, and G. London, "Increased stiffness of radial artery wall material in end-stage renal disease," *Hypertension*, vol. 30, no. 6, pp. 1425–1430, 1997.

[35] E. I. C. Fischer, D. Bia, R. Valtuille, S. Craf, C. Galli, and R. L. Armentano, "Vascular access localization determines regional changes in arterial stiffness," *Journal of Vascular Access*, vol. 10, no. 3, pp. 192–198, 2009.

[36] D. Bia, E. I. Cabrera-Fischer, Y. Zócalo et al., "Vascular accesses for haemodialysis in the upper arm cause greater reduction in the carotid-brachial stiffness than those in the forearm: study of gender differences," *International Journal of Nephrology*, vol. 2012, Article ID 598512, 10 pages, 2012.

[37] E. Hur, M. Usta, H. Toz et al., "Effect of fluid management guided by bioimpedance spectroscopy on cardiovascular parameters in hemodialysis patients: a randomized controlled trial," *American Journal of Kidney Diseases*, vol. 61, no. 6, pp. 957–965, 2013.

[38] Y.-P. Lin, W.-C. Yu, T.-L. Hsu, P. Y.-A. Ding, W.-C. Yang, and C.-H. Chen, "The extracellular fluid-to-intracellular fluid volume ratio is associated with large-artery structure and function in hemodialysis patients," *The American Journal of Kidney Diseases*, vol. 42, no. 5, pp. 990–999, 2003.

[39] S. Hogas, S. Ardeleanu, L. Segall et al., "Changes in arterial stiffness following dialysis in relation to overhydration and to endothelial function," *International Urology and Nephrology*, vol. 44, no. 3, pp. 897–905, 2012.

14

Glycaemic Control Impact on Renal Endpoints in Diabetic Patients on Haemodialysis

Danielle Creme and Kieran McCafferty

Royal London Hospital, Whitechapel Road, London E1 1BB, UK

Correspondence should be addressed to Danielle Creme; dcreme@gmail.com

Academic Editor: Alessandro Amore

Objective. To identify the number of haemodialysis patients with diabetes in a large NHS Trust, their current glycaemic control, and the impact on other renal specific outcomes. *Design.* Retrospective, observational, cross-sectional study. *Methods.* Data was collected from an electronic patient management system. Glycaemic control was assessed from HbA1c results that were then further adjusted for albumin (Alb) and haemoglobin (Hb). Interdialytic weight gains were analysed from weights recorded before and after dialysis, 2 weeks before and after the most recent HbA1c date. Amputations were identified from electronic records. *Results.* 39% of patients had poor glycaemic control (HbA1c > 8%). Adjusted HbA1c resulted in a greater number of patients with poor control (55%). Significant correlations were found with interdialytic weight gains ($P < 0.02$, $r = 0.14$), predialysis sodium ($P < 0.0001$, $r = -1.9$), and predialysis bicarbonate ($P < 0.02$, $r = 0.12$). Trends were observed with albumin and C-reactive protein. Patients with diabetes had more amputations (24 versus 2). *Conclusion.* Large number of diabetic patients on haemdialysis have poor glycaemic control. This may lead to higher interdialytic weight gains, larger sodium and bicarbonate shifts, increased number of amputations, and possibly increased inflammation and decreased nutritional status. Comprehensive guidelines and more accurate long-term tests for glycaemic control are needed.

1. Introduction

Diabetes and renal disease are both long-term conditions prevalent in the adult UK population at 14% and 7.5%, respectively [1]. The single most common aetiology of CKD is diabetic nephropathy. It is estimated that a quarter of all people with diabetes will develop end stage renal failure (ESRF), causing 21% and 11% of all deaths in type 1 and type 2 diabetes, respectively [2].

For people with diabetes requiring dialysis, one-year mortality rate was 17% compared with 11% for nondiabetic dialysis patients [3]. Other factors influence mortality such as old age, male gender, South Asian ethnicity, and lower socioeconomic status [4].

Slowing progression to ESRF in this patient group is the main treatment strategy for patients with diabetic nephropathy. While there is a plethora of research and evidence on methods and treatment to achieve this, outcomes and care once RRT (renal replacement therapy) has been initiated are less well defined.

It has been suggested that this patient group has a higher risk of complications such as cardiovascular disease, vascular calcification, infection, lower limb amputation, peripheral neuropathy, retinopathy, difficulties with vascular access, depression, and generalized decrease in quality of life (QoL) [5]. The severity of these complications could be mediated with better glycaemic control even after RRT initiation.

Aims. Aims of the study were to assess the prevalence of diabetes in the haemodialysis population to categorise the glycaemic control of the HD population into high and low risk categories and investigate the impact of poor glycaemic control on other renal specific outcomes.

2. Methods

Ethical approval was provided by the Clinical Effectiveness Unit and Audit Unit at Barts Health NHS Trust (registration number 5413). All patients on haemodialysis (HD) in August

2014 were included. Data was extracted from electronic data records (Renalware).

Inclusion criteria were patients >18 years, currently on HD at Barts Health NHS Trust. Patients without diabetes or an HbA1c were excluded from the biochemical analysis.

The most recent recorded HbA1c was used to quantify glycaemic control. The patients were then stratified into HbA1c ranges to assess glycaemic control. Stratification was based on available published evidence. All other biochemistry and amputation data was extracted from Renalware at the time of the individuals HbA1c date.

Interdialytic weight gains (IDWG) were calculated using weights before and after dialysis, 2 weeks before and after HbA1c date. Nonparametric data was analyzed using the Kruskal-Wallis test statistic with Dunn's postcomparison test while correlations were quantified using the Spearman correlation coefficients with GraphPad Prism 6 software (San Diego, CA, USA).

HbA1c was further adjusted for HD accounting for changes in albumin (Alb) and haemoglobin (Hb)

(i) $AG^* = 104.8 + 29.7 \times HbA1c - 18.4 \times Alb - 4.7 \times Hb$ [6]

*Average glucose.

3. Results

Out of 979 patients receiving HD at the time, 42% had Diabetes Mellitus (DM). Total number of diabetic patients receiving HD, $n = 412$ (42% of all HD patients). There was a significantly higher number of South Asians and older people with diabetes compared to the nondiabetic HD cohort ($p < 0.0001$) (Table 1).

39% of patients Trust wide had poorly controlled diabetes defined as HbA1c <5.4% (36 mmol/mol) or >8% (64 mmol/mol). 7% of these were at high risk defined as HbA1c >10% (86 mmol/mol).

Significant differences were seen with various biochemical and clinical parameters (ALP, Hb, sodium, and pre-HD systolic BP) when comparing each HbA1c category (Table 2). However, when each at-risk category (HbA1c outside the target range of 5.4%–7.9%) was compared to the optimally controlled group (HbA1c 5.4%–7.9%) using Dunn's multiple comparison testing, there were no significant differences seen between the groups.

There was an increase of 16% of patients with poorly controlled diabetes with HbA1c adjusted for Alb and Hb (Figure 1).

3.1. Correlations. Higher HbA1c is associated with larger fluid gains as there is a small ($r = 0.14$) but statistically and clinically significant ($p < 0.02$) positive correlation between IDWG and poorly controlled diabetes (Figure 2). There is a significant increase in systolic blood pressure with higher HbA1c values. There is a weak significant ($p < 0.0001$) negative correlation ($r = -1.9$) between poor glycaemic control and predialysis sodium (Figure 3). There is a weak ($r = 0.12$) but statistically significant ($p < 0.02$)

TABLE 1: Demographics.

	Diabetes present ($n = 412$)	No diabetes present ($n = 567$)
Ethnicity n (%)		
White	90 (22)	203 (36)
Black	114 (28)	176 (31)
South Asian	179 (43)	125 (22)
Other	29 (7)	63 (11)
Age (years)	65 (57–73)	56 (45–70)
Dialysis vintage (years)	2.6 (1.3–4.9)	2.9 (1.1–5.5)
Male gender n (%)	228 (55)	334 (59)
Diabetic cohort only		
Type of diabetes		
Type 1 n (%)	15 (4)	
Type 2 n (%)	397 (96)	
Insulin treated n (%)	260 (63)	
Kt/V	1.5 (1.4–1.7)	

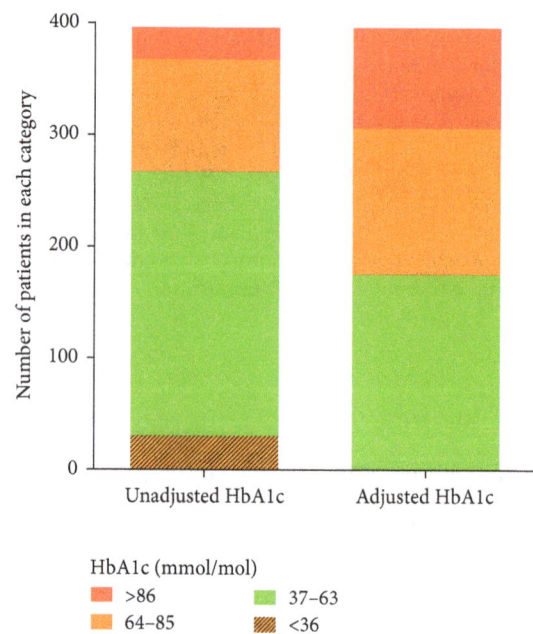

FIGURE 1: Glycaemic control assessment using HbA1c adjusted for albumin and haemoglobin.

correlation between poor glycaemic control and an increase in bicarbonate (Figure 4). There is a trend between poor glycaemic control, raised CRP, and reduced Alb which is not significant ($p = 0.07$ and $p = 0.08$, resp.). The proportion of patients with amputation who have diabetes is greater than those who do not, with 24 versus 2 patients, respectively, with 46% (11 patients) having an HbA1c >8% (65 mmol/mol). No other correlations between poor glycaemic control and other biochemical markers were observed (haemoglobin, ferritin, TSAT, WCC, potassium, phosphate, PTH, and vitamin D).

TABLE 2: Comparison of biochemistry of diabetic cohort according to glycaemic control.

Variable	<5.4% <36 mmol/mol	5.4–7.9% 37–63 mmol/mol	8–9.9% 64–85 mmol/mol	>10% >86 mmol/mol	p value
Urea (mmol/L)	18.5 (10.8–21.5)	16.8 (13.2–22.9)	17.5 (12.8–21.3)	17.5 (9.4–23.8)	0.98
Creatinine (μmol/L)	682 (570–839)	706 (571–845)	710 (558–853)	728 (624–854)	0.77
Albumin (g/L)	40 (37–43)	40 (38–42)	41 (38–43)	40 (37–41)	0.09
CRP (mg/L)	6 (5–15)	6 (5–20)	6 (5–14)	6 (5–17)	0.87
Hb (g/dL)	10.3 (8.9–11.2)	10.6 (9.6–11.5)	10.9 (10–11.7)	11 (9.8–11.9)	0.02
Ferritin (mcg/L)	394 (195–571)	445 (279–623)	458 (291–647)	496 (277–837)	0.69
TSAT (%)	22 (17–29)	25 (21–32)	26 (21–34)	26 (21–35)	0.2
Calcium (mmol/L)	2.3 (2.2–2.4)	2.3 (2.2–2.4)	2.3 (2.2–2.4)	2.2 (2.1–2.3)	0.06
Phosphate (mmol/L)	1.5 (1.3–1.9)	1.4 (1.1–1.7)	1.5 (1.2–1.9)	1.5 (1.3–1.9)	0.2
PTH (pmol/L)	44 (36–91)	40 (20–52)	34 (16–57)	41 (32–65)	0.1
ALP (unit/L)	99 (64–138)	117 (85–162)	104 (80–145)	134 (91–224)	0.01
Sodium (mmol/L)	139 (138–141)	138 (136–140)	139 (137–141)	138 (135–140)	0.002
Bicarbonate (mmol/L)	22 (20–23)	22 (20–24)	22 (20–24)	22 (22–24)	0.4
Potassium (mmol/L)	5.1 (4.6–5.7)	4.8 (4.5–5.5)	4.9 (4.4–5.4)	4.8 (4.5–5.5)	0.5
Kt/V	1.4 (1.4–1.8)	1.5 (1.3–1.7)	1.6 (1.4–1.7)	1.4 (1.4–1.6)	0.61
Pre-HD systolic BP (mm/Hg)	141 (131–159)	158 (138–175)	150 (132–170)	179 (133–202)	0.02

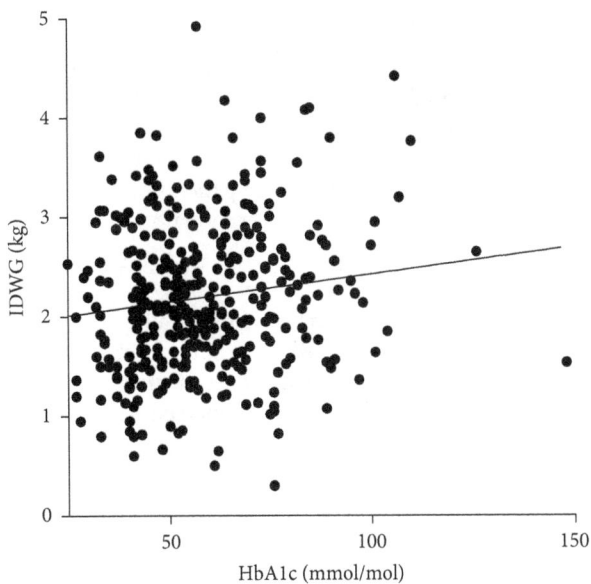

FIGURE 2: Correlation between glycaemic control and interdialytic weight gains.

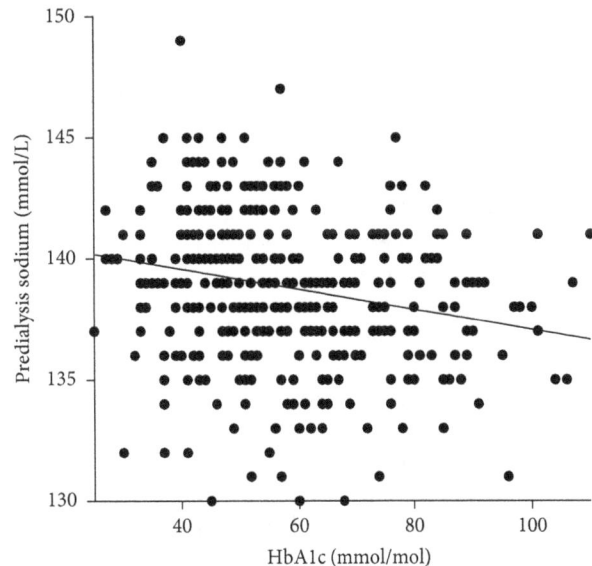

FIGURE 3: Correlation between glycaemic control and predialysis sodium.

4. Discussion

There is scant information published nationally or internationally on glycaemic control in HD-dependent diabetic patients. The renal registry has no data on glycaemic control of RRT patients.

4.1. Assessment of Glycaemic Control. There are several challenges in accurately assessing glycaemic control in this patient group. In the diabetic population without diabetic nephropathy and before RRT, HbA1c test is the gold standard test used to assess long-term glycaemic control. An HbA1c test will reflect the average amount of glucose a red blood cell (RBC) was exposed to during its life span.

There are several issues affecting the accuracy of HbA1c tests with ESRF. Urea derived isocyanate results in carbamylated Hb which is indistinguishable from glycated Hb, giving a false elevation in readings. Other inaccuracies arise from disruptions to RBC life span on which the test is based. Iron deficiency, B$_{12}$, or folate deficiencies also give falsely high readings as they extend RBC life span. Reduced RBC life span as a consequence of dialysis, recent transfusions and accelerated erythropoiesis result in falsely low results due to shorter periods of exposure to glucose.

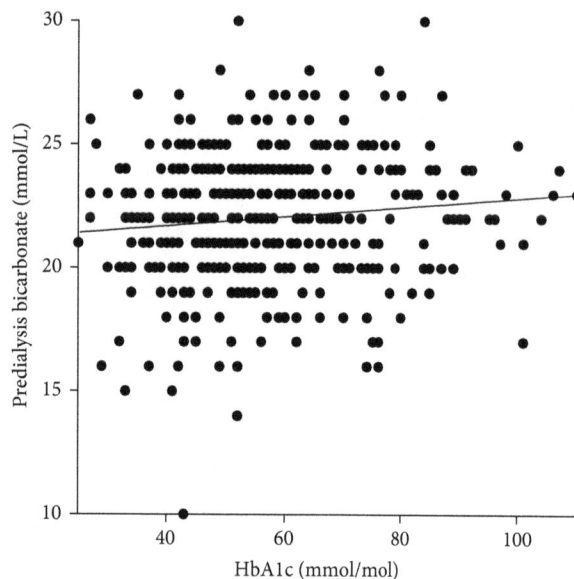

FIGURE 4: Correlation between glycaemic control and predialysis bicarbonate.

Other tests are available such as glycated albumin or glycated fructosamine. These reflect control over a shorter time period and are less affected by the unstable haemodynamic environment as HbA1c. Other factors such as increased protein turnover and malnutrition can affect the accuracy and validity of these tests. Their advantages and disadvantages have been discussed in several papers [7–9]. There are scant long-term trials looking at glycated albumin and chronic complications of diabetes, although one small long-term study found that glycated albumin correlated well with cardiovascular mortality [10]. A consensus on the best methods for assessing long-term glycaemic control in this patient cohort has yet to be reached. Clearly, there is a need for longer, more extensive research in this area. While there are good arguments for using these tests over HbA1c, at present, HbA1c remains the test used most often to monitor and determine glucose control in HD patients.

4.2. Adjusted HbA1c. A recent large study ($n = 11,986$) [6], having recognized anaemia, malnutrition, and inflammation's impact on survival in this patient cohort, has developed equation models adjusting for these confounding factors including Alb (model 3, $R^2 = 0.483$), Alb + Hb (model 4, $R^2 = 0.486$), and Alb + Hb + age + race (model 5, $R^2 = 0.491$). These all showed a stronger association than the DCCT A_{1c} derived average glucose equation did ($R^2 = 0.468$) with daily blood glucose. As this study was based in the USA, where ethnicity is very different to the present cohort, we applied model 4 to the data.

Following this adjustment, the number of patients with poor glycaemic control rose from 39% to 55%, eliminating those who appeared to have very low HbA1c. This highlights the concern of using tests which are inaccurate in this patient cohort. Using standard HbA1c results misclassifies

patients into lower risk categories; care therefore is not being efficiently or effectively targeted.

The most accurate method of assessing glucose control is regular self-monitoring of plasma glucose with finger prick tests. Target glucose levels for diabetic patients on HD suggested by one study were fasting <7.8 mmol/L and postprandial <11.1 mmol/L [11], giving an average HbA1c reading of <9%. Compliance and adherence are issues with this method as they involve regular pre- and postprandial daily tests which some patients find difficult to manage.

4.3. HbA1c Targets. While target HbA1c levels for diabetic population without CKD or ESRF are clearly defined based on large-scale studies (DCCT/EDIC, ACCORD, ADVANCE, and VADT), a consensus on HbA1c levels for the diabetic population receiving RRT has not been established. Current advice is centered around the prevention of hyperglycaemia and microvascular complications of diabetes.

   (i) *Dialysis Outcomes and Practice Patterns Study (DOPPS).* It is 7%-8% (53–64 mmol/mol), suggesting lower end for younger patients with fewer comorbidities and higher end for older patients with greater number of comorbidities [12].

  (ii) *Kidney Disease Outcomes Quality Initiative (KDOQI).* CKD population is 7% (53 mmol/mol), although in their rationale they mention that HbA1c levels of 7–9% are associated with better outcomes for survival, hospitalization, and CVD in patients on haemodialysis in most but not all observational studies [13].

 (iii) *Renal association.* It is <7.5% (<58 mmol/mol) [14].

Using survival and cardiovascular mortality as outcomes, several studies have attempted to stratify optimal and suboptimal glucose control. The most recent meta-analysis of observational studies suggested a J shaped curve relationship where an increase in mortality was associated with HbA1c <5.4% and >8.5% [15].

Ricks et al. [16], looking at >54,000 patient, also found increased mortality risks with HbA1c below and above 7%-7.9%, with <5% yielding hazard ratio of 1.35, >8% HR of 1.06 and >10% HR of 1.19.

There are no published national data looking at glycaemic control for diabetic patients on HD; therefore, it is difficult to assess whether the glycaemic control of the present cohort is better or worse than others. Irrespective, poor control in over half of the patients indicates that more directed and effective care is needed.

As noted by O'Toole et al. [17], besides the inherent problems with using HbA1c as a measure of glycaemic control in this population, there are several further confounding factors that must be considered when using HbA1c levels as a target outcome. Patients with very poor glycaemic control at the outset of dialysis are likely to have worse outcomes. In addition, poor glycaemic control is a surrogate for other factors contributing to poor self-care such as smoking and reduced adherence with medication, fluid restriction, and dietary recommendations.

4.4. Correlations and Additional Complications. Fluid management is one of the main challenges in HD with increased complexity in diabetic patients. Hyperglycaemia triggers osmoreceptors to stimulate thirst, leading to fluid consumption. Large IDWG and fluid overload lead to volume expansion and cardiac hypertrophy [18, 19] exacerbating pulmonary and cardiovascular symptoms. There are several methods for assessing IDWG, either in kilograms calculated from postdialysis weight to the following predialysis weight or by percentage weight change from dry weight. There are positives and negatives for each method; the first while being easier to calculate does not include dry weight in its estimation, while the second, allowing for proportional fluid to body mass estimations, relies on an estimated dry weight which may also be inaccurate.

In our study, we defined undesirable IDWG according to the KDOQI rationale of >2.5 kg between dialysis sessions [20] and observed a clinically and statistically significant ($p < 0.02$) if weak ($r = 0.14$) correlation between glycaemic control and IDWG (Figure 2). A recent prospective, 3-year follow-up study looking at >10,000 patients, found an increase in all cause and cardiovascular mortality rate in patients who had >2 kg IDWG from target weight in >30% of dialysis sessions [21]. The effect of glycaemia on IDWG was also reported by Davenport [22] who noted absolute and percentage IDWG was the lowest in the group with the best diabetic control classified as <6% versus poor control at >8% (2.0 ± 1 kg and 2.76 ± 1.5% versus 2.5 ± 1.1 kg and 3.3 ± 1.3% ($p < 0.05$), resp.). Our study supports the association of poor glycaemic control with excessive fluid intake; therefore, in a diabetic cohort where cardiovascular disease is already more prevalent, it is pertinent to prevent further exacerbation by undesirable IDWG by attempting to control hyperglycaemia.

Recent studies have elucidated an association between low predialysis Na and all cause and cardiovascular mortality [23, 24]. A further recent paper that looked at the relationship between predialysis Na levels, IDWG, and nutritional status found that low Na (<136.2 mlEq/L) was associated with increased IDWG and decreased lean body mass [25]. Our study shows that hyperglycaemia may exacerbate low Na as revealed, a statistically significant association between elevated HbA1c and low Na ($p < 0.0001$) (Figure 3). Predialysis sodium decreases with worsening glycaemic control due to translocational hyponatraemia. In marked hyperglycemia, extracellular fluid (ECF) osmolality rises and exceeds that of intracellular fluid (ICF). Glucose penetrates cell membranes slowly in the absence of insulin, resulting in movement of water out of cells into the ECF. Serum Na^+ concentration falls in proportion to the dilution of the ECF and therefore poor glycaemic control may be an additional contributing factor to hyponatraemia, increased mortality risk, high IDWG, and malnutrition.

The statistically significant correlation with elevated bicarbonate levels and raised HbA1c ($p < 0.002$) (Figure 4) was more difficult to explain, as hyperglycaemia usually increases acidosis due to hyperosmolality and release of free fatty acids and ketones, resulting in reduced pH; as such one would expect a lower bicarbonate level with poor glycaemic control. One explanation may be that patients with well controlled glycaemia are better nourished, choosing protein rich foods over carbohydrates. The increased protein intake may result in increased systemic acidity, therefore giving an inverse bicarbonate relationship. A recent paper looking at pH and bicarbonate association with mortality in HD patients noted that predialysis elevated pH was associated with increased risk of mortality but not before or after bicarbonate [26] which may render the association observed clinically insignificant.

Many observational studies have noted that HD patients are chronically inflamed. Insulin resistance and diabetes are also known to increase inflammatory cytokines although the precise mechanism remains unclear. In addition, there may be a reciprocal relationship present where inflammation and infection precipitate hyperglycaemia which in turn exacerbates and prolongs the inflammatory response. Hyperglycaemia is a known driving force for ischemia and poor wound healing which may also explain the far greater number of patients with amputations in the diabetic versus nondiabetic population, with 46% of patients with amputations having an HbA1c >8% (65 mmol/mol). A recent meta-analysis corroborated the increased risk of foot ischemia and lower limb amputation with higher HbA1c values [27].

While not a hard outcome like mortality, amputations have a major impact on a patient's QoL. A small interventional study ($n = 83$) by McMurray et al. [28] found that intensive glycaemic control intervention resulted in decreased need for amputations and hospitalisation and increase in QoL.

There may be a relationship between hyponatraemia, inflammation, and nutritional status in HD patients, which the study by Poulikakos et al. [25] tried to explore, although, as with our own study, the associations with CRP and albumin, while showing a positive trend, were not statistically significant.

The strengths of this paper lie in the attempt to stratify diabetic patients on HD into risk categories and observe impact on renal specific clinical parameters such as electrolyte imbalances and IDWG, which has not been done previously in the UK. Study design is a limitation as cross-sectional observational studies cannot prove causative effects and the reliance on a single measure of HbA1c to quantify glycaemic control may not be an accurate representation of a patient's long-term glycaemic control.

Nevertheless, while most studies focus on hard outcomes such as mortality, there are many other factors in the patient's journey which are important. Achieving euglycaemia in patients with diabetes in the context of ESRD and HD is complex and multifactorial; however, it is essential for improving their clinical progress and QoL.

5. Conclusion

Glycaemic control in many HD dependent patients with diabetes is poor and may lead to additional complications such as high IDWG, electrolyte imbalance, and amputations. Current tests for long-term glycaemic control are inaccurate and may result in misclassification of patients into lower risk categories leading to misdirected management. There is an urgent need for further research to provide more accurate tests for long-term monitoring of glycaemic control and long-term prospective studies into interventions for alternative outcomes such as improvement with amputations, inflammation, undesirable IDWG, nutritional status, and QoL.

Conflict of Interests

The authors declare that there is no conflict of interests.

Acknowledgments

This work forms part of the research themes contributing to the research portfolio of the Barts Health "Diabetic Kidney Disease Centre," supported and funded by the Barts and the London Charity.

References

[1] NHS, *Diabetes with Kidney Disease: Key Facts*, 2011, http://www.yhpho.org.uk/resource/view.aspx?RID=105786.

[2] Diabetes UK, "Diabetes facts and stats," 2014, http://www.diabetes.org.uk/Documents/About%20Us/Statistics/Diabetes-key-stats-guidelines-April2014.pdf.

[3] D. Ansell, J. Feehally, D. Fogarty et al., "UK renal registry 2009: the twelfth annual report of the renal association," *Nephron Clinical Practice*, vol. 115, supplement 1, 2010.

[4] F. Caskey, A. Davenport, A. Dawnay et al., "UK renal registry 2013 16th annual report of the renal association," *Nephron Clinical Practice*, vol. 125, no. 1-4, 2013.

[5] W. Schrag, "Diabetes: the dialysis outcomes practice patterns study (DOPPS) results and innovative patient care programs," *The Journal Of Nephrology Social Work*, vol. 26, 2007.

[6] J. Hoshino, M. Z. Molnar, K. Yamagata et al., "Developing an HbA1c-based equation to estimate blood glucose in maintenance hemodialysis patients," *Diabetes Care*, vol. 36, no. 4, pp. 922–927, 2013.

[7] M. Speeckaert, W. Van Biesen, J. Delanghe et al., "Are there better alternatives than haemoglobin A1c to estimate glycaemic control in the chronic kidney disease population?" *Nephrology Dialysis Transplantation*, vol. 29, no. 12, pp. 2167–2177, 2014.

[8] C.-M. Zheng, W.-Y. Ma, C.-C. Wu, and K.-C. Lu, "Glycated albumin in diabetic patients with chronic kidney disease," *Clinica Chimica Acta*, vol. 413, no. 19-20, pp. 1555–1561, 2012.

[9] F. E. Vos, J. B. Schollum, and R. J. Walker, "Glycated albumin is the preferred marker for assessing glycaemic control in advanced chronic kidney disease," *NDT Plus*, vol. 4, no. 6, pp. 368–375, 2011.

[10] K. Fukuoka, K. Nakao, H. Morimoto et al., "Glycated albumin levels predict long-term survival in diabetic patients undergoing haemodialysis," *Nephrology*, vol. 13, no. 4, pp. 278–283, 2008.

[11] R. H. K. Mak, "Impact of end-stage renal disease and dialysis on glycemic control," *Seminars in Dialysis*, vol. 13, no. 1, pp. 4–8, 2000.

[12] S. P. B. Ramirez, K. P. McCullough, J. R. Thumma et al., "Hemoglobin A$_{1c}$ levels and mortality in the diabetic hemodialysis population: findings from the Dialysis Outcomes and Practice Patterns Study (DOPPS)," *Diabetes Care*, vol. 35, no. 12, pp. 2527–2532, 2012.

[13] National Kidney Foundation, *KDOQI Clinical Practice Guideline for Diabetes and CKD: 2012 Update*, 2012, https://www.kidney.org/sites/default/files/docs/diabetes-ckd-update-2012.pdf.

[14] The Renal Association, "Detection, Monitoring and Care of Patients with CKD," 2011, http://www.renal.org/Clinical/GuidelinesSection/Detection-Monitoring-and-Care-of-Patients-with-CKD.

[15] C. J. Hill, A. P. Maxwell, C. R. Cardwell et al., "Glycated hemoglobin and risk of death in diabetic patients treated with hemodialysis: a meta-analysis," *American Journal of Kidney Diseases*, vol. 63, no. 1, pp. 84–94, 2014.

[16] J. Ricks, M. Z. Molnar, C. P. Kovesdy et al., "Glycemic control and cardiovascular mortality in hemodialysis patients with diabetes: a 6-year cohort study," *Diabetes*, vol. 61, no. 3, pp. 708–715, 2012.

[17] S. M. O'Toole, S. L. Fan, M. M. Yaqoob, and T. A. Chowdhury, "Managing diabetes in dialysis patients," *Postgraduate Medical Journal*, vol. 88, no. 1037, Article ID 130354, pp. 160–166, 2011.

[18] C. Zoccali, F. A. Benedetto, G. Tripepi, and F. Mallamaci, "Cardiac consequences of hypertension in hemodialysis patients," *Seminars in Dialysis*, vol. 17, no. 4, pp. 299–303, 2004.

[19] N. Sharpe, "Left ventricular remodeling: pathophysiology and treatment," *Heart Failure Monitor*, vol. 4, no. 2, pp. 55–61, 2003.

[20] KDOQI, *Clinical Practice Guidelines for Cardiovascular Disease in Dialysis Patients*, 2005, http://www2.kidney.org/professionals/KDOQI/guidelines_cvd/.

[21] J. E. Flythe, A. V. Kshirsagar, R. J. Falk, and S. M. Brunelli, "Associations of posthemodialysis weights above and below target weight with all-cause and cardiovascular mortality," *Clinical Journal of the American Society of Nephrology*, vol. 10, no. 5, pp. 808–816, 2015.

[22] A. Davenport, "Interdialytic weight gain in diabetic haemodialysis patients and diabetic control as assessed by glycated haemoglobin," *Nephron: Clinical Practice*, vol. 113, no. 1, pp. c33–c37, 2009.

[23] S. S. Waikar, G. C. Curhan, and S. M. Brunelli, "Mortality associated with low serum sodium concentration in maintenance hemodialysis," *The American Journal of Medicine*, vol. 124, no. 1, pp. 77–84, 2011.

[24] M. Hecking, A. Karaboyas, R. Saran et al., "Predialysis serum sodium level, dialysate sodium, and mortality in maintenance hemodialysis patients: the Dialysis Outcomes and Practice Patterns Study (DOPPS)," *American Journal of Kidney Diseases*, vol. 59, no. 2, pp. 238–248, 2012.

[25] D. Poulikakos, V. Marks, N. Lelos, and D. Banerjee, "Low serum sodium is associated with protein energy wasting and increased interdialytic weight gain in haemodialysis patients," *Clinical Kidney Journal*, vol. 7, no. 2, pp. 156–160, 2014.

[26] T. Yamamoto, S. Shoji, T. Yamakawa et al., "Predialysis and postdialysis ph and bicarbonate and risk of all-cause and cardiovascular mortality in long-term hemodialysis patients," *American Journal of Kidney Diseases*, vol. 66, no. 3, pp. 469–478, 2015.

[27] M. Kaminski, A. Raspovic, L. McMahon et al., "Risk factors for foot ulceration and lower extremity amputation in adults with end-stage renal disease on dialysis: a systematic review and meta-analysis," *Nephrology Dialysis Transplantation*, 2015.

[28] S. D. McMurray, G. Johnson, S. Davis, and K. McDougall, "Diabetes education and care management significantly improve patient outcomes in the dialysis unit," *American Journal of Kidney Diseases*, vol. 40, no. 3, pp. 566–575, 2002.

15

Decreased Serum 25-hydroxyvitamin D Level Causes Interventricular Septal Hypertrophy in Patients on Peritoneal Dialysis: Cardiovascular Aspects of Endogenous Vitamin D Deficiency

Bennur Esen,[1] **Irfan Sahin,**[2] **Ahmet Engin Atay,**[3] **Emel Saglam Gokmen,**[3]
Ozlem Harmankaya Kaptanogullari,[4] **Mürvet Yılmaz,**[4] **Suat Hayri Kucuk,**[5]
Serdar Kahvecioglu,[6] **and Nurhan Seyahi**[7]

[1]*Department of Internal Medicine and Nephrology, Bagcilar Education and Research Hospital, Istanbul, Turkey*
[2]*Department of Cardiology, Bagcilar Education and Research Hospital, Istanbul, Turkey*
[3]*Department of Internal Medicine, Bagcilar Education and Research Hospital, Istanbul, Turkey*
[4]*Department of Internal Medicine and Nephrology, Bakırkoy Sadi Konuk Education and Research Hospital, Istanbul, Turkey*
[5]*Department of Biochemistry, Bagcilar Education and Research Hospital, Istanbul, Turkey*
[6]*Department of Internal Medicine and Nephrology, Sevket Yılmaz Education and Research Hospital, Bursa, Turkey*
[7]*Department of Internal Medicine and Nephrology, Cerrahpasa School of Medicine, Istanbul University, Istanbul, Turkey*

Correspondence should be addressed to Ahmet Engin Atay; aeatay@hotmail.com

Academic Editor: Alessandro Amore

Introduction. In the present study, we aimed to analyze the relation of vitamin D with echocardiographic indexes in patients with end stage renal disease (ESRD) receiving renal replacement therapy (RRT). *Methods*. A total of 98 patients, 64 patients on hemodialysis (HD) (29F/35M, mean age 56.75 ± 18.63 years) and 34 age matched patients on peritoneal dialysis (PD) (21F/13M, mean age 58.11 ± 10.63 years), with similar duration of ESRD and RRT were enrolled into this cross-sectional study. Echocardiographic examination was performed after dialysis session at normovolemic status. Fasting blood samples were obtained before dialysis session. *Results*. Patients on PD and female patients in both groups had significantly lower level of 25-OH-D3 level when compared to patients on HD or male patients (p: 0.0001 and p: 0.0001). When all participants were considered, there was no significant association between 25-OH-D3 and echocardiographic parameters; however, in patients on PD, a significant negative correlation was determined between 25-OH-D3 and diastolic blood pressure, interventricular septal hypertrophy (ISH), and left ventricular mass index (LVMI) (r: −0.424, p: 0.012; r: −0.508, p: 0.004; r: 0.489, p: 0.04, resp.). *Conclusion*. Low serum 25-hydroxyvitamin D levels is associated with ISH and LVMI in PD patients.

1. Introduction

Besides its action on bone-mineral metabolism, vitamin D has numerous physiologic effects including cell growth and differentiation of immune system [1]. Also vitamin D deficiency (VDD) has a well-known association with endothelial dysfunction [2]. In vitro studies indicated a favourable antiproliferative effect of vitamin D replacement on relaxation of cardiomyocytes and diastolic functions of heart [3, 4].

Cardiovascular disorders (CVD) account most common cause of mortality in ESRD. On the other hand, chronic kidney disease (CKD) is associated with accelerated development of CVD [5]. Patients with CKD tend to have accelerated atherosclerosis, valvular calcification, asymmetric septal hypertrophy, and arrhythmias when compared to general population. Innovations in renal replacement procedures prolong survival in ESRD patients and consequent increase in CVD risk [6].

Vitamin D receptors have been identified in several extrarenal organ systems including cardiac myocytes and endothelial cells [7]. In animal studies, researchers have demonstrated an association between VDD and increased contractility and deteriorated systolic functions, both leading to myocardial hypertrophy [8]. Mose et al. showed that active vitamin D therapy for 6 months improved end-diastolic volume of left ventricule [9]. Similarly, active vitamin D and vitamin D receptor activators (paricalcitol) are related to decreased mortality and better cardiovascular risk profile. Low serum vitamin D level cause hypocalcemia and secondary hyperparathyroidism that are related to coronary artery calcification, cardiac failure, and mortality [8].

There is a strict relationship between VDD and CVD-related mortality; however exact mechanism is not clearly understood. We aimed to examine the effect of 25-OH-D3 on echocardiographic indices and cardiac functions in ESRD patients receiving RRT.

2. Material-Method

A cross-sectional study on 98 ESRD patients receiving RRT was conducted between January 2015 and March 2015 in Bagcilar Education and Research Hospital. Patients were divided into 2 subgroups: 64 patients on hemodialysis (HD) and 34 age matched patients on peritoneal dialysis (PD) with similar duration of ESRD and RRT. Ethics committee of Bagcilar Education and Research Hospital approved the study. Written informed consent was obtained from all participants.

Entire patients in each group were under dietary restrictions that is recommended by K/DOQI for patients on dialysis therapy [10]. Patients on PD and HD were regularly followed up in Dialysis Center and Nephrology outpatient service of Bagcilar Education and Research Hospital. Serum potassium, sodium, calcium, and hemogram analysis were performed by monthly intervals, and parathormon level was analyzed by 3-month intervals. Patients were informed about the results and, consequently, recommendations were updated by special dietitian. Also their first-degree relatives (parents, husbands, wives, or children) were integrated to follow-up procedure to augment patient's continuity and accommodation. Similarly, patients in both groups were advised with exposure to sunlight not less than 1 hour/day. The study was performed between January and March 2015 in Istanbul to eliminate variations of seasonal exposure to sunlight. All the patients have the same ethnic background and were residents of the same region in European side of Istanbul city. All the patients survived during the study period

Exclusion criteria were anemia, obesity, acute inflammatory or infectious disease, malignancy, immobility, ongoing treatment with immunosuppressive agents, severe hypertension, hypohyperparathyroidism, pregnancy, left ventricular ejection fraction (LVEF) <50%, moderate-to-severe valvular disease, or age younger than 18 years. Data regarding demographic features and physical examination were recorded.

Blood samples were collected after 8-hour fasting period. Serum levels of calcium (Ca), phosphorus (P), albumin, alkalen phosphatase (ALP), and low density lipoprotein (LDL) were analyzed by photometric method in Siemens

Advia 1800 device. Electrochemiluminescence immunoassay (ECLIA) method was used to analyze serum levels of parathormon (PTH) and 25-hydroxyvitamin D3. Vitamin D deficiencies were classified as severe, <5 ng/mL; moderate, 5–15 ng/mL; and mild, 15–29 ng/mL [11]. Vitamin D replacement was instituted on the basis of achieving a PTH level of <300 IU/L as recommended by K/DOQI [10]. The use of vitamin D replacement was recorded for each patient.

Echocardiographic examination was performed after dialysis session at normovolemic status. Normovolemia or dry weight was defined as postdialysis weight where the patient shows no sign of pulmonary or peripheral edema and do not have hypotension [12]. Fasting blood samples were obtained before dialysis session. All cases were examined by iE33 Echocardiography system to detect left ventricular end-diastolic dimension (LVEDD), left atrial diameter (LAD), left ventricular posterior wall thickness in diastole (LVPWT), interventricular septum thickness in diastole (IVST), and left ventricular ejection fraction (LVEF). Left ventricular mass was calculated according to the American Society of Echocardiography formula. Body mass index (BMI) was calculated by dividing weight into the square of height, body surface area (BSA) was calculated as ([height (cm) × weight (kg)]/3600)$^{1/2}$, and LV mass index was calculated by dividing LV mass into the BSA. Left ventricular hypertrophy was defined as LV mass index >115 g/m^2 (for men) and >95 g/m^2 (for women) [13]. The use of angiotensin converting enzyme (ACE) inhibitors and angiotensin receptor blockers (ARB) was recorded for each patient.

2.1. Statistical Analysis. SPSS 22.0 (SPSS, Chicago, Illinois, USA) package programme was used for statistical analysis. Parametric variables were compared with independent t-test, ordinal data were compared with Mann–Whitney U test, and nonparametric variables were compared with chi-square test. Quantitative parameters were compared with Kruskal Wallis test. Spearman's rho correlation test was used to evaluate the relation of parametric variables. A p value <0.05 was considered significant.

3. Results

Group 1 consists of 64 patients on HD with a mean age of 56.42 ± 18.37 years and mean RRT duration of 38.12 ± 15.62 months. In group 2, there were 34 patients on PD with a mean age of 53.11 ± 10.63 years and mean RRT duration of 34.64 ± 14.59 months. The mean age and RRT duration of both groups were similar. Creatinine levels were similar in both groups. In most of the patients, daily urine output was below 200 mL/day; therefore renal clearance was negligible.

Serum levels of Ca, P, PTH, and alkalen phosphatase (ALP) were similar between patients on HD and PD. Lipid profile including LDL-c, HDL-c, and triglyceride level were similar between patients on HD and PD. Serum 25-OH-D3 level of patients on PD (4.68 ± 2.93 ng/mL) was significantly lower than patients on HD (9.29 ± 7.47 ng/mL) (p: 0.0001). Women in both groups had low 25-OH-D3 level when compared to male participants (p: 0.0001). Table 1 shows the biochemical and demographic data of both groups.

TABLE 1: Comparison of biochemical variables between groups.

	HD	PD	p
25-OH-D vitamin (ng/dL)	9.29 ± 7.47	4.68 ± 2.93	**0.0001**
Age (years)	56.42 ± 18.37	53.35 ± 10.49	NS
Mean duration of RRT (months)	38.12 ± 15.62	34.64 ± 14.59	NS
Kt.V	1.45 ± 0.17	2.35 ± 0.35	**NS**
Urea (mg/dL)	119.45 ± 40.19	116.34 ± 39.86	**NS**
Creatinine (mg/dL)	7.61 ± 2.71	7.47 ± 3.14	NS
Calcium (mg/dL)	8.79 ± 0.87	8.20 ± 1.33	NS
Phosphorus (mg/dL)	4.94 ± 1.67	5.30 ± 1.47	NS
PTH (pg/mL)	490.07 ± 644.92	541.4 ± 545.3	NS
Uric acid (mg/dL)	5.79 ± 1.48	6.11 ± 1.17	NS
AST (U/L)	13.98 ± 10.18	14.21 ± 9.86	**NS**
ALT (U/L)	13.79 ± 16.11	14.12 ± 9.23	**NS**
ALP (mg/dL)	119.34 ± 49.72	103.03 ± 46.86	NS
LDH (U/L)	197.14 ± 48.75	202.46 ± 53.21	**NS**
Triglyceride (mg/dL)	169.86 ± 73.57	178.45 ± 79.28	NS
Total cholesterol (mg/dL)	189.43 ± 48.52	191.36 ± 45.97	**NS**
HDL (mg/dL)	39.36 ± 14.11	41.16 ± 13.85	**NS**
LDL (mg/dL)	105.67 ± 37.68	113.23 ± 37.53	**NS**
Na (mmol/L)	137.46 ± 3.96	140.06 ± 4.7	**NS**
K (mmol/L)	4.76 ± 0.69	4.59 ± 0.71	**NS**
BMI (kg/m^2)	26 ± 4	24 ± 5	**NS**
Systolic BP (mmHg)	117 ± 21	122 ± 17	**NS**
Diastolic BP (mmHg)	70 ± 15	72 ± 14	**NS**

Two patients in PD group and 3 patients in HD group were receiving statin therapy. The mean ± SD systolic blood pressure of patients on HD and PD was 118 ± 21 mmHg and 122 ± 17 mmHg, respectively. The mean ± SD diastolic blood pressure of patients on HD and PD was 70 ± 15 mmHg and 72 ± 14 mmHg, respectively. Both mean systolic and diastolic pressure of patients on HD and PD were statistically similar. The ratio of antihypertensive drug use in PD and HD group was similar. Frequency of ACE-inhibitor or ARB use was 8.2% and 6.9% for HD and PD patients respectively. Also vitamin D was administered according to parathormon level of patients as recommended by K/DOQI clinical practice guidelines for bone metabolism and disease in CKD. Frequency of active vitamin D use was 91.8% and 93.1% for HD and PD patients, respectively.

Echocardiographic parameters were similar in HD and PD group (Table 2). When all patients were considered, correlation analysis indicated a significant association between 25-OHD3 and age (r: −0.226, p: 0.028). However, there was no significant association between 25-OHD3 and echocardiographic parameters.

In HD group, there was no significant association between 25-OH-D3 and echocardiographic parameters (Table 3). In PD group, a significant inverse correlation was determined between 25-OH-D3 and diastolic blood pressure, aortic velocity (Aovel), pulmonary velocity (Pvel), aortic regurgitation (AR), interventricular septal hypertrophy (IVSH), and left ventricular mass index (r: −0.424, p: 0.012; r: −0.433, p: 0.024; r: −0.498, p: 0.006; r: −0.430, p: 0.022; r: −0.508, p: 0.004; r: 0.489, p: 0.04; resp.) (Table 4).

4. Discussion

Our study indicates that female participants and patients on PD have lower 25-OH-D3 level. Additionally, PD patients but not HD patients with low 25-OH-D3 level have structural cardiovascular changes which may be related to high diastolic blood pressure, ISH, and LVMI.

CVD-related mortality risk of patients with CKD varies between 40% and 50% [14]. Low serum 25-OH-D3 levels are frequently seen in CKD patients. In a study by Taskapan et al., mild, moderate, and severe VDD was observed in 43,9%, 48,4%, and 4,4%, respectively, similar to our study [15]. A growing body of evidence indicates the relation of VDD with morbidity and mortality in patients with CKD. Ravani et al. showed that 25-OH-D3 independently and more accurately predicts progression of CKD and mortality in 168 patients with stages 2–5 CKD when compared to 1,25-OH-D3 [16]. Wang and Wells demonstrated a high CV event risk in a study on 230 PD patients with low serum 25-OH-D3 level [17]. Pekkanen et al. determined a relation between decreased LVEF and low serum 25-OH-D3 level [18].

Drechsler et al. showed a 3 times increased sudden cardiac death among patients with severe VDD (<25 nmol/L) when compared to patients with adequate vitamin D status (>75 nmol/L) [19]. In "Framingham Offspring Study," patients with low serum 25-OH-D3 and without a history of CVD have high mortality rates [20]. All cause and CV related mortality rates were significantly higher in patients with low 25-OH-D level than normal 25-OH-D in patients that underwent coronary angiography and were followed up for 7.7 years [21].

TABLE 2: Echocardiographic indices of both groups.

	HD	PD	p
LVD, mm	47.4 ± 6.5	47.6 ± 7.4	0.878
LVS, mm	31.3 ± 6	30.2 ± 8.2	0.479
IVS, mm	12.7 ± 2.5	12.2 ± 2.4	0.310
PW, mm	12.3 ± 2.5	15.8 ± 2.36	0.212
EF, %	61.24 ± 7.09	63.77 ± 9.02	0.146
FS, %	33.3 ± 5.02	34.72 ± 5.91	0.235
EDV, ml	106.27 ± 31.99	111.27 ± 42.88	0.542
ESV, ml	41.64 ± 16.52	42.93 ± 34.5	0.815
Ao, mm	26.8 ± 2.7	26.1 ± 2.4	0.215
As.Aort, mm	32.7 ± 4.2	33.6 ± 5	0.360
LA, mm	37.2 ± 7.8	35.2 ± 6.9	0.231
Em, cm/s	59 ± 16	66 ± 24	0.175
Am, cm/s	71 ± 15	81 ± 21	**0.021**
E', cm/s	98 ± 12	79 ± 31	0.606
Aovel, m/s	1.32 ± 0.42	1.4 ± 0.39	0.452
Pvel, m/s	0.86 ± 0.16	0.9 ± 0.16	0.291
TAPSE, cm/s	19.46 ± 4.29	18.69 ± 3.6	0.408
MR	0.8 ± 0.62	0.72 ± 0.59	0.610
AR	0.31 ± 0.5	0.41 ± 0.57	0.398
TR	1.04 ± 0.19	1.07 ± 0.25	0.506
PAPs, mmhg	27.82 ± 8.81	27.73 ± 7.89	0.964

LVD: left ventricular end-diastolic dimension, LVSD: left ventricular end-systolic dimension, IVS: interventricular septal thickness, PW: posterior wall thickness, EF: ejection fraction, FS: fractional shortening, EDV: end-diastolic volume, ESV: end-systolic volume, Ao: aortic root, As.Aort: ascendant aorta, LA: LA end-systolic dimension, Em: mitral annular early diastolic velocity, Am: mitral annular late diastolic velocity, E: tissue Doppler early diastolic mitral annular velocity, Aovel: aortic valve velocity, Pvel: pulmonary valve velocity, TAPSE: tricuspid annular plane systolic excursion, MR: mitral regurgitation, AR: aortic regurgitation, TR: tricuspid regurgitation, and PAPs: estimated pulmonary artery systolic pressure.

TABLE 3: The relation of 25-OH-D3 with echocardiographic indices in HD group.

	25-OH-D	
	r	p
LVD (mm)	−0.160	0.235
LVS (mm)	−0.089	0.516
IVS (mm)	−0.037	0.784
PW(mm)	−0.043	0.750
LV mass index	−0.210	0.230
EF (%)	−0.056	0.680
Ao (mm)	0.053	0.693
As.aort (mm)	0.165	0.248
LA (mm)	−0.082	0.546
Em (cm/s)	0.120	0.373
Am (cm/s)	0.027	0.847
E (cm/s)	−0.042	0.761
Aovel (m/s)	0.010	0.939
Pvel (m/s)	−0.063	0.649
TAPSE (cm/s)	−0.214	0.117
AR	−0.042	0.765
TPAPs (mmHg)	−0.009	0.950

LVD: left ventricular end-diastolic dimension, LVSD: left ventricular end-systolic dimension, IVS: interventricular septal thickness, PW: posterior wall thickness, EF: ejection fraction, Ao: aortic root, As.Aort: ascendant aorta, LA end-systolic dimension: Em: mitral annular early diastolic velocity, Am: mitral annular late diastolic velocity, E: tissue Doppler early diastolic mitral annular velocity, Aovel: aortic valve velocity, Pvel: pulmonary valve velocity, TAPSE: tricuspid annular plane systolic excursion, AR: aortic regurgitation, and PAPs: estimated pulmonary artery systolic pressure.

Vitamin D metabolites have renoprotective effect by antiproteinuric, anti-inflammatory, and immunomodulatory properties and by suppression of renin-angiotensin-aldosterone system (RAAS) [22]. Low serum 25-OH-D level activates (RAAS) and increases fibroblast growth factor which are associated with progression of renal injury [23, 24]. Decreased serum 25-hydroxyvitamin D level leads to IVSH which is a significant predictor of cardiovascular morbidity in ESRD in pediatric population [25]. Additionally, low serum 25-OH-D3 have been related to increased inflammatory state which is involved in atherosclerosis and CVD [26, 27].

Hypertension, DM, dyslipidemia, age, volume-nutritional status, and dialysis adequacy are well-known CVD risk factors that are frequently seen in CKD patients [27]. All these factors are correlated with echocardiographic indexes including left ventricular diastolic diameter (LVdD), LVED, and ejection fraction (EF) [27]. Because calcium-phosphorus equilibrium as well as fluid and glycemic control has significant impact on cardiac myocytes (trophic effect of PTH on cardiac myocytes), echocardiographic examinations were performed after dialysis session at normovolemic status. In the Framingham Offspring Study, individuals with low

25-OH-D3 level had a hazard ratio of 1.62 for CVD risk [27]. Because fluid control is better in HD patients, PD patients have increased CVD and mortality risk [28].

Although it is out of our study object, vitamin D replacement has favourable impact on cardiac functions and diastolic dysfunction and is associated with regression of myocardial hypertrophy [29–31]. However authors of two large scaled human studies (PRIMO and OPERA trials) and an experimental animal study failed to demonstrate a beneficial effect of vitamin D therapy on structural and functional changes in myocardium [32–34]. It would be reasonable to state that maintaining an accurate vitamin D level has vital importance in ESRD because excessive vitamin D replacement may cause hypercalcemia and hyperphosphatemia where high CaxP level is also related to calciphylaxis and vascular or valvular calcification.

Low sample size and single point measurement of variables were two major limitations of the study. A large number of dialysis patients that have exclusion criteria mentioned in the material-method section were excluded. Additionally patients with low dialysis adequacy were also excluded to eliminate the effect of hypervolemia and electrolyte imbalance on echocardiographic indices. Cross-sectional design of the study was another major limitation that should be confirmed by RCTs. To the best of our knowledge, this was the first report that indicates the association of low endogenous

TABLE 4: The relation of echocardiographic variables with 25-OH-D3 in PD group.

	25-OH-D	
	r	*p*
LVD (mm)	0.081	0.669
LVS (mm)	0.103	0.590
IVS (mm)	−0.508	0.004
PW (mm)	−0.321	0.089
LV mass index (gr/m²)	−0.489	0.004
EF (%)	0.116	0.543
Ao (mm)	0.115	0.554
As.aort (mm)	0.195	0.301
LA (mm)	−0.119	0.539
Em (cm/s)	−0.114	0.565
Am (cm/s)	−0.213	0.258
E (cm/s)	0.352	0.061
Aovel (m/s)	−0.433	0.024
Pvel (m/s)	−0.498	0.006
TAPSE (cm/s)	−0.130	0.511
AR	−0.430	0.022
TPAPs (mmHg)	−0.221	0.250

LVD: left ventricular end-diastolic dimension, LVSD: left ventricular end-systolic dimension, IVS: interventricular septal thickness, PW: posterior wall thickness, EF: ejection fraction, Ao: aortic root, As.Aort: ascendant aorta, LA end-systolic dimension: Em: mitral annular early diastolic velocity, Am: mitral annular late diastolic velocity, E: tissue Doppler early diastolic mitral annular velocity, Aovel: aortic valve velocity, Pvel: pulmonary valve velocity, TAPSE: tricuspid annular plane systolic excursion, AR: aortic regurgitation, and PAPs: estimated pulmonary artery systolic pressure.

vitamin D status with diastolic dysfunction and ventricular hypertrophy in PD patients. In contrast to majority of previous studies, our study participants were similar in terms of CVD risk factors including blood pressure, dyslipidemia, serum glucose, age, obesity, uric acid level, and dialysis adequacy that provided us with elimination of effect of these factors on echocardiographic indices. Possible explanation of correlation between vitamin D and echocardiographic indices in PD is that fluid control and volume status were better in HD patients that have significant impact on both cardiovascular health and echocardiographic indices. Also intravenous or oral administration of vitamin D may affect serum level and echocardiographic indices. Owing to the fact that CKD patients on RRT have predisposition to CVD, 25-OH-D3 may become a candidate marker to predict future CV events. Regular follow-up of serum 25-OH-D3 may provide complementary data on cardiovascular health status of dialysis patients. Large scaled studies would clarify the exact role of vitamin D on cardiovascular morbidity and mortality in CKD patients.

References

[1] S. Chen, G. P. Sims, X. X. Chen, Y. Y. Gu, S. Chen, and P. E. Lipsky, "Modulatory effects of 1,25-dihydroxyvitamin D₃ on human B cell differentiation," *The Journal of Immunology*, vol. 179, no. 3, pp. 1634–1647, 2007.

[2] K. A. Nibbelink, D. X. Tishkoff, S. D. Hershey, A. Rahman, and R. U. Simpson, "1,25(OH)₂-vitamin D3 actions on cell proliferation, size, gene expression, and receptor localization, in the HL-1 cardiac myocyte," *Journal of Steroid Biochemistry and Molecular Biology*, vol. 103, no. 3-5, pp. 533–537, 2007.

[3] T. D. O'Connell, J. E. Berry, A. K. Jarvis, M. J. Somerman, and R. U. Simpson, "1,25-Dihydroxyvitamin D3 regulation of cardiac myocyte proliferation and hypertrophy," *American Journal of Physiology—Heart and Circulatory Physiology*, vol. 272, no. 4, pp. H1751–H1758, 1997.

[4] J. J. Green, D. A. Robinson, G. E. Wilson, R. U. Simpson, and M. V. Westfall, "Calcitriol modulation of cardiac contractile performance via protein kinase C," *Journal of Molecular and Cellular Cardiology*, vol. 41, no. 2, pp. 350–359, 2006.

[5] A. S. Go, G. M. Chertow, D. Fan, C. E. McCulloch, and C.-Y. Hsu, "Chronic kidney disease and the risks of death, cardiovascular events, and hospitalization," *The New England Journal of Medicine*, vol. 351, no. 13, pp. 1296–1370, 2004.

[6] T.-H. Kuo, D.-C. Yang, W.-H. Lin et al., "Compliance index, a marker of peripheral arterial stiffness, may predict renal function decline in patients with chronic kidney disease," *International Journal of Medical Sciences*, vol. 12, no. 7, pp. 530–537, 2015.

[7] H. F. Deluca and M. T. Cantorna, "Vitamin D: its role and uses in immunology," *FASEB Journal*, vol. 15, no. 14, pp. 2579–2585, 2001.

[8] S. Pilz, A. Tomaschitz, C. Drechsler, and R. A. de Boer, "Vitamin D deficiency and heart disease," *Kidney International Supplements*, vol. 1, no. 4, pp. 111–115, 2011.

[9] F. H. Mose, H. Vase, T. Larsen et al., "Cardiovascular effects of cholecalciferol treatment in dialysis patients—a randomized controlled trial," *BMC Nephrology*, vol. 15, article 50, 2014.

[10] "K/DOQI clinical practice guidelines for bone metabolism and disease in chronic kidney disease," *American Journal of Kidney Diseases*, vol. 42, pp. S1–S201, 2003.

[11] G. A. Block and F. K. Port, "Re-evaluation of risks associated with hyperphosphatemia and hyperparathyroidism in dialysis patients: recommendations for a change in management," *American Journal of Kidney Diseases*, vol. 35, no. 6, pp. 1226–1237, 2000.

[12] J. K. Leypold and A. K. Cheung, "Evaluating volume status in hemodialysis patients," *Advances in Renal Replacement Therapy*, vol. 5, pp. 64–74, 1998.

[13] R. M. Lang, M. Bierig, R. B. Devereux et al., "Recommendations for chamber quantification: a report from the American Society of Echocardiography's Guidelines and Standards Committee and the Chamber Quantification Writing Group, developed in conjunction with the European Association of Echocardiography, a branch of the European Society of Cardiology," *Journal of the American Society of Echocardiography*, vol. 18, no. 12, pp. 1440–1463, 2005.

[14] "Causes of death," *American Journal of Kidney Diseases*, vol. 34, no. 2, supplement 1, pp. S87–S94, 1999.

[15] H. Taskapan, I. Sahin, P. Tam, and T. Sikaneta, "Vitamin D and kidney," *International Journal of Endocrinology*, vol. 2013, Article ID 164103, 2 pages, 2013.

[16] P. Ravani, F. Malberti, G. Tripepi et al., "Vitamin D levels and patient outcome in chronic kidney disease," *Kidney International*, vol. 75, no. 1, pp. 88–95, 2009.

[17] T. J. Wang and Q. S. Wells, "Vitamin D deficiency and heart failure risk. Not so black and white?" *JACC: Heart Failure*, vol. 3, no. 5, pp. 357–359, 2015.

[18] M. P. Pekkanen, O. Ukkola, P. Hedberg et al., "Serum 25-hydroxyvitamin D is associated with major cardiovascular risk factors and cardiac structure and function in patients with coronary artery disease," *Nutrition, Metabolism and Cardiovascular Diseases*, vol. 25, no. 5, pp. 471–478, 2015.

[19] C. Drechsler, M. Verduijn, S. Pilz et al., "Vitamin D status and clinical outcomes in incident dialysis patients: results from the NECOSAD study," *Nephrology Dialysis Transplantation*, vol. 26, no. 3, pp. 1024–1032, 2011.

[20] V. Xanthakis, D. M. Enserro, J. M. Murabito et al., "Ideal cardiovascular health: associations with biomarkers and subclinical disease and impact on incidence of cardiovascular disease in the Framingham Offspring Study," *Circulation*, vol. 130, no. 19, pp. 1676–1683, 2014.

[21] G. N. Thomas, B. Ó. Hartaigh, J. A. Bosch et al., "Vitamin D levels predict all-cause and cardiovascular disease mortality in subjects with the metabolic syndrome: the Ludwigshafen risk and cardiovascular health (LURIC) study," *Diabetes Care*, vol. 35, no. 5, pp. 1158–1164, 2012.

[22] D. Santoro, D. Caccamo, S. Lucisano et al., "Interplay of vitamin D, erythropoiesis, and the renin-angiotensin system," *BioMed Research International*, vol. 2015, Article ID 145828, 11 pages, 2015.

[23] K. Yokoyama, A. Nakashima, M. Urashima et al., "Interactions between serum vitamin D levels and vitamin D receptor gene foki polymorphisms for renal function in patients with type 2 diabetes," *PLoS ONE*, vol. 7, no. 12, article e51171, 2012.

[24] K. Khademvatani, M. H. Seyyed-Mohammadzad, M. Akbari, Y. Rezaei, R. Eskandari, and A. Rostamzadeh, "The relationship between vitamin D status and idiopathic lower-extremity deep vein thrombosis," *International Journal of General Medicine*, vol. 7, pp. 303–309, 2014.

[25] S. Uysal, A. G. Kalayci, and K. Baysal, "Cardiac functions in children with vitamin D deficiency rickets," *Pediatric Cardiology*, vol. 20, no. 4, pp. 283–286, 1999.

[26] J. Donate-Correa, V. Domínguez-Pimentel, M. L. Méndez-Pérez et al., "Selective vitamin D receptor activation as anti-inflammatory target in chronic kidney disease," *Mediators of Inflammation*, vol. 2014, Article ID 670475, 6 pages, 2014.

[27] B. Esen, A. E. Atay, I. Sahin et al., "The relation of serum 25-hydroxy vitamin D3 with inflammation and indirect markers of thrombotic activity in patients with end stage renal disease," *Journal of Clinical and Experimental Nephrology*, vol. 1, pp. 1–6, 2016.

[28] S. Lai, A. Molfino, G. E. Russo et al., "Cardiac, inflammatory and metabolic parameters: hemodialysis versus peritoneal dialysis," *Cardiorenal Medicine*, vol. 5, no. 1, pp. 20–30, 2015.

[29] A. N. Kiani, H. Fang, L. S. Magder, and M. Petri, "Vitamin D deficiency does not predict progression of coronary artery calcium, carotid intima-media thickness or high-sensitivity C-reactive protein in systemic lupus erythematosus," *Rheumatology*, vol. 52, no. 11, pp. 2071–2076, 2013.

[30] S. Lemmilä, H. Saha, V. Virtanen, I. Ala-Houhala, and A. Pasternack, "Effect of intravenous calcitriol on cardiac systolic and diastolic function in patients on hemodialysis," *American Journal of Nephrology*, vol. 18, no. 5, pp. 404–410, 1998.

[31] N. P. Singh, V. Sahni, D. Garg, and M. Nair, "Effect of pharmacological suppression of secondary hyperparathyroidism on cardiovascular hemodynamics in predialysis CKD patients: a preliminary observation," *Hemodialysis International*, vol. 11, no. 4, pp. 417–423, 2007.

[32] C. W. Park, Y. S. Oh, Y. S. Shin et al., "Intravenous calcitriol regresses myocardial hypertrophy in hemodialysis patients with secondary hyperparathyroidism," *American Journal of Kidney Diseases*, vol. 33, no. 1, pp. 73–81, 1999.

[33] R. Thadhani, E. Appelbaum, Y. Pritchett et al., "Vitamin D therapy and cardiac structure and function in patients with chronic kidney disease: the PRIMO randomized controlled trial," *The Journal of the American Medical Association*, vol. 307, no. 7, pp. 674–684, 2012.

[34] A. Y.-M. Wang, F. Fang, J. Chan et al., "Effect of paricalcitol on left ventricular mass and function in CKD-the OPERA trial," *Journal of the American Society of Nephrology*, vol. 25, no. 1, pp. 175–186, 2014.

High Prevalence of Cardiovascular Disease in End-Stage Kidney Disease Patients Ongoing Hemodialysis in Peru: Why Should We Care About It?

Katia Bravo-Jaimes,[1,2] Alvaro Whittembury,[2] and Vilma Santivañez[2]

[1]*University of Rochester Medical Center, 601 Elmwood Avenue, Box MED, Rochester, NY 14642, USA*
[2]*Facultad de Medicina de San Fernando, Universidad Nacional Mayor de San Marcos (UNMSM), Lima, Peru*

Correspondence should be addressed to Katia Bravo-Jaimes; katia_bravo-jaimes@urmc.rochester.edu

Academic Editor: Alessandro Amore

Purpose. To determine clinical, biochemical, and pharmacological characteristics as well as cardiovascular disease prevalence and its associated factors among end-stage kidney disease patients receiving hemodialysis in the main hemodialysis center in Lima, Peru. *Methods*. This cross-sectional study included 103 patients. Clinical charts were reviewed and an echocardiogram was performed to determine prevalence of cardiovascular disease, defined as the presence of systolic/diastolic dysfunction, coronary heart disease, ventricular dysrhythmias, cerebrovascular disease, and/or peripheral vascular disease. Associations between cardiovascular disease and clinical, biochemical, and dialysis factors were sought using prevalence ratio. A robust Poisson regression model was used to quantify possible associations. *Results*. Cardiovascular disease prevalence was 81.6%, mainly due to diastolic dysfunction. It was significantly associated with age older than 50 years, metabolic syndrome, C-reactive protein levels, effective blood flow ≤ 300 mL/min, severe anemia, and absence of mild anemia. However, in the regression analysis only age older than 50 years, effective blood flow ≤ 300 mL/min, and absence of mild anemia were associated. *Conclusions*. Cardiovascular disease prevalence is high in patients receiving hemodialysis in the main center in Lima. Diastolic dysfunction, age, specific hemoglobin levels, and effective blood flow may play an important role.

1. Introduction

Chronic kidney disease is a public health problem around the world. It is increasing over time mainly due to an increasing number of diabetic patients, and with nearly 30% of the 170 million diabetic patients eventually developing diabetic nephropathy [1]. Worldwide, most patients with end-stage kidney disease (ESKD) who can access renal replacement therapy are receiving hemodialysis (HD) [2]. In 2013, there were 1,222 patients per million population (pmp) receiving hemodialysis in the USA [2], while, in 2006, there were 280 patients pmp in Latin America [3] and, in 2012, there were 300 patients pmp receiving hemodialysis in Peru [4].

Cardiovascular disease (CVD) is the main cause of death in patients with ESKD [2, 3]. It is estimated that ESKD patients are 5 to 20 times more likely to die because of cardiovascular causes than the general population [5]. Traditional cardiovascular risk factors do not completely explain higher mortality rates among hemodialysis patients [6], and nontraditional risk factors such as anemia, bone mineral disease, hyperhomocysteinemia, inflammation, hypercoagulability, and left ventricular hypertrophy (LVH) [7] have been demonstrated to play an important role in this population. The prevalence of CVD in hemodialysis patients varies across countries; that is, in the USA, ischemic heart disease, heart failure, peripheral vascular disease, and cerebrovascular disease were found in 41% [8], 40% [9], 22% [10], and 13% [11] of these patients, while, in Spain, they were found in 17%, 14%, 6%, and 2% [12] of HD patients.

It is estimated that 300,000 patients have chronic kidney disease in Peru, and more than 9,000 of them require renal replacement therapy [4]. The incidence of ESKD patients receiving hemodialysis is increasing over time [4]; however the prevalence of CVD in these patients remains to be estimated. Thus, this study had the following goals: (1) to determine clinical, biochemical, and pharmacological characteristics among ESKD patients receiving hemodialysis in the main hemodialysis center in Lima, the "Centro Nacional de Salud Renal" (CNSR), (2) to determine CVD prevalence in these patients, and (3) to determine the association between CVD and clinical, biochemical, and dialysis factors in these patients.

2. Methods

This cross-sectional study included one hundred and three prevalent HD patients (three sessions of hemodialysis a week for more than three months) from the largest HD center in Lima, Peru (CNSR, EsSalud), using a convenience sampling approach. All patients were adults and had never received renal transplantation or peritoneal dialysis. An informed consent was obtained before enrollment in the study. Ethics Committees from Universidad Nacional Mayor de San Marcos and Centro Nacional de Salud Renal reviewed and approved the study.

Using a standardized form, clinical charts were reviewed to gather the following information: age, gender, prescribed dry weight, cause of ESKD, hypertension status, diabetes status, latest electrocardiogram results, time on hemodialysis, effective blood flow, and current prescription of statins, aspirin, angiotensin-converting enzyme inhibitors (ACE-I), and angiotensin II receptor blockers (ARB). To determine history of CVD (coronary heart disease, cerebrovascular disease, peripheral vascular disease, and ventricular dysrhythmias) and comorbid medical conditions (chronic pulmonary obstructive disease, cancer, dementia, inability to ambulate, peptic ulcer disease, liver disease, HIV status, hepatitis C infection, and hepatitis B infection), chart reviews were supplemented by interviews with the patients, family members, and dialysis staff as necessary.

Patients underwent an evaluation that included (1) anthropometric measurements, (2) blood sample collection, and (3) an echocardiogram. Height and waist circumference were measured after dialysis; the latter was obtained to the nearest centimeter, midway between the lower limit of the rib cage and the iliac crest, with the subject standing, using a flexible and nondistensible tape. Blood samples were obtained before dialysis as part of the routine protocol in the hemodialysis center (a postdialysis sample was used to determine KT/V urea only), without specific instructions to the patients. Blood sample specimens were analyzed for total cholesterol, low-density lipoprotein cholesterol (LDL-C), high-density lipoprotein cholesterol (HDL-C), triglycerides, hemoglobin, calcium, phosphorus, C-reactive protein (CRP), parathyroid hormone, and KT/V urea. A two-dimensional and M-mode echocardiogram was performed using a M2540A model Philips echocardiograph by a single cardiologist at a private clinic using American Society of Echocardiography guidelines for wall thickness and chamber dimensions [13]. The echocardiographic measurements included ejection fraction, left ventricular filling pattern,

mitral E/A ratio, and left ventricular mass (calculated from the corrected American Society of Echocardiography method using end diastolic parameters: LV mass = $0.8\{1.04[(IVS + PWT + LVEDD)^3 - (LVEDD)^3]\} + 0.6$).

Charlson comorbidity index and metabolic syndrome status (according to the International Diabetes Federation criteria [14]) were calculated based on the clinical and laboratory results.

Cardiovascular disease (CVD) was defined as the presence of any of the following:

(i) Coronary heart disease: myocardial infarction or stable angina or unstable angina or coronary artery bypass graft or percutaneous coronary intervention.

(ii) Diastolic dysfunction: abnormal left ventricular filling pattern and/or mitral E/A ratio out of the range 0.7–3.1 if 64 years or under, or 0.5–1.7 if over 64 years [15] found on echocardiogram.

(iii) Systolic dysfunction: ejection fraction less than 55% found on echocardiogram.

(iv) Cerebrovascular disease: atherothrombotic cerebral infarction or carotid endarterectomy or transient ischemic attack.

(v) Peripheral vascular disease: renal artery stenosis or lower limbs revascularization or any limb amputation.

(vi) Ventricular dysrhythmias: electrocardiographic evidence of ventricular tachycardia or fibrillation.

Data are presented as mean ± SD for continuous variables (median (interquartile range), when not normally distributed) and as fractions for categorical variables. Bivariate analysis searching for associations between CVD and other variables was done using prevalence ratios (PR). Multivariate analysis was performed using a Poisson regression model with robust variance estimation in order to calculate adjusted prevalence ratios (aPR); an enter method was used. Variables included in the multivariate analysis were age, sex, hypertension, metabolic syndrome, CRP levels, severe anemia, absence of mild anemia, and effective blood flow. A p value <0.05 was considered statistically significant. All statistical analysis was done using STATA v. 13.0 for Windows.

3. Results

3.1. Study Patients. A total of 103 patients were included in the study (a third of the population receiving HD at CNSR). Patients were mainly male (n = 73, 71%). The mean age was 54.0 ± 14.6 years. The main causes of ESKD were hypertension (30%), glomerulonephritis (22%), and diabetes mellitus (12%). Miscellaneous causes accounted for 30% of the patients (including obstructive uropathy, systemic lupus erythematosus, nephrolithiasis, renal tuberculosis, and polycystic kidney disease). The cause of ESKD could not be determined in 6% of the patients. The mean time on hemodialysis, effective blood flow, and KT/V were 9.7 ± 4.6 years, 326.8 ± 38.1 mL/min, and 1.5 ± 0.3, respectively. The KT/V was less than 1.3 in 9% of patients.

TABLE 1: Clinical and biochemical data in the population at CNSR categorized by cardiovascular disease.

	With CVD N = 84 (82%)	Without CVD N = 19 (18%)	p value
Age (years)*	56.7 ± 13.6	40.4 ± 11.4	<0.001
Waist circumference (cm)*	94.3 ± 13.5	90.0 ± 13.2	0.162
Effective blood flow (mL/min)*	321.6 ± 33.1	341.1 ± 36.3	0.006
Total cholesterol (mg/dL)**	163.5 (49.7)	169.0 (26.5)	0.814
LDL-C (mg/dL)**	98.0 (33.7)	101.0 (23.5)	0.927
HDL-C (mg/dL)**	40.0 (9.7)	42.0 (7.5)	0.277
Triglycerides (mg/dL)**	150.0 (130.5)	136.0 (113.0)	0.652
Calcium (mg/dL)**	9.5 (2.5)	9.3 (1.6)	0.217
Hemoglobin (mg/dL)**	12.0 (1.4)	11.4 (5.1)	0.084
CRP (mg/dL)**	0.5 (0.8)	0.4 (0.4)	0.015
PTH (pg/mL)**	356.9 (427.3)	475.2 (50.0)	0.235

CNSR: Centro Nacional De Salud Renal; CRP: C-reactive protein; PTH: parathyroid hormone.
* Mean ± SD ** Median (interquartile range).

3.2. Comorbidities.

Ninety-five percent of the patients were hypertensive, 14% were diabetic, 64% had hepatitis C infection, 9% had inability to ambulate, 4% had COPD, 4% had HIV infection, and 1% had hepatitis B infection. The average waist circumference for men and women was 93.0 ± 13.4 cm and 86.0 ± 12.4 cm, respectively. There were 59% of men with waist circumference values above 90 cm and 76% of women with values above 80 cm. Metabolic syndrome was found in 50% of the patients. The average Charlson comorbidity index was 3.5 (range 2–11), and 71% of the patients had an index above 3.

3.3. Biochemical Profile.

Calcium-phosphorus product above 55 was found in 37% of the patients. Parathyroid hormone levels above 300 pg/mL were found in 54% of the patients. 7.8% of the subjects had albumin levels under 3.6 g/dL. 56% had CRP levels above 0.3 mg/dL. 63% of women had HDL-C level under 50 mg/dL and 41% of men had these levels under 40 mg/dL.

3.4. Pharmacological Profile.

Three percent of the patients received statins, with 66% of those patients having had a prior cardiovascular event. 60% of patients with coronary heart disease were not prescribed this medication and none of the patients with hypercholesterolemia were prescribed a statin. There were 15% of the subjects receiving aspirin, but just 20% of those with coronary heart disease were prescribed aspirin. ACE-I and ARB were prescribed in 44% and 18% of the patients, respectively.

3.5. Echocardiographic Evaluation.

Echocardiogram evaluations demonstrated diastolic dysfunction in 75% of the subjects and systolic dysfunction in 10% of them. LVH was noted in 55% of the patients, and amongst these patients 35% were not receiving ACE-I or ARB.

3.6. Cardiovascular Disease.

CVD was found in 81.6% of the patients (95% CI 73.6–89.5%). Diastolic dysfunction

TABLE 2: Cardiovascular disease: robust Poisson regression model.

Model	aPR	Robust std. err.	p value	95% CI
Age older than 50 years	1.3	0.132	0.005	1.1–1.6
EBF ≤ 300	1.2	0.106	0.036	1.0–1.4
Absence of mild anemia	1.5	0.249	0.023	1.1–2.1

Variables included in the initial analysis that did not reach statistical significance were: sex, hypertension, metabolic syndrome, CRP and severe anemia.

was found in 75% of the subjects, systolic dysfunction in 10%, cerebrovascular disease in 8%, coronary heart disease in 5%, peripheral vascular disease in 1%, and ventricular dysrhythmias in 1%. Clinical and biochemical differences between the patients with and without CVD are shown in Table 1.

3.7. CVD Associated Factors.

In the bivariate analysis, CVD was significantly associated with age older than 50 years (PR = 1.4; 95% CI 1.1–1.8; $p = 0.002$), metabolic syndrome (PR = 1.2; 95% CI 1.0–1.5; $p = 0.029$), CRP levels (PR = 1.0; 95% CI 1.0–1.1; $p = 0.015$), effective blood flow less than or equal to 300 mL/min (PR = 1.2; 95% CI 1.1–1.3; $p < 0.001$), severe anemia (hemoglobin lesser than 8 g/dL) [16] (PR = 1.2; 95% CI 1.1–1.4; $p < 0.001$) and absence of mild anemia (hemoglobin lesser than 11 g/dL or greater than 11.9 g/dL in females or 12.9 g/dL in males) [16] (PR = 1.6; 95% CI 1.0–2.3; $p = 0.016$). There was a tendency towards significant results for waist circumference greater than 82 cm (PR = 1.3; 95% CI 0.9–1.7; $p = 0.093$). However, the Poisson regression analysis (Table 2) showed that CVD was associated with age older than 50 years (aPR = 1.3; 95% CI 1.1–1.6; $p = 0.005$), effective blood flow less than or equal to 300 mL/min (aPR = 1.2; 95% CI 1.0–1.4; $p = 0.036$), and absence of mild anemia (aPR = 1.5; 95% CI 1.1–2.1; $p = 0.023$).

4. Discussion

This study has found an extremely high burden of CVD amongst Peruvian long-term HD patients at CNSR, representing an alarming prevalence that is not substantially different from higher-income countries. Some important associations between CVD disease and clinical, biochemical, and dialysis factors have also been found and potentially represent a challenge for Peruvian nephrologists, especially in the public healthcare system.

CVD prevalence in this study was found to be higher than 80%. When compared to Latin American countries, our sample had higher prevalence of diastolic dysfunction than Argentina (75% versus 40%) [17] and higher prevalence of cerebrovascular disease than Chile (8% versus 7%) [18]. When compared to countries outside Latin America, our sample had higher prevalence of cerebrovascular disease than Spain (8% versus 2%) and lower prevalence of coronary heart disease (5%) and peripheral vascular disease (1%) than Spain (16% and 5%) and the USA (41% and 31.6%) [11, 12].

The main component of CVD in this sample was diastolic dysfunction, which was detected *de novo* in 59% of the patients. This alteration has been recognized as the most common echocardiographic alteration in asymptomatic ESKD patients on HD [19] and is considered a predictor of cardiovascular events in these patients as well [20]. There is evidence suggesting that the severity of diastolic dysfunction and LVH might be ameliorated by adequate correction of anemia and hypertension [21, 22]. For these reasons, it is crucial to detect these problems in a timely fashion, performing an echocardiogram and involving a cardiologist in the multidisciplinary care of patients with CKD [7].

Unfortunately, most of the patients in our sample were not offered an echocardiogram in early stages of kidney disease or at admission to hemodialysis, most likely due to a demand-offer imbalance on the social security health system. The consequences of this disproportion are exemplified by the fact that more than one-third of patients with LVH were not receiving ACE-I or ARB. However there are other situations in which medication prescription status in this cohort was found to be concerning. There was aspirin underuse in patients with coronary heart disease; however specific patient factors, such as increased bleeding risk, may be involved in the low prescription rate and are beyond the scope of this study. Also, statins were not being used in patients with hypercholesterolemia, despite its efficacy to reduce LDL-C levels in this special population [23]. Nevertheless, it is important to note that though these drugs have demonstrated benefit at decreasing stroke incidence and lowering LDL-C levels, respectively, there is no evidence they can reduce mortality in this specific population [1, 2, 24].

As has been previously described in different CKD populations [25–29], we also found that CVD was associated with metabolic syndrome; however this was not confirmed with aPR test. The principal component of this syndrome, abdominal obesity, expressed by waist circumference, has demonstrated to be a predictor of cardiovascular events in ESKD patients [30], and in this study it showed a trend towards significant results. For these reasons we propose that a simple measurement such as waist circumference could potentially denote CVD in this population. However, prospective cohorts are required to evaluate the clinical consequences of these risk factors in Peruvian patients.

The association found between CVD and tight levels of hemoglobin is interesting and thought provoking. Not only patients with severe anemia were found to have higher prevalence of CVD, but also those without mild anemia. This means that patients with hemoglobin levels lower than 11 g/dL or higher than 12.9 g/dL in men or 11.9 g/dL in women had higher prevalence of CVD. These levels are somewhat compatible with those previously reported in the CHOIR study [31], where adverse outcomes were associated with hemoglobin levels higher than 13.0 g/dL. The novel finding in this study is the potential gender-specific difference in hemoglobin targets associated with CVD in this sample. Whether or not this difference is a reflection of the Peruvian population remains to be determined in larger studies. Furthermore, taking into account the varied geography of Peru, further research to determine the appropriate hemoglobin targets in patients with CKD living at high altitude is necessary and will help in determining a possible benefit in adjusting Peruvian Nephrology practice guidelines.

Other associated CVD factors included elevated CRP levels and lower effective blood flow. Elevated CRP levels, defined as above 0.3 mg/dL due to better association with cardiovascular mortality [32], were common in our sample (more than 50%), confirming previous findings in other Peruvian HD cohorts [33]. This demonstrates the underlying inflammatory status that these patients have and could be the resultant of metabolic syndrome. The potential use of CRP as a cardiovascular mortality predictor has been demonstrated in some studies [34] and its use in the Peruvian population should be encouraged. Conversely, effective blood flow seems to be a consequence rather than a predisposing factor in this sample. It might be explained by the fact that patients with CVD may not be able to tolerate elevated blood flows on hemodialysis. Alternatively, another explanation may be that HD techniques mostly applied in Peru use low flux dialyzers, which limits dialysis efficacy.

Unlike other studies where diabetes was the main cause of ESKD [1, 3], the most common cause in this sample was hypertension. This difference in demographics might be explained either by a higher mortality of diabetics at CNSR or that patients with multiple comorbidities receive hemodialysis at other centers better able to care for more complex patients. Another important characteristic of this sample is the high prevalence of hepatitis C virus infection (64%), which is greater than the rates reported by other countries like the USA (5.5–10%) [35], Italy (13.5–31%) [36], France (42%) [37], or Syria (49%) [38], but is comparable to Moldavia (75%) [39]. This may be explained by the long time these patients have lived on hemodialysis (9.7 ± 4.6 years). Filter reuse, dialysate processing, and infection control practices are other possible factors that may explain this increased hepatitis C infection rate [38, 39].

Our study has several limitations, including the sampling approach and sample size which does not allow extrapolating results to the Peruvian population. Additionally, the cross-sectional design does not allow making causal associations. It is important to remark that it was not possible to determine how the CVD prevalence changed with the time under HD, especially considering that for some patients this study provided their first lifetime echocardiogram and thus unrecognized diastolic dysfunction could have not been determined at the time of HD initiation. However several steps were taken to overcome these limitations, including (1) sampling the biggest hemodialysis center in Lima, which has a captive and stable population throughout the years, (2) calculating prevalence ratios instead of odds ratios to not overestimate associations, and (3) including a robust regression analysis to avoid confounding factors.

In conclusion, this study represents the first approach to CVD burden in HD patients in Peru and raises the concern about CVD diagnosis and management in this specific population. Age, effective blood flow, and hemoglobin levels outside a tight target are associated with high prevalence of diastolic dysfunction and CVD in this sample.

Ethical Approval

All procedures performed in studies involving human participants were in accordance with the ethical standards of the institutional and/or national research committee and with the 1964 Helsinki declaration and its later amendments or comparable ethical standards. Ethics Committees from Universidad Nacional Mayor de San Marcos and Centro Nacional de Salud Renal reviewed and approved the study.

Acknowledgments

The authors acknowledge Juana Hinostroza, Carlos Tumialán, Luis Segura, and Diego Yanqui for their commitment to research. Special thanks are due to William Borden and Rebeca Monk for revising the paper. Thesis Development Grant at Universidad Nacional Mayor de San Marcos, Office of the Vice-President for Research, is acknowledged.

References

[1] A. Schieppati and G. Remuzzi, "Chronic renal diseases as a public health problem: epidemiology, social, and economic implications," *Kidney International, Supplement*, vol. 68, no. 98, pp. S7–S10, 2005.

[2] U.S.RDS, *USRDS 2013 Annual Data Report: Atlas of Chronic Kidney Disease and End Stage Renal Disease in the United States*, National Institutes of Health, National Institute of Diabetes and Digestive and Kidney Diseases, 2013.

[3] A. M. Cusumano, M. C. G. Bedat, G. García-García et al., "Latin American dialysis and renal transplant registry: 2008 report (data 2006)," *Clinical Nephrology*, vol. 74, supplement 1, pp. S3–S8, 2010.

[4] I. Montalvo-Roel, *Estado Situacional de los Pacientes con Enfermedad Renal Crónica y la Aplicación de Diálisis como Tratamiento en el Perú*, Departamento de Investigaciones y Documentación Parlamentaria (DIDP), 2012.

[5] A. S. Levey, J. A. Beto, B. E. Coronado et al., "Controlling the epidemic of cardiovascular disease in chronic renal disease: what do we know? What do we need to learn? Where do we go from here? National Kidney Foundation Task Force on Cardiovascular Disease," *The American Journal of Kidney Diseases*, vol. 32, no. 5, pp. 853–906, 1998.

[6] A. K. Cheung, M. J. Sarnak, G. Yan et al., "Atherosclerotic cardiovascular disease risks in chronic hemodialysis patients," *Kidney International*, vol. 58, no. 1, pp. 353–362, 2000.

[7] K/DOQI Workgroup, "K/DOQI clinical practice guidelines for cardiovascular disease in dialysis patients," *American Journal of Kidney Diseases*, vol. 45, no. 4, supplement 3, pp. S1–S153, 2005.

[8] P. S. Parfrey and R. N. Foley, "The clinical epidemiology of cardiac disease in chronic renal failure," *Journal of the American Society of Nephrology*, vol. 10, no. 7, pp. 1606–1615, 1999.

[9] R. N. Foley, P. S. Parfrey, and M. J. Sarnak, "Clinical epidemiology of cardiovascular disease in chronic renal disease," *American Journal of Kidney Diseases*, vol. 32, no. 5, supplement 3, pp. S112–S119, 1998.

[10] M. J. Sarnak and A. S. Levey, "Cardiovascular disease and chronic renal disease: a new paradigm," *American Journal of Kidney Diseases*, vol. 35, no. 4, pp. S117–S131, 2000.

[11] K. Kundhal and C. E. Lok, "Clinical epidemiology of cardiovascular disease in chronic kidney disease," *Nephron: Clinical Practice*, vol. 101, no. 2, pp. c47–c52, 2005.

[12] J. Portolés, J. M. López-Gómez, P. Aljama, and A. M. Tato, "Cardiovascular risk in hemodialysis in Spain: prevalence, management and target results (MAR Study)," *Nefrologia*, vol. 25, no. 3, pp. 297–306, 2005.

[13] S. H. Park, C. Shub, T. P. Nobrega, K. R. Bailey, and J. B. Seward, "Two-dimensional echocardiographic calculation of left ventricular mass as recommended by the American Society of Echocardiography: correlation with autopsy and M-mode echocardiography," *Journal of the American Society of Echocardiography*, vol. 9, no. 2, pp. 119–128, 1996.

[14] K. G. Alberti, P. Zimmet, and J. Shaw, "Metabolic syndrome—a new world-wide definition. A consensus statement from the International Diabetes Federation," *Diabetic Medicine*, vol. 23, no. 5, pp. 469–480, 2006.

[15] H. Rimington, *Echocardiography: A Practical Guide for Reporting*, Informa Healthcare, 2nd edition, 2007.

[16] WHO, "Haemoglobin concentrations for the diagnosis of anaemia and assessment of severity. Vitamin and Mineral Nutrition Information System," Tech. Rep. WHO/NMH/NHD/MNM/111, World Health Organization, Geneva, Switzerland, 2011.

[17] G. Moretta, A. J. Locatelli, L. Gadola et al., "Rio de La Plata study: a multicenter, cross-sectional study on cardiovascular risk factors and heart failure prevalence in peritoneal dialysis patients in Argentina and Uruguay," *Kidney International. Supplement*, no. 108, pp. S159–S164, 2008.

[18] M. E. Sanhueza Villanueva, A. Cotera, L. Elgueta et al., "Assessment and follow up of diabetic patients in hemodialysis," *Revista Medica de Chile*, vol. 136, no. 3, pp. 279–286, 2008.

[19] R. J. Glassock, R. Pecoits-Filho, and S. H. Barberato, "Left ventricular mass in chronic kidney disease and ESRD," *Clinical Journal of the American Society of Nephrology*, vol. 4, supplement 1, pp. S79–S91, 2009.

[20] B. Quiroga, M. Villaverde, S. Abad, A. Vega, J. Reque, and J. M. López-Gómez, "Diastolic dysfunction and high levels of new cardiac biomarkers as risk factors for cardiovascular events and mortality in hemodialysis patients," *Blood Purification*, vol. 36, no. 2, pp. 98–106, 2013.

[21] F. U. Dzgoeva, T. M. Gatagonova, Z. K. Kadzaeva et al., "Diastolic dysfunction in different types of left ventricular hypertrophy in patients with end-stage renal failure: impact of long-term erythropoietin therapy," *Terapevticheskii Arkhiv*, vol. 85, no. 6, pp. 44–50, 2013.

[22] R. Pecoits-Filho, S. Bucharles, and S. H. Barberato, "Diastolic heart failure in dialysis patients: mechanisms, diagnostic approach, and treatment," *Seminars in Dialysis*, vol. 25, no. 1, pp. 35–41, 2012.

[23] B. C. Fellström, A. G. Jardine, R. E. Schmieder et al., "Rosuvastatin and cardiovascular events in patients undergoing hemodialysis," *The New England Journal of Medicine*, vol. 360, no. 14, pp. 1395–1407, 2009.

[24] C. W. Nemerovski, J. Lekura, M. Cefaretti, P. T. Mehta, and C. L. Moore, "Safety and efficacy of statins in patients with end-stage renal disease," *Annals of Pharmacotherapy*, vol. 47, no. 10, pp. 1321–1329, 2013.

[25] S. Bevc, A. Potočnik, and R. Hojs, "Lipids, waist circumference and body mass index in haemodialysis patients," *Journal of International Medical Research*, vol. 39, no. 3, pp. 1063–1074, 2011.

[26] K. Al Saran, S. Elsayed, A. Sabry, and M. Hamada, "Obesity and metabolic syndrome in hemodialysis patients: single center experience," *Saudi Journal of Kidney Diseases and Transplantation*, vol. 22, no. 6, pp. 1193–1198, 2011.

[27] M. Jalalzadeh, R. Mohammadi, F. Mirzamohammadi, and M. H. Ghadiani, "Prevalence of metabolic syndrome in a hemodialysis population," *Iranian Journal of Kidney Diseases*, vol. 5, no. 4, pp. 248–254, 2011.

[28] A. I. Q. Alfonso, R. F. Gallegos, R. F. Castillo, F. J. G. Jimenez, M. C. G. Rios, and I. G. Garcia, "Study of the metabolic syndrome and obesity in hemodialysis patients," *Nutrición Hospitalaria*, vol. 31, no. 1, pp. 286–291, 2015.

[29] A. P. de José, Ú. Verdalles-Guzmán, S. Abad et al., "Metabolic syndrome is associated with cardiovascular events in hemodialysis," *Nefrologia*, vol. 34, no. 1, pp. 69–75, 2014.

[30] C.-C. Wu, H.-H. Liou, P.-F. Su et al., "Abdominal obesity is the most significant metabolic syndrome component predictive of cardiovascular events in chronic hemodialysis patients," *Nephrology Dialysis Transplantation*, vol. 26, no. 11, pp. 3689–3695, 2011.

[31] A. K. Singh, L. Szczech, K. L. Tang et al., "Correction of anemia with epoetin alfa in chronic kidney disease," *The New England Journal of Medicine*, vol. 355, no. 20, pp. 2085–2098, 2006.

[32] T. Kawaguchi, L. Tong, B. M. Robinson et al., "C-reactive protein and mortality in hemodialysis patients: the Dialysis Outcomes and Practice Patterns Study (DOPPS)," *Nephron—Clinical Practice*, vol. 117, no. 2, pp. c167–c178, 2011.

[33] M. T.-R. Valdivia-Mazeyra, L.-Q. Cesar, and M. Teresa, "Asymptomatic cerebrovascular lesions and their relationship to vascular risk factors in patients with end stage renal disease on hemodialysis program," *Revista de la Sociedad Peruana de Medicina Interna*, vol. 25, no. 4, pp. 163–170, 2012.

[34] J. Zimmermann, S. Herrlinger, A. Pruy, T. Metzger, and C. Wanner, "Inflammation enhances cardiovascular risk and mortality in hemodialysis patients," *Kidney International*, vol. 55, no. 2, pp. 648–658, 1999.

[35] L. Finelli, J. T. Miller, J. I. Tokars, M. J. Alter, and M. J. Arduino, "National surveillance of dialysis-associated diseases in the United States, 2002," *Seminars in Dialysis*, vol. 18, no. 1, pp. 52–61, 2005.

[36] A. Di Napoli, P. Pezzotti, D. Di Lallo, N. Petrosillo, C. Trivelloni, and S. Di Giulio, "Epidemiology of hepatitis C virus among long-term dialysis patients: a 9-year study in an Italian region," *American Journal of Kidney Diseases*, vol. 48, no. 4, pp. 629–637, 2006.

[37] A.-M. Courouce, F. Bouchardeau, P. Chauveau et al., "Hepatitis C virus (HCV) infection in haemodialysed patients: HCV-RNA and anti-HCV antibodies (third-generation assays)," *Nephrology Dialysis Transplantation*, vol. 10, no. 2, pp. 234–239, 1995.

[38] B. Othman and F. Monem, "Prevalence of antibodies to hepatitis C virus among hemodialysis patients in Damascus, Syria," *Infection*, vol. 29, no. 5, pp. 262–265, 2001.

[39] A. Covic, L. Iancu, C. Apetrei et al., "Hepatitis virus infection in haemodialysis patients from Moldavia," *Nephrology Dialysis Transplantation*, vol. 14, no. 1, pp. 40–45, 1999.

Clinical Utility of Urinary β2-Microglobulin in Detection of Early Nephropathy in African Diabetes Mellitus Patients

U. E. Ekrikpo,[1] E. E. Effa,[2] E. E. Akpan,[1] A. S. Obot,[1] and S. Kadiri[3]

[1]University of Uyo and University of Uyo Teaching Hospital, Uyo, Nigeria
[2]University of Calabar, Calabar, Nigeria
[3]University College Hospital, Ibadan, Nigeria

Correspondence should be addressed to U. E. Ekrikpo; udemeekrikpo@uniuyo.edu.ng

Academic Editor: Franca Anglani

Background. Studies have indicated that diabetic tubulopathy may occur earlier than glomerulopathy, therefore providing a potential avenue for earlier diagnosis of diabetic nephropathy. Urinary beta-2-microglobulin (β2m) was investigated in this study as a potential biomarker in the detection of early nephropathy in type 2 diabetics. *Methods.* One hundred and two diabetic subjects and 103 controls that met the inclusion criteria had data (sociodemographic, medical history, physical examination, and laboratory) collected. Urinary β2m levels and urinary albumin concentration (UAC) were determined. *Results.* Elevated urinary β2m was more frequent among the diabetics (52%, 95% CI: 42.1–61.8%) than among the controls (32%, 95% CI: 22.9–41.2%). The frequency of microalbuminuria was higher in the diabetics (35.3%, 95% CI: 25.9–44.7%) than in the controls (15.5%, 95% CI: 8.4–22.6%). There was a positive correlation between urinary β2m and UAC (rho = 0.38, $p < 0.001$). Multivariate analysis showed BMI (OR: 1.23, 95% CI: 1.05–1.45), eGFR (OR: 0.97, 95% CI: 0.94–0.99), and presence of microalbuminuria (OR: 3.94, 95% CI: 1.32–11.77) as independent predictors of elevated urinary beta-2-microglobulin among the diabetics. *Conclusion.* Urinary β2m may be useful, either as a single test or as a component of a panel of tests, in the early detection of diabetic nephropathy.

1. Introduction

Diabetic nephropathy is the single most common cause of end stage renal disease (ESRD) in adults worldwide [1–3]. In North America, diabetes mellitus accounts for 45% and 15% of incident dialysis patients in the USA and Canada, respectively [4, 5]. Diabetes mellitus comprised 51% of incident patients started on renal replacement therapy in Canada [5]. Data from European renal registries show a 12% increase in DM related ESRD with a primary diagnosis of DM in 20–44% of patients [2, 3]. In Japan, more than 40% of incident ESRD patients have diabetes mellitus [6]. In Africa, reports from Tunisia indicate an annual increase of 16% in the rate of diabetes mellitus as a cause of ESRD [7]. Congo's experience shows that about 39% of the diabetics in Kinshasa have chronic kidney disease coming second only to hypertension as a major risk factor for developing chronic kidney disease [8].

The chronic kidney disease picture in Nigeria is somewhat different. Hospital based studies in various parts of Nigeria have shown diabetes mellitus as the third commonest cause of end stage renal disease following chronic glomerulonephritis and hypertensive nephrosclerosis [9–11], but it may not remain so for long. With the ongoing epidemiologic transition [12] in sub-Saharan Africa, the prevalence of diabetes mellitus and other chronic noncommunicable diseases may be on the rise [13]. There are already reports of increased DM prevalence related to a constellation of risk factors including overweight individuals, family history of diabetes mellitus, and heavy alcohol consumption [14, 15] which in themselves are CKD risks.

Associated with the increasing prevalence of diabetes mellitus is a concomitant increase in the incidence of diabetic nephropathy [16]. We may soon see diabetic nephropathy as the commonest cause of end stage renal disease in Nigeria, resembling the scenario in the developed world. This has already occurred in other parts of Africa like Egypt where the prevalence of diabetic ESRD steadily increased from 8.9% in

1996 to 14.5% in 2001 with a coincident increased mortality risk [17].

Clinical evaluation of renal function in diabetics, for many years, had involved the use of serum creatinine and the various estimations of the glomerular filtration rate using creatinine based formulae. This has its accuracy limitations as it will only detect more advanced cases of diabetic nephropathy [18]. Other methods for the assessment of GFR are either too cumbersome or too expensive to be used in a clinical setting. Renal biopsy is not routinely done and the finding of classical Kimmelstiel-Wilson lesions and other structural lesions like glomerular basement membrane thickening from a biopsy specimen may actually indicate an advanced disease stage.

More recently, attention has been focused on the use of persistent microalbuminuria to define the presence of incipient diabetic nephropathy [19] and initial work on microalbuminuria attributed excretion of >30 mg/day of albumin in urine to increased glomerular filtration of albumin. Though the glomerular origin of microalbuminuria has not been contested, studies in rodents and man have shown that impaired tubular reabsorption of albumin at the proximal convoluted tubule is partly responsible for microalbuminuria [20, 21]. One study suggests that the initial renal damage resulting in microalbuminuria is the loss of charge-dependent tubular protein reabsorption occurring prior to the damage of the glomerular charge barrier in diabetics [22] while another has shown in diabetic children that tubular proteinuria actually predates microalbuminuria [23]. We have previously demonstrated early tubular dysfunction in African diabetics using urinary NAG suggesting that tubular dysfunction may precede glomerular damage [24].

The foregoing suggests that investigations targeting the tubular function in diabetics may be of immense clinical benefit in detecting early diabetic nephropathy, possibly earlier than the occurrence of persistent microalbuminuria. This study investigates the clinical utility of urinary beta-2-microglobulin levels in detecting early nephropathy in African diabetics.

2. Methods

This was a single centre, observational cross-sectional study involving patients with diabetes mellitus seen in the medical outpatient clinic of the University of Uyo Teaching Hospital, Uyo. One hundred and thirteen diabetic patients who met the inclusion criteria and did not have any of the exclusion criteria described below were recruited using simple random sampling into the study. Exclusion criteria included individuals with end stage kidney disease [25], a history of urinary tract infection in the one month preceding the interview, renal ultrasound features suggestive of structural urinary tract abnormalities [26], diseases associated with increased serum beta-2-microglobulin (HIV disease [27], lymphomas, multiple myeloma, and connective tissue disease [28]), and history of aminoglycoside use in the two weeks preceding the day of the interview [26]. A group of 113 nondiabetic individuals who did not have any of the conditions listed in the exclusion criteria were also recruited. Height, weight, waist and hip circumference, and blood pressure were measured using standard techniques.

The urinary β2-microglobulin (β2m) level in the participants was assayed using the beta-2-microglobulin ELISA kit, EIA 3609, from DRG Diagnostics International Inc., USA, which has precision of 0.1 μg/mL. The average coefficient of variation for the plate control means was 10.4%. The proportion of participants with a urinary β2-microglobulin level >0.3 μg/mL (upper limit of normal for urinary β2m from ELISA kit information) was adjudged to have elevated urinary β2-microglobulin level. The presence of albuminuria was measured using MICROALBUMIN™, an immunoturbidimetric assay from Fortress Diagnostics Limited, Antrim Technology Park, United Kingdom. The patients were to have 3 urine samples collected monthly over a 3-month period. Those with at least 2 out of the 3 samples were deemed to have persistent microalbuminuria. Individuals who did not have all their samples collected were excluded from the analysis.

Creatinine estimation was determined using Jaffe's alkaline picrate kinetic method. The glomerular filtration rate was computed using the Cockroft-Gault, 4-variable MDRD and CKD-EPI formulae [29–31]. HbA1c levels were determined using the glycohemoglobin reagent colorimetric set from TECO Diagnostics, Anaheim, California 92807, USA. Total cholesterol, triglycerides, and HDL were assayed using RANDOX kits while LDL was derived from the Friedewald equation [32].

Data analysis was performed using STATA 10 (StataCorp, College Station, TX, USA). The baseline sociodemographic and clinical characteristics of the participants were analyzed. Mean ± standard deviation was computed for normally distributed continuous variables and median and their corresponding interquartile range for continuous variables that are not normally distributed. Pearson's Chi-square test (or Fisher's exact test) was used to compare categorical variables while Student's t-test (or its nonparametric equivalent) was employed in comparing quantitative variables. Univariate logistic regression was used to identify factors associated with elevated urinary β2-microglobulin. Factors with a p value of the Wald statistic <0.25 and those found in the literature review to be risk factors for diabetic nephropathy were included in the multivariate logistic regression. The assumption of linearity in the model was assessed by including polynomial functions of the continuous variables into the final model. A Receiver Operator Characteristic (ROC) curve for the model was used to assess the fit of the model. Ethical clearance was obtained from the University of Uyo Teaching Hospital Human Research Ethics Committee.

3. Results

One hundred and thirteen subjects and 113 controls were recruited into the study. Twenty-one [11 (9.7%) of the subjects and 10 (8.8%) controls] were lost to follow-up. Data from 102 subjects and 103 controls was available for analysis after excluding individuals who were lost to follow-up. Tables 1 and 2 show the sociodemographic, clinical, and laboratory characteristics of the study participants.

TABLE 1: Comparison of sociodemographic/clinical characteristics of subjects and controls.

(a)

	Subjects ($n = 102$)	Controls ($n = 103$)	p
Age (years, mean ± SD)	54.8 ± 10.1	53.2 ± 12.0	0.30[*]
Female gender, n (%)	64 (62.8)	59 (58.1)	0.43[†]
Married individuals, n (%)	90 (90.9)	83 (93.3)	0.69[†]
Educational status, n (%)			
No formal education	8 (8.2)	18 (20.2)	
Primary	19 (19.4)	22 (24.7)	0.02[†]
Secondary	11 (11.2)	3 (3.4)	
Tertiary	60 (61.2)	46 (51.7)	

[*]Student's t-test. [†]Chi-square test.

(b)

	Subjects ($n = 102$)	Controls ($n = 103$)	p
Family history of diabetes mellitus	43 (42.2%)	11 (10.7%)	<0.001
Family history of hypertension	27 (26.5%)	26 (25.2%)	0.94
Family history of kidney disease	8 (7.8%)	3 (2.9%)	<0.001
History of frothy urine	46 (45.1%)	5 (4.9%)	<0.001
History of hematuria	7 (6.9%)	1 (0.9%)	0.03[†]
Body mass index (kg/m^2)[**]	26.9 ± 4.5	26.2 ± 6.1	0.34[Δ]
Waist circumference (cm)[**]	95.8 ± 12.6	89.0 ± 15.3	0.007[Δ]
Hip circumference (cm)[**]	99.6 ± 13.6	96.2 ± 14.6	0.09
Waist-to-hip ratio[$]	0.94 (0.88–1.01)	0.93 (0.88–0.99)	0.17[*]
Systolic blood pressure (mmHg)[**]	134.2 ± 22.4	139.3 ± 22.1	0.10
Diastolic blood pressure (mmHg)[**]	82.3 ± 11.5	80.4 ± 13.7	0.29
mABP (mmHg)[$]	100.5 (93.3–108.3)	97.3 (86.3–109.3)	0.15

[†]Fisher's exact test. [*]Wilcoxon rank sum test. [Δ]Student's t-test. [$]Median (IQR). [**]Mean (SD). mABP: mean arterial blood pressure.

TABLE 2: Comparison of laboratory findings in both groups.

	Diabetics ($n = 102$)	Controls ($n = 103$)	p
Serum creatinine (μmol/L)[$]	91 (74–102)	84 (69–98)	0.03
Serum urea (mmol/L)[$]	4.6 (3.5–5.1)	3.7 (2.6–4.9)	0.003
Hemoglobin (g/dL)[$]	13.8 (13–14.8)	14.2 (13.6–14.8)	0.14
Serum uric acid (mmol/L)[**]	5.6 ± 1.5	5.0 ± 1.5	0.01
Random plasma glucose (mmol/L)[**]	12.0 ± 3.9	6.0 ± 1.6	<0.001
Glycated hemoglobin (%)[$]	7.1 (5.3–8.1)	4.6 (3.9–5.2)	<0.001
Total cholesterol (mg/dL)[**]	5.0 ± 1.4	3.5 ± 1.3	<0.001
Triglycerides (mg/dL)[**]	2.13 ± 0.93	1.40 ± 0.81	<0.001
LDL-cholesterol (mg/dL)[$]	3.0 (1.4–3.9)	1.4 (1.02–1.7)	<0.001
HDL-cholesterol (mg/dL)[$]	1.1 (0.86–1.2)	0.98 (0.86–1.2)	0.83
Atherogenic ratio (total cholesterol/HDL)[$]	4.4 (3.2–6.9)	3.3 (2.4–4.6)	<0.001
UAC (mg/L)[$]	23 (10–100)	0.36 (0.3–10.2)	<0.001
Estimated GFR$_{CG}$ (mL/min)[$]	68 (54–87)	81 (58–104)	0.02
Estimated GFR$_{MDRD}$ (mL/min/1.73 m^2)[$]	82.7 (67.1–97.9)	88.7 (76.2–117.8)	0.01
Estimated GFR$_{CKD-EPI}$ (mL/min/1.73 m^2)[$]	82.5 (67.4–97.3)	90.0 (75.7–109.8)	0.004
Urinary β2m (μg/mL)[$]	0.41 (0.1–0.99)	0.1 (0.1–0.41)	0.002

UAC: urinary albumin concentration; β2m: beta-2-microglobulin. [**]Mean (SD). [$]Median (IQR).

TABLE 3: Correlation of β2m with selected parameters in subjects and controls.

	Total ($N = 205$)		Subjects ($n = 102$)		Controls ($n = 103$)	
	Rho	p	Rho	p	Rho	p
Age	0.04	0.59	0.08	0.41	−0.03	0.80
Urinary albumin concentration	0.38	<0.001	0.34	0.004	0.28	0.004
eGFR$_{(CG)}$	−0.19	0.01	−0.31	0.002	−0.02	0.84
Serum creatinine	0.43	<0.001	0.45	<0.001	0.37	0.001
Serum urea	0.14	0.04	0.13	0.18	0.11	0.28
Serum uric acid	0.16	0.02	0.17	0.08	0.04	0.71
Total cholesterol	0.32	<0.001	0.33	0.001	0.14	0.15
Triglycerides	0.21	0.002	0.22	0.02	0.007	0.94
LDL-cholesterol	0.30	0.002	0.21	0.17	−0.06	0.64
HDL-cholesterol	−0.03	0.71	−0.12	0.21	0.04	0.71
Glycated hemoglobin	0.22	0.002	0.15	0.12	0.06	0.55

The subjects (diabetics) had a significantly higher proportion of individuals with tertiary and secondary levels of education compared to the controls. The age and gender distributions were similar for both groups and the proportion of married individuals in both groups was similar. The subjects had a significantly higher proportion of individuals with a family history of diabetes mellitus (42.2% versus 10.7%, $p < 0.001$). There was no significant difference in the proportion of individuals in both groups who had a positive family history of hypertension (25.2% for the subjects versus 26.5% for the controls, $p = 0.94$) but a family history of kidney disease was more prevalent among the subjects (7.8% compared to 2.9%) than the controls.

The hemoglobin levels and high-density lipoprotein were similar for both groups. The other laboratory parameters were found to be significantly different. The subjects had higher serum creatinine, urea, uric acid, glycated hemoglobin, and random plasma glucose compared to the control group. The LDL-cholesterol, total cholesterol, triglycerides, and atherogenic ratio were significantly higher in the subjects than in the controls. Among the subjects, 80.4% had at least one fraction of the lipid profile being deranged. This proportion increased to 86.8% among the diabetics with elevated urinary beta-2-microglobulin. This consisted of high LDL-cholesterol in 55.9%, high triglycerides in 70.6%, high total cholesterol in 40.2%, and low HDL-cholesterol in 48.0%. There were 65 (63.7%) subjects with poor long-term glycemic control defined as glycated hemoglobin greater than 6.5%.

4. Frequency of Elevated Urinary β2m

The subjects had median urinary β2m of 0.41 μg/mL (interquartile range: 0.1–0.99 μg/mL) while the controls had median urinary β2m of 0.1 μg/mL (IQR: 0.1–0.41). This difference was statistically significant. The proportion of subjects who had elevated urinary β2m was 52.0% (95% CI: 42.1–61.8%) compared to the 32.0% (95% CI: 22.9–41.2%) of the controls, $p = 0.004$. There was no gender difference in elevated urinary β2m among the subjects [50.0% (19) of males versus 53.1% of the female diabetics, $p = 0.76$]. There were 19 (43.2%) male controls with elevated urinary β2m compared to 14 (23.7%) female controls, $p = 0.03$.

There was no difference in the proportion of subjects with elevated urinary β2m between those with DM and hypertension and those with DM only. Fourteen (46.7%) of the 30 in the "DM only" group had elevated urinary β2m compared to 39 (54.2%) of the 72 with diabetes and hypertension, $p = 0.49$. Finally, among the controls, of the 49 with hypertension, 20 (40.8%) had elevated urinary β2m compared to 13 (24.1%) of the 54 controls without hypertension, $p = 0.07$.

Table 3 shows the correlations and p values for the associations with β2m and UAC, systolic and diastolic blood pressure, estimated GFR, the components of the lipid profile, and serum uric acid.

5. Predictors of Elevated β2m among the Diabetics

Univariate and multivariate regression models (Table 4) were used to investigate factors that independently predict the occurrence of elevated β2m in the diabetic population. At the univariate level, diabetics with microalbuminuria were 5 times more likely to have elevated β2m. Other significant associations with elevated urinary β2m at the univariate level included BMI (6% increased risk), eGFR (2% reduced risk), LDL (46% increased risk), triglycerides (93% increased risk), and increased atherogenic ratio (20% increased risk).

At the multivariate level, diabetics with persistent microalbuminuria had a nearly 4-fold increased risk of having tubular dysfunction as measured by elevation in urinary β2m excretion after adjusting for the effects of changes in eGFR, presence of hypertension, age, gender differences, dyslipidemia, BMI, waist circumference, HbA1c levels, and duration of diabetes mellitus.

6. Comparison of the Utility of Urinary β2m and Microalbuminuria in Detecting Early Diabetic Nephropathy

Table 5 shows comparable correlation parameters between albumin creatinine ratio and eGFR and between urinary β2m and eGFR among the subjects.

TABLE 4: Univariate and multivariate logistic regression models for factors predicting elevated β2m.

| | Univariate | | Multivariate* | |
	Odds ratio (95% CI)	p value	Odds ratio (95% CI)	p value
Age (years)	1.01 (0.97–1.04)	0.75	0.99 (0.95–1.05)	0.89
Male gender	0.84 (0.38–1.86)	0.67	1.17 (0.36–3.79)	0.80
Positive hypertension status	1.3 (0.56–2.99)	0.54	0.60 (0.20–1.80)	0.36
Duration of DM	1.00 (0.99–1.01)	0.82	0.99 (0.98–1.03)	0.17
Waist circumference	1.00 (0.97–1.03)	0.97	0.98 (0.93–1.03)	0.39
BMI	1.06 (0.97–1.16)	0.19	1.23 (1.05–1.45)	0.01**
Positive microalbuminuria	5.79 (2.30–14.59)	<0.001	3.94 (1.32–11.77)	0.01**
eGFR	0.98 (0.97–0.99)	0.04	0.97 (0.94–0.99)	0.04**
LDL-C	1.46 (1.08–1.99)	0.02	1.32 (0.71–2.43)	0.38
Total cholesterol/HDL	1.20 (1.03–1.41)	0.02	0.93 (0.71–1.24)	0.64
Triglycerides	1.93 (1.16–3.22)	0.01	1.85 (0.96–3.54)	0.06
HbA1c	1.18 (0.98–1.42)	0.07	1.09 (0.86–1.38)	0.47

*The area under the Receiver Operator Characteristic (ROC) curve of the model was 0.80. **Statistically significant after adjusting for other variables.

TABLE 5: Comparison of correlation of β2m with eGFR versus UAC with eGFR in subjects and controls.

| | Subjects ($n = 102$) | | Controls ($n = 103$) | |
	Rho	p	Rho	p
UAC	−0.29	0.01	−0.19	0.06
β2m	−0.31	0.01	−0.02	0.84

TABLE 6: Comparison of urinary β2m and microalbuminuria in detecting early DN.

| | Microalbuminuria | |
	Positive	Negative
Elevated urinary β2m		
Positive	28 (77.8%)	25 (37.9%)
Negative	8 (16.3%)	41 (62.1%)

McNemar $X = 8.76$, $p = 0.003$.

Among the normoalbuminuric subjects, 25 (37.9%) already had elevated urinary β2m detected while elevated urinary β2m was seen in 27.6% of the normoalbuminuric controls. This difference was statistically significant, $p < 0.001$.

Among the subjects with normal urinary β2m, only 8 (16.3%) had microalbuminuria. Only 7 (10.0%) of the controls with normal urinary β2m had microalbuminuria. The comparison of urinary β2m and microalbuminuria in the detection of early DN is shown in Table 6.

There was a significantly greater proportion of normoalbuminuric diabetics with elevated urinary β2m than normal urinary β2m with microalbuminuria.

7. Discussion

This study examines the clinical utility of urinary β2m excretion, a measure of renal tubular dysfunction, in the early diagnosis of diabetic nephropathy.

The median level of urinary β2m as well as the proportion of diabetics with elevated urinary β2m was significantly higher in the diabetics than in controls. Indeed, over half of the diabetics had elevated urinary β2m suggesting the presence of tubulopathy. Increased β2m levels in diabetics have been reported by other studies [33, 34] just as other studies have found proportions of diabetic tubulopathy in type 2 diabetes in the range of 55 to 57% using urinary β2m as a measure of tubulopathy [35]. We observed a linear relationship between urinary β2m and serum creatinine as well as a significant inverse relationship between GFR and urinary β2m in this diabetic population. These findings suggest that urinary β2m mirrors reasonably well increases in serum creatinine as renal function declines. This has been demonstrated elsewhere [36]. Apakkan Aksun et al. documented a significant positive correlation between urinary β2m and serum creatinine and a negative correlation with GFR estimated from the uptake phase of 99m technetium diethylenetriaminepentacetate renogram (GFR-DTPA) and creatinine clearance [34]. As serum creatinine increases and eGFR reduces, there is a concomitant worsening of diabetic tubulopathy manifesting itself as a rise in urinary β2m. Since this is a cross-sectional study, it is difficult to conclude whether the glomerulopathy leading to rising serum creatinine and reducing GFR occurred earlier than the tubulopathy or whether the tubulopathy led to the glomerular dysfunction. It is also likely that both lesions occurred concurrently. Both questions would best be addressed by a cohort study.

Multivariate analysis showed BMI as a predictor of elevated urinary β2m levels leading to a 23% increased risk of tubular dysfunction for every one unit increase in BMI among the diabetics after adjusting for all the other factors in the model. There have been arguments for and against the role of BMI in the progression of diabetic nephropathy. A retrospective cohort study refuted the idea of a significant effect of BMI on diabetic nephropathy after a 3-year follow-up period of type 2 diabetics [37] when analysis showed no association between eGFR and BMI. Many other workers believe obesity encourages progression of nephropathy of most aetiologies because of its strong association with albuminuria and nephrosclerosis. Waist circumference, a measure of abdominal obesity, did not have a significant influence on the development of diabetic tubulopathy in this study. It is therefore difficult to conclude from this study that higher BMI can encourage progression of diabetic nephropathy. Larger longitudinal studies on the effect of BMI on diabetic nephropathy among Blacks may help answer this question as this was not the primary aim of this study.

The other significant factors predisposing to high urinary β2m included eGFR and microalbuminuria. After adjusting for the effect of age, gender, duration since diagnosis of diabetes mellitus, lipid profile, BMI, waist circumference, hypertension, and glycated hemoglobin levels, there was a 3% reduction in the risk of developing elevated urinary β2m for every one unit increase in the eGFR. This suggests that as renal function worsens (declining eGFR), the amount of urinary β2m increases. This inverse relationship was also observed at the univariate analysis level of this study. This strong relationship between GFR and microalbuminuria has led to a suggestion that urinary β2m could be used either alone or as part of a panel of tests in the early diagnosis of diabetic nephropathy [34].

The subjects with microalbuminuria had a demonstrably significant fourfold increased likelihood of also having elevated urinary β2m compared to those with normoalbuminuria after adjusting for all the other factors in the multivariate model. The rising levels of urinary albumin concentration as urinary β2m increases may not be solely because of simultaneous tubular and glomerular dysfunction in diabetics but may possibly also be due to an earlier tubular dysfunction resulting in impaired reabsorption at the proximal tubules of albumin filtered through normal glomeruli [38]. This is one of the reasons why some consider tubular dysfunction to possibly occur earlier than glomerular dysfunction in diabetics.

More than a third of the normoalbuminuric diabetics in this study had already developed elevated levels of urinary β2m. On the other hand, only 16.3% of diabetics with normal urinary β2m had microalbuminuria. This difference in proportions was statistically significant suggesting that increases in urinary β2m may occur earlier than microalbuminuria. This finding appears to be in support of the newer pathogenetic theories of diabetic nephropathy that suggest that diabetic tubulopathy occurs earlier than diabetic glomerulopathy [38]. A study had documented up to 55% of normoalbuminuric diabetics with elevated urinary β2m [35]. Several explanations have been put forward including a strong correlation between glomerular hyperfiltration (one of the earliest features of glomerular dysfunction) in normoalbuminuric patients and fractional reabsorption of sodium at the proximal tubules [39]; secondly, the finding of a higher risk of progression to microalbuminuria from normoalbuminuria in individuals with increased kidney volume which is mainly due to tubular hypertrophy and interstitial expansion; and thirdly, the occurrence of increased proximal tubule reabsorption leading to glomerular hyperfiltration as a result of glomerulotubular feedback. Glomerulotubular feedback may explain the reduction in GFR after an initial rise in

early diabetic nephropathy whereas tubulointerstitial damage (especially atrophic proximal tubules) leads to reduced reabsorption of sodium and therefore reduced GFR.

Another factor to consider in the relationship between β2m and microalbuminuria is the relatively smaller molecular weight of β2m compared to albumin (one-sixth of albumin's molecular weight). This property encourages free filtration of β2m across the nondamaged filtration barrier. Smaller quantities of albumin are filtered across the "normal" filtration barrier and may require glomerular damage for larger quantities to be seen in urine. In the setting of tubulopathy, reabsorption of β2m is impaired and urinary β2m becomes elevated early in the course of diabetes mellitus. Moreover, for microalbuminuria to occur, the tubular mechanisms for reabsorption of proteins must have been overwhelmed by large quantities of albumin presented to the proximal tubules as a result of glomerulopathy [40]. This means microalbuminuria is not entirely a result of glomerular dysfunction but also has a tubular component to it.

It may be difficult from the findings of this study to conclude that elevated urinary β2m occurs earlier than microalbuminuria but one can safely say that elevated urinary β2m occurs at least as early as microalbuminuria in the course of diabetic nephropathy and there is a suggestion that urinary β2m elevation may occur earlier. This has led to the proposal to use a panel of urinary markers (including beta-2-microglobulin) to increase the chances of detecting early nephropathy in diabetics.

Additional Points

Limitation. The cross-sectional design of this study has limited our ability to document the temporal profile of the studied biomarkers in the evolution of diabetic nephropathy. A prospective cohort study of initially normoalbuminuric diabetic patients would have answered this question better.

References

[1] F. Shaheen and A. Al-Khader, "Epidemiology and causes of end stage renal disease (ESRD)," *Saudi Journal of Kidney Diseases and Transplantation*, vol. 16, pp. 277–281, 2005.

[2] P. C. W. Van Dijk, K. J. Jager, B. Stengel, C. Grönhagen-Riska, T. G. Feest, and J. D. Briggs, "Renal replacement therapy for diabetic end-stage renal disease: data from 10 registries in Europe (1991–2000)," *Kidney International*, vol. 67, no. 4, pp. 1489–1499, 2005.

[3] M. E. Williams, "Diabetic CKD/ESRD 2010: a progress report?" *Seminars in Dialysis*, vol. 23, no. 2, pp. 129–133, 2010.

[4] U.S. Renal Data System UADR, *Atlas of Chronic Kidney Disease and End-Stage Renal Disease in the United States*, National Institutes of Health, National Institute of Diabetes and Digestive and Kidney Diseases, Bethesda, Md, USA, 2008.

[5] C. E. Lok, M. J. Oliver, D. M. Rothwell, and J. E. Hux, "The growing volume of diabetes-related dialysis: a population based study," *Nephrology Dialysis Transplantation*, vol. 19, no. 12, pp. 3098–3103, 2004.

[6] K. Iseki, "Chronic kidney disease in Japan," *Internal Medicine*, vol. 47, no. 8, pp. 681–689, 2008.

[7] É. Counil, N. Cherni, M. Kharrat, A. Achour, and H. Trimech, "Trends of incident dialysis patients in Tunisia between 1992 and 2001," *American Journal of Kidney Diseases*, vol. 51, no. 3, pp. 463–470, 2008.

[8] E. K. Sumaili, E. P. Cohen, C. V. Zinga, J.-M. Krzesinski, N. M. Pakasa, and N. M. Nseka, "High prevalence of undiagnosed chronic kidney disease among at-risk population in Kinshasa, the Democratic Republic of Congo," *BMC Nephrology*, vol. 10, no. 1, article 18, 2009.

[9] O. R. Adetunji, J. O. Adeleye, N. O. Agada, and B. L. Salako, "Microalbuminuria and clinical correlates in black African patients with type 2 diabetes," *West African Journal of Medicine*, vol. 25, no. 4, pp. 279–283, 2006.

[10] C. O. Alebiosu, "Clinical diabetic nephropathy in a tropical African population," *West African Journal of Medicine*, vol. 22, no. 2, pp. 152–155, 2003.

[11] C. O. Alebiosu, O. O. Ayodele, A. Abbas, and I. A. Olutoyin, "Chronic renal failure at the Olabisi Onabanjo university teaching hospital, Sagamu, Nigeria," *African Health Sciences*, vol. 6, no. 3, pp. 132–138, 2006.

[12] A. R. Omran, "The epidemiologic transition: a theory of the epidemiology of population change," *Milbank Quarterly*, vol. 83, no. 4, pp. 731–757, 2005.

[13] N. Unwin, F. Mugusi, T. Aspray et al., "Tackling the emerging pandemic of non-communicable diseases in sub-Saharan Africa: the essential NCD health intervention project," *Public Health*, vol. 113, no. 3, pp. 141–146, 1999.

[14] E. E. Owoaje, C. N. Rotimi, J. S. Kaufman, J. Tracy, and R. S. Cooper, "Prevalence of adult diabetes in Ibadan, Nigeria," *East African Medical Journal*, vol. 74, no. 5, pp. 299–302, 1997.

[15] E. A. Nyenwe, O. J. Odia, A. E. Ihekwaba, A. Ojule, and S. Babatunde, "Type 2 diabetes in adult Nigerians: a study of its prevalence and risk factors in Port Harcourt, Nigeria," *Diabetes Research and Clinical Practice*, vol. 62, no. 3, pp. 177–185, 2003.

[16] C. O. Alebiosu and O. E. Ayodele, "The increasing prevalence of diabetic nephropathy as a cause of end stage renal disease in Nigeria," *Tropical Doctor*, vol. 36, no. 4, pp. 218–219, 2006.

[17] A. Afifi, M. El Setouhy, M. El Sharkawy et al., "Diabetic nephropathy as a cause of end-stage renal disease in Egypt: a six-year study," *Eastern Mediterranean Health Journal*, vol. 10, no. 4-5, pp. 620–626, 2004.

[18] R. Star, T. Hostetter, and G. L. Hortin, "New markers for kidney disease," *Clinical Chemistry*, vol. 48, no. 9, pp. 1375–1376, 2002.

[19] J. L. Gross, M. J. De Azevedo, S. P. Silveiro, L. H. Canani, M. L. Caramori, and T. Zelmanovitz, "Diabetic nephropathy: diagnosis, prevention, and treatment," *Diabetes Care*, vol. 28, no. 1, pp. 164–176, 2005.

[20] F. N. Ziyadeh and S. Goldfarb, "The renal tubulointerstitium in diabetes mellitus," *Kidney International*, vol. 39, no. 3, pp. 464–475, 1991.

[21] A. Tojo, M. Onozato, H. Ha et al., "Reduced albumin reabsorption in the proximal tubule of early-stage diabetic rats," *Histochemistry and Cell Biology*, vol. 116, no. 3, pp. 269–276, 2001.

[22] K. Kunika, T. Yamaoka, and M. Itakura, "Damage of charge-dependent renal tubular reabsorption causes diabetic microproteinuria," *Diabetes Research and Clinical Practice*, vol. 36, no. 1, pp. 1–9, 1997.

[23] F. Ginevri, E. Piccotti, R. Alinovi et al., "Reversible tubular proteinuria precedes microalbuminuria and correlates with the metabolic status in diabetic children," *Pediatric Nephrology*, vol. 7, no. 1, pp. 23–26, 1993.

[24] F. P. Udomah, U. E. Ekrikpo, E. Effa, B. Salako, A. Arije, and S. Kadiri, "Association between urinary N-acetyl-beta-D-glucosaminidase and microalbuminuria in diabetic black Africans," *International Journal of Nephrology*, vol. 2012, Article ID 235234, 5 pages, 2012.

[25] J. Floege and M. Ketteler, "β2-microglobulin-derived amyloidosis: an update," *Kidney International, Supplement*, vol. 59, no. 78, pp. S164–S171, 2001.

[26] L. W. S. Van Eps and G. H. C. Schardijn, "Value of determination of β2-microglobulin in toxic nephropathy and interstitial nephritis," *Wiener Klinische Wochenschrift*, vol. 96, no. 18, pp. 673–678, 1984.

[27] B. Hofmann, Y. X. Wang, W. G. Cumberland, R. Detels, M. Bozorgmehri, and J. L. Fahey, "Serum beta2-microglobulin level increases in HIV infection: relation to seroconversion, CD4 T-cell fall and prognosis," *AIDS*, vol. 4, no. 3, pp. 207–214, 1990.

[28] V. Henne, P. Frei, and P. Bürgisser, "Beta-2-microglobulin—a rapid and automated determination for a broad range of clinical applications," *Anticancer Research*, vol. 17, no. 4, pp. 2915–2918, 1997.

[29] D. W. Cockcroft and M. H. Gault, "Prediction of creatinine clearance from serum creatinine," *Nephron*, vol. 16, no. 1, pp. 31–41, 1976.

[30] A. S. Levey, J. Coresh, T. Greene et al., "Expressing the modification of diet in renal disease study equation for estimating glomerular filtration rate with standardized serum creatinine values," *Clinical Chemistry*, vol. 53, no. 4, pp. 766–772, 2007.

[31] A. S. Levey, L. A. Stevens, C. H. Schmid et al., "A new equation to estimate glomerular filtration rate," *Annals of Internal Medicine*, vol. 150, no. 9, pp. 604–612, 2009.

[32] W. T. Friedewald, R. I. Levy, and D. S. Fredrickson, "Estimation of the concentration of low-density lipoprotein cholesterol in plasma, without use of the preparative ultracentrifuge," *Clinical Chemistry*, vol. 18, no. 6, pp. 499–502, 1972.

[33] O. Kordonouri, R. Hartmann, C. Müller, T. Danne, and B. Weber, "Predictive value of tubular markers for the development of microalbuminuria in adolescents with diabetes," *Hormone Research*, vol. 50, supplement 1, pp. 23–27, 1998.

[34] S. Apakkan Aksun, D. Özmen, B. Özmen et al., "β2-microglobulin and cystatin C in type 2 diabetes: assessment of diabetic nephropathy," *Experimental and Clinical Endocrinology and Diabetes*, vol. 112, no. 4, pp. 195–200, 2004.

[35] A. Tanaka, K. Shima, M. Fukuda, Y. Tahara, Y. Yamamoto, and Y. Kumahara, "Tubular dysfunction in the early stage of diabetic nephropathy," *Medical Journal of Osaka University*, vol. 38, no. 1-4, pp. 57–63, 1989.

[36] J. Dauzat, S. Moinade, and G. Gaillard, "Beta 2 microglobulin in diabetic patients. Apropos of 190 subjects," *La Semaine des Hopitaux*, vol. 60, no. 11, pp. 745–748, 1984.

[37] A. Khedr, E. Khedr, and A. A. House, "Body mass index and the risk of progression of chronic kidney disease," *Journal of Renal Nutrition*, vol. 21, no. 6, pp. 455–461, 2011.

[38] M. C. Thomas, W. C. Burns, and M. E. Cooper, "Tubular changes in early diabetic nephropathy," *Advances in Chronic Kidney Disease*, vol. 12, no. 2, pp. 177–186, 2005.

[39] C. J. Magri and S. Fava, "The role of tubular injury in diabetic nephropathy," *European Journal of Internal Medicine*, vol. 20, no. 6, pp. 551–555, 2009.

[40] L. M. Russo, R. M. Sandoval, S. B. Campos, B. A. Molitoris, W. D. Comper, and D. Brown, "Impaired tubular uptake explains albuminuria in early diabetic nephropathy," *Journal of the American Society of Nephrology*, vol. 20, no. 3, pp. 489–494, 2009.

18

Malignancy in Membranous Nephropathy: Evaluation of Incidence

Basil Alnasrallah,[1] **John F. Collins,**[1] **and L. Jonathan Zwi**[2]

[1]*Department of Nephrology, Auckland City Hospital, 2 Park Drive, Grafton, Auckland 1023, New Zealand*
[2]*Department of Pathology, Auckland City Hospital, 2 Park Drive, Grafton, Auckland 1023, New Zealand*

Correspondence should be addressed to Basil Alnasrallah; polbeas@yahoo.com

Academic Editor: Anil K. Agarwal

Background. Membranous nephropathy (MN) can be associated with malignancy. However, the relative risk for malignancy remains unclear. It has been reported that higher numbers of inflammatory cells seen in the glomeruli at biopsy correlate with the occurrence of malignancy in patients with MN and might be used to direct screening. *Methods.* We examined the occurrence of malignancy in 201 MN patients in Auckland, New Zealand. We also examined the pathology of renal biopsies from 17 MN patients with malignancies and compared the number of inflammatory cells per glomerulus with matched control patients with MN but no malignancy. *Results.* 40 malignancies were identified in 37 patients, 28 of which occurred after the MN diagnosis. The standardized incidence ratio (SIR) was 2.1 (95% CI, 1.3–2.85) which was similar between patients ≥ 60 years and those <60 years. The median number of inflammatory cells per glomerulus did not differ between MN patients with and without malignancy at 1.86 (IQR, 1.17–2.7) and 2.07 (IQR, 1.17–3.65), respectively (*p* value 0.56). *Conclusions.* The relative risk of malignancy in MN patients was similar across different age groups. The number of inflammatory cells per glomerulus did not differentiate between MN patients with and without malignancies.

1. Introduction

Membranous nephropathy (MN) is a pathologic term that defines a specific glomerular lesion characterized by thickened glomerular capillary walls due to subepithelial deposition or in situ formation of immune-complex deposits [1]. The formation of these immune deposits leads to injury and impairment of glomerular basement membrane [2].

MN remains one of the most frequent glomerular diseases that cause nephrotic syndrome, accounting for around a third of renal biopsies in nondiabetic adults [3, 4]. About 75% of MN cases are idiopathic with no identifiable immunological stimulus and the remaining cases are secondary to a wide variety of primary causes, including neoplasia, infections, autoimmunity, and drugs [5, 6].

The link between MN and malignancy has been reported as early as 1966 by Lee et al. [7] and this association was confirmed later in a number of observational studies. However, the actual risk of malignancy has been shown to be quite variable between different studies, ranging from 2- to 10-fold increase relative to a matched population [8–11]. The malignancies most frequently associated with MN are solid tumors, including lung, gastrointestinal, and prostate carcinomas [9, 10, 12, 13].

This association has led to recommendations for regular screening for malignancy in MN patients around the time of diagnosis, especially when no obvious primary cause is identified [14]. The risk of malignancy in the following years is even less clear. In a population based analysis, the increased risk of malignancy associated with glomerulonephritis diminished after the first year of diagnosis and was not seen beyond 5 years [11].

A more recent study reported a significantly high annual risk of malignancy in patients with MN, which persisted up to 15 years after the diagnosis of MN [9]. This finding could impact on clinical practice and patients' outcomes, as more rigorous screening for malignancy during follow-up might be warranted. Identifying risk factors for malignancy can assist targeting at risk patients for future screening. However, only older age has been consistently found to be associated with malignancy risk [8–10]. Histological findings such as strong immunofluorescence staining with anti-immunoglobulin (Ig) G1 and G2 antibodies have been linked to malignancy-associated membranous nephropathy whereas IgG4 deposits were found predominantly in the idiopathic form of the disease [15, 16]. However, both of these findings have been challenged [17] and a recent review did not find a reliable immunoglobulin glomerular deposition pattern to differentiate between the two groups [18]. The high number of inflammatory cells infiltrating the glomeruli has been previously reported to be strongly associated with malignancy in MN patients compared to those without malignancy [10]. To our knowledge this has not been further validated or challenged. However, if true it could be a useful additional guide for clinicians to target their screening without the need for further staining.

We undertook a retrospective study of 201 MN patients to try to clarify the incidence of malignancies in patients with MN in Auckland, New Zealand, at the time of diagnosis and during follow-up and to examine the associated factors.

2. Materials and Methods

Ethical approval was obtained through the Northern B Health and Disability Ethics Committee of the Ministry of Health in New Zealand. Ethics approval number is *15/NTB/196*.

2.1. Identification of Patients. Patients were identified from the renal biopsy records of the Department of Pathology in Auckland City Hospital. All adult patients (≥18 years old) in whom the diagnosis of MN was made on renal biopsy between January 2003 and December 2013 were included. Baseline data at the time of renal biopsy were collected which included the following: age, sex, eGFR (4-variable Modification of Diet in Renal Disease Study equation), serum albumin level by BCG dye-binding method, degree of haematuria (as per urine RBC $* 10^6$/L, no haematuria if <10, microscopic haematuria if between 10 and 100, and gross haematuria if >100), and proteinuria (g/day) or protein/creatinine ratio (mgs/mmol).

2.2. Definition of Observation Period. The observation period of patients was defined as the time between kidney biopsy and December 31, 2015; death; or loss to follow-up.

2.3. Data for Kidney Biopsies. The pathology slides of renal biopsies in MN patients with malignancy diagnosed around the time of MN (from 1 year before to 5 years after renal biopsy) were reviewed, excluding patients with nonmalignant primary causes of MN. A group of idiopathic MN patients without malignancy were matched in age and gender at a rate of 2 : 1 to the cases and reviewed. All the renal biopsies were examined by a renal pathologist (LJZ) who was blinded to the clinical and laboratory data of the patients. The diagnosis of MN was confirmed histologically and the number of inflammatory cells per glomerulus was reported.

2.4. Identification of Malignancy in Patients with MN. We linked the patients' records using the New Zealand National Health Index number with the New Zealand Cancer Registry (NZCR), which is a register established in 1948 of all primary malignant diseases diagnosed in New Zealand, excluding squamous and basal cell skin cancers. In addition, the clinical records of all patients were systematically reviewed by a Renal Fellow (BA) to confirm the presence or absence of malignancy. All malignancies diagnosed from 1998 (5 years before the first renal biopsy) to December 2015 (end of observation period) were recorded.

At the time of conducting the study, NZCR had full data of malignancies to the end of 2013. For the years 2014 and 2015, malignancies were recorded based only on systematic review of the clinical records.

32 malignancies were reported on NZCR between 1998 and 2013 in 29 patients and confirmed on clinical records (6 malignancies in 3 patients, 2 each). In addition, on review of clinical records for the same period, 2 malignancies in 2 patients were identified and had not been reported by NZCR.

For the years 2014 and 2015, 6 more malignancies in 6 patients were identified on clinical records and therefore we report on 40 malignancies in 37 patients.

2.5. Statistical Analyses. Standardized incidence ratios (SIRs) were calculated as ratios between observed and expected numbers for site-specific malignancies and all malignancies. For the SIR for all malignancies and their subanalyses, the individual annual expected rate for a matched population in gender and in 5-year age groups was added for every year of follow-up using the rate of that particular year as a reference.

For example, for a 64-year-old male who is followed up for 10 years from 2004, the expected national malignancy rate of the year 2004 for males aged 60 to 65 years was used for the first year, for the second year, the national rate of the year 2005 of the same group was used, and, for the third year, the 2006 rate for males aged 65 to 70 years was used and so on. This was to provide the best representation of the expected malignancy risk and to minimize underestimation of the expected risk of malignancy, as malignancy risk increases with age.

Independent-samples t-test was used with continuous variables and chi-square test was used with categorical variables. Median and interquartile ranges (IQR) are reported by the weighted average method.

3. Results

The clinical records of 201 MN patients were reviewed, MN was classified by the treating nephrologist to be idiopathic in 158 patients (78.6%), and this was made after excluding primary causes of MN. Investigations for malignancy, immunological disorders, and hepatitis B and C were universal in this cohort. However, the details of some of the tests were not available to us for many of the patients. Testing for phospholipase A2 receptor (PLA2R) antibodies was not available in New Zealand at the period of patients' diagnoses (2003–2013) and therefore was not done in any of the patients. The diagnosis of secondary MN was made in 43 patients (21.4%). MN was classified as related to malignancy in 4

TABLE 1: Cohort characteristics at time of MN diagnosis.

Age (years)	56 (41–65)
Male	117 (58.2%)
Follow-up (months)	88 (45–117)
Serum albumin g/L	29 (23–35)
Proteinuria g/d	5 (2.6–9.55)
eGFR ml/min	70 (43.2–97.5)
Haematuria	84, no haematuria (43.3%)
	51, microscopic haematuria (26.3%)
	59, gross haematuria (30.4%)

Results are expressed as median (interquartile range) or as percentage.

TABLE 2: Clinical and laboratory data at time of kidney biopsy in patients with and without malignancy.

	Without malignancy	With malignancy	p value
Age (years)	53 (38.5–63.5)	65.5 (58.5–72)	<0.001
Proteinuria (g/d)	5 (2.7–8.85)	6.7 (2.05–10)	NS
Albumin (g/L)	30 (23–36)	26.5 (21.25–35)	NS
eGFR (ml/min)	70 (43–97)	65 (43.4–99.5)	NS
Haematuria			
(i) Nil	68 (43%)	16 (44.4%)	
(ii) Microscopic	41 (26%)	10 (27.8%)	NS
(iii) Gross	49 (31%)	10 (27.8%)	

Results are expressed as median (interquartile range) or as percentage; NS: p value > 0.05.

patients (2%) and to nonmalignant primary causes in 39 patients (19.4%) (30 patients, systemic lupus erythematosus; 5 patients, hepatitis B; 2 patients, graft-versus-host disease, 1 patient; visceral leishmaniasis, 1 patient; connective tissue disease-NOS). It should be emphasized that there is no clear definition for malignancy related MN in the literature; few criteria have been proposed to confirm a truly causal relationship between the two [12, 13].

The overall follow-up period from the date of biopsy was 1384 patient-years. Baseline characteristics at the time of renal biopsy are shown in Table 1.

3.1. Malignancies. 40 malignancies were identified in 37 patients (6 malignancies in 3 patients, 2 each) with a prevalence of 18.4%. Of the patients with nonmalignant primary causes of MN, only one had a malignancy during the observation period.

12 out of the 40 malignancies (30%) had been diagnosed before the diagnosis of MN in 10 patients (2 malignancies in each of 2 patients). The median time from diagnosis of these malignancies to renal biopsy was 65 months (IQR, 8.75–76.25). 28 malignancies were diagnosed after MN diagnosis in 27 patients, 4 of these were in malignancy related MN and were diagnosed within 6 months after renal biopsies. The median time from the diagnosis of MN to the diagnosis of malignancy was 40 months (IQR, 14–67.5). When the 4 cases of malignancy related MN were excluded, the median time to the diagnosis of malignancy was 44 months (IQR, 29–73.25). A de novo malignancy after MN was not diagnosed in any of the patients with malignancy prior to MN.

3.2. Risk Factors. Only age was a significant risk factor for malignancy as in Table 2.

3.3. Immunosuppressive Therapy. The use of *immuno-suppressive* therapy (cyclophosphamide and/or calcineurin inhibitors and/or mycophenolate and/or azathioprine) for more than 3 months was not different between MN patients who did and did not develop malignancy at 42.9% (9 patients) and 42.7% (50 patients), respectively. However, when only looking at the use of cyclophosphamide, more patients had 3 months or more of therapy in the malignancy group at 20.5% (8 patients) compared to 13.8% (13 patients), respectively,

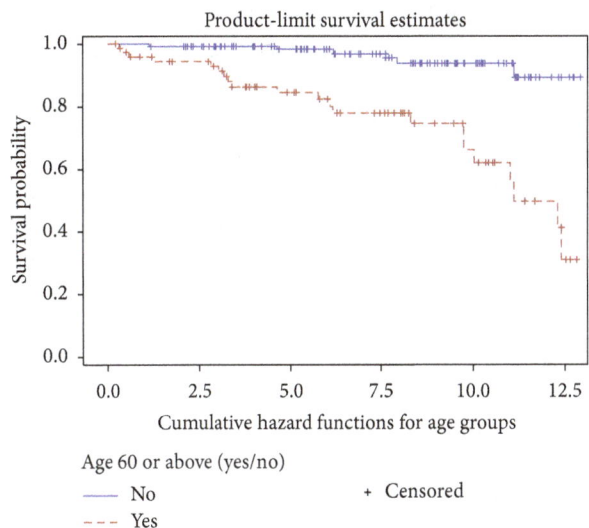

FIGURE 1: Malignancy-free survival in patients ≥ 60 years of age and those <60 years.

p value < 0.001. The mean cumulative dose to cyclophosphamide was 19.8 grams (SD +/− 12.2), with no significant difference between the 2 groups.

3.4. During Follow-Up. After excluding patients with malignancy prior to MN diagnosis, the follow-up period was 1284 person years from the date of renal biopsy. The Standardized Incidence Ratio (SIR) for cancer was significantly raised at *2.1 (95% CI, 1.3–2.85)*, it was *1.925 (95% CI, 1.06–2.79)* in males and *2.51 (95% CI, 0.87–4.15)* in females. When the cases of malignancy related MN were excluded, the SIR remained significantly elevated at *1.78 (95% CI, 1.06–2.49)* in the follow-up period.

Interestingly, the SIRs for patients who are ≥60 years and those <60 years were similar at *2.08 (95% CI, 1.16–2.99)* and *2.06 (95% CI, 0.63–3.49)*, respectively. This is despite a higher risk of malignancies in the older group and subsequently a significantly lower malignancy-free survival rate (*p < 0.001*), as seen in Figure 1.

When broken down by time from biopsy to 0–5 years and >5 years, the SIR was significantly high for the first 5 years at

TABLE 3: Types of malignancy and symptoms in new malignancies after MN.

localization of tumour	Histology	Age	Sex	Months after renal biopsy	Symptoms before malignancy diagnosis (Y: yes/N: no)
Rectal C20	Adenocarcinoma	66	m	1	Y, rectal bleeding
Pancreatic C259	Adenocarcinoma	65	f	1	Y, abdominal pain
Lung NSCLC C349	Not done	75	f	4	Y, dyspnea
Lung NSCLC C343	SCC	57	f	6	N
Cervical D069	CIN III	34	f	7	Y, vaginal bleeding
Colon C187	Adenocarcinoma	82	m	12	Y, symptomatic anaemia
Lung NSCLC C341	SCC	68	m	14	Y, haemoptysis
Prostate C61	Adenocarcinoma	62	m	17	Unknown
Left upper back C435	Metastatic melanoma	72	m	18	Y, skin lump
Lung NSCLC C341	SCC	74	m	27	Y, dry cough and dyspnea
Lung NSCLC C340	Adenocarcinoma	80	m	36	Y, chronic cough
Colon C19	Adenocarcinoma	74	m	37	Y, obstructive bowel symptoms
Lung NSCLC C343	Not done	74	m	37	Y, weight loss
Intestine C179	Neuroendocrine	72	f	41	Y, breast nodule
Unknown	Metastatic melanoma	79	f	41	Y, Dyspnea
Prostate C61	Adenocarcinoma	64	m	45	Y, Urinary voiding symptoms
Prostate C61	Adenocarcinoma	58	m	46	unknown
Intestinal C494	Liposarcoma	54	m	47	Y, Bloody diarrhoea
Unknown primary C269	metastatic adenocarcinoma	51	m	48	Y, Lower groin pain
Prostate C61	Adenocarcinoma	51	m	61	Y, Urinary voiding symptoms
Prostate C61	Adenocarcinoma	68	m	66	Y, Urinary voiding symptoms
Bile duct C240	Adenocarcinoma	64	f	69	Y, Jaundice
CLL C9110	CLL	55	f	76	Y, Cervical lymphadenopathy
Lung NSCLC C341	Adenocarcinoma	64	m	76	Y, Chest wall pain
Colon C182	Adenocarcinoma	61	m	101	Y, Change of bowel habit
Kidney C64	Clear cell carcinoma	55	f	108	N
Lung NSCLC C349	Adenocarcinoma	60	m	117	Y, Dry cough and dyspnea
Prostate C61	Adenocarcinoma	61	m	143	Y, Macroscopic haematuria

2.3 (95% CI, 1.29–3.4) and lost statistical significance after that at 1.7 (95% CI, 0.58–2.77).

3.5. Symptoms. For the 27 patients who were found to have malignancy after the MN diagnosis, the symptomatic status prior to the diagnostic test for malignancy was known in 26 of the 28 malignancies (92.9%). 24 of 26 malignancies (92.3%) were symptomatic prior to investigations. The list of symptoms is shown in Table 3.

3.6. SIR for Types of Malignancies. The SIR for lung malignancy was significantly increased at 8.9 (95% CI, 2.73–15). All of these happened in patients with a history of heavy smoking. The median time from MN diagnosis to the diagnosis of lung malignancy was 35 months (IQR. 14.5–61.5). The SIRs for colorectal and prostate malignancies in males were also high but not statistically significant at 4 (95% CI, 0.08–7.92) and 2.51 (95% CI, 0.5–4.5), respectively.

3.7. Review of Renal Biopsy Tissue. There were 20 patients with malignancy diagnosed between 1 year before and 5 years after MN diagnosis on renal biopsy. Two of these patients had the malignancy diagnosed prior to the biopsy and 18 had the malignancy diagnosed after. We attempted to obtain the pathology slides of these patients and compare them with matched controls with no malignancy at a ratio of 1 : 2.

17 biopsies from patients with malignancies were reviewed (3 could not be retrieved). All of these patients had 10 or more glomeruli on the biopsy with a median interval between the biopsy and the malignancy of 18 months (IQR, 4.5–41). 37 biopsies from patients with no malignancies were reviewed (3 could not be retrieved). The median numbers of glomeruli per biopsy in patients with and without malignancies were similar at 15 (IQR, 13–25.5) and 15 (IQR, 9–23), respectively. The median number of inflammatory cells per glomerulus was not different between the 2 groups at 1.86 (IQR, 1.17–2.7) in patients with malignancy and 2.07 (IQR, 1.17–3.65) in those without, p value 0.56, as in Figure 2.

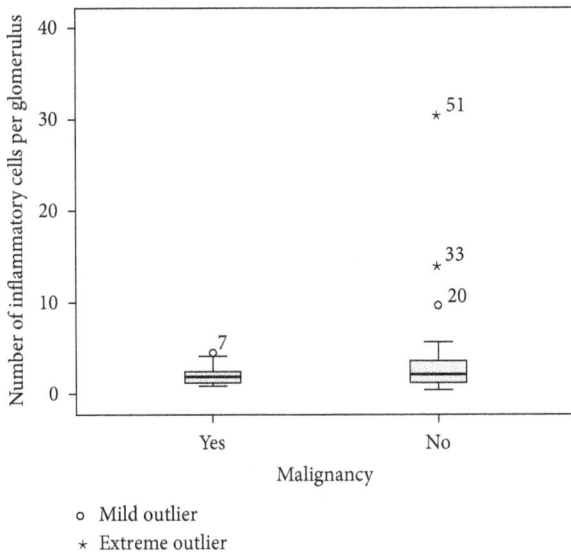

FIGURE 2: The median number of inflammatory cells per glomerulus in patients with and without malignancies.

The number of glomeruli analyzed on different levels was 917 (311 in the malignancy group and 606 in the control group).

A univariate analysis on Pearson test showed no correlation between the number of inflammatory cells per glomerulus and the period between cancer diagnosis and renal biopsy, p value 0.44. The median number of inflammatory cells per glomerulus was not different in the 6 patients with malignancies within 12 months of renal biopsy compared to the remaining 11 patients with malignancies at 1.01 (IQR, 0.87–1.95) and 2 (IQR 1.8–3), respectively, p value 0.3. No correlation between the total number of inflammatory cells in the biopsy or the inflammatory cells per glomerulus has been identified with any of the clinical variables (age, proteinuria, haematuria, eGFR, or serum albumin).

4. Discussion

This study provides strong evidence for a twofold increased risk of malignancy in MN patients in the follow-up years when compared to a matched population. The SIR of 2.1 is similar to that reported by Bjørneklett et al. at 2.25 who had a median follow-up of 6.2 years [9]. The minor disparity might be related to the different methods used. In the present study, the expected risk was calculated taking into account the annual change of risk, which minimized overestimation of the SIR.

MN patients are regularly screened for malignancy around the time of their diagnosis, and given the known association there might be a lower threshold for future screening compared to general population, which raises the possibility of detection bias. Lefaucheur et al. attempted to address this by identifying those patients with symptomatic malignancies and found that 11 patients (52%) were symptomatic, and the SIRs were raised at 7.1 (95% CI: 3.4–13) in males and 4.4 (95% CI: 0.5–16) in females [10]. However, this was a subsidiary

analysis of a group with a very high risk at the start (10-fold). During the follow-up after MN diagnosis in our study of 88 months, the number of symptomatic malignancies before diagnostic testing was high at 24 (92.3%). This might relate to the long follow-up as MN patients usually have screening for malignancy around the time of MN diagnosis, especially if no primary cause is found [1], but not routinely investigated during follow-up unless indicated or symptomatic. Therefore, the detected malignancies in our study are likely to be representative of the actual risk in these patients and not of better surveillance.

The data on long-term risk of malignancy in MN patients remains limited. In the present study, the risk of new malignancies decreased and lost significance beyond 5 years after the diagnosis of MN. After excluding patients with previous malignancies we had 1284 patient-years, which makes this study the largest of its kind.

Older age (≥60 years) has again been shown to be a strong risk factor for malignancy in MN patients; however, the SIRs were almost identical between old and younger patients. This should be emphasized to patients and clinicians when describing the malignancy risk in MN patients.

In the patients receiving cyclophosphamide for more than 3 months in our study, there was a higher rate of malignancy in the follow-up years. van den Brand et al. reported a significant increase in malignancy risk in MN patients receiving cyclophosphamide from 0.3% to 1% [19]. Cyclophosphamide has been linked historically to bladder malignancy [20] and haematological malignancies [21] especially when the mean cumulative dose is >36 g. However, none of the 44 MN patients who had cyclophosphamide in this study developed either. This might be partly explained by the fact that the mean cumulative dose in our cohort was not particularly high at 19.6 g, which falls within the current recommendations for managing idiopathic MN [14].

Lung malignancy has been reported to be the commonest malignancy in MN patients at 26% [8]. In our study the SIR was high at 8.9 and this was within the range of previously reported rates, 3.33 (95% CI: 0.91–8.52) [3] and 31.9 (95% CI: 12.8–65.7) [10]. All lung malignancies in our cohort were in heavy smokers. We thus support the recommendation that a Computed Tomography of the chest be undertaken for smokers with MN as proposed by Pani et al. [22]. However its value has not been prospectively examined.

Efforts have been made to identify histological markers in renal biopsies of MN patients which predict malignancy. Earlier papers suggested that different IgG subclass pattern of deposition could be helpful. Ohtani et al. reported a significantly more intense IgG1 and IgG2 deposition in malignancy-associated MN compared with idiopathic MN [15]. Later on, Qu et al. found no significant difference in IgG1 deposition and a small but significantly more intense IgG2 deposition in malignancy related MN compared to idiopathic MN [16]. Qu et al. also found that the IgG4 deposition was significantly different between the 2 groups, being absent in 88% of malignancy related MN compared to 14% of idiopathic MN. More recently, Lönnbro-Widgren et al. showed no difference between idiopathic MN and malignancy related MN in IgG1 or IgG2 deposition and reported a difference only in the IgG4 deposition between the two at 65% and 31%, respectively [17]. Murtas and Ghiggeri reported on a recent review that there was no reliable deposition pattern to differentiate between the two entities [18].

In their paper, Lefaucheur et al. reported that MN patients with malignancies had a significantly higher number of inflammatory cells in the glomeruli compared with matched idiopathic MN patients. The number of inflammatory cells was on average more than double that of the matched controls, and 8 inflammatory cells was the best cut-off value to distinguish between the 2 groups, with a specificity of 75% and a sensitivity of 92% ($p = 0.001$). This has not been further examined.

In the present study, there was no relation of the number of inflammatory cells in the glomeruli to the malignancy status or to the interval between the renal biopsy and the malignancy diagnosis. We had 3 patients in our cohort with 8 inflammatory cells or more per glomerulus on their renal biopsies and none of these patients had malignancy.

The exact mechanism underlying the association between MN and malignancy remains a matter of debate. Nevertheless, few mechanisms have been proposed [23, 24]. Antibodies may be generated against an antigen on the malignant tissues similar to an endogenous podocyte antigen, thereby leading to in situ glomerular immune-complex formation. Alternatively, shed tumor antigens may form circulating immune complexes that become trapped in the capillary wall. These complexes may initially form in a subendothelial location where the immune clearance is limited [25], dissociate, and reform in a subepithelial position. Another possibility is an extrinsic process such as an oncogenic virus or an altered immune function that causes both malignancy and MN.

A major argument against a causal association between malignancy and MN stems from the fact that they are both more common in older individuals which might merely represent two coincidental disease processes [24]. However, in our study we demonstrated clearly that this association persists across the age groups.

5. Conclusion

The relative risk for malignancy after the diagnosis of MN is more than twice that of a matched population and is similar across age groups. This increased risk is only found in the first 5 years of follow-up. The increased risk does not appear to relate to better surveillance, as it remains significantly high even for patients only with malignancy-specific symptoms prior to investigations. The risk of lung malignancy is particularly high at almost 9-fold. The number of inflammatory cells per glomerulus was not a helpful tool to differentiate between MN patients with and without malignancy.

Acknowledgments

This work was supported by the Renal Department in Auckland City Hospital, Auckland, New Zealand.

References

[1] C. Ponticelli and R. J. Glassock, "Glomerular diseases: membranous nephropathy-a modern view," *Clinical Journal of the American Society of Nephrology*, vol. 9, no. 3, pp. 609–616, 2014.

[2] W. L. Lai, T. H. Yeh, P. M. Chen et al., "Membranous nephropathy: a review on the pathogenesis, diagnosis, and treatment," *Journal of the Formosan Medical Association*, vol. 114, no. 2, pp. 102–111, 2015.

[3] M. Haas, S. M. Meehan, T. G. Karrison, and B. H. Spargo, "Changing etiologies of unexplained adult nephrotic syndrome: a comparison of renal biopsy findings from 1976–1979 and 1995–1997," *American Journal of Kidney Diseases*, vol. 30, no. 5, pp. 621–631, 1997.

[4] G. L. Braden, J. G. Mulhern, M. H. O'Shea, S. V. Nash, A. A. Ucci Jr., and M. J. Germain, "Changing incidence of glomerular diseases in adults," *American Journal of Kidney Diseases*, vol. 35, no. 5, pp. 878–883, 2000.

[5] R. J. Glassock, "Diagnosis and natural course of membranous nephropathy," *Seminars in Nephrology*, vol. 23, no. 4, pp. 324–332, 2003.

[6] A. G. Wasserstein, "Membranous glomerulonephritis," *Journal of the American Society of Nephrology*, vol. 8, no. 4, pp. 664–674, Apr 1997.

[7] J. C. Lee, H. Yamauchi, and J. Hopper Jr., "The association of cancer and the nephrotic syndrome.," *Annals of Internal Medicine*, vol. 64, no. 1, pp. 41–51, 1966.

[8] N. Leeaphorn, P. Kue-A-Pai, N. Thamcharoen, P. Ungprasert, M. B. Stokes, and E. L. Knight, "Prevalence of cancer in membranous nephropathy: A systematic review and meta-analysis of observational studies," *American Journal of Nephrology*, vol. 40, no. 1, pp. 29–35, 2014.

[9] R. Bjørneklett, B. E. Vikse, E. Svarstad et al., "Long-Term Risk of Cancer in Membranous Nephropathy Patients," *American Journal of Kidney Diseases*, vol. 50, no. 3, pp. 396–403, 2007.

[10] C. Lefaucheur, B. Stengel, and D. Nochy, "Membranous nephropathy and cancer: epidemiologic evidence and determinants of high-risk cancer association," *Kidney International*, vol. 70, no. 8, pp. 1510–1517, 2006.

[11] S. A. Birkeland and H. H. Storm, "Glomerulonephritis and malignancy: a population-based analysis," *Kidney International*, vol. 63, no. 2, pp. 716–721, 2003.

[12] J. Bacchetta, L. Juillard, P. Cochat, and J.-P. Droz, "Paraneoplastic glomerular diseases and malignancies," *Critical Reviews in Oncology/Hematology*, vol. 70, no. 1, pp. 39–58, 2009.

[13] P. M. Ronco, "Paraneoplastic glomerulopathies: new insights into an old entity," *Kidney International*, vol. 56, no. 1, pp. 355–377, 1999.

[14] G. Eknoyan, N. Lameire, K.-U. Eckardt et al., "Kidney disease: improving global outcomes (KDIGO) glomerulonephritis work group. KDIGO clinical practice guideline for glomerulonephritis," *Kidney International Supplements*, vol. 2, pp. 139–274, 2012.

[15] H. Ohtani, H. Wakui, A. Komatsuda et al., "Distribution of glomerular IgG subclass deposits in malignancy-associated membranous nephropathy," *Nephrology Dialysis Transplantation*, vol. 19, no. 3, pp. 574–579, 2004.

[16] Z. Qu, G. Liu, J. Li et al., "Absence of glomerular IgG4 deposition in patients with membranous nephropathy may indicate malignancy," *Nephrology Dialysis Transplantation*, vol. 27, no. 5, pp. 1931–1937, 2012.

[17] J. Lönnbro-Widgren, K. Ebefors, J. Mölne, J. Nyström, and B. Haraldsson, "Glomerular IgG subclasses in idiopathic and malignancy-associated membranous nephropathy," *Clinical Kidney Journal*, vol. 8, no. 4, pp. 433–439, 2015.

[18] C. Murtas and G. M. Ghiggeri, "Membranous glomerulonephritis: histological and serological features to differentiate cancer-related and non-related forms," *Journal of Nephrology*, vol. 29, no. 4, pp. 469–478, 2016.

[19] J. A. J. G. van den Brand, P. R. van Dijk, J. M. Hofstra, and J. F. M. Wetzels, "Cancer risk after cyclophosphamide treatment in idiopathic membranous nephropathy," *Clinical Journal of the American Society of Nephrology*, vol. 9, no. 6, pp. 1066–1073, 2014.

[20] M. Faurschou, I. J. Sorensen, L. Mellemkjaer et al., "Malignancies in wegener's granulomatosis: incidence and relation to cyclophosphamide therapy in a cohort of 293 patients," *Journal of Rheumatology*, vol. 35, no. 1, pp. 100–105, 2008.

[21] S. Bernatsky, R. Ramsey-Goldman, L. Joseph et al., "Lymphoma risk in systemic lupus: effects of disease activity versus treatment," *Annals of the Rheumatic Diseases*, vol. 73, no. 1, pp. 138–142, 2014.

[22] A. Pani, C. Porta, L. Cosmai et al., "Glomerular diseases and cancer: evaluation of underlying malignancy," *Journal of Nephrology*, vol. 29, no. 2, pp. 143–152, 2016.

[23] J. F. Cambier and P. Ronco, "Onco-nephrology: glomerular diseases with cancer," *Clinical Journal of the American Society of Nephrology*, vol. 7, no. 10, pp. 1701–1712, 2012.

[24] L. H. Beck Jr., "Membranous nephropathy and malignancy," *Seminars in Nephrology*, vol. 30, no. 6, pp. 635–644, 2010.

[25] M. Mannik, S. A. Stapleton, M. W. Burns, C. E. Alpers, and V. J. Gauthier, "Glomerular subendothelial and subepithelial immune complexes, containing the same antigen, are removed at different rates," *Clinical & Experimental Immunology*, vol. 84, no. 2, pp. 367–372, 1991.

19

Association of Poor Social Support and Financial Insecurity with Psychological Distress of Chronic Kidney Disease Patients Attending National Nephrology Unit in Sri Lanka

Ramya Hettiarachchi[1] and Chrishantha Abeysena (iD)[2]

[1]Community Medicine, Postgraduate Institute of Medicine, University of Colombo, Colombo, Sri Lanka
[2]Department of Public Health, Faculty of Medicine, University of Kelaniya, Colombo, Sri Lanka

Correspondence should be addressed to Chrishantha Abeysena; chrishanthaabeysena@yahoo.com

Academic Editor: David B. Kershaw

Background. Chronic kidney disease (CKD) is associated with high morbidity and mortality. Hence, CKD patients are often in chronic psychological distress. The objective of the study was to describe factors associated with psychological distress of CKD patients attending National Nephrology Unit. *Methods.* A descriptive cross-sectional study was conducted among 382 CKD patients above 18 years of age applying systematic sampling. The data was collected using self-administered questionnaires to assess the psychological distress (GHQ-12), social support (SSQ6), coping strategies (BRIEFCOPE), pain (0 to 10 numeric pain rating scale), and physical role limitation due to ill health (SF36QOL). Sociodemographic and disease-related data were collected using an interviewer administered questionnaire and a data extraction sheet. Multiple logistic regression was applied for determining the associated factors. The results were expressed as adjusted odds ratio (AOR) and 95% confidence intervals (95% CI). *Results.* Percentage of psychological distress was 55.2% (95% CI: 48.4% to 62%). Poor social support (AOR = 1.81, 95% CI: 1.14–2.88), low satisfaction with the social support received (AOR = 4.14, 95% CI: 1.59–10.78), stages IV and V of CKD (AOR = 2.67, 95% CI: 1.65–4.20), presence of comorbidities (AOR = 2.38, 95% CI: 1.21–4.67), within one year of diagnosis (AOR = 2.23, 95% CI: 1.36–3.67), low monthly income (AOR = 2.26, CI: 1.26–4.06), higher out-of-pocket expenditure per month (AOR = 1.75, 95% CI: 1.75–1.99), and being a female (AOR = 2.95, 95% CI: 1.79–4.9) were significantly associated with psychological distress. *Conclusions.* More than half of the CKD patients were psychologically distressed. Factors such as financial and social support will be worth considering early because of their modifiability.

1. Background

Chronic kidney disease (CKD) is reported as a major global public health problem due to growing number of patients and heavy cost [1, 2]. Around 10% of global population suffers from CKD similar to the burden of diabetes [2, 3]. Significant number of new CKD patients is being reported throughout Sri Lanka since recent past. CKD is the 7th cause of death and 3500 deaths occurred due to kidney disease in Sri Lanka in year 2012 [4]. Therefore, more attention must be paid to improve the wellbeing and reduce the mortality of these patients [5].

The physical discomfort due to the illness as well as treatment modalities such as oral medications, hemodialysis, renal transplantation, dietary, and fluid restrictions hamper the psychological wellbeing of CKD patients. High prevalence of psychological issues associated with CKD led to the introduction of Psychonephrology [6, 7]. Researchers have identified female gender, living alone, loss of employment, high out-of-pocket expenditure and reduced economic productivity, multimorbidity, increasing severity of illness, and stages four and five of the disease as factors significantly associated with psychological distress among CKD patients [8, 9], while social support and coping strategies are known to reduce the distress [10, 11].

Improper adherence to medical advice leads to increased morbidity and mortality in CKD [12, 13]. Further, patients with end stage renal failure, a deadly incurable illness, need to undergo dialysis or a renal transplant for survival. This will further aggravate the psychological distress [14, 15].

Therefore, periodical assessment of psychological status of CKD patients is needed [7]. Psychological distress among CKD patients had not been assessed previously in Sri Lanka. Therefore, the aim of the study was to describe the factors associated with psychological distress of CKD patients attending National Institute of Nephrology Unit in Sri Lanka.

2. Methods

A hospital-based cross-sectional study was carried out at the National Institute of Nephrology Unit, Colombo, Sri Lanka, during April to September 2015. All the CKD patients registered in the clinic with evidence of chronic renal disease documented in a diagnosis card or in a clinic book participated in the study irrespective of cause and duration of illness. We excluded patients with depleted neurological state (Glasgow coma scale of <15), patients with a psychiatric illness.

A total final sample size of 420 was calculated with the critical value as 1.96 which corresponds to 95% confidence limit, precision as 5%, and an expected prevalence as 55% [16] with 10% nonresponse. Systematic sampling technique was used to enroll patients to the study. Source for the sampling frame was the clinic attendance register. Every third patient was invited to participate in the study until the total sample size was achieved.

The questionnaire comprised two sections. Section one was an interviewer administered questionnaire comprising variables on sociodemographic, economic, and disease-related factors. Section two was a self-administered questionnaire. It included a short form of social support questionnaire (SSQ6) to measure social support [17], BRIEFCOPE to assess coping strategies [18], 0–10 pain rating scale to assess pain [19], and GHQ 12 to assess psychological distress [20].

The SSQ6 consists of six items to measure perceived social support and satisfaction for the received support for each item. It was translated and culturally adapted. A panel of experts provided judgmental validity for the instrument. With regard to provision of perceived social support, the maximum number of people for each item was confined to nine while minimum was zero. SSQ6 score ranged from 54 to zero. Total SSQ6 score was categorized into two for bivariate analysis: as poor social support when SSQ6 score was ≤25th percentile (≤13 people to give support) and as high social support when SSQ6 score was >25th percentile (>13). Satisfaction for the received social support from people was measured by six-point Likert scale. Minimum satisfaction score was six and maximum satisfaction score was 36. Total satisfaction score was categorized into two at 75th centile for bivariate analysis. Score < 75th (≤22.5) was considered low satisfaction and ≥75th was considered as higher social satisfaction over received support.

BRIEF COPE [18] was validated to Sri Lanka [21], with a reliability of Cronbach's alpha of 0.75. It was scored with four-point Likert scale. Coping strategies were categorized into three in BRIEF COPE as dysfunctional coping, problem focused coping, and emotion focused coping. Total coping score was calculated for each category. Each coping score was subcategorized into three as low, moderate, and high at 15th and 85th centiles. Number of patients with moderate and high coping responses were amalgamated for bivariate analysis.

Financial insecurity was assessed in terms of per capita monthly income and out-of-pocket expenditure for health per month. We obtained per capita monthly income of CKD patients in Sri Lankan rupees as a continuous variable. Monthly income of less than 10,000 Sri Lankan rupees per month was defined as low monthly income. Out-of-pocket expenditure for health per month was calculated adding total expenditure for drugs, medical investigations, transport, bystanders, doctor charges, and treatments such as for dialysis. More than 6000 Sri Lankan rupees were defined as high out-of-pocket expenditure per month.

CKD patients suffer from joint pain and perceived bodily muscular skeletal pain. Therefore, we measured pain in a severity scale of zero to ten (severe pain) [19]. Score of ≥four was taken as the cut-off value which indicates significant pain interfering with activities [19]. The life events over the last three months were measured using an instrument containing eight items [22]. We assigned a minimum score of zero and maximum score of eight. If a patient had experienced at least one life event during the last three months, they were categorized under "stress group."

Problems faced with the work and other regular daily activities due to the physical ill health were assessed with relevant questions (physical functioning component) extracted from the Short Form 36 quality of life questionnaire [23]. Minimum score was zero and maximum score was four. The total score of ≤1 was considered minimum physical role limitation and total score of four was considered as the maximum physical role limitation due to ill health.

Accurate knowledge on prognosis of CKD was assessed by inquiring whether they agree to the statement "CKD is a controllable disease and has to undergo renal transplant or dialysis at the end stage." Perceived knowledge on prognosis of CKD was assessed by inquiring whether they agree to the statement "CKD is progressive and incurable or non-progressive and curable disease."

General Health Questionnaire Item 12 (GHQ12) which was validated to Sri Lanka [20] was used to assess the psychological distress of CKD patients. The total GHQ score of ≥2 was considered as psychological distress.

A record sheet was used to collect secondary data such as serum creatinine, stage of CKD, treatment modality, and comorbidities from patient's clinic records. Pretest of the questionnaire was carried out among ten CKD patients. Eligible patients were invited to participate after their clinic activities. The questionnaire was given to patients in a separate room with a view to maintain privacy and confidentiality in the absence of any person other than the patient and the data collector.

Data was analyzed using SPSS version 16. Psychological distress of CKD patients was assessed with the univariate analysis expressed as percentages and confidence intervals. Bivariate analysis was applied for assessing the association between the factors and psychological distress of CKD patients. All variables at bivariate analysis with P value < 0.2

TABLE 1: Percentage of psychological distress according to selected factors.

| Factors | Sample size | Psychological distress | | 95% confidence interval |
		Number	Percentage	
Age in years				
18–40	60	33	55.0	52.1 to 57.9
41–60	149	87	58.4	57.3 to 59.3
61–80	162	85	52.5	51.4 to 53.6
≥81	6	3	50.0	17.3 to 52.7
Sex				
Male	166	104	49.3	48.4 to 50.2
Female	211	104	62.7	61.8 to 63.6
Ethnicity				
Sinhalese	327	175	53.5	54.1 to 52.9
Non-Sinhalese	50	33	66.0	62.8 to 69.2
Religion				
Buddhists	278	144	51.8	52.5 to 51.1
Non-Buddhists	99	64	64.6	66.1 to 63.1
Marital status				
Unmarried	48	25	52.1	48.2 to 56.0
Ever married	329	183	55.6	55.0 to 56.1
Stage of the illness				
Stage 01	42	21	50.0	54.7 to 45.3
Stage 02	58	22	37.9	33.6 to 42.2
Stage 03	114	58	50.2	52.6 to49.2
Stage 04	71	42	59.2	56.9 to 61.5
Stage 05	89	64	71.9	70.5 to 73.3
Total	377	208	55.2	54.8 to 55.8

were eligible for multiple logistic regression analysis which was applied for controlling confounding factors. Results were expressed as adjusted odds ratios (OR) and 95% confidence intervals (CI).

Permission to conduct the study was obtained from the Director of the National Institute of Nephrology and from the respective consultant nephrologists. All eligible patients were explained regarding the study. Informed written consent was obtained from those who were eligible and willing.

3. Results

We invited 420 eligible CKD patients. Nonresponse rate was 9.1%. Therefore, 382 patients participated in the study. Mean age of the study population was 54.5 years (SD: +/−31.6). Majority of CKD patients were males (212, 55.5%), Sinhalese (329, 86.1%), and Buddhists (279, 73%) from Gampaha District (138, 36.1%), studied up to ordinary level examination (237, 62%), and in end stage renal failure (125, 32.7%).

3.1. Percentage of Psychological Distress. Response rate for the GHQ12 was 89.7% (377). Of them, 55.2% (CI: 54.7%–55.7%) had psychological distress. The percentage of psychological distress was higher among patients aged between 61 and 80 years (57.8%) and among females (62.7%), non-Sinhalese (66%), and non-Buddhists (64.6%) and who were in stage V of the illness (71.9%) (Table 1).

3.2. Factors Associated with Psychological Distress. As shown in Table 2, psychological distress of CKD patients was significantly associated with demographic and economic factors such as female gender, patients educated up to ordinary level, currently unemployed, out-of-pocket expenditure of >6000 rupees per month, and distance to the nephrology clinic from living place of >150 km.

Of all social and disease-related factors, duration of illness < 12 months, visiting the nephrology clinic > 1 per month, maximum physical role limitation due to ill health, perceived knowledge regarding prognosis of chronic kidney disease, poor social support, low satisfaction for the received social support, stages IV and V of the disease, currently undergoing dialysis, and having comorbidities (one or more) were significantly associated with psychological distress of CKD patients (Table 3).

A statistically significant association was observed between psychological distress of CKD patients with poor social support, less satisfaction over received social support, presence of comorbidities, out-of-pocket expenditure for

TABLE 2: Unadjusted odds ratios of demographic and economic factors and psychological distress.

Factors	Psychological distress		Odds ratio	95% confidence interval	P value
	Yes n (%)	No n (%)			
Age: <60 years	121 (58.2)	89 (52.7)	1.25	0.83 to 1.88	0.28
Sex: females	104 (50.0)	61 (36.7)	1.73	1.14 to 0.64	0.01
Ethnicity: Sinhala	175 (84.1)	152 (89.9)	0.59	0.31 to 1.10	0.09
Province of living: western	140 (67.3)	120 (71.0)	0.84	0.54 to 1.30	0.44
Educational status: ≤O/L	89 (42.8)	53 (31.4)	1.64	1.07 to 2.50	0.02
Religion: Buddhists	144 (69.2)	134 (79.3)	0.58	0.37 to 0.94	0.03
Marital status: unmarried	25 (12.0)	23 (13.6)	0.87	0.47 to 1.6	0.64
Living alone	24 (11.5)	22 (13.0)	0.87	0.47 to 1.61	0.64
Currently employed	121 (58.7)	73 (43.2)	1.87	1.24 to 2.81	0.003
Low monthly income	52 (25.0)	28 (16.6)	1.68	1.0 to 2.8	0.05
High out-of-pocket expenditure	108 (51.9)	67 (39.6)	1.64	1.09 to 2.48	0.01
Distance to nephrology unit from residence: >150 Km	32 (15.4)	13 (7.7)	2.18	1.1 to 4.3	0.02

health more than 6000 rupees per month, low monthly income, female gender, duration since diagnosis 12 months or less, and stages IV or V renal disease (Table 4).

4. Discussion

The present study found that 55.2% of CKD patients attending Maligawatta nephrology clinic suffered from psychological distress. The percentage of psychological distress among CKD patients was higher than the general population (5%–27%) as well as cancer patients (30%) [24, 25]. The present study finding was compatible with two other studies [9, 16]. Sumanathissa reported prevalence of psychological distress as 55% in the Anuradhapura nephrology clinic [16] in Sri Lanka. Another study conducted in Sweden to measure psychological distress among CKD patients revealed it as 53.5% [9].

The present study revealed that female CKD patients were almost three times more psychologically distressed than male CKD patients. According to Sumanathissa, depression was associated with female CKD patients in Anuradhapura nephrology clinic [16]. Similarly, Sfyrkou in Sweden reported that women have high psychological distress compared to men [9].

In the present study, CKD patients who had a low monthly income were more likely to be distressed than CKD patients who earned adequate monthly income. This finding was consistent with two other studies, a 12-year cohort study done by Orpana et al. in USA [26] and another in UK [27] by Kosidou et al., which have detected low income as significantly associated with psychological distress when adjusted for sociodemographic characteristics and baseline health characteristics.

CKD patients who spend more than >6000 rupees as out-of-pocket expenditure for health per month were significantly distressed than CKD patients who spend ≤6000 rupees per month. Some CKD patients of the study sample received only limited number of free dialysis sessions. Thereafter, they had

to bear the cost for the rest of dialysis sessions. And some of the patients from faraway places get their investigations done from private sector as well. However, findings of a study done in Australia [28] in 2015 were contrary to ours. High out-of-pocket expenditure was not associated with depression among CKD patients when adjusted for confounding factors such as household income, occupation, and government concessions.

In our study, presence of one or more comorbidities was significantly associated with psychological distress of CKD patients. A hospital-based study done by Jayasinghe on CKD patients in Badulla found that poor mental functioning score was significantly associated with the presence of one or more comorbidities [22]. A similar finding has been reported by Sfyrkou in Sweden [9].

It was noted that CKD patients in stages IV and V were having significantly higher psychological distress compared to CKD patients in stage one to three. Similar findings have been described by Chiang et al. in 2013 [8]. A meta-analysis, carried out by Palmar et al., found that stage five CKD patients were having significant depressive symptoms compared to patients in stage one to four [29].

Emotions sharing, financial aid, and any kind of support for the diseased patient relieve psychological distress. Therefore, social support has a public health importance because this is a modifiable factor. In the present study, social support was measured in two ways: number of people available to give support and the satisfaction over received support. Poor social support in both the domains was significantly associated with high psychological distress. In the study by Patel et al. among end stage renal disease patients, a higher depression score with perceived lower social support was found [10]. A study done by Kimmel et al. describes that social support leads to good mental health score and even increases the survival as well [7, 15]. Cukor et al. describe that social support improves the quality of life by acting as a protective factor against psychological ill health and stress [6].

TABLE 3: Unadjusted odds ratios of social and disease related factors and psychological distress.

Factors	Psychological distress		Odds ratio	95% confidence interval	P value
	Yes n (%)	No n (%)			
Duration of illness since diagnosis: <12 months	83 (39.9)	48 (28.4)	1.67	1.08 to 2.58	0.02
Frequency of hospital visits per month: >once a month	75 (36.1)	41 (24.3)	1.76	1.12 to 2.76	0.01
Presence of maximum physical role limitation due to ill health	146 (70.2)	99 (58.6)	1.66	1.08 to 2.55	0.02
Significant pain interfering with activities	104 (50.0)	68 (40.2)	1.48	0.98 to 2.24	0.06
Perceived knowledge regarding the prognosis of CKD	106 (51.0)	56 (33.1)	2.1	1.38 to 3.19	0.001
Accurate knowledge on prognosis of CKD	148 (71.2)	115 (68.0)	1.15	0.74 to 1.8	0.51
Social support					
Number of people giving support ≤13 (poor social support)	124 (59.6)	72.0 (42.6)	1.99	1.31 to 3.0	0.001
Satisfaction over social support received ≤22.5 (low satisfaction)	31 (14.9)	7 (4.1)	3.94	1.68 to 9.21	0.001
Disease severity: stages IV and V	129 (62.9)	66 (39.1)	2.55	1.68 to 3.87	0.001
Treatment modality: dialysis	68 (32.7)	20 (11.8)	3.61	2.09 to 6.27	0.001
Presence of comorbidities	183 (88.0)	135 (79.9)	1.84	1.05 to 0.23	0.03
Experience of at least one life event	136 (65.4)	99 (68.6)	1.34	0.88 to 2.03	0.17
Coping strategies					
Dysfunctional coping: low	13.0 (6.5)	11.0 (6.9)	0.96	0.42 to 2.21	0.93
Problem focused coping: low	9.0 (4.4)	6.0 (3.6)	1.24	0.43 to 3.54	0.93
Emotion focused coping: low	174 (83.7)	133 (78.7)	1.38	0.82 to 2.33	0.23

TABLE 4: Adjusted odds ratios of the factors associated with psychological distress of CKD patients.

Factors	B	Standard error	OR	95% CI for OR		P value
Poor social support	0.59	0.24	1.81	1.14	2.88	0.01
Low satisfaction over received social support	1.42	0.49	4.13	1.59	10.78	0.004
Presence of at least one comorbidity	0.87	0.34	2.38	1.21	4.67	0.01
High out-of-pocket expenditure	0.56	0.24	1.75	1.09	2.82	0.001
Low monthly income	0.81	0.3	2.26	1.26	4.06	0.007
Sex: female	1.09	0.26	2.96	1.79	4.9	0.006
Duration of illness since diagnosis ≤12 months	0.80	0.25	2.23	1.36	3.67	0.001
Distance to nephrology unit from residence: >150 Km	0.71	0.38	2.03	0.97	4.25	0.06
Presence of maximum physical role limitation due to ill health	0.41	0.25	1.50	0.93	2.43	0.1
Disease severity: stages IV and V	0.98	0.24	2.66	1.65	4.29	0.001

B = beta coefficient; OR = odds ratio; and CI = confidence interval.

5. Conclusion

More than half of the CKD patients (55.2%) were psychologically distressed. More attention should be paid to the factors associated with psychological distress. Activities should be taken especially on the modifiable factors like improvement of quality and quantity of social support, reduction of out-of-pocket expenditure, establishment of social security system, and increase of the income level of CKD patients. Because the study is a hospital-based one extrapolation of results to the broader population should be done with caution.

References

[1] V. Jha, G. Garcia-Garcia, K. Iseki et al., "Chronic kidney disease: global dimension and perspectives," *The Lancet*, vol. 382, no. 9888, pp. 260–272, 2013.

[2] "The global issue of kidney disease," *The Lancet*, vol. 382, no. 9887, p. 101, 2013.

[3] C. O. Alebiosu and O. E. Ayodele, "The global burden of chronic kidney disease and the way forward," *Ethnicity & Disease*, vol. 15, no. 3, pp. 418–423, 2005.

[4] P. G. Mahipala, "Chronic kidney disease financial and economic costs, (2013)".

[5] "Weekly epidemiological report. Screening guidelines for chronic kidney disease in Sri Lanka, WER ,epidemiology unit, (2014)".

[6] D. Cukor, S. D. Cohen, R. A. Peterson, and P. L. Kimmen, "Psychosocial aspects of chronic disease: ESRD as a paradigmatic illness," *Journal of the American Society of Nephrology*, vol. 18, no. 12, pp. 3042–3055, 2007.

[7] P. L. Kimmel, R. A. Peterson, K. L. Weihs et al., "Multiple measurements of depression predict mortality in a longitudinal study of chronic hemodialysis outpatients," *Kidney International*, vol. 57, no. 5, pp. 2093–2098, 2000.

[8] H.-H. Chiang, H. Livneh, M.-L. Yen, T.-C. Li, and T.-Y. Tsai, "Prevalence and correlates of depression among chronic kidney disease patients in Taiwan," *BMC Nephrology*, vol. 14, no. 1, article no. 78, 2013.

[9] C. Sfyrkou, "Psychological distress and multimorbidity in patients with chronic kidney disease".

[10] S. S. Patel, R. A. Peterson, and P. L. Kimmel, "Psychosocial factors in patients with chronic kidney disease: The impact of social support on end-stage renal disease," *Seminars in Dialysis*, vol. 18, no. 2, pp. 98–102, 2005.

[11] S. P. Ramirez, D. S. Macêdo, P. M. G. Sales et al., "The relationship between religious coping, psychological distress and quality of life in hemodialysis patients," *Journal of Psychosomatic Research*, vol. 72, no. 2, pp. 129–135, 2012.

[12] L. R. Martin, S. L. Williams, K. B. Haskard, and M. R. DiMatteo, "The challenge of patient adherence," *Therapeutics and Clinical Risk Management*, vol. 1, no. 3, pp. 189–199, 2005.

[13] J. Lin, G. E. Sklar, V. M. S. Oh, and S. C. Li, "Factors affecting therapeutic compliance: a review from the patient's perspective," *Therapeutics and Clinical Risk Management*, vol. 4, no. 1, pp. 269–286, 2008.

[14] P. L. Kimmel, S. L. Emont, J. M. Newmann, H. Danko, and A. H. Moss, "ESRD patient quality of life: Symptoms, spiritual beliefs, psychosocial factors, and ethnicity," *American Journal of Kidney Diseases*, vol. 42, no. 4, pp. 713–721, 2003.

[15] P. L. Kimmel and R. A. Peterson, "Depression in patients with end-stage renal disease treated with dialysis: has the time to treat arrived?" *Clinical Journal of The American Society of Nephrology : CJASN*, vol. 1, no. 3, pp. 349–352, 2006.

[16] M. Sumanathissa, *Prevalence of Major Depressive Episode among (Pre-Dialysis) Patients, with Choronic Kidney Disease in The North Central Province of Sri Lanka*, Institute of Medicine, University of Colombo, Sri Lanka, 2010.

[17] I. G. Sarason, H. M. Levine, R. B. Basham, and B. R. Sarason, "Assessing social support: the social support questionnaire," *Journal of Personality and Social Psychology*, vol. 44, no. 1, pp. 127–139, 1983.

[18] N. Yusoff, W. Y. Low, and C. H. Yip, "Reliability and validity of the brief COPE scale (english version) among women with breast cancer undergoing treatment of adjuvant chemotherapy: A Malaysian study," *Medical Journal of Malaysia*, vol. 65, no. 1, pp. 41–44, 2010.

[19] M. McCaffery and C. Pasero, "Using the 0-to-10 pain rating scale: Nine common problems solved," *American Journal of Nursing*, vol. 101, no. 10, pp. 81–82, 2001.

[20] H. Abeysena, P. Jayawardana, U. Peiris, and A. Rodrigo, "Validation of the sinhala version of the 12-item general health questionnaire," *Journal of the Postgraduate Institute of Medicine*, vol. 1, 2014.

[21] N. F. Indika Pathiraja, "Psychosocial correlates of burnout among public health midwives in Sri," https://www.copsoq-network.org/assets/pdf/2013/Pathiraja-Indika-burnout-in-midwives.pdf.

[22] A. Jayasinghe, *Quality of life and its associated factors among patients with Chronic Kidney Disease attending the Provincial General Hospital Badulla*, Post Graduate Institute of Medicine, University of Colombo, Sri Lanka, 2012.

[23] N. S. Gunawardena, *Factors affecting functional outcome of lower limb amputee soldiers in two Districts of Sri Lanka*, University of Colombo, 2002.

[24] A. Drapeau, A. Marchand, and D. Beaulieu-Prévost, "Epidemiology of psychological distress," in *Mental Illnesses-Understanding, Prediction And Control*, pp. 105–134, InTech Open Access Publisher, 2012.

[25] J. R. Zabora, C. G. Blanchard, E. D. Smith et al., "Prevalence of psychological distress among cancer patients across the disease continuum," *Journal of Psychosocial Oncology*, vol. 15, no. 2, pp. 73–87, 1997.

[26] H. M. Orpana, L. Lemyre, and R. Gravel, "Income and psychological distress: the role of the social environment," *Health reports*, vol. 20, no. 1, pp. 21–28, 2009.

[27] K. Kosidou, C. Dalman, M. Lundberg, J. Hallqvist, G. Isacsson, and C. Magnusson, "Socioeconomic status and risk of psychological distress and depression in the stockholm public health cohort: A population-based study," *Journal of Affective Disorders*, vol. 134, no. 1-3, pp. 160–167, 2011.

[28] B. M. Essue, G. Wong, J. Chapman, Q. Li, and S. Jan, "How are patients managing with the costs of care for chronic kidney disease in Australia? A cross-sectional study," *BMC Nephrology*, vol. 14, no. 1, article no. 5, 2013.

[29] S. Palmer, M. Vecchio, J. C. Craig et al., "Prevalence of depression in chronic kidney disease: Systematic review and meta-analysis of observational studies," *Kidney International*, vol. 84, no. 1, pp. 179–191, 2013.

20

Acute Kidney Injury in Diabetes Mellitus

D. Patschan and G. A. Müller

Clinic of Nephrology and Rheumatology, University Hospital of Göttingen, Göttingen, Germany

Correspondence should be addressed to D. Patschan; d.patschan@gmail.com

Academic Editor: Laszlo Rosivall

Diabetes mellitus (DM) significantly increases the overall morbidity and mortality, particularly by elevating the cardiovascular risk. The kidneys are severely affected as well, partly as a result of intrarenal athero- and arteriosclerosis but also due to noninflammatory glomerular damage (diabetic nephropathy). DM is the most frequent cause of end-stage renal disease in our society. Acute kidney injury (AKI) remains a clinical and prognostic problem of fundamental importance since incidences have been increased in recent years while mortality has not substantially been improved. As a matter of fact, not many studies particularly addressed the topic "AKI in diabetes mellitus." Aim of this article is to summarize AKI epidemiology and outcomes in DM and current recommendations on blood glucose control in the intensive care unit with regard to the risk for acquiring AKI, and finally several aspects related to postischemic microvasculopathy in AKI of diabetic patients shall be discussed. We intend to deal with this relevant topic, last but not least with regard to increasing incidences and prevalences of both disorders, AKI and DM.

1. Introduction and Aim

The incidence and prevalence of diabetes mellitus (DM) have continuously been increased over the last 20 years. Meanwhile an estimated number of 387 million people worldwide suffer from DM [1]. Morbidity and mortality of diabetic patients are substantially aggravated by cardiovascular complications including coronary artery, cerebrovascular, and peripheral artery disease. In addition, DM may significantly affect kidneys and urinary tract. The disease accounts for most cases of end-stage renal disease in Western-Europe and in the US. Approximately 40% of all patients requiring dialysis therapy on a regular basis suffer from diabetes mellitus as respective cause [2]. Chronic renal insufficiency results from both, extra- and intrarenal atherosclerosis, and from diabetes-associated glomerular damage (diabetic nephropathy). In addition, diabetic kidneys are characterized by severe interstitial inflammation [3]. Finally, patients are at higher risk for developing contrast-induced nephropathy (CIN) [4] and frequently suffer from bacterial infections, often involving urinary tract and renal tissue *per se*.

Acute kidney injury (AKI) on the other hand remains a fundamental problem in hospitalized patients worldwide. As a matter of fact, incidences have also increased steadily in recent years, reaching almost 20% in middle-Europe.

This most likely results from ageing of the population in general, accompanied by an overall increased morbidity [5]. A meta-analysis from 2013 that evaluated more than 300 studies showed an average AKI world-incidence of even more than 30% in adults [6]. Nevertheless, mortality rates have only mildly been improved since the early 1990s. Zeng and colleagues reported dramatical differences in AKI mortality, depending on the severity of the syndrome [7]. If related to the AKIN criteria [8] overall in-hospital mortality rates were as follows: no AKI 0.6%, AKIN stage I 5.3%, AKIN stage II 13.4%, and AKIN stage III 35.4%. The lowest survival rates have been reported in patients suffering from a malignant disorder and from sepsis-associated AKI with the need for renal replacement therapy. In this particular group, mortality can exceed even 90% [9].

Regarding not only the individual but also the epidemiological and economical consequences of both disorders, DM and AKI, it is somehow surprising how few studies addressed the topic "AKI in diabetes mellitus." This article is intended to summarize the current knowledge of three aspects related to the field. Firstly, we will give an epidemiological overview: how does diabetes affect AKI risk and survival? Do diabetic patients suffer from an overall higher morbidity after AKI? Secondly, we will discuss the importance of blood glucose control at the intensive care unit (ICU) with special attention to AKI incidences and survival. Finally, several experimental investigations will be discussed. We will especially focus on microvascular or endothelial dysfunction which may emerge early during the course of the disease, thus potentially increasing ischemia-vulnerability of the organ.

2. AKI Epidemiology in Diabetes Mellitus

Several studies evaluated AKI epidemiology in diabetic patients. Mehta and colleagues [10] performed a retrospective analysis, based on the *Society of Thoracic Surgeons National Database*. All patients included between 2002 and 2004 were analyzed, with a total number of 449,524 individuals. The total prevalence of DM was 33%. Dialysis treatment became mandatory in 6,451 patients after surgery. In individuals requiring dialysis, diabetes was diagnosed more frequently than in those without renal replacement therapy (49 versus 33%, $p < 0.0001$). In addition, more detailed analysis using a multivariate logistic regression model revealed diabetes as independent risk factor for developing AKI after cardiac surgery. Another study published by Oliveira and colleagues [11] prospectively evaluated patients undergoing aminoglycoside treatment ($n = 980$). The primary endpoint was a reduction in the glomerular filtration rate (GFR) of 20% or more. The diabetes prevalence was 19.6% in patients that fulfilled the endpoint versus 9.3% without GFR reduction ($p = 0.007$). Comparable to the study by Mehta et al. [10] Oliveira and colleagues performed logistic regression analyses as well. These showed several independent AKI risk factors: baseline GFR of $<60 \, \text{mL/min/1.73 m}^2$, the use of iodinated contrast media, hypotension, concomitant use of nephrotoxic drugs, and diabetes (OR, 2.13; 95% CI, 1.01 to 4.49; $p = 0.046$). Girman et al. [12] retrospectively performed a survey of the *General Practice Research Database* (UK), comparing 119,966 type 2 DM patients with 1,794,516 nondiabetic individuals. The yearly AKI incidence was 198 versus 27/100,000 subjects, and the difference remained statistically significant even after adjustment for other well-known AKI risk factors and comorbidities. At this point it needs however to be mentioned that diabetic patients displayed an overall higher cumulative morbidity in general. They differed in the following categories: obesity, congestive heart failure, hypertension, alcohol and tobacco exposure, past AKI episodes, CKD prevalence, therapy with ACE inhibitors/angiotensin receptor blockers, therapy with other antihypertensive drugs, statin treatment, and NSAID use (*p* values in every category below 0.001). Hsu and colleagues compared 1,746 hospitalized adults (*Kaiser Permanente Northern California*) that developed dialysis-requiring AKI with over 600,000 individuals without such a complication [13]. The following parameters were identified as independent AKI risk factors: preadmission diabetes mellitus, arterial hypertension, and preexisting proteinuria.

The study by Thakar, performed in a prospective manner, somehow differed from the other investigations since it exclusively evaluated type 2 diabetic patients (*VA healthcare system*). The primary endpoint was progression towards CKD stage 4, depending on several risk factors and in particular depending on the presence of AKI during the observational period (01/1999–12/2004). General risk factors for CKD progression were arterial hypertension, obesity, and higher average age. Kidney-related risk factors were initial proteinuria, a lower mean GFR at the beginning of the study, and AKI *per se*. It also became apparent that survival probability gradually decreased with increasing number of AKI episodes. Finally, mortality increased further with lower initial mean GFR. Recently, Venot et al. [14] published an investigation designed as prospective case-control study. Three-hundred and eighteen diabetic patients were compared with 746 nondiabetic controls, and patients in both groups suffered from either severe sepsis or from septic shock. Interestingly, AKI incidences did not differ between the two groups but surviving subjects with diabetes more often required dialysis at discharge, showed higher mean serum creatinine levels, and did recover less efficiently than nondiabetics. The study by Venot et al. has several limitations which were discussed in the original manuscript in detail. First, the diagnosis of diabetes was made according to the medical history available from patients/relatives/consultants, HBA1C levels were not incorporated neither were diabetic long-term complications. Next, preexisting CKD was not defined as exclusion criterion since in some patients exact information about the initial status of kidney function was missing. Third, the diagnosis of AKI was made according to the KDIGO criteria [15] but without including urine output rates which were not documented. Finally, the need for dialysis treatment was not determined according to standardized criteria but was evaluated by clinicians from different sites in individual manners. Together, these confounding factors may potentially account for the lack of differences between diabetic and nondiabetic patients.

Two additional investigations confirmed these findings [16, 17]. Table 1 summarizes the results of the mentioned studies related to the topic. In summary the current data, although not consistently acquired in a controlled and prospective manner, indicate a higher AKI risk in the presence of (type 2) DM and they suggest a higher AKI-morbidity and mortality risk if patients suffer from the diabetic disease. An additional remark may be allowed with regard to all of the studies discussed above: they (almost) all investigated patients treated in the intensive care unit. By far not every patient who develops AKI during in-hospital treatment is being transferred to the intensive care unit. Therefore, a vast amount of outcome data may be missing in these investigations.

Another aspect that needs to be discussed is AKI risk in relation to preexisting diabetic nephropathy and to other coexisting morbidities. The currently available data suggest a higher AKI risk in diabetic individuals as compared to nondiabetic persons but it remains unclear whether this association is attributable to the hyperglycemic milieu *per se* or if it potentially results from end-organ damage such as generalized and intrarenal atherosclerosis. Only very few studies evaluated this particular aspect. Vallon [18] brought up the question whether changes in tubular homeostasis in diabetic nephropathy may increase AKI risk or not. In the end, any mechanistic relationship between diabetes-induced upregulation of TGF-β, (premature) senescence, and inflammation could only be suggested.

TABLE 1: Selected studies that evaluated AKI incidences and outcomes in diabetic patients. For detailed description see text.

Study/year	Design	Results
Mehta et al., 2006 [10]	Retrospective, data-based analysis (*Society of Thoracic Surgeons National Database*), DM prevalence in AKI patients after cardiac surgery; included individuals: 449,524	DM prevalence 49 versus 33% in AKI versus no AKI ($p < 0.0001$)
Oliveira et al., 2009 [11]	Prospective single-center analysis, DM prevalence in aminoglycoside-induced AKI; included individuals: 980	DM prevalence 19.6 versus 9.3% in AKI versus no AKI ($p = 0.007$)
Girman et al., 2012 [12]	Retrospective, data-based analysis (*General Practice Research Database*), AKI in DM versus no DM; included individuals: 119,966 type 2 DM patients and 1,794,516 nondiabetic individuals	Yearly AKI incidence in DM versus no DM: 198 versus 27/100,000 subjects
Venot et al., 2015 [14]	Prospective case-control study, AKI incidences and outcomes of patients with severe sepsis/septic shock, DM versus no DM; included individuals: 318 diabetic and 746 nondiabetic controls	AKI incidences not different but dialysis frequency and serum creatinine at discharge higher in DM
Kheterpal et al., 2009 [16]	Retrospective, data-based analysis (American College of *Surgeons National Surgical Quality Improvement Program*), AKI incidence after general surgery; included individuals: 75,952	Identification of DM as independent preoperative risk factor
Mittalhenkle et al., 2008 [17]	Prospective case-control study (*Cardiovascular Health Study*), AKI incidence in the elderly; included individuals: 5,731	Association of DM with incident acute renal failure (AKI)

To conclude the whole section, it has to be realized that AKI risk is most likely being increased in diabetic individuals. Nevertheless, the pathophysiological determinants responsible for such association are currently unknown. It needs to be elucidated more in detail how diabetic and nondiabetic comorbidities potentially increase the risk for acute kidney injury in diabetes mellitus.

3. Blood Glucose Control at the Intensive Care Unit: Impact on AKI Incidence and Survival

Chronic hyperglycemia is a well-known risk factor for atherosclerosis. Elevated blood glucose levels have nevertheless also been associated with impaired outcomes in acute situations such as myocardial infarction and stroke [19–21]. The mechanisms responsible may include hyperglycemia-induced release of free fat acids, the inactivation of nitric oxide (NO), and increased production of reactive oxygen species (ROS) [19], respectively. A number of studies compared glucose control in the intensive care unit by either conventional or intensified (continuously administered) insulin therapy with regard to AKI incidences. Thomas et al. reviewed the results in a 2007 published meta-analysis [22]. Three controlled, randomized, and prospective and 2 noncontrolled, prospective studies were included [23–27]. In all included studies, the AKI risk-ratio (RR) was below 1 in patients undergoing intensified insulin therapy (0.74 [24], 0.66 [23], 0.15 [27], 0.25 [26], and 0.67 [25]). Nevertheless, in two of the above mentioned (randomized controlled) studies [23, 25] the 95% confidence intervals were up to 0.99, respectively. Thus, differences between conventional and intensified insulin treatment regimens were only mild. One study in contrast showed significant AKI protection under intensified glucose control [27]. However, it may in

addition not be concluded that stricter protocols for glucose control exclusively improve outcomes of ICU patients. The NICE-SUGAR [28] trial compared ICU patients receiving glucose control in a strict (81–108 mg/dL) versus a liberal (>108 and below 180 mg/dL) manner. Three thousand fifty-four patients were assigned to the first and 3,050 individuals to the second group in a prospective manner. As a matter of fact, AKI incidences did not differ between the two categories but survival was significantly lower in those receiving a stricter insulin therapy (n = 829—27.5% versus 751—24.9% with $p = 0.02$). It needs to be noted that severe hypoglycemia, defined as blood glucose levels of below 40 mg/dL, occurred in 206 (6.8%) patients in the first versus 15 (0.5%) patients in the second group ($p < 0.001$). The 2012 published version of the "KDIGO clinical practice guidelines for acute kidney injury" [15] therefore recommended target glucose levels of 110–149 mg/dL to be achieved in ICU patients. Thus, AKI incidences may be reduced without further aggravating mortality.

4. Microvascular Dysfunction and AKI in Diabetes Mellitus

Hyperglycemia is a well-known risk factor for endothelial dysfunction [29]. Even quite early after being exposed to a hyperglycemic milieu, for instance, induced by the administration of "advanced glycation end-products" (AGEs), cultured endothelial cells show impaired production of nitric oxide which reflects the loss of cellular competence [29]. In addition, hyperglycemia has also been proven as inductor of premature endothelial senescence (stress-induced premature senescence—SIPS) [30]. The term "senescence" describes the process of functional and structural ageing of cells. Its first description was made by Hayflick and Moorhead who observed inhibition of fibroblast proliferation during cell culturing for several weeks [31]. Such "replicative type" of cellular senescence must be differentiated from another process of ageing that results from pathological stimuli such as oxidative stress [32], poor cell culture conditions [30], and/or the activation of certain (proto)oncogenes [33]. This second type has been defined as "stress-induced premature senescence" or SIPS [34]. According to current concepts, SIPS results from intracellular accumulation of telomeres, ultimately leading to DNA damage [35]. At the end of this section we will address potential pathophysiological consequences of DM-induced endothelial SIPS in AKI.

The importance of microvascular dysfunction in AKI has been highlighted by numerous experimental investigations. In most cases AKI ensues from transient renal hypoperfusion or ischemia [5]. The hallmark in ischemic AKI (iAKI) is tubular cell dysfunction and damage. The respective cellular and molecular mechanisms have extensively been studied and reviewed in the past [29–32]. In addition, ischemia also induces significant interstitial inflammation and functional impairment/structural damage of small peritubular and glomerular blood vessels [29, 30, 33–35]. The inflammatory response is being initiated by both tubular and vascular malfunction and encompasses the activation of virtually all components of the innate and acquired immune system [30]. The topic "postischemic inflammation" should meanwhile be recognized as a separate area in the field [35]. Microvascular damage on the other hand significantly affects the kidney in the short- and the long-term. Short-term effects involve endothelial cell expansion and apoptosis/necrosis, both resulting in microvascular obstruction. Thus, postischemic reperfusion is inhibited and kidney regeneration is prolonged [36, 37]. In addition, every ischemic insult diminishes the intrarenal total vascular surface area, subsequently followed/accompanied by endothelial-to-mesenchymal transdifferentiation (EndoMT) [38–40]. The ultimate consequence is aggravated fibrosis and an increased risk for CKD [33, 41, 42]. Nevertheless, the impact of diabetes-induced endothelial dysfunction (ED) on ischemia-vulnerability of the kidney has only sporadically been investigated in the past. Goor and colleagues [43] analyzed a model of type I DM. Rats were repeatedly injected with streptozotocin, followed by oral supplementation with the substance N-omega-nitro-L-arginine, a well-known nitric oxide synthase inhibitor. Fourteen days later, animals were subjected to ischemia-reperfusion injury. Postischemic creatinine clearance was significantly higher in nondiabetic animals (163 ± 30 versus 90 ± 22 μL/min/100 g; p < 0.005). In addition, only nondiabetic rats showed increased serum and urinary levels of nitric oxide (NO) despite pharmacological NO synthesis inhibition. Finally, animals from both groups were provided with the NO donor L-arginine. This measure exclusively improved kidney function in nondiabetic rats. Taken together, this study has several important implications. Firstly, nondiabetic animals were capable of producing NO even after exogenous NO synthesis inhibition, most likely by alternative mechanisms. Secondly, nondiabetic animals still showed sensitivity towards NO which predominantly acts on the microvascular level. In other words, quite early after diabetes induction (14 days),

animals displayed severe endothelial dysfunction (reduced NO synthesis and diminished NO sensitivity) resulting in aggravated postischemic kidney damage. Another study of interest was published by Shi and colleagues in 2007 [44]. By using Laser-Doppler Flowmetry, postischemic kidney reperfusion was analyzed in both compartments, the renal medulla and the cortex. Two parameters were of interest: postischemic flow acceleration and time until complete normalization of capillary flow. In contrast to the study by Goor et al. [43] diabetes was not induced by pharmacological measures but the authors used a well-established genetic model of type II diabetes, db/db mice [45]. These animals suffer from severe insulin resistance and obesity. As a matter of fact, both outcome parameters were significantly impaired in db/db as opposed to db/m and to wildtype control mice: postischemic flow acceleration was reduced and time until flow normalization was significantly longer in both compartments. It has to be noted that animals were only 10–12 weeks old. In summary, this study also points towards microvascular or endothelial dysfunction to occur quite *early* during the diabetic disease and it indicates that DM-induced ED alone may significantly affect ischemia-vulnerability of the kidney.

Another study also revealed diabetes as "fast-acting" risk factor for AKI, although it did not focus on diabetes-associated endothelial dysfunction. Rats were subjected to renal ischemia at week 2 after finishing a diabetes induction protocol using the substance streptozotocin [46]. Animals were analyzed 4 and 8 weeks later. Nondiabetic rats almost completely recovered from functional impairment and tissue damage while diabetic rats showed extensive inflammation and tubulointerstitial fibrosis at week 4. At week 8, diabetic kidneys were even reduced in mass, resulting from severe tubular loss. It may however not be forgotten that increased ischemia-sensitivity of the renal tissue in diabetes does exclusively result not only from impaired vascular (endothelial) function but also from aggravated inflammation. This particular topic shall however not be discussed at the moment. We would rather like to refer to some excellent manuscripts on the subject [35, 47, 48].

Finally, we would like to briefly mention a study recently published by Peng and colleagues [49]. Streptozotocin- (STZ-) treated mice showed higher ischemia-vulnerability than nondiabetic controls, although ischemia was applied quite early (3 weeks) after finishing the STZ protocol. Even though this model cannot truly be defined as model of diabetic nephropathy which usually evolves years after onset of diabetes in humans, it became apparent that hyperglycemia substantially induced p53 both, *in vivo* and *in vitro*. Subsequently, mitochondrial release of cytochrome C was increased as well. The ischemic damage decreased upon p53 silencing using siRNA. Together, the study offered a new mechanistic perspective on processes responsible for increased ischemia-sensitivity of the kidney in diabetes [50].

Finally, we would like to discuss possible implications of DM-induced endothelial SIPS in AKI. Although it must be understood as a rather pathological event, the hallmark of SIPS is faster or premature ageing of cells. The functional consequences more or less correspond to those that occur during normal ageing of tissues/organs. As pointed out

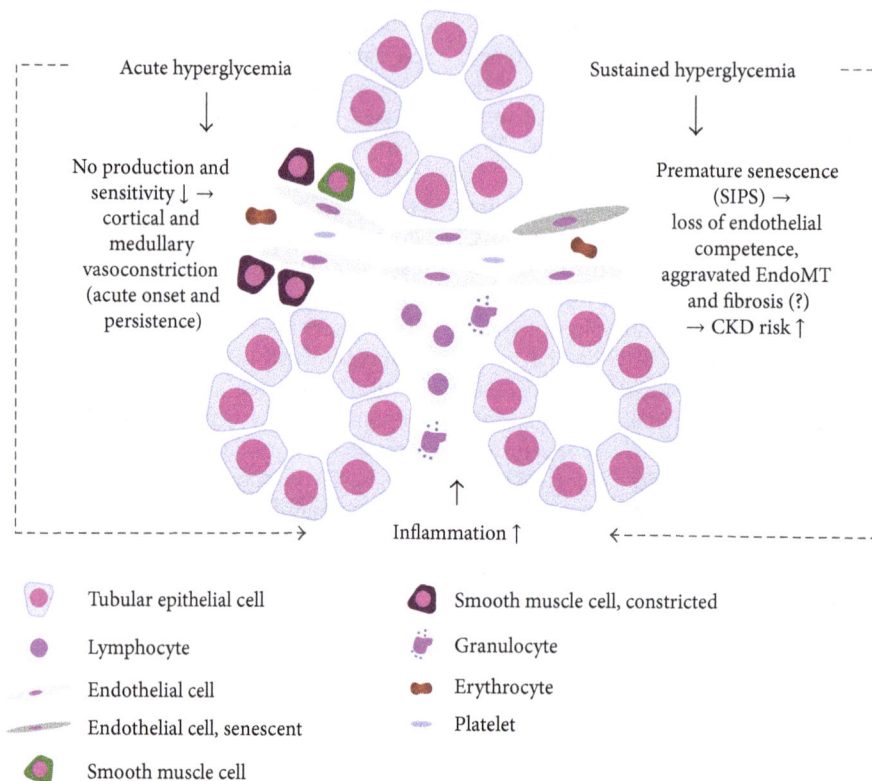

FIGURE 1: Pathophysiological consequences of DM on postischemic MV in AKI.

earlier, AKI incidences have steadily increased in recent years, significantly resulting from ageing of the population in general [5]. Higher age-related susceptibility of the kidney has been reported by several investigators [49, 50]. Schmitt and Cantley [51] reviewed the mechanisms that may increase kidney vulnerability in older individuals in an excellent manner [50]. Numerous processes were discussed including declined capacity of renal epithelial cells to proliferate, impaired function of certain types of stem and progenitor cells, and alterations of renal growth factor profiles. Clements and colleagues demonstrated exacerbation of vascular rarefication and CKD risk in aged mice following ischemia-reperfusion injury [52]. Nevertheless, the investigation was not performed under diabetic circumstances. A dynamic cascade of hyperglycemia-associated endothelial SIPS, accompanied by reduced autophagy, has been reported by Goligorsky and colleagues [53]. Autophagy (AP) is widely regarded as endogenous mechanism of self-protection/repair [54]. Own studies showed that TGF-beta-induced SIPS of cultured early endothelial progenitor cells goes in parallel with diminished AP as well [55]. As a matter of fact, intrarenal endothelial autophagy stimulation by pharmacological measures reduced mesenchymal transition of endothelial cells (EndoMT) after AKI [55]. EndoMT has been repeatedly reported to aggravate kidney fibrosis [38, 39]. One may therefore argue that endothelial SIPS, induced either by ischemia *per se* or by prolonged hyperglycemia, promotes EndoMT and fibrosis while increased AP mediates the opposite. Recently, we reported increased EndoMT and endothelial SIPS to occur in diabetic nephropathy. However, no investigation published so far analyzed endothelial SIPS in AKI under diabetic circumstances. We therefore recently initiated a project related to this particular topic. We intend to reduce endothelial SIPS by pharmacological AP stimulation after AKI. We sincerely hope to identify stress-induced cellular senescence as hallmark of aggravated postischemic endothelial damage within the diabetic microenvironment. Thus, antisenescent therapeutic strategies should be tested and hopefully established in order to improve microvasculopathy and AKI outcomes in the short- and long-term.

Figure 1 summarizes pathophysiological aspects of DM-associated microvasculopathy in AKI.

5. Conclusions

(i) In summary, we conclude that DM potentially increases AKI risk and long-term mortality/morbidity of AKI.

(ii) In the intensive care unit, blood glucose levels should be adjusted to high-normal/mildly increased levels. Thus, AKI risk may be minimized without elevating mortality rates.

(iii) Finally, DM should be recognized as "fast-acting" risk factor for kidney vulnerability to ischemia. The tissue susceptibility increases as a result of significant microvasculopathy and of interstitial inflammation. The latter effects can occur even in nondiabetic patients in whom acute blood glucose deterioration is not efficiently controlled.

Acknowledgments

The studies were supported by *Else Kröner-Fresenius-Stiftung*, *Jackstädt-Stiftung*, and *Deutsche Forschungsgemeinschaft*.

References

[1] Z. Aziz, P. Absetz, J. Oldroyd, N. P. Pronk, and B. Oldenburg, "A systematic review of real-world diabetes prevention programs: learnings from the last 15 years," *Implementation Science*, vol. 10, article 172, 2015.

[2] A. Mima, "Diabetic nephropathy: protective factors and a new therapeutic paradigm," *Journal of Diabetes and Its Complications*, vol. 27, no. 5, pp. 526–530, 2013.

[3] J. Hoshino, K. Mise, T. Ueno et al., "A pathological scoring system to predict renal outcome in diabetic nephropathy," *American Journal of Nephrology*, vol. 41, no. 4-5, pp. 337–344, 2015.

[4] R. Mehran, E. D. Aymong, E. Nikolsky et al., "A simple risk score for prediction of contrast-induced nephropathy after percutaneous coronary intervention: development and initial validation," *Journal of the American College of Cardiology*, vol. 44, no. 7, pp. 1393–1399, 2004.

[5] A. Bienholz, B. Wilde, and A. Kribben, "From the nephrologist's point of view: diversity of causes and clinical features of acute kidney injury," *Clinical Kidney Journal*, vol. 8, no. 4, pp. 405–414, 2015.

[6] P. Susantitaphong, D. N. Cruz, J. Cerda et al., "World incidence of AKI: a meta-analysis," *Clinical Journal of the American Society of Nephrology*, vol. 8, no. 9, pp. 1482–1493, 2013.

[7] X. Zeng, G. M. McMahon, S. M. Brunelli, D. W. Bates, and S. S. Waikar, "Incidence, outcomes, and comparisons across definitions of AKI in hospitalized individuals," *Clinical Journal of the American Society of Nephrology*, vol. 9, no. 1, pp. 12–20, 2014.

[8] S. Duan, Q. Liu, P. Pan et al., "RIFLE and AKIN criteria for mortality and risk factors of acute kidney injury in hospitalized patients," *Zhong Nan Da Xue Xue Bao Yi Xue Ban*, vol. 38, no. 12, pp. 1243–1252, 2013.

[9] M. Heeg, A. Mertens, D. Ellenberger, G. A. Müller, and D. Patschan, "Prognosis of AKI in malignant diseases with and without sepsis," *BMC Anesthesiology*, vol. 13, article 36, 2013.

[10] R. H. Mehta, J. D. Grab, S. M. O'Brien et al., "Bedside tool for predicting the risk of postoperative dialysis in patients undergoing cardiac surgery," *Circulation*, vol. 114, no. 21, pp. 2208–2216, 2006.

[11] J. F. P. Oliveira, C. A. Silva, C. D. Barbieri, G. M. Oliveira, D. M. T. Zanetta, and E. A. Burdmann, "Prevalence and risk factors for aminoglycoside nephrotoxicity in intensive care units," *Antimicrobial Agents and Chemotherapy*, vol. 53, no. 7, pp. 2887–2891, 2009.

[12] C. J. Girman, T. D. Kou, K. Brodovicz et al., "Risk of acute renal failure in patients with Type 2 diabetes mellitus," *Diabetic Medicine*, vol. 29, no. 5, pp. 614–621, 2012.

[13] C. Y. Hsu, J. D. Ordõez, G. M. Chertow, D. Fan, C. E. McCulloch, and A. S. Go, "The risk of acute renal failure in patients with chronic kidney disease," *Kidney International*, vol. 74, no. 1, pp. 101–107, 2008.

[14] M. Venot, L. Weis, C. Clec'h et al., "Acute kidney injury in severe sepsis and septic shock in patients with and without diabetes mellitus: A Multicenter Study," *PLoS ONE*, vol. 10, no. 5, article e0127411, 2015.

[15] A. Zarbock, S. John, A. Jörres, D. Kindgen-Milles, and Kidney Disease: Improving Global Outcome, "New KDIGO guidelines on acute kidney injury. Practical recommendations," *Anaesthesist*, vol. 63, no. 7, pp. 578–588, 2014.

[16] S. Kheterpal, K. K. Tremper, M. Heung et al., "Development and validation of an acute kidney injury risk index for patients undergoing general surgery: results from a national data set," *Anesthesiology*, vol. 110, no. 3, pp. 505–515, 2009.

[17] A. Mittalhenkle, C. O. Stehman-Breen, M. G. Shlipak et al., "Cardiovascular risk factors and incident acute renal failure in older adults: The Cardiovascular Health Study," *Clinical Journal of the American Society of Nephrology*, vol. 3, no. 2, pp. 450–456, 2008.

[18] V. Vallon, "Do tubular changes in the diabetic kidney affect the susceptibility to acute kidney injury?" *Nephron Clinical Practice*, vol. 127, no. 1-4, pp. 133–138, 2014.

[19] F. Angeli, G. Reboldi, C. Poltronieri et al., "Hyperglycemia in acute coronary syndromes: from mechanisms to prognostic implications," *Therapeutic Advances in Cardiovascular Disease*, vol. 9, no. 6, pp. 412–424, 2015.

[20] P. Seners, G. Turc, C. Oppenheim, and J.-C. Baron, "Incidence, causes and predictors of neurological deterioration occurring within 24 h following acute ischaemic stroke: a systematic review with pathophysiological implications," *Journal of Neurology, Neurosurgery and Psychiatry*, vol. 86, no. 1, pp. 87–94, 2015.

[21] E. Rostami, "Glucose and the injured brain-monitored in the neurointensive care unit," *Frontiers in Neurology*, vol. 5, article 91, 2014.

[22] G. Thomas, M. C. Rojas, S. K. Epstein, E. M. Balk, O. Liangos, and B. L. Jaber, "Insulin therapy and acute kidney injury in critically ill patients—a systematic review," *Nephrology Dialysis Transplantation*, vol. 22, no. 10, pp. 2849–2855, 2007.

[23] G. Van den Berghe, A. Wilmer, G. Hermans et al., "Intensive insulin therapy in the medical ICU," *The New England Journal of Medicine*, vol. 354, no. 5, pp. 449–461, 2006.

[24] G. Van Den Berghe, P. Wouters, F. Weekers et al., "Intensive insulin therapy in critically ill patients," *The New England Journal of Medicine*, vol. 345, no. 19, pp. 1359–1367, 2001.

[25] B. Van Vlem, P. Lecomte, and K. Van Varenbergh, "Strict perioperative glucose control is renoprotective in patients undergoing cardiac surgery," *Journal of the American Society of Nephrology*, vol. 17, p. 769A, 2006.

[26] J. S. Krinsley, "Effect of an intensive glucose management protocol on the mortality of critically Ill adult patients," *Mayo Clinic Proceedings*, vol. 79, no. 8, pp. 992–1000, 2004.

[27] L. Wang, S. Lei, Y. Wu et al., "Intensive insulin therapy in critically ill patients," *Zhongguo Wei Zhong Bing Ji Jiu Yi Xue Chin. Crit. Care Med. Zhongguo Weizhongbing Jijiuyixue*, vol. 18, no. 12, pp. 748–750, 2006.

[28] S. Finfer, R. Bellomi, D. Blair et al., "Intensive versus conventional glucose control in critically Ill patients," *The New England Journal of Medicine*, vol. 360, no. 13, pp. 1283–1297, 2009.

[29] D. P. Basile, M. D. Anderson, and T. A. Sutton, "Pathophysiology of acute kidney injury," *Comprehensive Physiology*, vol. 2, no. 2, pp. 1303–1353, 2012.

[30] P. Devarajan, "Update on mechanisms of ischemic acute kidney injury," *Journal of the American Society of Nephrology*, vol. 17, no. 6, pp. 1503–1520, 2006.

[31] A. Kribben, C. L. Edelstein, and R. W. Schrier, "Pathophysiology of acute renal failure," *Journal of Nephrology*, vol. 12, supplement 2, pp. S142–S151, 1999.

[32] A. Kribben, S. Herget-Rosenthal, F. Pietruck, and T. Philipp, "Acute renal failure—an update," *Deutsche Medizinische Wochenschrift*, vol. 128, no. 22, pp. 1231–1236, 2003.

[33] D. P. Basile, D. Donohoe, K. Roethe, and J. L. Osborn, "Renal ischemic injury results in permanent damage to peritubular capillaries and influences long-term function," *American Journal of Physiology—Renal Physiology*, vol. 281, no. 5, pp. F887–F899, 2001.

[34] D. P. Basile, J. L. Friedrich, J. Spahic et al., "Impaired endothelial proliferation and mesenchymal transition contribute to vascular rarefaction following acute kidney injury," *American Journal of Physiology—Renal Physiology*, vol. 300, no. 3, pp. F721–F733, 2011.

[35] S. R. Mulay, A. Holderied, S. V. Kumar, and H.-J. Anders, "Targeting inflammation in so-called acute kidney injury," *Seminars in Nephrology*, vol. 36, no. 1, pp. 17–30, 2016.

[36] T. Yamamoto, T. Tada, S. V. Brodsky et al., "Intravital videomicroscopy of peritubular capillaries in renal ischemia," *American Journal of Physiology—Renal Physiology*, vol. 282, no. 6, pp. F1150–F1155, 2002.

[37] S. V. Brodsky, T. Yamamoto, T. Tada et al., "Endothelial dysfunction in ischemic acute renal failure: rescue by transplanted endothelial cells," *American Journal of Physiology—Renal Physiology*, vol. 282, no. 6, pp. F1140–F1149, 2002.

[38] E. M. Zeisberg, S. E. Potenta, H. Sugimoto, M. Zeisberg, and R. Kalluri, "Fibroblasts in kidney fibrosis emerge via endothelial-to-mesenchymal transition," *Journal of the American Society of Nephrology*, vol. 19, no. 12, pp. 2282–2287, 2008.

[39] E. O'Riordan, N. Mendelev, S. Patschan et al., "Chronic NOS inhibition actuates endothelial-mesenchymal transformation," *American Journal of Physiology—Heart and Circulatory Physiology*, vol. 292, no. 1, pp. H285–H294, 2007.

[40] D. Patschan, K. Loddenkemper, and F. Buttgereit, "Molecular mechanisms of glucocorticoid-induced osteoporosis," *Bone*, vol. 29, no. 6, pp. 498–505, 2001.

[41] D. P. Basile, "The endothelial cell in ischemic acute kidney injury: implications for acute and chronic function," *Kidney International*, vol. 72, no. 2, pp. 151–156, 2007.

[42] C. Basile, "The long-term prognosis of acute kidney injury: acute renal failure as a cause of chronic kidney disease," *Journal of Nephrology*, vol. 21, no. 5, pp. 657–662, 2008.

[43] Y. Goor, G. Peer, A. Iaina et al., "Nitric oxide in ischaemic acute renal failure of streptozotocin diabetic rats," *Diabetologia*, vol. 39, no. 9, pp. 1036–1040, 1996.

[44] H. Shi, D. Patschan, T. Epstein, M. S. Goligorsky, and J. Winaver, "Delayed recovery of renal regional blood flow in diabetic mice subjected to acute ischemic kidney injury," *American Journal of Physiology—Renal Physiology*, vol. 293, no. 5, pp. F1512–F1517, 2007.

[45] B. Betz and B. R. Conway, "Recent advances in animal models of diabetic nephropathy," *Nephron—Experimental Nephrology*, vol. 126, no. 4, pp. 191–195, 2014.

[46] J. Melin, O. Hellberg, L. M. Akyürek, Ö. Källskog, E. Larsson, and B. C. Fellström, "Ischemia causes rapidly progressive nephropathy in the diabetic rat," *Kidney International*, vol. 52, no. 4, pp. 985–991, 1997.

[47] J. K. Kim, "Fat uses a TOLL-road to connect inflammation and diabetes," *Cell Metabolism*, vol. 4, no. 6, pp. 417–419, 2006.

[48] G. Gao, B. Zhang, G. Ramesh et al., "TNF-α mediates increased susceptibility to ischemic AKI in diabetes," *American Journal of Physiology—Renal Physiology*, vol. 304, no. 5, pp. F515–F521, 2013.

[49] J. Peng, X. Li, D. Zhang et al., "Hyperglycemia, p53, and mitochondrial pathway of apoptosis are involved in The susceptibility of diabetic models to ischemic acute kidney injury," *Kidney International*, vol. 87, no. 1, pp. 137–150, 2015.

[50] S. J. Allison, "Acute kidney injury: mechanism of AKI sensitivity in diabetic nephropathy," *Nature Reviews Nephrology*, vol. 10, no. 9, p. 484, 2014.

[51] R. Schmitt and L. G. Cantley, "The impact of aging on kidney repair," *American Journal of Physiology—Renal Physiology*, vol. 294, no. 6, pp. F1265–F1272, 2008.

[52] M. E. Clements, C. J. Chaber, S. R. Ledbetter, and A. Zuk, "Increased cellular senescence and vascular rarefaction exacerbate the progression of kidney fibrosis in aged mice following transient ischemic injury," *PLoS ONE*, vol. 8, no. 8, Article ID e70464, 2013.

[53] M. S. Goligorsky, J. Chen, and S. Patschan, "Stress-induced premature senescence of endothelial cells: a perilous state between recovery and point of no return," *Current Opinion in Hematology*, vol. 16, no. 3, pp. 215–219, 2009.

[54] D. J. Klionsky, K. Abdelmohsen, A. Abe et al., "Guidelines for the use and interpretation of assays for monitoring autophagy (3rd edition)," *Autophagy*, vol. 12, no. 1, pp. 1–222, 2016.

[55] D. Patschan, K. Schwarze, E. Henze, S. Patschan, and G. A. Müller, "Endothelial autophagy and Endothelial-to-Mesenchymal Transition (EndoMT) in eEPC treatment of ischemic AKI," *Journal of Nephrology*, vol. 29, no. 5, pp. 637–644, 2016.

21

Characteristics of the Relationship of Kidney Dysfunction with Cardiovascular Disease in High Risk Patients with Diabetes

Attilio Losito,[1] Loretta Pittavini,[1] Ivano Zampi,[2] and Elena Zampi[3]

[1]*Renal Unit, Santa Maria Della Misericordia Hospital, Perugia, Italy*
[2]*Institute of Geriatrics and Gerontology, Department of Clinical and Experimental Medicine, University of Perugia, Ospedale S. Maria della Misericordia, Perugia, Italy*
[3]*Department of Medicine, Hospital of Pantalla, Todi, Italy*

Correspondence should be addressed to Attilio Losito; atlosito@tin.it

Academic Editor: Franca Anglani

We aimed at comparing the relationship of reduced estimated glomerular filtration rate (eGFR) with cardiovascular disease (CVD) and mortality between high risk patients with and without type 2 diabetes mellitus (T2DM). The cross-sectional study evaluated 16,298 participants (1,627 T2DM) acutely admitted to hospital. The longitudinal study comprised 7,508 patients (673 with diabetes and 6,835 without). eGFR was categorized into 6 stages from >90 to <15 mL/min/1.73 m^2. Kidney dysfunction was defined by an eGFR < 60 mL/min/1.73 m^2. Patients with T2D showed a higher prevalence of CVD (37.9% versus 23.6%; $P < 0.001$) and kidney dysfunction (25% versus 13.2%; $P < 0.001$) than in the general population. An association with CVD was found with eGFR stages from 30 to 90 mL/min/1.73 m^2 in T2D and from <15 to 90 mL/min/1.73 m^2 in general population, in whom the association of eGFR with coronary heart disease was in an inverse relationship ($P < 0.01$ for trend). Survival, in diabetes, was lower ($P = 0.037$) but not associated with kidney dysfunction. *Conclusions.* In a high risk population, patients admitted to hospital, the relationship of kidney function with CVD is different between T2D and the general population. Competing mortality and the presence of other major risk factors in diabetes may be responsible for this difference.

1. Introduction

People with type 2 diabetes mellitus (T2DM) are at high risk for cardiovascular disease (CVD) [1]. The higher prevalence of CVD in diabetes than in the general population was shown many years ago in the Framingham study and has been regularly confirmed by many studies [2, 3]. The prevalence of cardiovascular complications is influenced by several factors, some linked to demography and personal history and some linked to associated conditions [4]. In the general population the reduction in renal function is associated with a parallel increase in CVD risk, with the highest risk being found in patients with lowest renal function [5]. Also in diabetes it has been shown that the reduction of renal function represents a CVD risk factor [6]. Yet, since in people with diabetes several risk factors for CVD operate at the same time, it is not easy to single out the role played by renal dysfunction. Recently, studies have addressed the association of kidney function with the

risk of different CVD in T2DM [7]. In these researches the specific role of renal dysfunction, separated from other diabetes associated risk factors, has not been investigated. Particularly, the magnitude of the association of reduced renal function with CVD has not been compared between T2DM and people without diabetes. Such a comparison might help to single out the specific role of diabetes in the complex relationship between kidney dysfunction and CVD. Patients at high risk, such as patients admitted to hospital, are a population particularly suited for an investigation on the association between kidney dysfunction and CVD, for, in these patients, CVD and renal dysfunction are highly prevalent as it is the associated mortality [8]. Most studies on the relationship between renal dysfunction and CVD in diabetes have been carried out on outpatient population and data on high risk patients are lacking. The present study was undertaken to assess the association of different degrees of reduction in renal function with CVD morbidity in T2DM comparison with a patients without diabetes. The study was carried out in people acutely admitted to hospital.

2. Material and Methods

2.1. Setting. The study was carried out at the Santa Maria Della Misericordia Hospital in Perugia, Italy, that collects all admissions of a catchment population of approximately 200,000 and is the core clinical facility for acute CVD events in the area.

2.2. Study Population and Data Sources. The study is composed by two parts, cross-sectional and survival analysis. The cross-sectional study included 16,298 consecutive Caucasian people, 1,627 with type 2 DM and 14,671 without, admitted to every department of the hospital from 1 January 2007 to 31 December 2007. Patients were identified by an electronic discharge diagnosis based on International Classification of Disease (ICD) codes. People with type 2 DM were singled out by the code 250. Type 1 diabetes people were excluded. CVD examined in the association study were coronary heart disease (CHD), codes 412, 413, and 414, acute myocardial infarction (MI) code 410, ischemic stroke (IS) codes 433, 434, and 436, and hemorrhagic stroke (HS) codes 430–432. Arterial hypertension was recorded by the codes 401–405. Patients with a diagnosis of acute renal failure (ICD-9: 584) and patients treated by dialysis (ICD-9: V45.1) were excluded from the analysis. The longitudinal study included 7,508 consecutive patients (673 with diabetes and 6,835 without) of the above cohort, who lived in the Perugia area. Their survival was periodically checked by electronic searches in the registry office of the personal social security code. The follow-up ended on 31 December 2009. Mortality data were obtained from the registry office of the local health authority.

2.3. Measurements. The value of serum creatinine measured on admission was used for the study. A Shimadzu CL-7300 autoanalyzer was used for all determinations of serum creatinine. The analysis was performed with the automated reaction-rate method of Jaffé (BioSystems SA Costa Brava, 30 08030 Barcelona, Spain). Calibration was performed at the start and at the end of every session with a serum-based calibrator (Biochemistry Calibrator, cod. 18011, BioSystems SA). Quality control was performed with Biochemistry Control Serum Levels I and II (BioSystems SA). The performances of the measurement procedure were as follows: linearity limit: 1768 μmol/L of creatinine; repeatability (within run): mean concentration 150.2 μmol/L, coefficient of variation (CV) 2.9%; mean concentration 468.5 mg/dL, CV 1.3%; reproducibility (run to run): mean concentration of 150.2 μmol/L, CV 3.9%; mean concentration 468 μmol/L, CV 2.9%. Normal values for laboratory were as follows: men, 79.6–114.9 μmol/L; women, 53.1–97.2 μmol/L. Creatinine values were recalibrated to isotope dilution mass spectrometry (IDMS) [9].

For the estimation of GFR, the Chronic Kidney Disease Epidemiology Collaboration (CKD-EPI) formula was used: GFR = 141 ×min(S_{cr}/κ, 1)$^{\alpha}$ × max(S_{cr}/κ, 1)$^{-1.209}$ × 0.993^{Age}× 1.018 [if female] × 1.159 [if black] [10].

2.4. Survival. The outcome was death from any cause. Survival was assessed for people with and without diabetes together and separately.

2.5. Statistical Analysis. Participants were categorized according to eGFR stages (≥90 [reference group], 60–89, 45–59, 30–44, 15–29, and <15 mL/min/1.73 m^2) following the classification recommended by National Kidney Foundation [11].

Participants' characteristics are presented as means with standard deviations or frequencies and percentage. Continuous and categorical variables were compared by ANOVA and chi-square test, respectively. Odds ratio (OR) and 95% confidence interval (CI) of the association of CVD with reduced GFR were estimated by logistic regression after adjusting for age and sex. eGFR was entered into the regression as a categorical variable. Different eGFR cutoffs were used. The first was set at 60 mL/min/1.73 m^2. In the next analysis eGFR was entered as the above described six separated stages with ≥90 mL/min as the reference group. Finally, the analysis was repeated with the cutoff set at 90 mL/min. To calculate the trend of significant ORs across eGFR stages we considered the discrete stages as continuous variables and analyzed by linear regression. CVD was the dependent variable in the logistic regression. CVD was entered either separately for each type of disease or pooled together. Participants with and without diabetes were analyzed separately. In all analysis P values > 0.05 were considered nonsignificant (NS).

Survival was estimated by the Kaplan-Meier procedure. Survival curves of diabetic and nondiabetic patients were compared by log-rank statistics.

Cox proportional hazard regression was used to assess the role of the different variables on survival. Hazard ratios (HRs), adjusted for age and sex, were calculated together with their 95% CIs. In the Cox model, eGFR was entered as a categorical variable in 6 groups using the >90 mL/min as a reference group. The proportional hazard assumption was tested by Schoenfeld's residuals.

Statistical analysis was performed with STATA 11 for Windows (Stata Corp LP, 4905 Lakeway Drive College Station, TX, USA).

3. Results

3.1. Baseline Demographic and Laboratory Characteristics. General characteristics of the study population are presented categorized by the presence of diabetes in Table 1. In people with diabetes, 407 discharge diagnoses of CVD were recorded (25%). In the remaining patients, CVD diagnoses were 1,943 (13.2%). The difference was significant (chi-square 186.7, $P <$ 0.001).

3.2. Renal Function. With respect to renal function the group with T2DM showed a significantly lower eGFR than the group without diabetes (Table 1). When the eGFR was adjusted for age, the mean was 74.6 (CI 73.4–75.9) mL/min/1.73 m^2 in diabetes and 75.4 (CI 75.0–75.8) mL/min/1.73 m^2 in the other patients. An eGFR < 60 mL/min/1.73 m^2

TABLE 1: Characteristics of studied patients.

	Diabetes	No diabetes	P
Number	1,627	14,671	
Sex (men%)	58.20%	50.3	<0.001
Age (years)	65.0 ± 19.8	57.0 ± 22.7	<0.001
Hypertension	509 (31.2%)	2037 (13.9%)	<0.001
MI	25 (1.5%)	102 (0.7%)	<0.001
CHD	211 (12.9%)	920 (6.2%)	<0.001
Angina	4 (0.2%)	40 (0.3%)	N.S.
TIA	27 (1.6%)	144 (0.9%)	0.009
IS	113 (6.9%)	536 (3.6%)	<0.001
HE	27 (1.6%)	201 (1.3%)	N.S.
S. creatinine (μmol/L)	111.4 ± 69.8	97.2 ± 53.0	<0.001
eGFR (mL min/1.73 m^2)	67.8 ± 30.1	76.1 ± 34.3	<0.001
eGFR 60 < mL min/1.73 m^2	617 (37.9%)	3477 (21.3%)	<0.001
eGFR stages	6	6	<0.001
>90 mL/min/1.73 m^2	255 (15.6%)	2956 (20.1%)	0.014
60–89 mL/min/1.73 m^2	734 (45.1%)	8238 (56.1%)	<0.001
45–59 mL/min/1.73 m^2	346 (21.2%)	3477 (23.7)	<0.001
30–44 mL/min/1.73 m^2	170 (10.4%)	2202 (15.0%)	<0.001
15–29 mL/min/1.73 m^2	70 (4.3%)	831 (5.7%)	<0.01
<15 mL/min/1.73 m^2	31 (1.9%)	124 (0.8%)	<0.001

MI: myocardial infarction; CIHD: chronic ischemic heart disease; TIA: transient ischemic attack; IS: ischemic stroke; HE: hemorrhagic stroke.

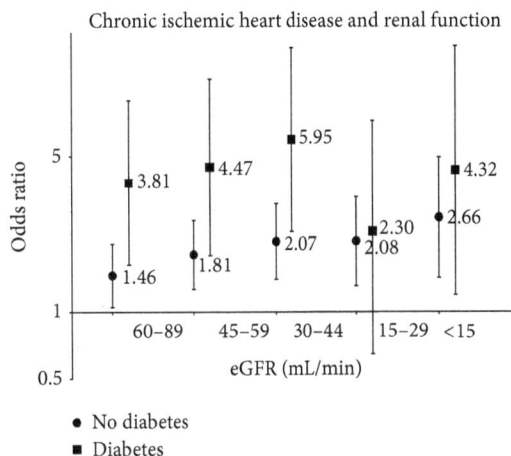

FIGURE 1: Association reduced of eGFR with CVD in patients with diabetes and patients without. The ORs for 5 different stages of eGFR are shown with their 95% CI. In patients without diabetes there is a significant linear increase in ORs for chronic ischemic heart disease as eGFR declines to <15 mL/min/1.73 m^2 ($P < 0.001$). In patients with diabetes the trend is not statistically significant.

was present in 617 (37.9%) people with T2DM and in 3,477 (23.6%) without diabetes (chi-square 168.7, $P < 0.001$).

3.3. Association of Pooled CVD with Kidney Dysfunction. The logistic regression, with pooled CVD as dependent variable, showed in the group without diabetes a significant association with eGFR < 60 mL/min/1.73 m^2 (Table 2). This association was absent in diabetes. When the eGFR cutoff for reduced kidney function was set at 90 mL/min/1.73 m^2, the regression showed an association of eGFR below that value with CVD both in people with diabetes (OR 3.505, CI 1.917–6.408, $P < 0.001$) and in those without (OR 2.173, CI 1.664–2.837, $P < 0.001$).

The analysis of the association between eGFR < 60 mL/min/1.73 m^2 and individual CVD showed a significant association with CHD only in the group without diabetes (OR 1.361, CI 1.171–1.581, $P < 0.001$). In the analysis with eGFR entered as 6 separate stages, different results between diabetes and nondiabetes were found (Table 3). In diabetes, a reduction of eGFR below 30 mL/min/1.73 m^2 was not associated with CVD, while in the group without diabetes a significant association was present across all stages of kidney function reduction.

3.4. Association of Individual CVD with Kidney Dysfunction. The logistic regression was also performed for the individual CVD with large enough numbers to allow a meaningful analysis. This analysis showed that, in patients with CHD, the relationship with reduced eGFR was different between people with diabetes and those without, in whom a significant

trend of increase in ORs from higher to lower eGFR was observed ($r^2 = 0.92$, $P = 0.009$) (Figure 1). This trend was not observed in T2DM. IS was associated only with eGFR 60–89 mL/min/1.73 m^2 in people with diabetes, while, in those without diabetes, the association was present with eGFR from 89 through 30 mL/min/1.73 m^2 (Table 4). Hemorrhagic stroke was not associated with reduced kidney function in either group.

3.5. Survival Analysis. During the follow-up (26.7 $\pm$ 8.9 months), 1,148 deaths were recorded, 120 in the group with diabetes and 1,028 in the group without diabetes. Median survival was 31.2 and 32.9 months in people with and without type 2 DM, respectively (log-rank 4.368, $P = 0.037$).

The Cox analysis, in absence of diabetes, produced a predictive model for mortality including age, sex, and eGFR (Table 5). In this model, patients with an eGFR 15–29 mL/min/1.73 m^2 showed a 43% higher risk of mortality than those with an eGFR > 90 mL/min/1.73 m^2. In presence of diabetes, the reduction of eGFR of any degree was not significantly associated with mortality.

4. Discussion

In our study, people with diabetes show a higher prevalence of reduced renal function and CVD than patients without diabetes. Diabetic patients in our study represent a high risk group. This is shown not only by the significant shorter survival than those without diabetes, but also for their causes for hospitalization. In fact during the 12 months of observation MI was detected in 1.5% of diabetic patients, twice the value of 0.82% per year found in recent epidemiological studies in [12]. The same goes for stroke, present in 6.9% in our cohort, a much higher finding compared to what is generally found in average risk diabetic patients [13].

TABLE 2: Association of pooled CV disease with eGFR < 60 mL/min.

	Diabetes, CV number: 407			No diabetes, CV number: 1,943		
	OR	95% CI	P	OR	95% CI	P
Age	1.033	1.024–1.042	<0.001	1.045	1.041–1.049	<0.001
Sex (M)	1.839	1.414–2.393	<0.001	1.976	1.762–2.217	<0.001
Hypertension	0.778	0.601–1.007	NS	1.654	1.458–1.876	<0.001
eGFR < 60 mL min^{-1} 1.73 m^{-2}	0.872	0.675–1.126	NS	1.29	1.141–1.459	0.013

TABLE 3: Association of grouped CV disease with stages of eGFR.

eGFR stages	Diabetes (407)				No diabetes (1,943)			
	n	OR	95% CI	P	n	OR	95% CI	P
≥90 mL/min/1.73 m^2	18	—	—	—	94	—	—	—
60–89 mL/min/1.73 m^2	211	3,379	1.841–6.201	<0.001	1024	1,908	1.471–2.475	<0.001
45–59 mL/min/1.73 m^2	105	3,105	1.604–6.014	<0.001	512	2,203	1.659–2.921	<0.001
30–44 mL/min/1.73 m^2	57	3,316	1.633–6.737	<0.001	213	2,027	1.475–2.781	<0.001
15–29 mL/min/1.73 m^2	10	1,226	0.481–3.123	NS	75	1,850	1.251–2.733	0.002
<15 mL/min/1.73 m^2	6	1,595	0.509–4.991	NS	25	2,116	1.219–3.672	0.008

*Obtained by logistic regression with eGFR ≥ 90 mL/min/1.73 m^2 as reference group.

TABLE 4: Association between stages of eGFR and ischemic stroke.

eGFR stages	Diabetes, IS number: 113			No diabetes, IS number: 536		
	OR	95% CI	P	OR	95% CI	P
60–89 mL/min/1.73 m^2	3.539	1.192–10.562	0.023	3.209	1.883–5.465	<0.001
45–59 mL/min/1.73 m^2	2.831	0.876–9.154	NS	3.44	1.956–6.052	<0.001
30–44 mL/min/1.73 m^2	2.873	0.825–1.001	NS	2.369	1.267–4.431	0.007
15–29 mL/min/1.73 m^2	0.96	0.160–5.762	NS	0.947	0.373–2.355	NS
<15 mL/min/1.73 m^2	°			1.860	0.599–5.771	NS

°Numbers too small for the analysis.

TABLE 5: HRs of AC mortality in different stages of reduction of eGFR*.

eGFR (mL/min/1.73 m^2)	Diabetes, patients number: 673			No diabetes, patients number: 6,835		
	HR	95% CI	P	HR		P
60–89	0.487	0.231–1.0281	NS	0.433	0.341–0.550	<0.001
45–59	0.580	0.266–1.265	NS	0.471	0.361–0.614	<0.001
30–44	1.157	0.524–2.552	NS	0.759	0.569–1.010	NS
15–29	0.849	0.318–2.269	NS	1.430	1.036–1.973	0.029
<15	2.665	0.965–7.360	NS	1.236	0.699–2.185	NS
Age	1.074	1.051–1.099	<0.001	1.071	1.065–1.077	<0.001
Sex (male)	0.810	0.551–1.190	NS	1.386	1.221–1.573	<0.001

*Obtained from Cox regression analysis.

We have found that diabetic patients present a different relationship of CVD with reduced renal function. In fact, using eGFR < 60 mL min^{-1} 1.73 m^{-2} as a cutoff, a commonly used index for reduced kidney function [14], in diabetes we did not find the association between kidney dysfunction and CVD shown in individuals without diabetes. Furthermore, in the analysis for individual CVD in patients without diabetes, ORs of the association with CHD increase progressively with the reduction of eGFR. In T2DM this trend was absent.

There were differences also in the survival analysis. This showed, in absence of diabetes, an association between certain degrees of reduction of kidney function and mortality. In diabetes the mortality was higher than in the group without T2 DM. Furthermore, at variance with this group, in diabetes no relationship of mortality with reduced eGFR was found.

These findings are new and broaden our knowledge on the association between kidney function and CVD complications in diabetes. Our results suggest that the risk factors present only in diabetic patients play a more important role than kidney dysfunction in the association. with CVD. Yet it must be underlined that the patients we studied represent a high risk group, as shown by the high mortality rate. This high risk state may explain the higher prevalence of reduced kidney function we have found, compared with that of previous Italian studies, dealing mostly with outpatients populations. While in US and UK, among adults with a diagnosis of diabetes, CKD prevalence was ~40% [14, 15], in Italy, a survey on a population of patients attending diabetes clinics reported a prevalence of ~19% [16]. We found that ~38% of people with T2DM and 21.3% of patients without diabetes, admitted to hospital, had an eGFR < 60 mL/min/1.73 m^2.

Also the prevalence of CVD in diabetes was much higher than in the group without diabetes: 25% versus 13.2%. This finding is close to the 23.2% reported in the recent Italian RIACE study, which was not limited to high risk diabetic patients [17]. In our study, to assess kidney function, we used only eGFR. This represents a limitation. In fact, in most of the above studies, eGFR was associated with albuminuria measurement. This increases the probability of detecting a renal dysfunction. The lack of data on albuminuria in our study may explain, at least in part, the difference in results with previous reports.

In our cohort, in T2DM, also the relationship between reduced kidney function and CVD was different from the group without diabetes. The results obtained with pooled CVD were confirmed in the analysis of individual CVD: IS and CHD. Particularly interesting are the findings in CHD, where the significant increase in the ORs of the association with different stages of reduction in eGFR was not observed in diabetes. Furthermore, in T2D, the association with reduced eGFR was much stronger in CHD than in IS. In the general population the association of kidney dysfunction with IS is an inconstant finding [18, 19]. In the present study in T2DM, eGFR < 60 mL/min was not associated with IS. In diabetes, a weaker relation of reduced eGFR to cerebrovascular disease than in the general population was shown previously in an Italian study [16]. This different relationship with kidney dysfunction between CHD and IS may be explained by the difference in involved vascular beds. In fact a maladaptive arterial remodeling has been suggested, consequence of kidney dysfunction, acting in coronary arteries and not at carotid artery level [18]. Previous reports have proposed that nonalbuminuric renal impairment, as a manifestation of prevailing renal macrovascular involvement, would be more frequently associated with coronary atherosclerosis or all-cause mortality [20, 21].

People with diabetes, in our cohort, represent a high risk sample. Therefore the difference in CVD association with the rest of population may be also explained by a competing mortality that, preceding the study, might have selected examined patients. The higher mortality, we found in diabetes, is in keeping with this hypothesis.

On the whole, our study suggests that, in a high risk population, the role of kidney dysfunction as a risk factor for CVD is different between diabetic and nondiabetic patients. The risk factors for CVD present only in diabetes may be responsible for this difference [22, 23]. Their presence may act either synergically or competitively with kidney function, altering its association with CVD.

4.1. Limitations. Although our results are strengthened by centralized laboratory measurements and homogeneous diagnostic criteria they are applicable only to high risk patients and not to the ordinary outpatients with diabetes. There is a large difference in the number of patients with and without diabetes, although it reflects the actual proportion of admitted patients. Age and sex differences between the two groups were taken into account performing the analysis after adjustment for these variables.

Furthermore there are limitations in the measurements and in the risk factors analyzed. The single value of serum creatinine is a limitation of our study since it may introduce bias in the assessment of the association of CVD with reduced kidney dysfunction [7]. Among cardiovascular risk factors, we analyzed only hypertension as a discrete variable. The lack of blood pressure values and pharmacological treatment represent another limitation of our study.

5. Conclusions

In summary, our study shows that in high risk patients with diabetes the reduction of eGFR is highly prevalent but the relationship of kidney dysfunction with CVD is different from that observed in people without diabetes.

References

[1] S. M. Grundy, I. J. Benjamin, G. L. Burke et al., "Diabetes and cardiovascular disease: a statement for healthcare professionals from the american heart association," *Circulation*, vol. 100, no. 10, pp. 1134–1146, 1999.

[2] W. B. Kannel and D. L. McGee, "Diabetes and glucose tolerance as risk factors for cardiovascular disease: the Framingham study," *Diabetes Care*, vol. 2, no. 2, pp. 120–126, 1979.

[3] C. S. Fox, S. Coady, P. D. Sorlie et al., "Increasing cardiovascular disease burden due to diabetes mellitus: The Framingham Heart Study," *Circulation*, vol. 115, no. 12, pp. 1544–1550, 2007.

[4] A. Becker, G. Bos, F. De Vegt et al., "Cardiovascular events in type 2 diabetes: comparison with nondiabetic individuals without and with prior cardiovascular disease: 10-Year follow-up of the Hoorn study," *European Heart Journal*, vol. 24, no. 15, pp. 1406–1413, 2003.

[5] A. S. Go, G. M. Chertow, D. Fan, C. E. McCulloch, and C.-Y. Hsu, "Chronic kidney disease and the risks of death, cardiovascular events, and hospitalization," *New England Journal of Medicine*, vol. 351, no. 13, pp. 1296–1370, 2004.

[6] T. Ninomiya, V. Perkovic, B. E. de Galan et al., "Albuminuria and kidney function independently predict cardiovascular and renal outcomes in diabetes," *Journal of the American Society of Nephrology*, vol. 20, no. 8, pp. 1813–1821, 2009.

[7] Y. Wang, P. T. Katzmarzyk, R. Horswell, W. Zhao, J. Johnson, and G. Hu, "Kidney function and the risk of cardiovascular disease in patients with type 2 diabetes," *Kidney International*, vol. 85, no. 5, pp. 1192–1199, 2014.

[8] A. Losito, L. Pittavini, C. Ferri, and L. De Angelis, "Kidney function and mortality in different cardiovascular diseases: relationship with age, sex, diabetes and hypertension," *Journal of Nephrology*, vol. 24, no. 3, pp. 322–328, 2011.

[9] A. Carobene, C. Ferrero, F. Ceriotti et al., "Creatinine measurement proficiency testing: assignment of matrix-adjusted ID GC-MS target values," *Clinical Chemistry*, vol. 43, no. 8, pp. 1342–1347, 1997.

[10] A. S. Levey, L. A. Stevens, C. H. Schmid et al., "A new equation to estimate glomerular filtration rate," *Annals of Internal Medicine*, vol. 150, no. 9, pp. 604–612, 2009.

[11] A. S. Levey, J. Coresh, E. Balk et al., "Foundation practice guidelines for chronic kidney disease: evaluation, classification, and stratification," *Annals of Internal Medicine*, vol. 139, no. 2, pp. 137–147, 2003.

[12] D. C. Burgess, D. Hunt, L. Li et al., "Incidence and predictors of silent myocardial infarction in type 2 diabetes and the effect of fenofibrate: an analysis from the Fenofibrate Intervention and Event Lowering in Diabetes (FIELD) study," *European Heart Journal*, vol. 31, no. 1, pp. 92–99, 2010.

[13] V. Kothari, R. J. Stevens, A. I. Adler et al., "UKPDS 60: risk of stroke in type 2 diabetes estimated by the UK prospective diabetes study risk engine," *Stroke*, vol. 33, no. 7, pp. 1776–1781, 2002.

[14] C. J. Hill, C. R. Cardwell, C. C. Patterson et al., "Chronic kidney disease and diabetes in the National Health Service: a cross-sectional survey of the UK National Diabetes Audit," *Diabetic Medicine*, vol. 31, no. 4, pp. 448–454, 2014.

[15] L. C. Plantinga, D. C. Crews, J. Coresh et al., "Prevalence of chronic kidney disease in US adults with undiagnosed diabetes or prediabetes," *Clinical Journal of the American Society of Nephrology*, vol. 5, no. 4, pp. 673–682, 2010.

[16] G. Pugliese, A. Solini, E. Bonora et al., "Distribution of cardiovascular disease and retinopathy in patients with type 2 diabetes according to different classification systems for chronic kidney disease: a cross-sectional analysis of the renal insufficiency and cardiovascular events (RIACE) Italian multicenter study," *Cardiovascular Diabetology*, vol. 13, article 59, 2014.

[17] A. Solini, G. Penno, E. Bonora et al., "Renal Insufficiency And Cardiovascular Events (RIACE) Study Group: diverging association of reduced glomerular filtration rate and albuminuria with coronary and noncoronary events in patients with type 2 diabetes: the renal insufficiency and cardiovascular events (RIACE) Italian multicentre study," *Diabetes Care*, vol. 35, no. 1, pp. 143–149, 2012.

[18] A. Losito, L. Pittavini, C. Ferri, and L. De Angelis, "Reduced kidney function and outcome in acute ischaemic stroke: relationship to arterial hypertension and diabetes," *Nephrology Dialysis Transplantation*, vol. 27, no. 3, pp. 1054–1058, 2012.

[19] M. J. Bos, P. J. Koudstaal, A. Hofman, and M. M. B. Breteler, "Decreased glomerular filtration rate is a risk factor for hemorrhagic but not for ischemic stroke: The Rotterdam Study," *Stroke*, vol. 38, no. 12, pp. 3127–3132, 2007.

[20] R. J. MacIsaac, S. Panagiotopoulos, K. J. McNeil et al., "Is non-albuminuric renal insufficiency in type 2 diabetes related to an increase in intrarenal vascular disease?" *Diabetes Care*, vol. 29, no. 7, pp. 1560–1566, 2006.

[21] W. Y. So, A. P. Kong, R. C. Ma et al., "Glomerular filtration rate, cardiorenal end points, and all-cause mortality in type 2 diabetic patients," *Diabetes Care*, vol. 29, no. 9, pp. 2046–2052, 2006.

[22] B. B. Dokken, "The pathophysiology of cardiovascular disease and diabetes: beyond blood pressure and lipids," *Diabetes Spectrum*, vol. 21, no. 3, pp. 160–165, 2008.

[23] G. Hu, P. Jousilahti, and J. Tuomilehto, "Joint effects of history of hypertension at baseline and type 2 diabetes at baseline and during follow-up on the risk of coronary heart disease," *European Heart Journal*, vol. 28, no. 24, pp. 3059–3066, 2007.

22

Acute Kidney Injury in Hematopoietic Stem Cell Transplantation

Vinod Krishnappa,[1] **Mohit Gupta,**[2] **Gurusidda Manu,**[3] **Shivani Kwatra,**[1] **Osei-Tutu Owusu,**[4] **and Rupesh Raina**[5]

[1]*Akron Nephrology Associates/Akron General Cleveland Clinic, Akron, OH, USA*
[2]*Department of Internal Medicine, Akron General Cleveland Clinic, Akron, OH, USA*
[3]*Onco-Hospitalist, Beth Israel Deaconness Medical Center, Boston, MA, USA*
[4]*Department Hematology/Medical Oncology, Akron General Cleveland Clinic, Akron, OH, USA*
[5]*Department of Nephrology/Internal Medicine, Akron General Cleveland Clinic, Akron, OH, USA*

Correspondence should be addressed to Rupesh Raina; rraina@chmca.org

Academic Editor: Kazunari Kaneko

Hematopoietic stem cell transplantation (HSCT) is a highly effective treatment strategy for lymphoproliferative disorders and bone marrow failure states including aplastic anemia and thalassemia. However, its use has been limited by the increased treatment related complications, including acute kidney injury (AKI) with an incidence ranging from 20% to 73%. AKI after HSCT has been associated with an increased risk of mortality. The incidence of AKI reported in recipients of myeloablative allogeneic transplant is considerably higher in comparison to other subclasses mainly due to use of cyclosporine and development of graft-versus-host disease (GVHD) in allogeneic groups. Acute GVHD is by itself a major independent risk factor for the development of AKI in HSCT recipients. The other major risk factors are sepsis, nephrotoxic medications (amphotericin B, acyclovir, aminoglycosides, and cyclosporine), hepatic sinusoidal obstruction syndrome (SOS), thrombotic microangiopathy (TMA), marrow infusion toxicity, and tumor lysis syndrome. The mainstay of management of AKI in these patients is avoidance of risk factors contributing to AKI, including use of reduced intensity-conditioning regimen, close monitoring of nephrotoxic medications, and use of alternative antifungals for prophylaxis against infection. Also, early identification and effective management of sepsis, tumor lysis syndrome, marrow infusion toxicity, and hepatic SOS help in reducing the incidence of AKI in HSCT recipients.

1. Introduction

Hematopoietic stem cell transplantation (HSCT) has emerged as one of the most popular therapies for management of neoplastic disorders primarily lymphoproliferative disorders and bone marrow failure states including aplastic anemia and thalassemias [1, 2]. Every year, a number of transplants are conducted across the globe. However, the use of HSCT has been limited by an increased number of side effects noticed after the procedure is done. In this review, we will be discussing one of the major complications related to HSCT, namely, acute kidney injury (AKI).

Several different studies comparing the incidence of AKI amongst various HSCT modalities have been reported. Most patients undergoing HSCT develop AKI within the course of 1 year. However, the definition of AKI used has varied significantly amongst studies. Hence, the exact incidence of AKI is difficult to estimate. Currently, the incidence of AKI has been reported anywhere from 20% to 73% [3]. However, some studies have reported statistics as high as 92% [4].

2. Types of HSCT

Various types of HSCT are currently being used in today's era. These include myeloablative allogeneic, nonmyeloablative allogeneic, and autologous HSCT.

Myeloablative allogeneic HSCT involves use of a conditioning regimen composed of chemotherapy and radiation prior to the infusion of human leucocyte antigen matched donor cells [1, 5]. Conditioning regimens used in myeloablative HSCT involve cyclophosphamide, busulfan, cytarabine, and total body irradiation. Variations in the conditioning regimen have been reported amongst different studies especially depending on the malignancy [6, 7].

Nonmyeloablative allogeneic HSCT involves the use of a reduced intensity-conditioning regimen prior to the infusion of the donor cells. This modality of HSCT is better suited for patients with significant comorbidities [1]. Conditioning regimens involved in nonmyeloablative HSCT include fludarabine, busulfan, and cyclosporine [6, 8].

Autologous HSCT involves extraction of patient's own stem cells prior to administration of chemotherapy and radiation followed by infusion of the same stem cells after processing [3].

3. Prophylaxis against Graft-versus-Host Disease and Infections

All allogeneic transplant recipients receive prophylaxis against graft-versus-host-disease (GVHD). Regimens for prophylaxis include cyclosporine A (CsA), mycophenolate mofetil (MMF), tacrolimus (FK), or even short-term methotrexate (MTX) [9, 10]. However, the use of the above regimens for prophylaxis against GVHD is limited to allogeneic transplants. Furthermore, most of the patients discussed in various studies received prophylaxis against infections with acyclovir and azoles [11].

4. Treatment of Graft-versus-Host Disease

GVHD can be classified into acute and chronic categories based on duration of onset after HSCT and clinical findings. Acute GVHD has great significance as it can independently serve as a risk factor for the development of AKI in HSCT recipients [12]. The contribution of GVHD to AKI can be twofold. It could either be related to cytokine-mediated inflammation affecting the tubules/glomeruli or indirectly related to the use of medications such as cyclosporine, which by itself can predispose to nephrotoxicity. Furthermore, the presence of GVHD promotes viral reactivation such as cytomegalovirus (CMV), which can also contribute to AKI. The use of prednisolone in GVHD also predisposes to AKI [12]. Medical treatment options for GVHD include prednisone, antithymocyte globulin, sirolimus, and mycophenolate mofetil [3].

5. Definitions and Classification Systems of AKI Used across Various Studies

The incidence of AKI reported has varied significantly amongst various studies primarily due to the variations in definitions used for AKI (Table 1). In a recent study performed by Hingorani et al. in 2015, AKI was defined as a rise in serum creatinine of 0.3 mg/dL within 48 hours and/or 1.5 times the previous creatinine within 7 days [9]. In a study performed by Kang et al. in 2012, AKI following HSCT was

defined as a rise in serum creatinine to 2-fold its initial value. Furthermore, severe AKI was defined as a rise in serum creatinine to the extent that it requires dialysis therapy [13]. In other studies performed by Yu et al. in 2010 and Caliskan et al. in 2006, AKI was graded on the basis of glomerular filtration rate (GFR) and requirement of dialysis, with grade 0 being a decrease in GFR to less than 25% of base value. Grade 1 was a fall of 25% or more in baseline GFR value and rise in serum creatinine less than 2-fold; grade 2 was a 2-fold or more increase in serum creatinine without requiring dialysis. Grade 3 on the other hand required dialysis with rise in serum creatinine to 2-fold or more [7, 14]. Prior to the above studies, analysis conducted by Zhou et al. and Lopes et al. defined AKI as doubling of serum creatinine in the first 100 days after transplantation [15, 16].

Acute Dialysis Quality Initiative (ADQI) group proposed AKI classification by the RIFLE criteria with R relating to risk, I to injury, F to failure, L to loss of kidney function, and E to end stage kidney disease. Three of these categories relate to severity, namely, risk, injury, and failure. Two of them relate to outcome, namely, loss and end stage kidney disease. AKI-R (risk) was defined as an increase in serum creatinine to 1.5 times base value or fall in GFR > 25% or decrease in urinary output to less than 0.5 mL/kg/h for 6 hrs. AKI-I (Injury) was defined as creatinine rise to 2 times the base value or fall in GFR > 50% or decrease in urine output to less than 0.5 mL/kg/h for 12 hrs. Furthermore, AKI-F (failure) was defined as rise in creatinine to 3 times the base value or fall in GFR by 75% or serum creatinine > 4 mg/dL or decrease in urine output to less than 0.3 mL/kg/h for 24 hrs or anuria for 12 hrs. Loss of renal functions was defined as total loss of kidney function requiring dialysis for >4 weeks and end stage renal disease was defined as requirement of dialysis for >3 months [17]. In 2007, the AKI network came out with a new staging system for AKI based on the previous RIFLE classification. It classified Stage 1 as rise in serum creatinine to >0.3 mg/dL or 1.5–2 times baseline value or fall in urine output to <0.5 mL/kg/h for >6 hrs, Stage 2 as rise in serum creatinine 2-3 times baseline value or fall in urine output to <0.5 mL/kg/h for >12 hrs, and Stage 3 as increase in serum creatinine > 3 times baseline value or fall in urine output to <0.3 mL/kg/h for 24 hrs or anuria for 12 hrs [18]. A comparative assessment study done by Ando et al. reflected that the AKI network criteria had lesser sensitivity in comparison to the RIFLE criteria to detect AKI in stem cell transplantation (SCT) patients especially in those with lower grades of AKI [6].

6. Incidence of AKI

Now that we have discussed the above variation in definitions of AKI, we will discuss the incidence of AKI reported across various studies for HSCT recipients. We will also analyze key differences in the incidence and risk factors of AKI amongst myeloablative allogeneic, nonmyeloablative allogeneic, and autologous transplant recipients (Table 2).

6.1. Myeloablative Allogeneic Transplant Recipients. The incidence of AKI reported in this subclass of transplant recipients

TABLE 1: Definitions and classification systems used for acute kidney injury.

Study/criteria	Classification	Definition
Hingorani et al. (2015)	AKI	Rise in Sr Cr of 0.3 mg/dL in <48 hrs and/or 1.5 times the previous level in <7 days
Kang et al. (2012)	AKI	Rise in Sr Cr to twice its initial value
	Severe AKI	Rise in Sr Cr to the level that requires dialysis
Yu et al. (2010) Caliskan et al. (2006)	Grade 0	Fall in GFR < 25% of the baseline value
	Grade 1	Fall in baseline GFR 25% or more and rise in Sr Cr < 2-fold
	Grade 2	More than or equal to 2-fold increase in Sr Cr without requiring dialysis
	Grade 3	More than or equal to 2-fold increase in Sr Cr requiring dialysis
Zhou et al. (2009) Lopes et al. (2006)	AKI	Doubling of Sr Cr in the first 100 days after transplantation
AKI network criteria (2007)	Stage 1	Rise in Sr Cr to >0.3 mg/dL or 1.5–2 times baseline value or fall in urine output to <0.5 mL/kg/h for >6 hrs
	Stage 2	Rise in Sr Cr 2-3 times baseline value or fall in urine output to <0.5 mL/kg/h for >12 hrs
	Stage 3	Rise in Sr Cr > 3 times baseline value or fall in urine output to <0.3 mL/kg/h for 24 hrs or anuria for 12 hrs
RIFLE criteria (2004) by ADQI group	AKI-R (risk)	Rise in Sr Cr 1.5 times baseline value or fall in GFR > 25% or fall in urine output to <0.5 mL/kg/h for 6 hrs
	AKI-I (injury)	Rise in Sr Cr 2 times the baseline value or fall in GFR > 50% or fall in urine output to <0.5 mL/kg/h for 12 hrs
	AKI-F (failure)	Rise in Sr Cr 3 times the baseline value or fall in GFR by 75% or Sr Cr > 4 mg/dL or fall in urine output to less than 0.3 mL/kg/h for 24 hrs or anuria for 12 hrs
	Persistent ARF	Total loss of kidney functions requiring dialysis > 4 weeks
	End stage renal disease	Requirement of dialysis for >3 months

AKI: acute kidney injury, Sr: serum, Cr: creatinine, GFR: glomerular filtration rate, ARF: acute renal failure, and ADQI: acute dialysis quality initiative.

TABLE 2: Incidence and risk factors for different types of HSCT.

Type of transplant	Incidence range	Risk factors
Myeloablative allogeneic transplantation	18.8–66%	Female sex, hypertension, sepsis, hepatic SOS, GVHD, amphotericin B
Nonmyeloablative allogeneic transplantation	29–53.6%	Diabetes mellitus, >3 prior lines of chemotherapy, acute GVHD, methotrexate use against GVHD prophylaxis
Myeloablative autologous transplantation	12–52%	Sepsis, amphotericin B toxicity, aminoglycoside (for sepsis) toxicity

HSCT: hematopoietic stem cell transplantation; Hepatic SOS: sinusoidal obstruction syndrome; GVHD: graft-versus-host disease.

lymphoblastic leukemia (ALL), and myelodysplastic syndrome (MDS) as 33% while using a conditioning regimen composed of busulfan and cyclophosphamide [19]. In a five-year study conducted by Kang et al. for patients receiving myeloablative allogeneic HSCT, incidence of AKI was reported at 18.8% [13]. However, some studies such as the one by Ando et al. have reported 66% incidence of AKI in patients receiving myeloablative allogeneic transplants [6]. Further more, a comparative study of AKI incidence between autologous and allogeneic transplant recipients revealed an incidence of 52% in the myeloablative autologous group versus 91% in the myeloablative allogeneic group [14].

Risk factors noted for the development of AKI in this subgroup include female sex, hypertension, sepsis, development of hepatic sinusoidal obstruction syndrome (SOS), GVHD, and use of amphotericin B. The conditioning regimen itself poses as a separate risk factor for the development of AKI [14, 19].

6.2. Nonmyeloablative Allogeneic Transplant Recipients. The incidence of AKI in this subclass is significantly lower in comparison to patients receiving myeloablative allogeneic transplants. In a multicenter retrospective study done by Liu et al. the incidence of AKI reported amongst patients

is considerably higher in comparison to other subclasses such as nonmyeloablative allogeneic or autologous transplant recipients. Studies conducted by Ataei et al. in 2015 reported an incidence of AKI amongst myeloablative allogeneic recipients having acute myeloid leukemia (AML), acute receiving nonmyeloablative allogeneic stem cell transplantation (NMA-SCT) was reported as 29% with the majority of them developing AKI grade 1. The mortality rate was also found to significantly increase from AKI grade 1 (54.5%) to AKI grade 3 (71.4%) [5]. In a single center study conducted by Piñana et al. in Barcelona, 188 patients underwent reduced intensity-conditioning allogeneic HSCT and were analyzed for the incidence and risk factors contributing towards AKI. The incidence was reported at 52% with median time to development of AKI at 31 days. The majority of patients developed AKI grade 1 in comparison to grades 2-3 [8]. In a retrospective study conducted by Lopes et al. in Lisbon, Portugal, analyzing 82 patients receiving reduced intensity-conditioning allogeneic HSCT, the incidence of AKI by RIFLE criteria was reported up to 53.6% out of which 4.8% required dialysis [20].

Risk factors associated with the development of AKI in a study by Piñana et al. were diabetes mellitus, having received >3 prior lines of chemotherapy and use of MTX for prophylaxis against GVHD. The development of acute GVHD served as a risk factor only after 100 days had elapsed from the time of HSCT. Furthermore, no correlation was found between cyclosporine levels and the development of acute renal failure (ARF) [8]. Interestingly enough, diabetes mellitus plays a much bigger role in the development of ARF in these patients especially when combined with cyclosporine. Diabetic nephropathy by itself is one of the prime causes of end stage renal disease (ESRD). Furthermore, cyclosporine when used in conjunction can impair glucose metabolism by reducing insulin secretion and promoting resistance in the tissues to the peripheral effects of insulin [21]. Hence, cyclosporine use in diabetic patients, along with steroids which are used most often in this setting, has a synergistic effect on kidney injury especially within the first 100 days after HSCT [8]. On the contrary, another study showed that there was no association between diabetes mellitus and development of renal failure, and necessity of mechanical ventilation in NMA-SCT patients has been shown to be a strong risk factor for AKI development [22].

6.3. Myeloablative Autologous Transplant Recipients. The incidence of AKI in patients receiving myeloablative autologous transplants has ranged from 12% to as high as 52% [14, 16]. In a prospective study conducted by Caliskan et al. 47 patients undergoing HSCT were analyzed for the development of AKI. Comparison between autologous and allogeneic transplant recipients revealed an incidence of 52% in the autologous group versus 91% in the allogeneic group. Moreover, higher grades of AKI were reported in the allogeneic group compared to the autologous group. Risk factors associated with the development of AKI in the autologous group were sepsis, amphotericin B, and aminoglycoside nephrotoxicity. Sepsis and use of antibiotics and antifungals for sepsis contributed to 85% of renal dysfunction in the autologous study group. Cyclosporine and development of GVHD were major contributing factors to the development of AKI in the allogeneic group but neither of these was seen in the autologous group [14].

7. Pathophysiology of Acute Kidney Injury in HSCT

Multiple factors have been implicated in the causation of AKI after HSCT, which are discussed in detail including management options and have been summarized in Table 3.

7.1. Sepsis and Acute Kidney Injury. The contribution of sepsis to the development of AKI in patients receiving HSCT is manifold but studies have shown mixed results. Sepsis is more likely to occur in patients receiving HSCT generally due to immunosuppression owing to the prior malignancy or immunosuppressive therapy. The inflammatory response in sepsis leads to vasodilatation of the arterioles leading to decrease in effective intravascular volume being delivered to the kidneys [3]. This is more along the lines of a prerenal type of AKI. Furthermore, inflammatory mediators such as cytokines released during the initial phase are capable of damaging the renal tubules directly that results in a more renal type of AKI picture [23]. In a study by Merouani et al., sepsis and resulting hypotension accounted for increased AKI and higher mortality rates. Besides, hypotension was more prevalent in subjects with higher grades of renal failure [24]. On the contrary, in a study by Caliskan et al., hypotension failed to show positive correlation in the causation of AKI in autologous HSCT, although sepsis has been strongly implicated as a major factor in the development of AKI and higher mortality rates [14]. Another study found no association between sepsis and AKI but venoocclusive disease (VOC) and age have been shown to be risk factors for AKI in allogeneic HSCT [25]. Sepsis, use of nephrotoxic antibiotics for sepsis and hypotension may all have a synergistic effect resulting in AKI [3, 14].

7.2. Nephrotoxic Medications and Acute Kidney Injury. Several medications such as antifungals and antibiotics used in the treatment of sepsis, antivirals, and immunosuppressants, which are toxic to the kidney, may pose a direct risk and contribute significantly to the development of AKI.

Amphotericin B is one of the most commonly implicated agents for the development of AKI in HSCT recipients. It is capable of inducing renal vasoconstriction, hence hypoperfusion of the kidney resulting in tubular epithelium damage [3]. Certain preparations such as lipid based (liposomal) amphotericin have been studied and found to have a lower risk of kidney injury compared to conventional amphotericin [26, 27]. Nevertheless, a study by Hingorani et al. showed significantly increased risk of AKI associated with both conventional and liposomal amphotericin preparations and suggested to limit its use only for documented fungal infections or in situations where there has been usage of other antifungals for prophylaxis [28]. Alternately, newer antifungal drugs such as itraconazole, fluconazole, and voriconazole that are equally effective and have a better side effect profile should be substituted wherever possible [28, 29]. Recently, a study by Rocha et al. analyzed the relationship between urinary levels of neutrophil gelatinase-associated lipocalin (UNGAL) and amphotericin induced AKI. UNGAL is a potential early biomarker for drug induced AKI and found

TABLE 3: Pathophysiology and management of AKI in HSCT.

Etiology	Pathophysiology	Management/potential therapeutic options
Sepsis	Vasodilatation and reduced renal blood flow resulting in ischemia and direct renal tubular insult by inflammatory cytokines	Treatment of sepsis with appropriate medication
Nephrotoxic medication		
Amphotericin B	Vasoconstriction of renal vasculature resulting in hypoperfusion and renal tubular epithelial damage	Measurement of urinary UNGAL levels may serve as early biomarker of AKI. Restricting amphotericin use only for documented fungal infections. Use of antifungals with minimal nephrotoxicity such as itraconazole, fluconazole, and voriconazole.
Acyclovir	Formation of crystals in renal tubules and collecting ducts resulting in obstruction especially with IV administration in high doses	Demonstration of birefringent needle shaped crystals in urinary sediment under polarizing microscopy helps in diagnosis. Slower IV administration, hydration, and renal dose adjustments are recommended
Aminoglycosides	Intracellular accumulation in proximal tubules and change in cellular permeability	Measurement of alanine aminopeptidase and N-acetyl-beta-D glucosaminidase in urine may serve as an early biomarker of nephrotoxicity. Reduction in dosage frequency is the mainstay of management
Cyclosporine A	Renal vasoconstriction secondary to renin-angiotensin system activation. Increased production of VEGF. Downregulation of renal Klotho and increased oxidative stress causing renal endothelial damage. Thrombotic microangiopathy. Impaired glucose metabolism	Potential treatment options are aliskiren, valsartan, and switching to alternative immunosuppressant such as sirolimus
Hepatic SOS	Damage to hepatic sinusoidal endothelial cells by chemotherapeutic agents and subendothelial deposition of fibrin and other blood products resulting in venular obstruction. Glutathione depletion due to chemotherapeutic drug detoxification by glutathione pathway resulting in hepatocellular necrosis and fibrosis	Circulating endothelial cells (CECs) and plasminogen activator inhibitor-1 are potential biomarkers. Modification of conditioning regimens and use of defibrotide
Thrombotic microangiopathy	Renal endothelial injury by cytokines released in GVHD. Decreased levels of VEGF. Exposure to calcineurin inhibitors, TBI, and infections	Measurement of serum NETs level may serve as early biomarker for TMA. Continuing acute GVHD treatment may be of benefit. Plasma exchange has a limited role. Eculizumab may be a potential treatment option
Marrow infusion toxicity	Exposure to cryoprecipitants causes hemolysis and heme precipitation in distal renal tubules resulting in tubular obstruction	Alkalinization of urine and mannitol induced diuresis
Tumor lysis syndrome	Lysis of tumor cells releasing intracellular products into circulation resulting in hyperuricemia, hyperphosphatemia, hyperkalemia, and hypocalcemia. Precipitation of calcium phosphate and urate crystals causes damage to renal tubules. Vasoconstriction of renal arterioles and exposure to inflammatory cytokines causes injury to renal tubules	Mainstay of management involves IV hydration, rasburicase, and allopurinol. Low phosphate diet and phosphate binders for hyperphosphatemia. Medical management of hyperkalemia and renal replacement therapy in resistant cases and severe AKI

TABLE 3: Continued.

Etiology	Pathophysiology	Management/potential therapeutic options
Infections		
BK virus	Immunosuppression reactivates dormant virus in urinary tract causing renal tubular injury and hemorrhagic cystitis	Reducing immunosuppression is the mainstay of treatment. Supportive care for cystitis.
Adenovirus	Tubulointerstitial nephritis and cystitis	Supportive care. Intravesical cidofivir is potential treatment option for cystitis

UNGAL: urinary neutrophil gelatinase-associated lipocalin; AKI: acute kidney injury; IV: intravenous; GVHD: graft-versus-host disease; VEGF: vascular endothelial growth factor; TBI: total body irradiation; TMA: thrombotic microangiopathy; SOS: sinusoidal obstruction syndrome; NETs: neutrophil extracellular traps.

in higher levels in the amphotericin group with AKI than in subjects without AKI. This may serve as an early predictor of drug induced AKI and warrants employment of alternate options in advance to prevent deterioration of renal functions [30]. However, large-scale studies are needed to establish concrete evidence of this association.

Antiviral medications such as acyclovir are used in patients receiving HSCT and can contribute to the development of AKI. Acyclovir can precipitate in the renal tubules and collecting ducts forming crystals resulting in obstruction. This occurs especially with intravenous administration in high doses. Preexisting renal disease, rapid infusion of acyclovir, and dehydration predispose to the drug toxicity and development of AKI [31]. Most often AKI is asymptomatic but rarely presents with nausea, vomiting, and flank pain in less than 48 hours of acyclovir use and urinalysis may show hematuria and pyuria [32]. Polarizing microscopy of urinary sediment demonstrates birefringent needle-shaped crystals inside the leukocytes [33]. Management involves slower infusion, adequate hydration, and dosage modification in preexisting renal disease [31–33].

Aminoglycosides have also been implicated as an important cause for the development of AKI in HSCT recipients. No studies have clearly demonstrated aminoglycosides as an independent risk factor for the development of AKI; however, when used in sepsis or preexisting renal disease or in conjunction with other nephrotoxic medications, they do play a significant role. The toxicity of aminoglycosides is primarily due to intracellular accumulation of the drug that leads to alterations in cellular permeability in proximal renal tubules [3]; hence reduction in the frequency of dosing may help in reducing the incidence of nephrotoxicity. This hypothesis is supported by Olsen et al. through his study that once daily dosing of tobramycin even with higher doses in critical care patients reduced the incidence of nephrotoxicity. Furthermore, the same study found elevated urinary excretion of enzymes such as alanine aminopeptidase and N-acetyl-beta-D glucosaminidase in patients receiving multiple daily dosing compared to once daily dosing subjects. This increase in urinary enzyme level preceded elevation of serum creatinine and may serve as early markers of nephrotoxicity [34]. A meta-analysis of once daily dosing of aminoglycosides versus multiple daily dosing showed no difference in efficacies and toxicity rates between two regimens, although 2 of 22

studies revealed decreased risk of nephrotoxicity with once daily dosing [35]. Recently an update on current literature by Stankowicz et al. concluded that once daily dosing of aminoglycoside is therapeutically effective and minimizes the risk of drug toxicity and monitoring [36].

Cyclosporine A (CsA) is a calcineurin inhibitor used frequently for prevention of GVHD in HSCT recipients. Hence, the use of CsA is restricted to allogeneic transplant recipients [1, 3]. The mechanism by which cyclosporine use leads to renal damage is manifold and poorly understood. Calcineurin inhibitors are capable of causing renin angiotensin system activation and vasoconstriction of renal arterioles. They also decrease renal Klotho expression and increase oxidative stress causing renal endothelial damage [37]. Calcineurin inhibitors are also implicated in the pathogenesis of thrombotic microangiopathy (TMA), which serves as an independent risk factor for the development of AKI [38, 39]. Recently, a study demonstrated that calcineurin inhibitors such as tacrolimus and CsA augment production of renin and vascular endothelial growth factor (VEGF) in renal collecting ducts that causes renal ischemia and periductal fibrosis resulting in calcineurin-induced nephropathy. Furthermore, this process was attenuated by aliskiren, a direct renin inhibitor that may have clinical uses in the prevention of calcineurin-induced nephrotoxicity [40]. Another recent study showed that angiotensin receptor blocker, valsartan, has beneficial effects in preventing CsA related nephrotoxicity. Valsartan has been shown to reduce CsA induced oxidative stress and Klotho downregulation by unknown mechanisms, thereby decreasing the risk of nephrotoxicity [37].

Several studies have however failed to demonstrate a statistically significant relationship between blood CsA levels and development of AKI. For example, a retrospective study performed by Zhou et al. failed to demonstrate a relationship between CsA levels and development of AKI in a group of 86 patients undergoing allogeneic HSCT [15]. In another prospective study conducted by Piñana et al., where 188 patients undergoing reduced intensity-conditioning allogeneic HSCT were analyzed, CsA was implicated as the cause of ARF in 71% of patients, but no correlation was found between the blood levels of CsA and development of ARF [8]. In contrast, a study by Caliskan et al. showed CsA nephrotoxicity as the main factor in the causation of kidney failure, especially during 20–33 days after HSCT when

CsA levels in blood starts declining. This indicates a time lag in the development of renal failure [14]. CsA can impair glucose metabolism and its use in diabetics may have a synergistic effect on kidney injury due to diabetes related nephropathy [8, 21]. Some studies in heart transplant recipients have demonstrated that replacing CsA by inhibitor of mammalian target of rapamycin such as sirolimus improves renal recovery; however further research is essential to assess its impact [41].

7.3. Hepatic Sinusoidal Obstruction Syndrome (SOS) and Acute Kidney Injury.

Hepatic sinusoidal obstruction syndrome (SOS) previously known as venoocclusive disease (VOD) is a commonly encountered complication after HSCT and has been implicated to be an independent risk factor for the development of AKI. Although the pathophysiology of AKI in the SOS setting is poorly defined, it appears to be a variant of hepatorenal syndrome (HRS), which is, in itself, multifactorial in nature. HRS appears to be primarily hemodynamic and does not result in structural and renal lesions or tubular dysfunction [42].

Hepatic SOS is characterized by painful hepatomegaly, hyperbilirubinemia, fluid retention, and ascites. It is generally seen within 30 days of HSCT and the incidence widely varies ranging from 0 to 62.3% with a mean of 13.7% [43]. Hepatic SOS is more common in myeloablative allogeneic transplant recipients in comparison to others and exact pathogenesis remains unclear. However, the most favored theory is that sinusoidal endothelial cells and hepatocytes located within zone 3 of the acinus are damaged by the myeloablative conditioning regimen resulting in subendothelial deposition of fibrin and other blood products in the affected venules. This leads to progressive venular narrowing and obstruction that causes intrahepatic portal hypertension [44]. Furthermore, release of cytokines due to tissue injury and glutathione depletion due to chemotherapeutic drug detoxification by glutathione pathway causes hepatocellular necrosis and fibrosis [43, 44]. Reduction in nitric oxide has also been shown to correlate with the development of SOS due to disruption in the sinusoidal perfusion [45].

In a prospective study conducted by Moiseev et al., the increased number of circulating endothelial cells (CECs) was found to be associated with the incidence of hepatic SOS in patients undergoing allogeneic HSCT. On the day of SOS, the number of CECs was significantly higher than in the rest of the group. The cutoff level established for this assay was >100 CECs/mL and may serve as a biomarker marker for the diagnosis of hepatic SOS [46]. Studies have also established the utility of plasminogen activator inhibitor-1 (PAI) as a marker for the diagnosis and also for predicting the severity of SOS [47, 48].

Risk factors that predispose to development of hepatic SOS include presence of preexisting liver disease, use of methotrexate for prophylaxis against GVHD, and use of TBI > 12 cGy [49]. One of the most important risk factors related to the development of hepatic SOS is the preconditioning regimen. In a study conducted by Qiao et al., the effects of TBI and busulfan/cyclophosphamide were compared with regard to the incidence of hepatic SOS in mice. It was reported that both regimens damaged hepatic sinusoidal endothelial cells; however, the incidence of hepatic SOS was higher with busulfan-cyclophosphamide regimen compared to TBI [50]. Other risk factors include total parenteral nutrition for >1 week, young age (due to small sinusoidal lumens predisposing to easy occlusion), thalassemia major, osteopetrosis, and hemophagocytic lymphohistiocytosis in children; all have been shown to increase the risk of hepatic endothelial injury and SOS [51].

7.3.1. SOS Diagnostic Criteria.

Two different criteria have been established for the diagnosis of hepatic SOS, namely, the Seattle and Baltimore criteria. The Seattle criteria require the presence of at lease two of the three manifestations: jaundice, painful hepatomegaly, and fluid retention or weight gain within 20 days of HSCT [44, 52]. The Baltimore criteria require bilirubin of 2 mg/dL or greater plus two or more of these manifestations: painful hepatomegaly, weight gain > 5%, or ascites, within 21 days of HSCT [53].

7.3.2. Grading of SOS.

Severity of hepatic SOS is graded as mild when the illness fulfills the diagnostic criteria but is self-limiting without necessity of treatment, moderate when SOS subsides with diuretic or analgesic treatment, and severe when SOS persists beyond 100 days or results in death [44].

7.3.3. Prevention of SOS.

As conditioning regimens have been implicated as the primary risk factor, modification in the regimen has been found to reduce the risk of developing hepatic SOS. Oral busulfan when metabolized in the hepatic endothelial cells causes depletion of glutathione, hence promoting more oxidative stress and hepatic damage. Use of intravenous busulfan bypasses hepatic metabolism and has been found to reduce the risk of SOS development [54]. Use of MTX and tacrolimus for GVHD prophylaxis has been found to have a decreased incidence of SOS in comparison to tacrolimus, methotrexate, and sirolimus regimen [55].

There are several pharmacological measures that have been recently introduced for the management of hepatic SOS. Earlier studies implicated the use of tissue plasminogen activator (tPA) as well as methylprednisolone for short periods of time for the management of SOS. A study conducted by Yoon et al. established that the use of t-PA was associated with an increased risk of bleeding complications and the risk being greater with higher cumulative doses of tPA. Furthermore, it was advised against the use of tPA dose escalating protocols for management of moderate-severe SOS [56]. Recent studies have shown promising results with the use of defibrotide, a mixture of ss-oligodeoxyribonucleotides derived from porcine DNA, for the treatment of SOS. It acts by increasing the activity of tPA and inducing prostaglandin I_2 and E_2 production thereby preventing platelet aggregation. Besides, defibrotide also has anti-inflammatory properties. Defibrotide has a greater beneficial effect if used within the first 2 days of HSCT [57]. A retrospective analysis conducted by Park et al. demonstrated the benefit of defibrotide for prophylaxis against SOS especially in high-risk patients [58]. More recently, phase 3 clinical trial concluded that defibrotide use is associated with significant survival benefit in hepatic SOS patients with multiorgan failure [59]. CART (Concentrated Ascites Reinfusion Therapy) is a novel technique involving the filtration, concentration, and reinfusion of drained ascites that has been shown to be a supportive care management option of tense ascites in SOS after HSCT [60].

7.4. Thrombotic Microangiopathy and Acute Kidney Injury. Thrombotic microangiopathy (TMA) such as thrombotic thrombocytopenic purpura (TTP) and hemolytic uremic syndrome (HUS) are not uncommon in HSCT, and the incidence has been reported anywhere from 0.5% to 63.6% [61]. TMA is primarily characterized by thrombocytopenia due to platelet aggregation, fragmentation of erythrocytes, and renal failure. However the cause of TMA in HSCT is different and is due to calcineurin inhibitors, total body irradiation (TBI), acute GVHD, and infections [38, 62]. The diagnosis of TMA in HSCT is often based on nonspecific laboratory features such as anemia, thrombocytopenia, and elevation in LDH and creatinine levels, which are commonly seen in patients receiving HSCT [62]. Hence, the true incidence of TMA may actually be underestimated. A retrospective study conducted by Changsirikulchai et al. on 314 patients who underwent hematopoietic cell transplant (HCT) revealed that development of acute GVHD grades II to IV, patient-donor sex mismatch, TBI > 1200 cGy, and adenovirus infections were risk factors for development of TMA. Further analysis revealed that cyclosporine did not contribute to the development of TMA [62]. On the contrary, studies done previously showed positive correlation between calcineurin inhibitor use and TMA in HSCT patients [38, 39]. The etiology of TMA in HSCT recipients was linked to endothelial injury either directly by GVHD or by cytokines released from GVHD occurring in other parts of the body [38, 62]. Also, some studies have revealed the role of VEGF in the pathogenesis of TMA and acute GVHD. Lower levels of VEGF were shown to be associated with severe forms of acute GVHD and TMA type glomerular injury [63, 64].

Management recommendations from the retrospective study were against adjustments in dosage or discontinuation of cyclosporine regimens, but favored continuing acute GVHD treatment. Plasma exchange is of limited use in treating HSCT associated TMA because the underlying etiology is not related to abnormal von Willebrand factor-cleaving protease. However, a case has been reported where CsA associated TMA and thrombocytopenia associated multiorgan failure were successfully treated with plasma exchange [65]. Eculizumab, a monoclonal antibody which prevents the production of membrane attack complex (MAC) by inhibiting conversion of C5 to C5a and C5b, has been successfully tried in the treatment of TMA secondary to calcineurin inhibitor and cytomegalovirus (CMV). Discontinuation of causative agents and early initiation of eculizumab therapy protects against further complement mediated host cell damage and also provides ample time for the treatment of infections [66, 67]. Recently, a retrospective study conducted by Arai et al. demonstrated that serum levels of neutrophil extracellular traps (NETs) were significantly elevated when compared to the pretransplantation level especially in patients developing TMA following HSCT. NETs may serve as an early biomarker for the detection of HSCT associated TMA [68].

7.5. Marrow Infusion Toxicity and Acute Kidney Injury. Marrow infusion toxicity has also been implicated in the pathogenesis of AKI amongst HSCT recipients. Patients can present with constellation of symptoms including hypotension, nausea, vomiting, and abdominal pain. Patients receiving harvested stem cells are often exposed to various cryoprecipitants such as dimethyl sulfoxide during the HSCT procedure. These toxic molecules are capable of causing hemolysis in the recipient resulting in precipitation of heme proteins in the distal tubule culminating in tubular obstruction [69]. A study demonstrated the presence of hemoglobin casts in renal tubules resulting in marked tubular dilatation and necrosis which was found at autopsy of patients who died after autologous bone marrow transplantation (BMT) [70]. Mainstays of management include alkalinization of urine, which increases heme solubility facilitating its excretion [71], and mannitol induced diuresis that prevents heme trapping in renal tubules [72].

7.6. Tumor Lysis Syndrome and Acute Kidney Injury. Anticancer therapy causes tumor cell lysis spilling intracellular contents in to the blood stream resulting in tumor lysis syndrome. As most patients undergoing HSCT are in remission at the time of transplantation, the incidence of tumor lysis contributing to AKI is very rare. However, certain malignancies, especially leukemias and lymphoproliferative disorders with high cell turnover, can undergo spontaneous tumor lysis [1, 3]. Newer chemotherapeutic regimens using flavopiridol to treat chronic lymphocytic leukemia (CLL) have been associated with a higher risk of tumor lysis syndrome [73]. Metabolic abnormalities in tumor lysis syndrome include hypocalcaemia, hyperphosphatemia, hyperuricemia, and hyperkalemia [74]. Renal injury is primarily due to precipitation of urate crystals and calcium phosphate in renal tubules [75]. Furthermore, hyperuricemia has been shown to be associated with crystal-independent renal damage by renal arteriolar vasoconstriction and release of proinflammatory cytokines that cause significant tubular injury [76]. The management of tumor lysis syndrome includes intravenous hydration and administration of agents such as rasburicase and allopurinol to reduce blood uric acid levels. Also, other management options are low phosphate diet and phosphate binders for hyperphosphatemia and renal replacement therapy for severe cases of AKI and resistant hyperkalemia [75].

7.7. Infectious Complications of HSCT and Acute Kidney Injury. Most patients after receiving HSCT are immunosuppressed and hence susceptible to a number of infectious complications. BK virus and adenovirus are common infections complicating HSCT, both of which are capable of inflicting damage to the kidneys.

BK virus is a member of the polyoma family and is generally seropositive in the majority of the population. Usually it is dormant in the urinary tract after primary infection in childhood; however, during times of immunosuppression, the virus reactivates. On reactivation, it causes damage to renal tubules and manifests either as nephritis or hemorrhagic cystitis with cystitis being the more common presentation [77]. The identification of BK virus infection is paramount in the course of the disease and most of the medications such as cidofovir, foscarnet, and leflunomide have not shown convincing data in the treatment. The major therapeutic option for BK virus nephritis is gradual reduction in immunosuppression. In a 5-year study by Hardinger et al., it was demonstrated that minimizing immunosuppression in patients with BK viremia improves graft survival and renal functions significantly [78]. Cystitis on the other hand resolves spontaneously and may only benefit from supportive care.

Adenovirus infection causes more commonly cystitis and rarely tubulointerstitial nephritis in HSCT recipients [79]. Adenovirus nephritis may manifest as fever, hematuria, and flank pain. Adenovirus cystitis has been reported to occur in a greater frequency especially amongst allogeneic transplant recipients and in patients with high grade GVHD and in those with severe immunosuppression [80, 81]. Management is supportive care but some case reports have proven that intravesical cidofivir therapy is superior to intravenous therapy against adenovirus cystitis; however, the data is very limited for now [82, 83].

8. Role of Albuminuria and Hypoalbuminemia in Acute Kidney Injury

Albuminuria has traditionally been defined as a urine albumin to urine creatinine ratio of 30 to 300 mg per gram of creatinine and has recently been identified in clinical studies to be a marker of endothelial damage in kidney and other organs [84]. In a prospective study conducted by Hingorani et al., 142 patients were analyzed for the development of albuminuria after receiving allogeneic and autologous HSCT. The incidence of albuminuria was more in patients with allogeneic HSCT compared to autologous HSCT. Albuminuria was found to be a useful marker of systemic inflammation and found to be associated with development of acute GVHD, hypertension, and progression of renal disease. However, this study did not establish any relationship between albuminuria and development of AKI [84].

Hypoalbuminemia, on the other hand, has a more significant relationship with the development of AKI in HSCT recipients. In a study by Caliskan et al., low baseline serum albumin levels correlated with the development of AKI. Possible explanation for this correlation is decreased oncotic pressure due to hypoalbuminemia results in intravascular volume contraction and renal ischemia. In addition, exposure to nephrotoxic drugs precipitates the condition. Hence, baseline serum albumin levels prior to HSCT may be an important risk factor for the development of AKI [14].

9. Novel Markers of Acute Kidney Injury in HSCT

One of the most traditional markers that have been used to establish the definition of AKI is serum creatinine. Although serum creatinine remains the gold standard, in this section we will discuss other biomarkers that have recently shown sensitivity for detection of kidney injury especially after HSCT. These may help guide us in the future to predict and treat AKI more aggressively.

Elafin is a protein that primarily produced by cellular elements such as epithelial cells and macrophages in response to injurious stimuli. It inhibits two key enzymes that mediate proteolysis, namely, proteinase 3 and neutrophil elastase. It has previously been identified as a marker in patients with GVHD. In a study conducted by Hingorani et al., increased urinary elafin levels were found to be associated with the development of albuminuria, AKI, progression to chronic kidney disease, and death in HSCT recipients [9].

Urinary Liver-Type Fatty Acid Binding Protein (L-FABP) was recently investigated as a marker for AKI after HSCT. In the study conducted by Shingai et al. involving 206 patients, the incidence of AKI was higher in patients with elevated baseline urinary L-FABP levels [85].

Urinary Alpha 1M is a urinary biomarker for predicting severe AKI. In a prospective study conducted by Morito et al., urinary alpha 1M was found to be useful for predicting severe AKI after HSCT [86].

10. Management of Acute Kidney Injury

AKI after HSCT has been found to be associated with an increased risk of mortality and decreased overall survival. Many studies have evaluated the utility of other therapeutic options for prevention of this complication. A recent randomized controlled trial conducted by Ataei et al. failed to demonstrate the benefit of N-acetyl cysteine in the prevention of AKI amongst myeloablative allogeneic transplant recipients [19]. Currently, avoidance of risk factors associated with the development of AKI remains the mainstay of management [3].

These would include the following:

(a) Use of the reduced intensity-conditioning regimen wherever possible

(b) Closer monitoring of nephrotoxic medications such as amphotericin or use of liposomal preparations

(c) Use of alternative antifungals such as fluconazole and voriconazole for prophylaxis against infection

(d) Early identification and management of sepsis

(e) Use of diuresis and alkalinization of urine in conditions such as tumor lysis syndrome or marrow infusion toxicity

(f) Early identification and management of hepatic SOS with defibrotide

(g) More importantly, early involvement of the nephrologist in the disease course is helpful in prevention of AKI and related complications.

11. Conclusion

One of the major limitations of HSCT in the management of lymphoproliferative disorders and bone marrow failure is

AKI. The identified risk factors are GVHD, use of nephrotoxic medications, sepsis, hepatic SOS, tumor lysis syndrome, TMA, and marrow infusion toxicity. The management of AKI in HSCT recipients is primarily directed at prevention of risk factors that contributes to the development of AKI. This includes avoiding nephrotoxic medications wherever possible, use of reduced intensity-conditioning regimen, and early identification and management of sepsis, tumor lysis syndrome, hepatic SOS, and marrow infusion toxicity. Nevertheless, early involvement of the nephrologist in the disease process is most important for effective management of AKI and related complications.

References

[1] D. Sawinski, "The kidney effects of hematopoietic stem cell transplantation," *Advances in Chronic Kidney Disease*, vol. 21, no. 1, pp. 96–105, 2014.

[2] F. Saddadi, I. Najafi, M. S. Hakemi, K. Falaknazi, F. Attari, and B. Bahar, "Frequency, risk factors, and outcome of acute kidney injury following bone marrow transplantation at Dr Shariati Hospital in Tehran," *Iranian Journal of Kidney Diseases*, vol. 4, no. 1, pp. 20–26, 2010.

[3] A. Kogon and S. Hingorani, "Acute kidney injury in hematopoietic cell transplantation," *Seminars in Nephrology*, vol. 30, no. 6, pp. 615–626, 2010.

[4] C. Clajus, N. Hanke, J. Gottlieb et al., "Renal comorbidity after solid organ and stem cell transplantation," *American Journal of Transplantation*, vol. 12, no. 7, pp. 1691–1699, 2012.

[5] H. Liu, Y.-F. Li, B.-C. Liu et al., "A multicenter, retrospective study of acute kidney injury in adult patients with nonmyeloablative hematopoietic SCT," *Bone Marrow Transplantation*, vol. 45, no. 1, pp. 153–158, 2010.

[6] M. Ando, J. Mori, K. Ohashi et al., "A comparative assessment of the RIFLE, AKIN and conventional criteria for acute kidney injury after hematopoietic SCT," *Bone Marrow Transplantation*, vol. 45, no. 9, pp. 1427–1434, 2010.

[7] Z.-P. Yu, J.-H. Ding, B.-A. Chen et al., "Risk factors for acute kidney injury in patients undergoing allogeneic hematopoietic stem cell transplantation," *Chinese Journal of Cancer*, vol. 29, no. 11, pp. 946–951, 2010.

[8] J. L. Piñana, D. Valcárcel, R. Martino et al., "Study of kidney function impairment after reduced-intensity conditioning allogeneic hematopoietic stem cell transplantation. A single-center experience," *Biology of Blood and Marrow Transplantation*, vol. 15, no. 1, pp. 21–29, 2009.

[9] S. Hingorani, L. S. Finn, E. Pao et al., "Urinary elafin and kidney injury in hematopoietic cell transplant recipients," *Clinical Journal of the American Society of Nephrology*, vol. 10, no. 1, pp. 12–20, 2015.

[10] J. Mori, K. Ohashi, T. Yamaguchi et al., "Risk assessment for acute kidney injury after allogeneic hematopoietic stem cell transplantation based on acute kidney injury network criteria," *Internal Medicine*, vol. 51, no. 16, pp. 2105–2110, 2012.

[11] Y. Kagoya, K. Kataoka, Y. Nannya, and M. Kurokawacorrespondence, "Pretransplant predictors and posttransplant sequels of acute kidney injury after allogeneic stem cell transplantation," *Biology of Blood and Marrow Transplantation*, vol. 17, no. 3, pp. 394–400, 2011.

[12] J. A. Lopes and S. Jorge, "Acute kidney injury following HCT: incidence, risk factors and outcome," *Bone Marrow Transplantation*, vol. 46, no. 11, pp. 1399–1408, 2011.

[13] S. H. Kang, H. S. Park, I. O. Sun et al., "Changes in renal function in long-term survivors of allogeneic hematopoietic stem-cell transplantation: single-center experience," *Clinical Nephrology*, vol. 77, no. 3, pp. 225–230, 2012.

[14] Y. Caliskan, S. K. Besisik, D. Sargin, and T. Ecder, "Early renal injury after myeloablative allogeneic and autologous hematopoietic cell transplantation," *Bone Marrow Transplantation*, vol. 38, no. 2, pp. 141–147, 2006.

[15] T. Zhou, X.-N. Cen, Z.-X. Qiu et al., "Clinical analysis of acute renal failure after allogeneic hematopoietic stem cell transplantation," *Zhongguo Shi Yan Xue Ye Xue Za Zhi*, vol. 17, no. 3, pp. 723–728, 2009.

[16] J. A. Lopes, S. Jorge, S. Silva et al., "Acute renal failure following myeloablative autologous and allogeneic hematopoietic cell transplantation," *Bone Marrow Transplantation*, vol. 38, no. 10, p. 707, 2006.

[17] R. Bellomo, C. Ronco, J. A. Kellum, R. L. Mehta, and P. Palevsky, "Acute renal failure—definition, outcome measures, animal models, fluid therapy and information technology needs: the Second International Consensus Conference of the Acute Dialysis Quality Initiative (ADQI) Group," *Critical Care*, vol. 8, no. 4, pp. R204–R212, 2004.

[18] R. L. Mehta, J. A. Kellum, S. V. Shah et al., "Acute kidney injury network: report of an initiative to improve outcomes in acute kidney injury," *Critical Care*, vol. 11, no. 2, p. R31, 2007.

[19] S. Ataei, M. Hadjibabaie, A. Moslehi et al., "A double-blind, randomized, controlled trial on *N*-acetylcysteine for the prevention of acute kidney injury in patients undergoing allogeneic hematopoietic stem cell transplantation," *Hematological Oncology*, vol. 33, no. 2, pp. 67–74, 2015.

[20] J. A. Lopes, S. Gonçalves, S. Jorge et al., "Contemporary analysis of the influence of acute kidney injury after reduced intensity conditioning haematopoietic cell transplantation on long-term survival," *Bone Marrow Transplantation*, vol. 42, no. 9, pp. 619–626, 2008.

[21] H. E. Wahlstrom, M. Lavelle-Jones, D. Endres, R. Akimoto, O. Kolterman, and A. R. Moossa, "Inhibition of insulin release by cyclosporine and production of peripheral insulin resistance in the dog," *Transplantation*, vol. 49, no. 3, pp. 600–604, 1990.

[22] C. R. Parikh, B. M. Sandmaier, R. F. Storb et al., "Acute renal failure after nonmyeloablative hematopoietic cell transplantation," *Journal of the American Society of Nephrology*, vol. 15, no. 7, pp. 1868–1876, 2004.

[23] R. W. Schrier and W. Wang, "Acute renal failure and sepsis," *The New England Journal of Medicine*, vol. 351, no. 2, pp. 159–169, 2004.

[24] A. Merouani, E. J. Shpall, R. B. Jones, P. G. Archer, and R. W. Schrier, "Renal function in high dose chemotherapy and autologous hematopoietic cell support treatment for breast cancer," *Kidney International*, vol. 50, no. 3, pp. 1026–1031, 1996.

[25] E. Gruss, C. Bernis, J. F. Tomas et al., "Acute renal failure in patients following bone marrow transplantation: prevalence, risk factors and outcome," *American Journal of Nephrology*, vol. 15, no. 6, pp. 473–479, 1995.

[26] P. Sorkine, H. Nagar, A. Weinbroum et al., "Administration of amphotericin B in lipid emulsion decreases nephrotoxicity: results of a prospective, randomized, controlled study in critically ill patients," *Critical Care Medicine*, vol. 24, no. 8, pp. 1311–1315, 1996.

[27] P. J. Cagnoni, "Liposomal amphotericin B versus conventional amphotericin B in the empirical treatment of persistently febrile neutropenic patients," *Journal of Antimicrobial Chemotherapy*, vol. 49, no. 1, pp. 81–86, 2002.

[28] S. R. Hingorani, K. Guthrie, A. Batchelder et al., "Acute renal failure after myeloablative hematopoietic cell transplant: incidence and risk factors," *Kidney International*, vol. 67, no. 1, pp. 272–277, 2005.

[29] K. A. Marr, "Empirical antifungal therapy-new options, new tradeoffs," *New England Journal of Medicine*, vol. 346, no. 4, pp. 278–280, 2002.

[30] P. N. Rocha, M. N. Macedo, C. D. Kobayashi et al., "Role of urine neutrophil gelatinase-associated lipocalin in the early diagnosis of amphotericin B-induced acute kidney injury," *Antimicrobial Agents and Chemotherapy*, vol. 59, no. 11, pp. 6913–6921, 2015.

[31] D. Brigden, A. E. Rosling, and N. C. Woods, "Renal function after acyclovir intravenous injection," *The American Journal of Medicine*, vol. 73, no. 1, pp. 182–185, 1982.

[32] M. A. Perazella, "Crystal-induced acute renal failure," *The American Journal of Medicine*, vol. 106, no. 4, pp. 459–465, 1999.

[33] M. H. Sawyer, D. E. Webb, J. E. Balow, and S. E. Straus, "Acyclovir-induced renal failure. Clinical course and histology," *The American Journal of Medicine*, vol. 84, no. 6, pp. 1067–1071, 1988.

[34] K. M. Olsen, M. I. Rudis, J. A. Rebuck et al., "Effect of once-daily dosing vs. multiple daily dosing of tobramycin on enzyme markers of nephrotoxicity," *Critical Care Medicine*, vol. 32, no. 8, pp. 1678–1682, 2004.

[35] T. C. Bailey, J. Russell Little, B. Littenberg, R. M. Reichley, and W. Claiborne Dunagan, "A meta-analysis of extended-interval dosing versus multiple daily dosing of aminoglycosides," *Clinical Infectious Diseases*, vol. 24, no. 5, pp. 786–795, 1997.

[36] M. S. Stankowicz, J. Ibrahim, and D. L. Brown, "Once-daily aminoglycoside dosing: an update on current literature," *American Journal of Health-System Pharmacy*, vol. 72, no. 16, pp. 1357–1364, 2015.

[37] S. Raeisi, A. Ghorbanihaghjo, H. Argani et al., "The effects of valsartan on renal klotho expression and oxidative stress in alleviation of cyclosporine nephrotoxicity," *Transplantation*, 2016.

[38] E. Holler, H. J. Kolb, E. Hiller et al., "Microangiopathy in patients on cyclosporine prophylaxis who developed acute graft-versus-host disease after HLA-identical bone marrow transplantation," *Blood*, vol. 73, no. 7, pp. 2018–2024, 1989.

[39] H. Nakamae, T. Yamane, T. Hasegawa et al., "Risk factor analysis for thrombotic microangiopathy after reduced-intensity or myeloablative allogeneic hematopoietic stem cell transplantation," *American Journal of Hematology*, vol. 81, no. 7, pp. 525–531, 2006.

[40] Á. Prókai, R. Csohány, E. Sziksz et al., "Calcineurin-inhibition results in upregulation of local renin and subsequent vascular endothelial growth factor production in renal collecting ducts," *Transplantation*, vol. 100, no. 2, pp. 325–333, 2016.

[41] C. A. Gleissner, A. Doesch, P. Ehlermann et al., "Cyclosporine withdrawal improves renal function in heart transplant patients on reduced-dose cyclosporine therapy," *American Journal of Transplantation*, vol. 6, no. 11, pp. 2750–2758, 2006.

[42] B. D. Humphreys, R. J. Soiffer, and C. C. Magee, "Renal failure associated with cancer and its treatment: an update," *Journal of the American Society of Nephrology*, vol. 16, no. 1, pp. 151–161, 2005.

[43] J. A. Coppell, P. G. Richardson, R. Soiffer et al., "Hepatic veno-occlusive disease following stem cell transplantation: incidence, clinical course, and outcome," *Biology of Blood and Marrow Transplantation*, vol. 16, no. 2, pp. 157–168, 2010.

[44] S. I. Bearman, "The syndrome of hepatic veno-occlusive disease after marrow transplantation," *Blood*, vol. 85, no. 11, pp. 3005–3020, 1995.

[45] L. D. DeLeve, X. Wang, G. C. Kanel et al., "Decreased hepatic nitric oxide production contributes to the development of rat sinusoidal obstruction syndrome," *Hepatology*, vol. 38, no. 4, pp. 900–908, 2003.

[46] I. S. Moiseev, E. V. Babenko, A. A. Sipol, V. N. Vavilov, and B. V. Afanasyev, "Measurement of circulating endothelial cells to support the diagnosis of veno-occlusive disease after hematopoietic stem cell transplantation," *International Journal of Laboratory Hematology*, vol. 36, no. 4, pp. e27–e29, 2014.

[47] C. Salat, E. Holler, H.-J. Kolb et al., "Plasminogen activator inhibitor-1 confirms the diagnosis of hepatic veno-occlusive disease in patients with hyperbilirubinemia after bone marrow transplantation," *Blood*, vol. 89, no. 6, pp. 2184–2188, 1997.

[48] M. Pihusch, H. Wegner, P. Goehring et al., "Diagnosis of hepatic veno-occlusive disease by plasminogen activator inhibitor-1 plasma antigen levels: a prospective analysis in 350 allogeneic hematopoietic stem cell recipients," *Transplantation*, vol. 80, no. 10, pp. 1376–1382, 2005.

[49] P. G. Richardson, V. T. Ho, S. Giralt et al., "Safety and efficacy of defibrotide for the treatment of severe hepatic veno-occlusive disease," *Therapeutic Advances in Hematology*, vol. 3, no. 4, pp. 253–265, 2012.

[50] J. Qiao, J. Fu, T. Fang et al., "Evaluation of the effects of preconditioning regimens on hepatic veno-occlusive disease in mice after hematopoietic stem cell transplantation," *Experimental and Molecular Pathology*, vol. 98, no. 1, pp. 73–78, 2015.

[51] M. Gökce, B. Kuskonmaz, M. Cetin, D. U. Cetinkaya, and M. Tuncer, "Coexisting or underlying risk factors of hepatic veno-occlusive disease in pediatric hematopoietic stem cell transplant recipients receiving prophylaxis," *Experimental and Clinical Transplantation*, vol. 11, no. 5, pp. 440–446, 2013.

[52] G. B. McDonald, M. S. Hinds, L. D. Fisher et al., "Veno-occlusive disease of the liver and multiorgan failure after bone marrow transplantation: a cohort study of 355 patients," *Annals of Internal Medicine*, vol. 118, no. 4, pp. 255–267, 1993.

[53] R. J. Jones, K. S. K. Lee, W. E. Beschorner et al., "Venoocclusive disease of the liver following bone marrow transplantation," *Transplantation*, vol. 44, no. 6, pp. 778–783, 1987.

[54] J.-H. Lee, S.-J. Choi, J.-H. Lee et al., "Decreased incidence of hepatic veno-occlusive disease and fewer hemostatic derangements associated with intravenous busulfan vs oral busulfan in adults conditioned with busulfan + cyclophosphamide for allogeneic bone marrow transplantation," *Annals of Hematology*, vol. 84, no. 5, pp. 321–330, 2005.

[55] C. Cutler, K. Stevenson, H. T. Kim et al., "Sirolimus is associated with veno-occlusive disease of the liver after myeloablative allogeneic stem cell transplantation," *Blood*, vol. 112, no. 12, pp. 4425–4431, 2008.

[56] J.-H. Yoon, W.-S. Min, H.-J. Kim et al., "Experiences of t-PA use in moderate-to-severe hepatic veno-occlusive disease after hematopoietic SCT: is it still reasonable to use t-PA?" *Bone Marrow Transplantation*, vol. 48, no. 12, pp. 1562–1568, 2013.

[57] M. Mohty, F. Malard, M. Abecassis et al., "Sinusoidal obstruction syndrome/veno-occlusive disease: current situation and perspectives—a position statement from the European Society for Blood and Marrow Transplantation (EBMT)," *Bone Marrow Transplantation*, vol. 50, no. 6, pp. 781–789, 2015.

[58] M. Park, H. J. Park, H.-S. Eom et al., "Safety and effects of prophylactic defibrotide for sinusoidal obstruction syndrome in hematopoietic stem cell transplantation," *Annals of Transplantation*, vol. 18, no. 1, pp. 36–42, 2013.

[59] P. G. Richardson, M. L. Riches, N. A. Kernan et al., "Phase 3 trial of defibrotide for the treatment of severe veno-occlusive disease and multi-organ failure," *Blood*, vol. 127, no. 13, pp. 1656–1665, 2016.

[60] H. Takahashi, R. Sakai, A. Fujita et al., "Concentrated ascites reinfusion therapy for sinusoidal obstructive syndrome after hematopoietic stem cell transplantation," *Artificial Organs*, vol. 37, no. 10, pp. 932–936, 2013.

[61] J. N. George, X. Li, J. R. McMinn, D. R. Terrell, S. K. Vesely, and G. B. Selby, "Thrombotic thrombocytopenic purpura-hemolytic uremic syndrome following allogeneic HPC transplantation: a diagnostic dilemma," *Transfusion*, vol. 44, no. 2, pp. 294–304, 2004.

[62] S. Changsirikulchai, D. Myerson, K. A. Guthrie, G. B. McDonald, C. E. Alpers, and S. R. Hingorani, "Renal thrombotic microangiopathy after hematopoietic cell transplant: role of GVHD in pathogenesis," *Clinical Journal of the American Society of Nephrology*, vol. 4, no. 2, pp. 345–353, 2009.

[63] V. Eremina, J. A. Jefferson, J. Kowalewska et al., "VEGF inhibition and renal thrombotic microangiopathy," *The New England Journal of Medicine*, vol. 358, no. 11, pp. 1129–1136, 2008.

[64] C.-K. Min, S. Y. Kim, M. J. Lee et al., "Vascular endothelial growth factor (VEGF) is associated with reduced severity of acute graft-versus-host disease and nonrelapse mortality after allogeneic stem cell transplantation," *Bone Marrow Transplantation*, vol. 38, no. 2, pp. 149–156, 2006.

[65] Ç. Ödek, T. Kendirli, A. Yaman, T. Ileri, Z. Kuloğlu, and E. Ince, "Cyclosporine-associated thrombotic microangiopathy and thrombocytopenia- associated multiple organ failure: a case successfully treated with therapeutic plasma exchange," *Journal of Pediatric Hematology/Oncology*, vol. 36, no. 2, pp. e88–e90, 2014.

[66] A. Java, A. Edwards, A. Rossi et al., "Cytomegalovirus-induced thrombotic microangiopathy after renal transplant successfully treated with eculizumab: case report and review of the literature," *Transplant International*, vol. 28, no. 9, pp. 1121–1125, 2015.

[67] E. Morales, C. Rabasco, E. Gutierrez, and M. Praga, "A case of thrombotic micro-angiopathy after heart transplantation successfully treated with eculizumab," *Transplant International*, vol. 28, no. 7, pp. 878–880, 2015.

[68] Y. Arai, K. Yamashita, K. Mizugishi et al., "Serum neutrophil extracellular trap levels predict thrombotic microangiopathy after allogeneic stem cell transplantation," *Biology of Blood and Marrow Transplantation*, vol. 19, no. 12, pp. 1683–1689, 2013.

[69] R. A. Zager, "Acute renal failure in the setting of bone marrow transplantation," *Kidney International*, vol. 46, no. 5, pp. 1443–1458, 1994.

[70] D. M. Smith, D. D. Weisenburger, P. Bierman, A. Kessinger, W. P. Vaughan, and J. O. Armitage, "Acute renal failure associated with autologous bone marrow transplantation," *Bone Marrow Transplantation*, vol. 2, no. 2, pp. 195–201, 1987.

[71] R. A. Zager, "Studies of mechanisms and protective maneuvers in myoglobinuric acute renal injury," *Laboratory Investigation*, vol. 60, no. 5, pp. 619–629, 1989.

[72] R. A. Zager, C. Foerder, and C. Bredl, "The influence of mannitol on myoglobinuric acute renal failure: functional, biochemical, and morphological assessments," *Journal of the American Society of Nephrology*, vol. 2, no. 4, pp. 848–855, 1991.

[73] K. A. Blum, A. S. Ruppert, J. A. Woyach et al., "Risk factors for tumor lysis syndrome in patients with chronic lymphocytic leukemia treated with the cyclin-dependent kinase inhibitor, flavopiridol," *Leukemia*, vol. 25, no. 9, pp. 1444–1451, 2011.

[74] A. Q. Lam and B. D. Humphreys, "Onco-nephrology: AKI in the cancer patient," *Clinical Journal of the American Society of Nephrology*, vol. 7, no. 10, pp. 1692–1700, 2012.

[75] T. I. Mughal, A. A. Ejaz, J. R. Foringer, and B. Coiffier, "An integrated clinical approach for the identification, prevention, and treatment of tumor lysis syndrome," *Cancer Treatment Reviews*, vol. 36, no. 2, pp. 164–176, 2010.

[76] M. Shimada, R. J. Johnson, W. S. May et al., "A novel role for uric acid in acute kidney injury associated with tumour lysis syndrome," *Nephrology Dialysis Transplantation*, vol. 24, no. 10, pp. 2960–2964, 2009.

[77] H. H. Hirsch and J. Steiger, "Polyomavirus BK," *The Lancet Infectious Diseases*, vol. 3, no. 10, pp. 611–623, 2003.

[78] K. L. Hardinger, M. J. Koch, D. J. Bohl, G. A. Storch, and D. C. Brennan, "BK-virus and the impact of pre-emptive immunosuppression reduction: 5-year results," *American Journal of Transplantation*, vol. 10, no. 2, pp. 407–415, 2010.

[79] M. Ito, N. Hirabayashi, Y. Uno, A. Nakayama, and J. Asai, "Necrotizing tubulointerstitial nephritis associated with adenovirus infection," *Human Pathology*, vol. 22, no. 12, pp. 1225–1231, 1991.

[80] I. Bil-Lula, M. Ussowicz, B. Rybka et al., "Hematuria due to adenoviral infection in bone marrow transplant recipients," *Transplantation Proceedings*, vol. 42, no. 9, pp. 3729–3734, 2010.

[81] B. Bruno, R. A. Zager, M. J. Boeckh et al., "Adenovirus nephritis in hematopoietic stem-cell transplantation," *Transplantation*, vol. 77, no. 7, pp. 1049–1057, 2004.

[82] P. Fanourgiakis, A. Georgala, M. Vekemans et al., "Intravesical instillation of cidofovir in the treatment of hemorrhagic cystitis caused by adenovirus type 11 in a bone marrow transplant recipient," *Clinical Infectious Diseases*, vol. 40, no. 1, pp. 199–201, 2005.

[83] M. Sakurada, T. Kondo, M. Umeda, H. Kawabata, K. Yamashita, and A. Takaori-Kondo, "Successful treatment with intravesical cidofovir for virus-associated hemorrhagic cystitis after allogeneic hematopoietic stem cell transplantation: a case report and a review of the literature," *Journal of Infection and Chemotherapy*, vol. 22, no. 7, pp. 495–500, 2016.

[84] S. R. Hingorani, K. Seidel, A. Lindner, T. Aneja, G. Schoch, and G. McDonald, "Albuminuria in hematopoietic cell transplantation patients: prevalence, clinical associations, and impact on survival," *Biology of Blood and Marrow Transplantation*, vol. 14, no. 12, pp. 1365–1372, 2008.

23

Pediatric Nephrology and Rheumatology Practice Patterns in Granulomatosis with Polyangiitis: A Midwest Pediatric Nephrology Consortium Study

Cristin D. W. Kaspar ⬤,[1] Keia Sanderson,[2] Seza Ozen,[3] Priya S. Verghese,[4] Megan Lo,[1] Timothy E. Bunchman,[1] Scott E. Wenderfer ⬤,[5] and Jason Kidd[6]

[1]*Virginia Commonwealth University, Children's Hospital of Richmond, Pediatric Nephrology, Virginia, USA*
[2]*University of North Carolina, Department of Medicine-Nephrology, North Carolina, USA*
[3]*Hacettepe University, Department of Pediatrics, Turkey*
[4]*University of Minnesota, Division of Pediatric Nephrology, Minnesota, USA*
[5]*Baylor College of Medicine, Pediatrics-Renal, Texas, USA*
[6]*Virginia Commonwealth University, Internal Medicine Nephrology, Virginia, USA*

Correspondence should be addressed to Cristin D. W. Kaspar; cristin.kaspar@vcuhealth.org

Academic Editor: David B. Kershaw

Objective. To assess practice pattern similarities and differences amongst pediatric rheumatologists and nephrologists in the management of pediatric Granulomatosis with Polyangiitis (GPA). *Methods.* A voluntary survey was distributed to the Midwest Pediatric Nephrology Consortium Group (MWPNC) and an international pediatric rheumatology email listserv in 2016-2017. Data were collected on general practice characteristics and preferences for induction management under three clinical scenarios (A-C): newly diagnosed GPA with glomerulonephritis, GPA with rapidly progressive glomerulonephritis, and GPA with pulmonary hemorrhage. In addition, individual preferences for GPA maintenance medications, disease monitoring, and management of GPA with end-stage renal disease were ascertained. *Results.* There was a 68% response rate from the MWPNC membership and equal numbers of rheumatology respondents. Survey results revealed Rituximab plus Cyclophosphamide is a more common induction choice for rheumatologists than nephrologists in induction Scenarios A and B, whereas Cyclophosphamide is more commonly chosen by nephrologists in Scenario A. Plasmapheresis rates increased for Scenarios A, B, and C for both specialties, but were overall low. There was no clear consensus on the duration of maintenance therapy nor diagnostic work-up. Rheumatologists more frequently chose Rituximab for maintenance and induction compared to nephrologists. There was also a higher than expected proportion of Mycophenolate Mofetil use for both specialties. *Conclusion.* This survey has revealed important differences in the way that rheumatologists and nephrologists manage this disease. It highlights the need for well-designed clinical trials in pediatric GPA patients and reveals that both specialties must be represented during consensus-building and clinical trial design efforts.

1. Introduction

ANCA-associated vasculitis (AAV) is a disease which includes Granulomatosis with Polyangiitis (GPA) (formerly known as Wegener Granulomatosis), Microscopic Polyangiitis (MPA), and Eosinophilic Granulomatosis with Polyangiitis (EoGPA, formerly known as Churg Strauss Syndrome). Despite the commonality of ANCA association, the epidemiology, pathophysiology, course, and prognosis of these diseases are not uniform [1]. GPA is the most common AAV and while the incidence is low, it is rising from 0.2 to 1.2 per 100,000 [2], a trend that is consistent with our local experience.

The median age of GPA disease onset in childhood ranges from 11.7 to 14 years in the European Vasculitis registry and the international ARCHiVE cohort study, respectively [1, 3, 4]. In the ARCHiVE registry, 83% of newly diagnosed pediatric GPA patients presented with glomerulonephritis.

The care of patients with GPA bridges the expertise of primarily two subspecialties, rheumatology and nephrology. It is presumed that current practice patterns of GPA amongst rheumatologists and nephrologists differ. To date there are no pediatric nephrology consensus guidelines supporting the management of the renal involvement of this disease. The European League Against Rheumatism (EULAR) released consensus statements in 2009 and updated in 2016 for AAV management, including recommendations for rapidly progressive glomerulonephritis (RPGN), pulmonary hemorrhage, and organ-threatening complications [5]. However these recommendations are not pediatric-specific and do not address management of end-stage renal disease in AAV, and it is unclear how familiar pediatric nephrologists are with the recommendations. Prompted by a recent increase in new pediatric GPA diagnoses in our local practice area and a lack of consensus guidance, we undertook a comparative survey to illustrate the practice patterns amongst pediatric nephrologists and rheumatologists for three different clinical presentations of pediatric GPA.

Pediatric GPA patients with renal involvement require a cooperative partnership between pediatric rheumatology and nephrology to care for the organ-threatening complications of this vasculitis and for the long-term management of immunosuppression. The goal of this survey is to identify commonalities in practice as well as to highlight disparate practice patterns that reveal specific education needs and areas that require further research.

2. Methods

This is an international descriptive survey of pediatric nephrologists and rheumatologists regarding the practice patterns of GPA. Members of the Midwest Pediatric Nephrology Consortium (MWPNC) and those of a pediatric rheumatology email listserv were asked to complete a voluntary survey on GPA practice patterns. The MWPNC is a collaborative clinical and translational research organization with 73 member centers represented across the United States, Puerto Rico, and Canada. The pediatric rheumatology listserv has an international email membership termed the "Pediatric Rheumatology Bulletin Board" hosted by McMaster University. A total of four email solicitations were sent between October 2016 and April 2017 to both memberships. Study objectives were presented to MWPNC members at a biannual research conference during this time period. Survey data were managed and collected using REDCap electronic data capture hosted at Virginia Commonwealth University (REDCap supported by Award Number UL1TR000058 from the NCRR). The full survey is available in Supplementary Materials 1 and included 5 sections.

Section 1 identified general characteristics such as the respondent's practice setting, the number of pediatric GPA patients currently followed, and whether their division had written consensus protocols for either the induction or maintenance treatment of GPA. In Section 2, respondents were asked to provide their first-line choice of induction medications depending on the presentation of a GPA patient

in three different scenarios. They were first asked to consider management choices in a new GPA patient presenting with glomerulonephritis (Scenario A), a new patient with rapidly progressive glomerulonephritis (RPGN, Scenario B) as diagnosed using site-specific criteria, and a new patient with pulmonary hemorrhage (Scenario C). After induction differences were ascertained for Scenarios B and C, respondents were instructed to frame their remaining responses under Scenario A, for a presentation of a new diagnosis GPA with glomerulonephritis. In Sections 3 and 4, preferences were ascertained for maintenance Cyclophosphamide versus Rituximab, maintenance Azathioprine versus Mycophenolate Mofetil use, Trimethoprim-Sulfamethoxazole use, and clinical tools used for assessing initial and relapse disease activity. Finally, Section 5 was directed towards understanding the management of end-stage renal disease, including choice of dialysis modality, the timing of renal transplant once in remission, and the preferred choice of transplant immunosuppressive medications in GPA.

Multiple group proportions were compared by χ^2 analysis, two sample proportions by Adjusted Wald test, with statistical significance level alpha <0.05. Statistical analysis was performed using JMP v.13.

3. Results

3.1. Survey Section 1: General Characteristics. Of the 145 responses to the survey, 7 were incomplete across all sections and excluded. The remaining 138 responses represented 42 unique rheumatology institutions and 3 unidentified, and 50 unique nephrology institutions and 2 unidentified which represented 68% of the MWPNC membership. Table 1 lists practice setting differences and characteristics of the respondents. The primary management responsibility differed by specialty: 27% of the nephrology respondents (Neph) claimed they had primary management responsibility, whereas no rheumatology respondents (Rheum) reported that nephrology primarily managed the patients. Seven Rheum and 9 Neph respondents completed Section 1, but failed to complete Sections 2-5 and were therefore censored from the remainder of the analysis.

3.2. Survey Section 2: Induction Medications. Respondents were asked to select their individual preference for first-line induction medications under the three clinical scenarios (Scenarios A-C). One or multiple answers could be selected from the following choices: Cyclophosphamide (IV or PO), Rituximab, steroid (IV or PO), plasmapheresis, or other. After Scenario A choices were made, respondents were asked if their induction preferences would differ from Scenario A when considering Scenarios B or C, and if affirmed would prompt a follow-up set of questions with the same answer choices. Table 2 summarizes the answer combinations and any significant specialty differences for each scenario.

Specialty-specific differences emerged for choice of induction agent across scenarios. Neph were more likely to choose Cyclophosphamide for Scenario A, whereas Rheum were more likely than Neph to use Rituximab together with

TABLE 1: General characteristics of survey respondents.

	Total N	Rheum %	Neph %
Identified as a Rheumatologist / Nephrologist	138	44.9	55.1
Experience Level	138		
In practice >5 years		61.8	79.1
In practice <5 years		27.3	17.9
Fellows-in-training		10.9	3
Mid-Level Providers		0	0
Practice Setting	138		
University/Tertiary care/Academic		90.9	98.5
Community Hospital / Non-teaching / Non-academic		1.8	1.5
Private Practice		7.3	0
Supervise fellows directly	136	44.4	54.5
Institution has a Pediatric Nephrology Division	138	98.2	100
Institution has a Pediatric Rheumatology Division	135	96.3	89.2
Management			
Who manages pediatric GPA patients primarily at your institution?	138		
Primary Rheum		44 *	9.5 *
Primary Neph		0 *	27 *
Co-Management		56 *	63.5 *
Your institution does NOT have a written induction protocol	138	87.3	92.5
Your institution does NOT have a written maintenance protocol	138	90.9	97.0
Number of GPA patients currently followed in practice	138		
0		3.6	14.9
1		7.3	13.4
2-4		40.0	35.8
5-7		20.0	23.9
8-10		16.4	4.5
11+		12.7	7.5

*Denotes significant difference by specialty p <0.0001.

Cyclophosphamide for both Scenarios A and B. Additionally there was an unique specialty difference for those who stated their induction agent would differ in Scenario C, a new diagnosis patient with pulmonary hemorrhage.

Experience level (categorized by <5 years including fellows in training, or ≥ 5 years) influenced Rheum responses for Cyclophosphamide and Rituximab in Scenario A only. Those with relatively more practice experience (≥5 years) chose Cyclophosphamide with more frequency (67.65% versus 23.81%, p=0.0008) and chose Rituximab with less frequency (78.18% versus 95.24%, p=0.0120). Plasmapheresis choice in Scenarios A-C and all other responses for Scenarios B and C were insignificant (p>0.05) when filtered by Rheum practice experience. There were no significant differences related to experience in Scenarios A-C for nephrologists. Next, induction responses were filtered for the number of GPA patients actively followed in the practice, categorized as 0-4 versus ≥ 5. There were no significant differences (p>0.05) for the induction agent chosen in either specialty when filtered by patient volume, except for Neph responses for Rituximab in Scenario C (pulmonary hemorrhage), where 64.29% of those with relatively higher patient volume chose Rituximab versus 35.71% with lower volume, p=0.02.

The remaining questions in Section 2 regarding dosing characteristics of the induction medications asked respondents to frame their answers in terms of Scenario A.

3.2.1. Cyclophosphamide. The majority (65.3%) of respondents chose ">3 to 6 months" as the typical duration of induction Cyclophosphamide whereas 21.3% chose ">2 to 3 months." The chosen interval was once per month in 78.5% whereas only 9.2% chose daily oral or every 2 weeks IV (specialty difference p>0.05). Both Rheum and Neph use an increasing dose protocol ending at 1000 mg/m^2 (85%, p>0.05), but more Neph start at 500 mg/m^2 (71.4%, specialty difference p=0.0358) whereas 36% of Rheum start at either 500 mg/m^2 or 750 mg/m^2. Conversely there was a consensus with no specialty difference for the starting dose, which was a median of 500 mg/m^2, amongst those that chose both Cyclophosphamide and Rituximab for induction. Finally, 46.1% of respondents (specialty difference p>0.05) routinely refer adolescent patients to fertility specialists, whereas another 10.8% only refer if the patient nears a maximum cumulative dose limit of 10-15 g/m^2.

TABLE 2: Characteristics of combination answer selections for Scenarios A-C.

	N	Overall % if no specialty difference	Rheum %	Neph %	*p-value of specialty difference
Scenario A	<u>122</u>				
Cyclophosphamide	77	*	**36.4**	**63.6**	**p=0.0114**
+ IV/PO Steroid	71	92.2			
+ Rituximab	26	*	61.5	38.5	p=0.001
+ Plasmapheresis	14	19.5			
+ Rituximab + Plasmapheresis	9	11.7			
Rituximab without Cyclophosphamide	39	**60**			
+ IV/PO Steroid	36	92.3			
+ IV/PO Steroid + Plasmapheresis	6	15.4			
IV/PO Steroid without Cyclophosphamide, Rituximab, or Plasmapheresis	6	*	**0**	**100**	**p<0.0001**
Scenario B My preferences would be different than that chosen in Scenario A	<u>75</u>	<u>61.5</u>			
Cyclophosphamide	61	**81.3**			
+ IV/PO Steroid	52	85.3			
+ Rituximab	23	*	65.2	34.8	p=0.0185
+ Plasmapheresis	40	65.6			
+ Rituximab + Plasmapheresis	17	27.8			
Rituximab without Cyclophosphamide	7	**9.3**			
+ IV/PO Steroid	0	0			
+ IV/PO Steroid + Plasmapheresis	7	100			
Plasmapheresis without Cyclophosphamide or Rituximab	6	*	**0**	**100**	**p<0.0001**
Other[i]	1	1.3			
Scenario C My preferences would be different than that chosen in Scenario A	<u>72</u>	*	<u>47.2</u>	<u>67.7</u>	<u>**p=0.0232**</u>
Cyclophosphamide	45	**63.4**			
+ IV/PO Steroid	40	88.9			
+ Rituximab	16	35.6			
+ Plasmapheresis	40	88.9			
+ Rituximab + Plasmapheresis	13	32.5			
Rituximab without Cyclophosphamide	13	**18.3**			
+ IV/PO Steroid	12	92.3			
+ IV/PO Steroid + Plasmapheresis	10	83.3			
Plasmapheresis without Cyclophosphamide or Rituximab	11	**13.4**			
Other[ii]	3	4.1			

[i]One subject chose 'other' but did not describe treatment in free text.

[ii]One subject chose 'other' but did not describe treatment in free text; two did not select any option.

3.2.2. Rituximab. The method of dosing induction Rituximab differed significantly by specialty in terms of duration (p=0.0054), interval (p=0.0217), starting dose (p=0.0386), and set maximum dose (p=0.0033). The majority of Rheum (51.4%) dose at 750 mg/m^2 every two weeks (35.1% dose at 375 mg/m^2), whereas most Neph (77.8%) dose at 375 mg/m^2 every four weeks. Rheum was more likely than Neph (84.6% versus 50%) to set a maximum dose of Rituximab of 1,000 mg, whereas 50% of Neph reported no set maximum dose.

3.2.3. Steroids. The form of steroid chosen for induction differed by specialty (p=0.0068): "IV Methylprednisolone always" was chosen by 47.7% of Rheum and 75.9% by Neph, whereas "IV Methylprednisolone usually, depending on severity" was chosen by 38.6% Rheum and 22.2% Neph. Only 1.9% of Neph and 13.6% Rheum chose "PO steroid usually" and none "PO steroid always." Three days of induction IV Methylprednisolone was the most common approach by both Rheum (89.5%) and Neph (88.5%). 92.2% overall dose IV Methylprednisolone using a mg/kg unit up to a set maximum amount of 1,000 mg (93.3%). Only 6 respondents (100% Neph) chose IV steroid as the lone induction agent for Scenario A, while none chose this as single therapy in Scenarios B or C.

3.2.4. Plasmapheresis. While approximately 60% of respondents stated their induction choice would differ in a RPGN (Scenario B) or pulmonary hemorrhage (Scenario C) presentation versus Scenario A, there were similarities in the proportions of Rituximab and Cyclophosphamide selections with no difference by specialty. The difference arose in a higher selection of plasmapheresis: in Scenarios A, B, and C, respectively, the percentage of Rheum that chose plasmapheresis increased from 11.4%, 36.7%, and 51.9% versus Neph 21.4%, 42.9%, and 35.7%. Six and 11 respondents chose plasmapheresis as the lone induction agent for Scenarios B and C, respectively, which differed by specialty only for Scenario B.

3.3. Survey Section 3: Maintenance Medications. Respondents were next asked about duration of maintenance therapy, presuming patients remain free of relapse during that time. Most commonly respondents chose ">18 months to 2 years" (34.5%), followed by ">2 to 3 years" (26.7%) and ">12 to 18 months" (19.8%) with no difference by specialty (p=0.3335).

3.3.1. Steroids. 74.6% of respondents "always" use prednisone as a part of maintenance therapy; 22.8% use it "depending on severity of illness at presentation" (no specialty difference, p>0.05). The duration did differ by specialty (p=0.0022): 49.1% of Rheum wean prednisone "as quickly as possible once in remission, no set duration" versus 18% of Neph. The next most common response was "wean off by 6 months" (Rheum 29.1%, Neph 27.9%) and "wean off by 1 year" (Rheum 12.7%, Neph 23%). 18% of Neph versus 1.8% Rheum preferred to "remain on prednisone for the duration of maintenance therapy."

3.3.2. Rituximab. 60% of Rheum versus 9.8% Neph chose Rituximab as first-line maintenance therapy (p<0.0001). Of note, 97% of Rheum and 60% Neph who chose Rituximab for first-line maintenance also chose Rituximab for first-line induction therapy (p=0.0403). The duration for maintenance Rituximab did not differ by specialty (p=0.3967): the most common response was ">6-12 months" (30.8%), followed by ">24 months" (23.1%) and ">18-24 months" (20.5%). Overall 61.5% of respondents dose Rituximab at intervals of once every 6 months, with some (25.6%) dosing it if the CD19 count rises above a set level (no specialty difference, p>0.05). Only 9 respondents described how they use this CD19 level in free text, and there was no consensus amongst the responses. 94.7% dose using mg/m^2 unit. Most Neph begin dosing at 375 mg/m^2 (83.3%), whereas Rheum start dosing at 750 mg/m^2

(44.8%), p=0.0419. A consensus maximum set dose of 1,000 mg was common amongst both groups (82.1%).

3.3.3. Azathioprine, Mycophenolate Mofetil, and Trimethoprim-Sulfamethoxazole. Overall 50.5% of respondents use Azathioprine over Mycophenolate Mofetil (MMF, 38.5%) for maintenance, and 11% overall chose "Other-not Azathioprine, MMF, or Rituximab primarily for maintenance." While there was no difference by specialty for Azathioprine versus MMF choice, p=0.0654, Neph chose MMF in greater proportions than Rheum (45.8% versus 30%). Free text options were provided by 10 out of 12 respondents who chose "Other": 3 reported using both Azathioprine and MMF simultaneously, 3 use Methotrexate, 3 stated they choose either Azathioprine or MMF situationally, and 1 misclassified and prefers Rituximab over Azathioprine/MMF. Of those that selected Rituximab for maintenance in the previous survey question (n=39), 47.1% also chose Azathioprine and 35.3% MMF with no difference by specialty (p>0.05).

The use of Trimethoprim-Sulfamethoxazole (TMP-SMX) for either *Pneumocystis jiroveci* (PJP) prophylaxis or as an additional component to maintenance therapy was next determined and did not differ by specialty (p>0.05). Overall, 81% of respondents use TMP-SMX in some way for GPA treatment: 37.1% of respondents use TMP-SMX purely for PJP prophylaxis, 37.1% use it for both PJP prophylaxis and to reduce relapse by decreasing sino-pulmonary carriage of staphylococcus or streptococcus bacteria, and 6.9% report using it to reduce the risk of relapse alone. The majority, 78%, do not monitor staphylococcus or streptococcus nasal carriage by nasal swab or culture, however, 10% check once at the start of treatment, and 12% test nasal swabs periodically. The TMP-SMX dosing interval did differ by specialty (p=0.0006), with Neph dosing it daily (48%, Rheum 11.4%), followed by three times a week (Neph 48%, Rheum 80%) and least common once per day on weekends only (Neph 4%, Rheum 9.1%).

3.4. Survey Section 4: Diagnostic Work-Up and Disease Monitoring

3.4.1. Diagnostic Work-Up. 88.3% of Neph "always" obtain a renal biopsy to confirm the diagnosis of GPA upon initial presentation, versus 47.3% of Rheum (p<0.0001). The extent of CT imaging to determine involvement of sino-pulmonary disease at the time of GPA diagnosis did not differ by specialty (p=0.0825). Most commonly a "LIMITED CT-scan depending on clinical presentation" (56.5%) was chosen, followed by "always obtain a FULL CT Head, Neck, Sinus, and Chest" (35.7%) or "no, never" (7.8%). Those that chose the limited CT-scan option were asked in follow-up whether they "always" obtained one or multiple specific organ systems: "head" (0%), "neck" (0%), "sinus" (Rheum 21%, Neph 79%, p=0.0266), "chest" (Rheum 37.1%, Neph 14.5%, p=0.0022), or "any combination of these but only if the patient has active symptoms" (24.6% overall, p=0.4934).

3.4.2. Disease Monitoring. To define a GPA relapse, 41.2% overall use "either clinical characteristics or serological marker elevation," 35.1% use "clinical characteristics and symptomatology only," and 23.7% require "both clinical and serological marker elevation simultaneously" with no specialty difference, p>0.05. Specific diagnostic tools routinely employed included the following: ESR or CRP (Rheum 75.8%, Neph 50%, p=0.0019), ANCA titer (63.0%, p=0.1473), hematuria and/or proteinuria (73.9%, p=0.1038), and 9.4% (p=0.4970) use the Birmingham Vasculitis Activity Score. Three respondents wrote in use of the Pediatric Vasculitis Activity Score to assess relapse. The majority of respondents monitor ANCA titers "every 3 months" (64.4%), followed by "every 6 months" (13.9%), "only at times when a clinical relapse is suspected" (9.6%), "other" (8.7%), or "never" (3.5%) without specialty difference.

3.5. Survey Section 5: Management of GPA with End-Stage Renal Disease (ESRD). The answer choices for the questions on dialysis and ESRD management included an option to select "unsure–I do not manage dialysis or transplant" (Rheum > Neph as expected, p<0.0001) and are reported in Table 3. It was expected that nearly all Rheum and some Neph would choose this 'unsure' option as ESRD management would be outside the scope of practice for some. However, there was variability in the proportion selecting the 'unsure' option for each question. Next, the 'unsure' responses were excluded from analysis. Once a GPA patient is declared ESRD, the time in remission considered 'safe' to receive a kidney transplant was "10-12 months" (34.7%), followed by "4-6 months" (25.0%) and "13-18 months" (23.6%) with no difference by specialty (p=0.2452). Although there was specialty difference in those that stated their transplant induction and maintenance choices would differ from non-GPA transplant recipients, proportions of the actual medications chosen were similar between groups. The majority (79.6%) chose anti-thymocyte globulin and IV steroid (81.5%) for induction, while majority for maintenance was MMF (98.2%), tacrolimus (94.5%), and PO steroid (67.3%).

4. Discussion

This survey revealed notably that, for GPA presenting with glomerulonephritis (Scenario A), an induction preference emerged for Rheum towards Rituximab + Cyclophosphamide and Neph towards Cyclophosphamide. The adult RAVE trial showed noninferiority of Rituximab to Cyclophosphamide for induction, as well as noninferiority in achieving complete remission rates at 6, 12, or 18 months in the follow-up RITUXVAS trial [6, 7]. However, the RAVE trial did not include dialysis-dependent patients at the time of presentation or those with serum creatinine >4 mg/dL, characteristics that might be seen in a presentation of RPGN as with Scenario B. No trial has compared combination therapy (Cyclophosphamide + Rituximab) versus monotherapy for induction to our knowledge. One possible reason for the preferred combination is perhaps a perception of a more severe disease in pediatric than adult patients with GPA and glomerulonephritis. An alternative explanation is that the combination choice may allow for a reduced dose of

Cyclophosphamide to decrease toxicity, which is suggested by these data which showed more Rheum chose a starting dose of 750 mg/m^2 for Cyclophosphamide alone but the median dose was 500 mg/m^2 for the combination Cyclophosphamide + Rituximab.

The percentage of those choosing induction plasmapheresis for Scenarios B and C (roughly 35-50%) is not as high as would be expected if individuals follow or agree with the EULAR recommendations, where it is stated that plasma exchange should be considered for patients with RPGN or pulmonary hemorrhage (Statement #6, grades of evidence 1B and C, respectively) [5]. The rationale for choosing IV steroid as the lone induction agent for a minority of Neph respondents is unclear, but perhaps reflects a misunderstanding of the question or area for further investigation. Practice experience level and patient volume did differ for some induction responses, but did not have a consistent effect to explain differences revealed by this study.

There was little consensus overall on maintenance therapies or strategies; for example, no consensus emerged for the total duration of maintenance therapy, duration of steroid, or reason for using TMP-SMX. The overall 50% use of Azathioprine for maintenance was lower than expected, considering the findings of the IMPROVE [8] and WEGENT [9] trials that showed Azathioprine is superior to MMF or Methotrexate with fewer adverse events in adult GPA studies. Most Rheum use Rituximab for maintenance (and first-line induction) in line with the findings of the adult MAINRITSAN trial [10], where Rituximab was found to be superior for major relapses over 28 months compared to maintenance Azathioprine. Despite the majority of Rheum choosing Rituximab for both induction and maintenance, there was no consensus on the total duration of maintenance therapy revealing an area for investigation. The specialty differences in induction and maintenance preference found by this survey may reflect subspecialty favor of the medications based on experience with other diseases. For example, Cyclophosphamide and MMF are commonly used in systemic lupus erythematosus and other conditions and may explain the Neph preference for these agents. Additionally, if a provider is expecting that a GPA patient will eventually need renal transplantation, they might choose MMF for maintenance of GPA in planning the continuation of this medication for maintenance after transplantation.

Finally, Section 5 of the survey revealed some areas for consensus building but also areas that require further investigation. Limited adult data exist on renal transplant outcomes in GPA, and it is not clear whether the findings in the literature can be extrapolated to pediatrics. It is not unexpected that the rates of Rheum answering "unsure–I do not manage dialysis or transplant" were higher than Neph; however the absolute numbers choosing this option varied by question in this section. This may indicate that some rheumatologists do have practice preferences for some ESRD/dialysis management questions but not others, and is worth exploring in future studies. For example, 42 out of 55 Rheum were unsure of dialysis modality choice when considering infection risk, but only 32 out of 55 were unsure

TABLE 3: Management of GPA with end-stage renal disease.

Survey Question	Specialty, N	Yes, %	No, %	Unsure, %	p-value
Aside from routine considerations of modality, do you PREFER Hemodialysis over Peritoneal Dialysis (PD) because of the risk of infection from immunosuppression on PD?	Rheum, 55	9.1	14.5	76.4	P=0.019
	Neph, 63	17.4	74.6	7.94	
Once a patient is on dialysis, do you try to taper off the immunosuppression earlier than a non-dialysis GPA patient?	Rheum, 55	5.5	36.4	58.2	<0.0001
	Neph, 60	28.3	70.0	1.7	
Do you wait for ANCA titer to become negative before listing for transplant?	Rheum, 55	3.6	16.4	80.0	<0.0001
	Neph, 59	30.5	55.9	13.6	
Do you believe ANCA titer positivity AT THE TIME OF RENAL TRANSPLANT influences graft survival or vasculitis relapse rate?	Rheum, 55	7.3	9.1	83.6	<0.0001
	Neph, 58	25.8	51.7	22.4	
Is your renal transplant INDUCTION immunosuppression for a patient with GPA any different than a non-GPA renal transplant patient?	Rheum, 54	3.7	3.7	92.6	<0.0001
	Neph, 59	18.6	64.4	17.0	
Is your renal transplant MAINTENANCE immunosuppression for a patient with GPA any different than a non-GPA renal transplant patient?	Rheum, 55	3.6	3.6	92.7	<0.0001
	Neph, 59	20.3	66.1	13.6	

whether immunosuppression should be tapered sooner than non-dialysis GPA patients. The variance in Rheum selection of the unsure option may reflect the cooperative management relationship between Neph and Rheum for these patients, even after a patient has developed ESRD. Overall, most respondents do not wait for ANCA to be negative at time of transplant nor believe it influences risk of relapse which is supported by a retrospective adult study [11]. However 25% of respondents in this survey would transplant at less than 12 months in remission, which in the same study was associated with graft loss. ANCA disease relapse is reported to be low once patients are on chronic dialysis, but rates of infectious episodes while on chronic dialysis are high at 1.92/person-year [12, 13]. Some experts recommend hemodialysis over peritoneal dialysis for this reason, but no trials have specifically addressed this. Our survey did not find a preference for hemodialysis when considering infection risk. Lee et al. recommended from their analysis that continued immunosuppression after 4 months in ESRD dialysis-dependent patients is unlikely to be individually beneficial weighing the risks and benefits [14]. While a comprehensive study addressing the risk of infection versus benefit of continued immunosuppression while on dialysis has not been undertaken, the 75.6% response rate (excluding unsure responses) that immunosuppression course would not be shortened conflicts with the prior recommendations, revealing an area for future study. Co-management of these children even after ESRD is warranted based on the lack of data and variability of practice patterns.

5. Conclusion

This survey has revealed differences in practice patterns between specialties, with a few trends noted. Rituximab + Cyclophosphamide is a more common induction choice for rheumatologists than nephrologists in Scenarios A and B, whereas Cyclophosphamide is more commonly chosen by nephrologists in Scenario A. Plasmapheresis rates increased for Scenarios A, B, and C for both specialties, but were not as frequently chosen as one would expect if EULAR recommendations were followed. Variability found in this survey may be explained by a multitude of reasons: pediatric GPA patients with glomerulonephritis may be perceived to be more ill or not fit the recommendations extrapolated from adult trials; specialists may not be familiar with the most recent study results or recommendations as they encounter pediatric GPA patients rarely with majority following 2-4 in the practice; specialists may apply knowledge of management of other conditions to management of GPA contrary to recommendations; and the lack of evidence-based consensus statements or clinical trials for pediatric-specific GPA leads to varied practice patterns.

This survey has revealed important differences in the way that rheumatologists and nephrologists manage this disease. It has identified a need for improved dissemination of evidence-based results to influence practice patterns and reveals that both specialties must be represented during consensus-building and clinical trial design efforts. This study

also underlines the need for well-designed controlled trials in pediatric GPA patients.

Abbreviations

MWPNC: Midwest Pediatric Nephrology Consortium
GPA: Granulomatosis with polyangiitis
AAV: ANCA-associated vasculitis
MMF: Mycophenolate Mofetil
TMP-SMX: Trimethoprim-sulfamethoxazole.

Disclosure

No direct funding source was used for this work.

Authors' Contributions

Dr. Kaspar conceptualized and designed the study, drafted the initial manuscript, and revised and reviewed the final manuscript. Drs. Kidd, Lo, and Bunchman contributed to the design of the study and revised and reviewed the final manuscript. Drs. Sanderson, Ozen, Verghese, and Wenderfer revised and reviewed the final manuscript. All authors approved the final manuscript as submitted and agree to be accountable for all aspects of the work.

Acknowledgments

Use of REDCap for data collection and management was supported by a VCU institutional Award no. UL1TR000058 from the NCRR. The authors thank Dr. Sarah Hoffmann, MD, Virginia Commonwealth University Health System, Children's Hospital of Richmond, Pediatric Rheumatology, USA, for her contributions to the survey design.

References

[1] D. A. Cabral, D. L. Canter, E. Muscal et al., "Comparing Presenting Clinical Features in 48 Children With Microscopic Polyangiitis to 183 Children Who Have Granulomatosis With Polyangiitis (Wegener's): An ARChiVe Cohort Study," *Arthritis Rheumatol*, vol. 68, no. 10, pp. 2514–2526, 2016.

[2] M. Twilt, S. Benseler, and D. Cabral, "Granulomatosis with polyangiitis in childhood," *Current Rheumatology Reports*, vol. 14, no. 2, pp. 107–115, 2012.

[3] M. Bohm, M. I. Gonzalez Fernandez, S. Ozen et al., "Clinical features of childhood granulomatosis with polyangiitis (wegener's granulomatosis)," *Pediatric Rheumatology*, vol. 12, article 18, 2014.

[4] S. Ozen, A. Pistorio, and S. M. Iusan, "EULAR/PRINTO/PRES criteria for Henoch-Schönlein purpura, childhood polyarteritis nodosa, childhood Wegener granulomatosis and childhood Takayasu arteritis: Ankara 2008. Part II: final classification criteria," *Annals of the Rheumatic Diseases*, vol. 69, no. 5, pp. 798–806, 2010.

[5]   M. Yates, R. A. Watts, I. M. Bajema et al., "EULAR/ERA-EDTA recommendations for the management of ANCA-associated vasculitis," *Annals of the Rheumatic Diseases*, vol. 75, no. 9, pp. 1583–1594, 2016.

[6]   D. Geetha, U. Specks, J. H. Stone et al., "Rituximab versus cyclophosphamide for ANCA-associated vasculitis with renal involvement," *Journal of the American Society of Nephrology*, vol. 26, no. 4, pp. 976–985, 2015.

[7]   R. B. Jones, S. Furuta, J. W. C. Tervaert et al., "Rituximab versus cyclophosphamide in ANCA-associated renal vasculitis: 2-year results of a randomised trial," *Annals of the Rheumatic Diseases*, vol. 74, no. 6, pp. 1178–1182, 2015.

[8]   T. F. Hiemstra, M. Walsh, A. Mahr et al., "Mycophenolate mofetil vs azathioprine for remission maintenance in antineutrophil cytoplasmic antibody-associated vasculitis: a randomized controlled trial," *The Journal of the American Medical Association*, vol. 304, no. 21, pp. 2381–2388, 2010.

[9]   C. Pagnoux, A. Mahr, M. A. Hamidou et al., "Azathioprine or methotrexate maintenance for ANCA-associated vasculitis," *The New England Journal of Medicine*, vol. 359, no. 26, pp. 2790–2803, 2008.

[10] L. Guillevin, C. Pagnoux, A. Karras et al., "Rituximab versus azathioprine for maintenance in ANCA-associated vasculitis," *The New England Journal of Medicine*, vol. 371, no. 19, pp. 1771–1780, 2014.

[11] M. A. Little, B. Hassan, S. Jacques et al., "Renal transplantation in systemic vasculitis: When is it safe," *Nephrology Dialysis Transplantation* , vol. 24, no. 10, pp. 3219–3225, 2009.

[12] R. Goupil, S. Brachemi, A.-C. Nadeau et al., "Lymphopenia and treatment-related infectious complications in ANCA-associated vasculitis," *Clinical Journal of the American Society of Nephrology*, vol. 8, no. 3, pp. 416–423, 2013.

[13] M. Romeu, C. Couchoud, J.-C. Delarozière et al., "Survival of patients with ANCA-associated vasculitis on chronic dialysis: Data from the French REIN registry from 2002 to 2011," *QJM: An International Journal of Medicine*, vol. 107, no. 7, Article ID hcu043, pp. 545–555, 2014.

[14] T. Lee, A. Gasim, V. K. Derebail et al., "Predictors of treatment outcomes in ANCA-associated vasculitis with severe kidney failure," *Clinical Journal of the American Society of Nephrology*, vol. 9, no. 5, pp. 905–913, 2014.

Undiagnosed Kidney Injury in Uninsured and Underinsured Diabetic African American Men and Putative Role of Meprin Metalloproteases in Diabetic Nephropathy

Lei Cao,[1] **Rashin Sedighi,**[1] **Ava Boston,**[1] **Lakmini Premadasa,**[1] **Jamilla Pinder,**[2] **George E. Crawford,**[1] **Olugbemiga E. Jegede,**[2] **Scott H. Harrison,**[1] **Robert H. Newman,**[1] **and Elimelda Moige Ongeri**[1]

[1]*Department of Biology, North Carolina A&T State University, Greensboro, NC 27411, USA*
[2]*Cone Health Community Health and Wellness Center, Greensboro, NC 27401, USA*

Correspondence should be addressed to Elimelda Moige Ongeri; eongeri@ncat.edu

Academic Editor: Jaime Uribarri

Diabetes is the leading cause of chronic kidney disease. African Americans are disproportionately burdened by diabetic kidney disease (DKD) and end stage renal disease (ESRD). Disparities in DKD have genetic and socioeconomic components, yet its prevalence in African Americans is not adequately studied. The current study used multiple biomarkers of DKD to evaluate undiagnosed DKD in uninsured and underinsured African American men in Greensboro, North Carolina. Participants consisted of three groups: nondiabetic controls, diabetic patients without known kidney disease, and diabetic patients with diagnosed DKD. Our data reveal undiagnosed kidney injury in a significant proportion of the diabetic patients, based on levels of both plasma and urinary biomarkers of kidney injury, namely, urinary albumin to creatinine ratio, kidney injury molecule-1, cystatin C, and neutrophil gelatinase-associated lipocalin. We also found that the urinary levels of meprin A, meprin B, and two kidney meprin targets (nidogen-1 and monocytes chemoattractant protein-1) increased with severity of kidney injury, suggesting a potential role for meprin metalloproteases in the pathophysiology of DKD in this subpopulation. The study also demonstrates a need for more aggressive tests to assess kidney injury in uninsured diabetic patients to facilitate early diagnosis and targeted interventions that could slow progression to ESRD.

1. Introduction

Diabetic kidney disease (DKD) is the leading cause of end stage renal disease (ESRD). Minority ethnic groups in the United States (e.g., African Americans, Native Americans, and Hispanics) are disproportionately affected by DKD. A 2008 US Renal Data Systems survey showed that ESRD rates associated with diabetes are three times higher in African Americans than in their Caucasian counterparts, with the percentage of new cases of kidney disease attributed to diabetes among young African Americans currently standing at 43%. The prevalence of type 2 diabetes is related to nutrition and sedentary lifestyles [1], which promote obesity and are associated with the metabolic syndrome. The most recent data on obesity in the US indicate that 40% of the adult population is obese [2]. Even more alarmingly, the same study shows a rising prevalence of obesity among the young, with 18.5% of children in the United States being obese. This trend in obesity is likely going to further exacerbate the current diabetes epidemic. Furthermore, the prevalence of obesity is significantly higher among Hispanics and African Americans of all age categories [2]. Other previous studies had shown that African Americans have greater adjusted odds of having diabetes compared to Caucasian Americans [3]. Other factors contributing to health disparities in diabetes include disparities in healthcare resource allocation [1, 4], healthcare utilization [4], quality of diabetes care, perceived self-efficacy, and susceptibility genes [5]. Minority men are at a markedly elevated risk for the receipt of low-quality healthcare. Studies have shown that the differences in ESRD care that African American and Caucasian American men have received are statistically significant [6], with African American men consistently receiving worse care.

While susceptibility genes are known to contribute to the disparities in DKD, the cellular and molecular mechanisms involved in its progression are not fully understood. Such knowledge is important for the development of therapies and diagnostic tools that are efficacious for people from diverse ethnic backgrounds. Recently, several protein biomarkers have been developed that may offer insights into the molecular mechanisms of disease pathology. These include the type I transmembrane glycoprotein, kidney injury marker-1 (KIM-1), the cysteine-protease inhibitor, cystatin C, and the ubiquitous lipocalin family member, neutrophil gelatinase-associated lipocalin (NGAL) [7–9]. Meprin zinc metalloproteases, which are abundantly expressed in the brush border membranes (BBM) of renal proximal tubules, have also emerged as susceptibility markers for DKD [10]. Meprins are also expressed in podocytes [11] and leukocytes (monocytes and macrophages) [12] and play a role in inflammation, an underlying cause of fibrosis as observed in DKD. Meprins are composed of two subunits, α and β, encoded by distinct genes on chromosomes 6 and 18, respectively, in humans [13, 14], and on chromosomes 17 and 18, respectively, in mice [15]. Oligomerization of meprins results in two protein isoforms, meprin A (α-α or α-β) and meprin B (β-β). Meprin β gene polymorphisms were associated with DKD in the Pima Indians, an ethnic group in the United States with an extremely high incidence of type 2 diabetes and subsequent ESRD [10]. Interestingly, both the expression and the activity of meprins decrease at the onset of diabetic kidney injury in rodent models [16].

Consistent with how decreased meprin activity relates to kidney injury, we recently showed that meprin $\alpha\beta$ double knockout mice exhibit more severe kidney injury upon streptozotocin-induced type 1 diabetes [17]. *In vitro* and *in vivo* studies have identified several kidney meprin targets that play a role in renal fibrosis. For example, meprins are capable of cleaving and/or degrading several extracellular matrix (ECM) proteins, such as procollagen III, collagen IV, laminin, fibronectin, and nidogen-1 [18–22]. Since renal pathological changes seen in DKD are a direct consequence of accumulation of ECM proteins [23–26] due to excess production and/or reduced degradation of ECM proteins, meprins could play a role in modulating this imbalance. Other studies have shown that meprins proteolytically process proteins involved in inflammation, an underlying process for renal fibrosis [27]. Such modulators of inflammation include proinflammatory cytokines (e.g., interleukin 1β (IL-1β) [28], IL-6 [29, 30], IL-18 [31]) and monocyte chemoattractant protein-1 (MCP-1 [32]) as well as the proteolytic release of the anti-inflammatory molecule, N-acetyl-seryl-aspartyl-lysyl-proline (Ac-SDKP) from thymosin β4 [33]. The objectives of the current study were to use recently developed protein biomarkers to evaluate undiagnosed kidney injury among uninsured and underinsured African American men in Greensboro, NC. We further sought to determine whether the levels of urinary meprins and their targets correlate with the existence and/or the severity of kidney injury.

2. Materials and Methods

2.1. Subjects. Diabetic African American men aged 18–65 years were recruited through the Cone Health Community Health and Wellness Center in Greensboro, North Carolina, a facility that primarily serves uninsured and underinsured patients. This study was approved by the North Carolina A&T State University and Cone Health Institutional Review Boards (IRB). Written informed consent was obtained from each study participant. Age-matched, nondiabetic controls were also recruited through the Community Health and Wellness Center and local faith-based organizations. Three groups were included: (i) diabetic patients without known kidney disease ($n = 76$); (ii) diabetic patients with diagnosed kidney disease ($n = 21$); and (iii) age-matched nondiabetic controls ($n = 75$). Surveys were administered to establish patient profiles and family medical history. Medical information was provided by participants through surveys and verified using medical records. Patients with ESRD and other chronic disease conditions were excluded. All patient data were deidentified prior to analysis.

2.2. Determination of Anthropometric Data Related to the Metabolic Syndrome. The height and body weight of each participant were measured during their visit and used to compute the body mass index. Additionally, blood pressure and waist circumference were measured.

2.3. Collection of Blood and Urine Samples. Fasting blood and urine samples were collected from the three groups of patients. The diabetic status for the nondiabetic control group was confirmed by measuring fasting glucose levels using a glucose meter (ReliOn®). Blood samples were obtained by trained phlebotomists via intravenous route, collected into heparin tubes, and stored on ice for an average of one hour before being processed to obtain plasma. To obtain plasma, the blood samples were centrifuged at 2,750 ×g for 15 minutes at 4°C using an Allegra X-14R centrifuge (Beckman Coulter, Brea, CA). The plasma was then aliquoted into microfuge tubes and stored at −80°C until proteomic analysis. Urine samples were also held on ice before being aliquoted and stored at −80°C until analysis.

2.4. Assessment of Kidney Injury. For biochemical assessment of kidney injury, we performed assays for traditional biomarkers of kidney injury, namely, urinary albumin and creatinine, which were then used to calculate the urinary albumin to creatinine ratio (UACR). The UACR is the current gold standard for clinical diagnosis of DKD. Albumin assays utilized Albuwell® ELISA kits from Exocell (Philadelphia, PA) while creatinine was measured using a calorimetric assay kit from Diazyme Laboratories (Poway, CA). We also determined the levels of three recently developed protein markers of kidney injury, namely, KIM-1, cystatin C, and

NGAL using enzyme-linked immunosorbent assay (ELISA) (R&D Systems, Minneapolis, MN). All of the assays were performed according to the manufacturers' instructions with absorbance being read at 450 nm using a F500 Pro multimode microplate reader (Tecan, USA). Standard curves for all biomarkers except albumin were generated using four parameter logistic (4-PL) curve fits (GraphPad Prism software). Standard curves for albumin were generated using log-log regression, according to the manufacturer's instructions. The urinary levels of each kidney injury marker were normalized to the urinary creatinine levels.

2.5. Western Blot Analysis for Urinary Meprins and Nidogen-1. Western blot analysis was used to determine the urinary levels of meprin A, meprin B, and nidogen-1, according to previously described protocols [34–36]. Briefly, 25 μl of the urine samples were combined with SDS loading buffer supplemented with β-mercaptoethanol and heated at 80°C for 5 minutes. Three or four representative samples from each group were then resolved on the same 8% polyacrylamide gel under denaturing conditions. Following electrophoresis, the proteins were transferred to a nitrocellulose membrane, blocked in blocking buffer (5% nonfat dry milk dissolved in tris-buffered saline, 0.05% Tween-20 (TBS-T)), and then probed with primary antibodies for meprin A (HMC14, rabbit polyclonal, diluted 1 : 3300 in blocking buffer), meprin B (HMC77, rabbit polyclonal diluted 1 : 5000 in blocking buffer), or nidogen-1 (Millipore; rat polyclonal diluted 1 : 1000 in blocking buffer). The HMC14 and HMC77 antibodies were a gift from Dr. Judith Bond (Penn State Hershey Medical Center). Following incubation with the primary antibody solution, membranes were washed three times in TBS-T for 15 min each and then incubated with corresponding secondary antibodies conjugated to horse radish peroxidase (Bio-Rad, diluted 1 : 10,000 in TBS-T). Finally, membranes were washed three times in TBS-T for 15 min each before the addition of chemiluminescence substrate (Thermo Scientific, Waltham, MA). Protein bands were detected by exposure to X-ray film or by exposure of the membrane to Amersham Imager 600 (GE Healthcare, Chicago, IL). The Western blots were repeated for a total of 9 or 12 samples from each subcategory. We first grouped samples based on self-reported and diagnosed diabetes status, with 4 representative samples from each group (diabetics, diabetics with DKD, and nondiabetic controls) included in each gel. Subsequent blots grouped the samples from diabetic patients without diagnosed kidney disease based on their UACR levels, with 3 samples from each group included in each gel, that is, (i) nondiabetic, (ii) normoalbuminuria (UACR < 30 mg/g), (iii) microalbuminuria (30 mg/g ≤ UACR ≤ 300 mg/g), and (iv) macroalbuminuria (UACR > 300 mg/g).

2.6. Assays for MCP-1. We performed assays for a second meprin target, monocyte chemoattractant protein 1 (MCP-1), using ELISA kits (R&D Systems) according to the manufacturer's instructions. Standard curves generated using 4-PL curve fits (GraphPad Prism) were used to determine the MCP-1 concentrations. Urinary MCP-1 levels were normalized to the urine creatinine levels in each sample.

2.7. Statistical Analysis. The data were analyzed by one-way ANOVA and Tukey's honest significant difference test (GraphPad Prism Software). Logarithmic transformation was conducted for the kidney injury biomarker values (i.e., UACR, KIM-1, Cystatin C, NGAL) and MCP-1 before statistical analysis. To identify the diabetic subjects with high risk for kidney injury, the mean, standard deviation, upper quartile (Q3), and interquartile range (IQR) from the nondiabetic group were calculated. Diabetic subjects with values greater than mean + 2SD and Q3 + 1.5IQR of the nondiabetic group were considered to be at high risk for DKD.

3. Results

3.1. Anthropometric Data Related to the Metabolic Syndrome. Since the metabolic syndrome is often associated with diabetes mellitus, we first assessed various measures of obesity and cardiovascular health among members of each group. Based on BMI measurements, the majority of the participants in our study were either overweight (25.0 ≤ BMI ≤ 29.9) or obese (BMI ≥ 30), with no significant differences between nondiabetic and diabetic participants (Table 1 and Figures 1(a) and 1(b)). On the other hand, significant differences were observed in the mean waist circumference of diabetic and nondiabetic patients (Table 1 and Figure 1(d); p=0.0002). Notably, a substantially larger proportion of diabetic patients (70.8%) had a waist circumference > 102 cm compared to nondiabetic patients (39.1%) (Figure 1(c)). Finally, 77.0% of nondiabetic and 85.1% of diabetic participants were prehypertensive (120 mm Hg ≤ systolic bp ≤ 139 mm Hg or 80 mm Hg ≤ diastolic BP ≤ 89 mm Hg), hypertensive stage 1 (140 mmHg ≤ systolic BP ≤ 159 mm Hg or 90 mm Hg ≤ diastolic BP ≤ 99 mm Hg), or hypertensive stage 2 (systolic BP ≥ 160 mm Hg, or diastolic BP ≥ 100 mm Hg) (Table 1 and Figures 2(a)–2(d)).

3.2. Undiagnosed Kidney Injury in Diabetic Patients. To assess the incidence of kidney injury within each group, we first determined the UACR for each participant based on his albumin and creatinine levels (Figure 3(a)). While the average UACRs of both the diabetic patients and the patients with diagnosed DKD were significantly higher than those of the nondiabetic controls, the average UACR in the diabetic group was significantly lower than that of patients with diagnosed DKD ($p = 0.01$ after transformation). Interestingly, there was a large degree of variation in UACRs among the diabetic patients, suggesting that members of this group may exhibit varying degrees of kidney injury (Figure 3(a), bottom panel). Therefore, in subsequent analyses, we used the UACRs to further subdivide the diabetic participants without known kidney disease into three subgroups: normoalbuminuria (UACR < 30 mg/g); microalbuminuria (30 mg/g ≤ UACR ≤ 300 mg/g); and macroalbuminuria (UACR > 300 mg/g) (Figure 3(b)). Among the diabetic patients, 54.0% (41/76) had an UACR characteristic of normoalbuminuria, 35.5% (27/76) had UACR indicative of microalbuminuria, and 10.5% (8/76) had UACR in the macroalbuminuria range. Moreover, five of the participants in the microalbuminuria subgroup (5/27, 18.5%) exhibited UACR levels between 200 and 300 mg/g, placing them near the borderline between micro- and

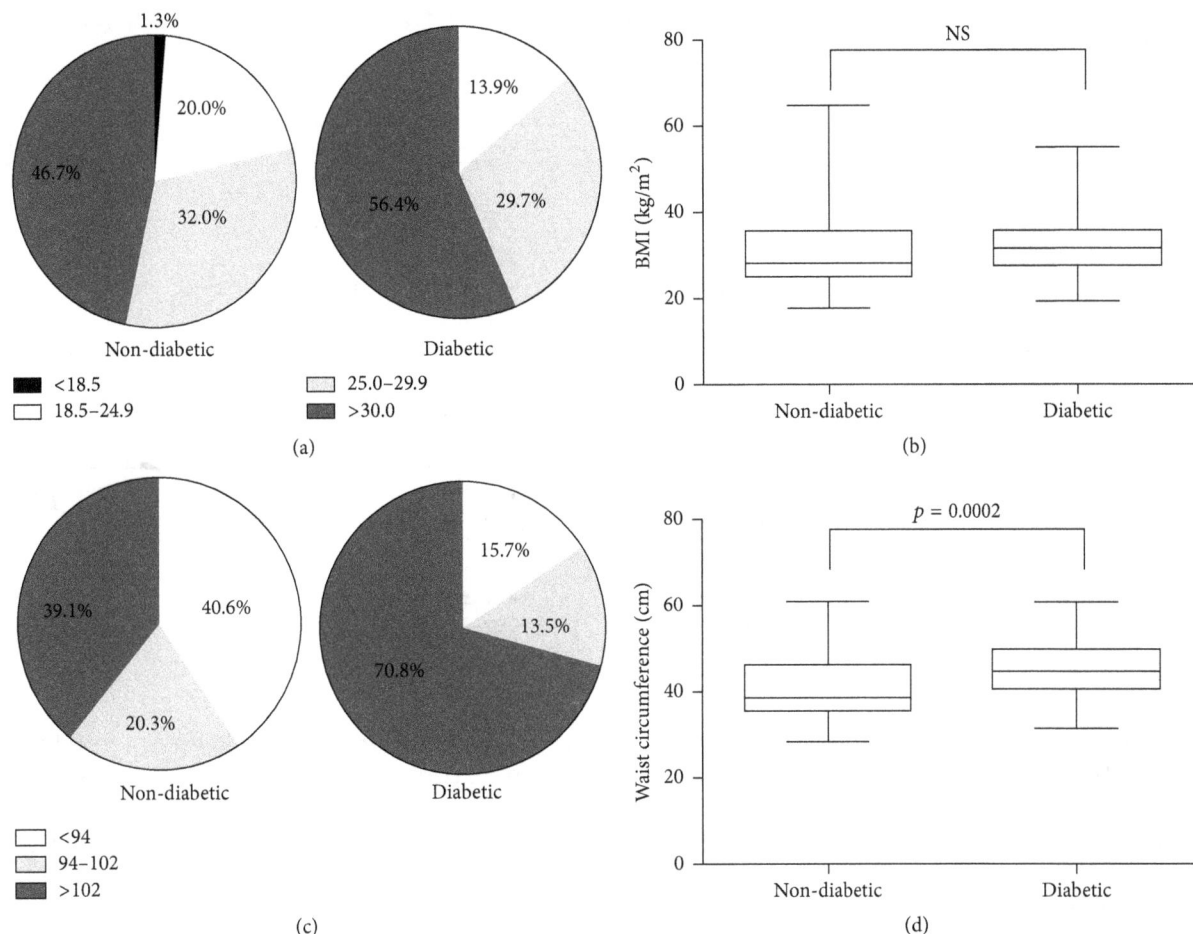

FIGURE 1: *Anthropometric data related to the metabolic syndrome.* (a) BMI distribution in nondiabetic and diabetic groups showing the proportion of underweight (BMI < $18.5 \, \text{kg/m}^2$), normal weight ($18.5 \, \text{kg/m}^2 \leq$ BMI $\leq 24.9 \, \text{kg/m}^2$), overweight ($25.0 \, \text{kg/m}^2 \leq$ BMI $\leq 29.9 \, \text{kg/m}^2$), and obese ($30.0 \, \text{kg/m}^2 \leq$ BMI) in nondiabetic ($n = 75$) and diabetic ($n = 85$) groups. (b) Box plots of BMI for nondiabetic and diabetic groups. The upper and lower whiskers indicate the maximum and minimum values. The upper and lower borders of the box indicate the 25th and the 75th percentile, respectively. The black line in each box indicates the median. (c) Waist circumference (WC) distribution in nondiabetic and diabetic groups showing the proportion of normal waist circumference (WC < 94 cm), increased health risk (94 cm $\leq$ WC $\leq$ 102 cm), and substantial health risk (102 cm < WC) in nondiabetic ($n = 69$) and diabetic ($n = 85$) groups. (d) Box plots of WC for nondiabetic and diabetic groups. The upper and lower whiskers indicate the maximum and minimum values, respectively. The upper and lower borders of the box indicate the 25th and the 75th percentile, respectively. The black line in each box indicates the median. NS indicates no significant difference.

macroalbuminuria. This distribution suggested that a significant proportion of the diabetic patients may have varying degrees of undiagnosed kidney injury. Therefore, we used a series of recently developed proteomic markers of kidney injury to further interrogate the kidney injury status of the participants (Figures 4–6). For instance, KIM-1 is a type I transmembrane glycoprotein that has recently been correlated with kidney tissue damage in models of acute kidney injury as well as DKD [37–39]. Analysis of plasma KIM-1 levels revealed that diabetic patients had significantly higher plasma KIM-1 levels ($p < 0.0001$) than nondiabetic controls (Figure 4(a)). Moreover, when plasma KIM-1 values were compared between the diabetic and nondiabetic groups, 52% of the diabetic subjects had plasma KIM-1 values that were at least two standard deviations above the mean of the

nondiabetic group (Table 2). Perhaps more strikingly, 45% of the patients in the diabetic group exhibited plasma KIM-1 levels that were three standard deviations above the mean, further suggesting that a large proportion of the patients in the diabetes group may be suffering from undiagnosed kidney disease. Indeed, comparison among diabetic patients with varying UACR levels revealed significant differences between the subgroups (Figure 4(c)). In fact, plasma KIM-1 levels appear to correlate with severity of kidney injury (as determined by UACR), with diabetic patients with macroalbuminuria exhibiting significantly higher levels than diabetic patients with microalbuminuria, which exhibited significantly higher levels than diabetic patients with normoalbuminuria, which exhibited significantly higher levels than nondiabetic controls (Figure 4(c)).

TABLE 1: Clinical characteristics of subjects. Data are mean ± SD. *Note.* *p* value is calculated between controls and diabetic patients with or without known kidney disease. Values without a common letter (a, b, or ab) are significantly different.

(a)

	Nondiabetic controls	Diabetics	*p* value
n	75	85	
Age (years)	45.3 ± 12.8	49.3 ± 10.1	0.0215
Body mass index (kg/m^2)	30.5 ± 8.3	32.7 ± 7.9	0.0695
Waist circumstance (cm)	101.0 ± 17.7	112.7 ± 17.3	0.0002
Blood pressure (mmHg)			
Systolic	135.9 ± 20.4	137.4 ± 19.8	0.6236
Diastolic	87.12 ± 12.8	86.2 ± 11.8	0.6224

(b)

	Nondiabetic controls	*Diabetics*			*DKD*
		Normoalbuminuria	Microalbuminuria	Macroalbuminuria	
n	75	41	27	8	9
Age (years)	45.8 ± 12.8[a]	50.3 ± 11.2[a]	49.7 ± 8.9[a]	46.3 ± 12.2[a]	44.2 ± 8.9[a]
BMI (kg/m^2)	30.5 ± 7.7[a]	32.9 ± 8.0[a]	32.9 ± 7.5[a]	30.3 ± 6.3[a]	27.5 ± 4.2[a]
WC (cm)	101.0 ± 17.7[b]	114.3 ± 16.8[a]	112.8 ± 17.5[a]	102.6 ± 16.1[ab]	101.3 ± 13.15[ab]
Blood pressure					
Systolic (mmHg)	135.9 ± 20.4[a]	135.2 ± 19.9[a]	135.5 ± 16.4[a]	141.5 ± 32.6[a]	144 ± 21.4[a]
Diastolic (mmHg)	87.12 ± 12.8[a]	85.2 ± 12.0[a]	86.1 ± 12.5[a]	86.1 ± 13.1[a]	89.6 ± 14.5[a]

TABLE 2: Biomarkers of kidney injury in diabetic patients with no known kidney disease, nondiabetic controls, and diabetics with diagnosed kidney disease. DM: diabetes mellitus; DKD: diabetic kidney disease; KIM-1: kidney injury molecule-1; NGAL: neutrophil gelatinase-associated lipocalin; MCP-1: monocyte chemoattractant protein-1; Q3: upper quartile; IQR: interquartile range.

Biomarker	Plasma KIM-1 (pg/ml)	Urine KIM-1 (μg/g Cr)	Plasma cystatin C (μg/ml)	Urine cystatin C (ng/g Cr)	Plasma NGAL (ng/ml)	Urine NGAL (ng/g Cr)
Range of nondiabetic group	(7.78, 63.44)	(0.16, 1.23)	(0.49, 1.21)	(5.29, 82.72)	(5.98, 76.64)	(0.43, 26.57)
Mean ± SD	30.39 ± 17.97	0.47 ± 0.30	0.87 ± 0.20	27.45 ± 20.74	41.75 ± 18.24	5.84 ± 5.71
>mean + 2SD in DM versus in DKD	52% versus 100%	23% versus 20%	17% versus 78%	19% versus 64%	17% versus 40%	24% versus 73%
>mean + 3SD in DM versus in DKD	45% versus 80%	12% versus 20%	11% versus 78%	14% versus 64%	13% versus 40%	21% versus 64%
Q3 ± IQR	46.56 ± 29.62	0.54 ± 0.31	0.97 ± 0.22	27.75 ± 11.95	55.44 ± 27.40	7.55 ± 5.04
>Q3 + 1.5 IQR in DM versus in DKD	40% versus 80%	25% versus 27%	17% versus 78%	43% versus 79%	13% versus 40%	24% versus 73%
>Q3 + 3 IQR in DM versus in DKD	24% v. 70%	10% versus 20%	11% versus 78%	21% versus 64%	6% versus 30%	21% versus 64%

We next investigated whether urinary KIM-1 levels also correlated with the extent of kidney injury among the participants in our study. To account for differences in urine concentration, during these analyses, we normalized urinary levels of KIM-1 to the creatinine levels for each subject. Though normalized urinary KIM-1 levels were elevated in diabetic patients compared to the nondiabetic controls, there was not a significant difference between the two groups (Figure 4(b)). However, subcategorization based on UACR revealed that diabetic patients with macroalbuminuria exhibited normalized urinary KIM-1 levels similar to those within the DKD group (Figure 4(d)). Importantly, the levels observed in the macroalbuminuria group were significantly higher than those of either the nondiabetic controls or the diabetic patients with normoalbuminuria (Figure 4(d)). Moreover, though the proportion of high urinary KIM-1 values among diabetic subjects was less than that observed for plasma KIM-1, 23% and 12% of the diabetic patients still exhibited urinary KIM-1 levels that were two and three standard deviations above the mean of the nondiabetic controls, respectively (Table 2). A similar distribution was also observed if the comparison was done using the upper quartile plus either 1.5

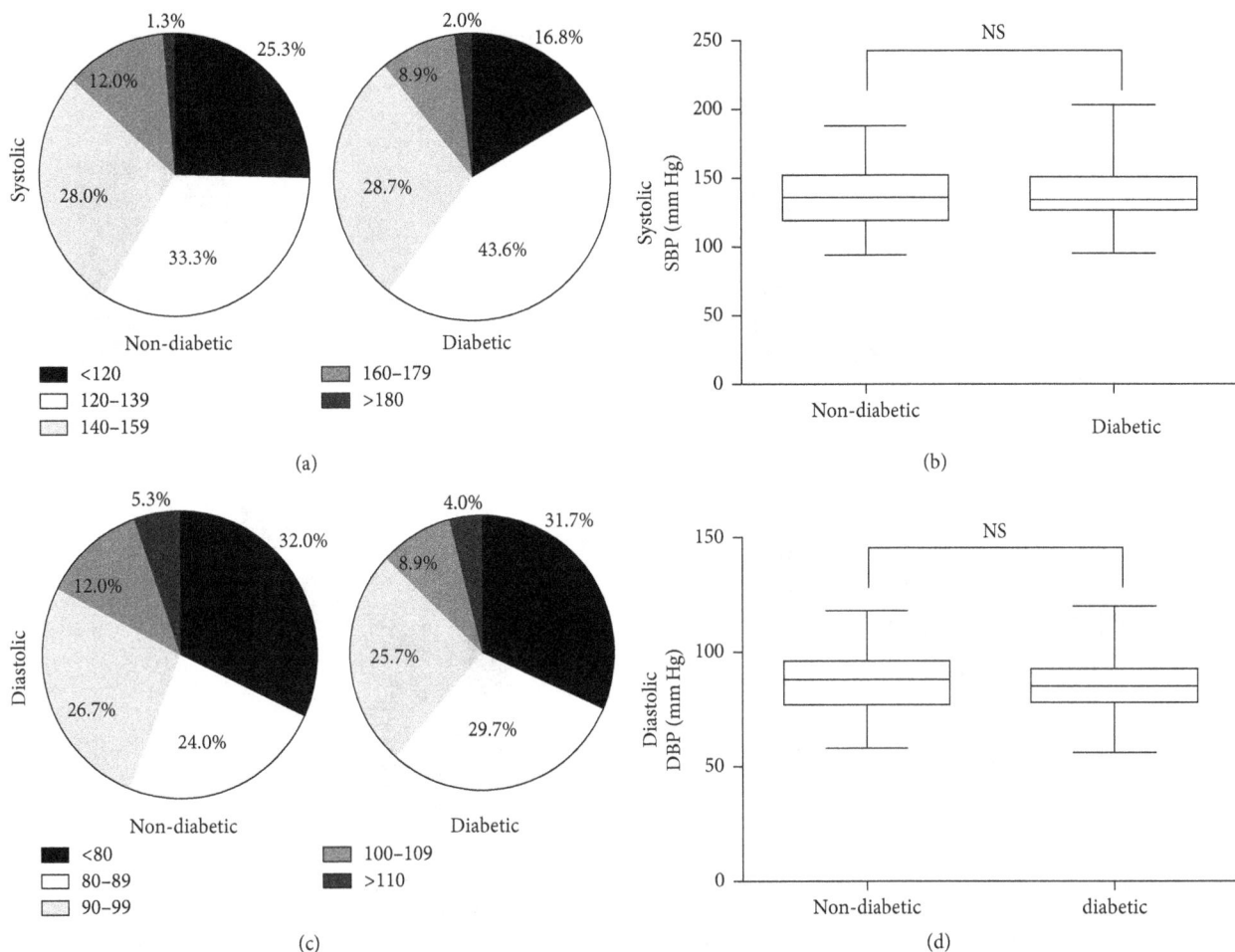

FIGURE 2: *Blood pressure measurements.* (a) Systolic blood pressure distribution in nondiabetic and diabetic groups showing the proportion of normal BP (80 mm Hg ≤ SBP < 119 mm Hg), prehypertension (120 mm Hg ≤ SBP ≤ 139 mm Hg), hypertension stage 1 (140 mm Hg ≤ SBP ≤ 159 mm Hg), and hypertension stage 2 (SBP ≤ 160 mm Hg) in nondiabetic ($n = 69$) and diabetic ($n = 85$) groups. (b) Box plot of systolic blood pressure for nondiabetic and diabetic groups. The upper and lower whiskers indicate the maximum and minimum values, respectively. The upper and lower borders of the box indicate the 25th and the 75th percentile, respectively, while the black line in each box indicates the median. (c) Diastolic blood pressure distribution in nondiabetic and diabetic groups showing the proportion of normal BP (60 mm Hg < DBP < 79 mm Hg), hypertension (80 mm Hg < DBP < 89 mm Hg), hypertension stage 1 (90 mm Hg ≤ DBP ≤ 99 mm Hg), and hypertension stage 2 (DBP ≤ 100 mm Hg). (d) Box plot of diastolic blood pressure for nondiabetic and diabetic groups. The upper and lower whiskers indicate the maximum and minimum values, respectively. The upper and lower borders of the box indicate the 25th and the 75th percentile, respectively. The black line in each box indicates the median. SBP: systolic blood pressure. DBP: diastolic blood pressure. NS indicates no significant difference.

times or 3 times the interquartile range (Table 2). Thus, KIM-1 appears to correlate well with the extent of kidney injury among the African American men in our study, with plasma KIM-1 showing a stronger correlation than urinary KIM-1.

Similar trends were also observed for two other emerging protein markers of kidney injury, namely, cystatin C and NGAL [38, 40]. For instance, both urinary and plasma cystatin C were significantly higher among patients with DKD compared to nondiabetic controls and diabetic patients without diagnosed DKD (Figures 5(a) and 5(b)). In contrast, only marginal increases were observed between the diabetic group and the nondiabetic controls (Figures 5(a) and 5(b)). However, within the diabetic group, patients with

macroalbuminuria exhibited significantly higher plasma cystatin C levels than either nondiabetic controls or diabetic patients with normoalbuminuria and microalbuminuria (Figure 6(a)). On the other hand, though normalized urinary cystatin C levels increased steadily as patients in the diabetic group progressed from normoalbuminuria to microalbuminuria to macroalbuminuria, the observed increases did not result in urinary cystatin C levels that were significantly higher than those observed in the nondiabetic group (Figure 6(b)). Indeed, only patients in the DKD group exhibited significantly higher levels of normalized urinary cystatin C. Interestingly, the percentage of participants whose cystatin C levels were two standard deviations above the mean of

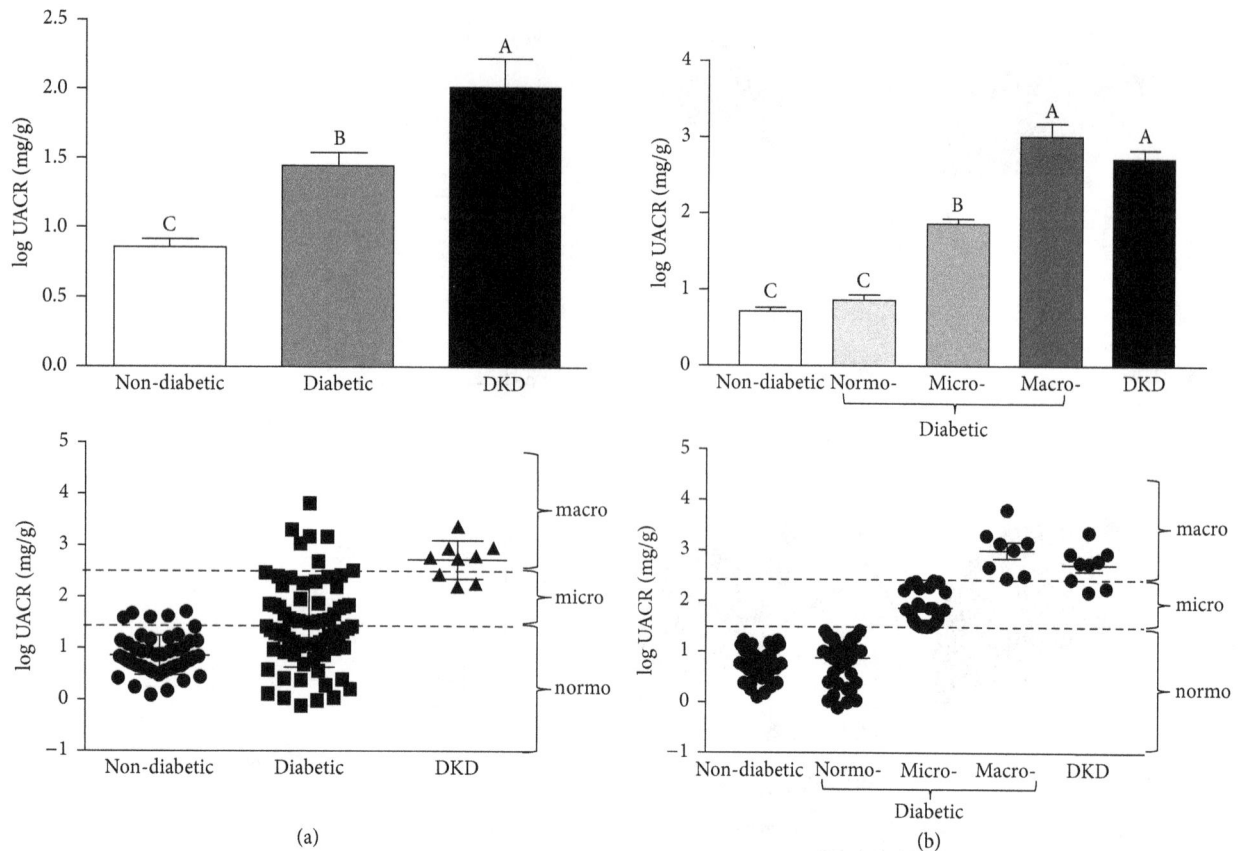

(a)   (b)

FIGURE 3: *Urinary albumin to creatinine ratios (UACRs).* (a) Log-transformed UACRs among nondiabetic controls, diabetic patients with no known kidney disease, and diabetic patients with diagnosed diabetic kidney disease (DKD). Data are represented as both a bar chart showing mean log UACR ± SEM within each group (top) and a scatter plot showing values for each individual within the group (bottom). UACR levels corresponding to normo- (log UACR < 1.47), micro- (1.47 < log UACR < 2.47), and macroalbuminuria (log UACR > 2.47) are indicated by dashed lines. (b) Log-transformed UACR as in (a), except that diabetic patients with no known kidney disease have been subdivided into normo-, micro-, and macroalbuminuria based on their UACRs. Labels without a common letter are significantly different from one another ($p < 0.05$) based on one-way ANOVA and Tukey's honest significant difference test.

the nondiabetic group was similar regardless of whether plasma or urinary cystatin C was considered (17% versus 19%, resp.) (Table 2). In contrast, when the interquartile range (IQR) was used to compare the groups, differences emerged between plasma and urinary cystatin C. For instance, while a similar percentage of subjects (17%) were found to be 1.5 IQR above the third quartile (Q3) when plasma cystatin C levels were used, a much larger percentage of subjects (43%) exhibited urinary cystatin C levels that were 1.5 IQR above Q3 (Table 2). Since IQR is more robust against outliers and nonnormal data, this may suggest that one or two outliers in the diabetic group may have resulted in a skewed or nonnormal distribution for the urinary cystatin C values. Like cystatin C, analysis of NGAL levels also revealed elevated levels in a subpopulation of the diabetic group. For example, though significantly higher levels of urine and plasma NGAL were only observed in patients with DKD when patients were grouped according to diabetic status alone (Figures 5(c) and 5(d)), closer examination revealed that diabetic patients with macroalbuminuria exhibited significantly higher NGAL levels than nondiabetic controls in both their plasma and

urine (Figures 6(c) and 6(d)). The percentages of diabetic subjects having plasma and urinary NGAL levels greater than two SD above the mean of nondiabetic subjects were 17% and 24%, respectively (Table 2). A similar distribution (13% and 24% for plasma and urinary NGAL, resp.) was observed if IQR was used for comparison. Together, the assays for proteomic markers of kidney function revealed undiagnosed kidney injury in a significant proportion of the diabetic patients (Table 2). This was true for assays utilizing traditional measures of kidney injury, that is, UACR (Figure 3), as well as a panel of recently developed proteomic markers of kidney injury (Table 2; Figures 4–6).

3.3. Elevated Urinary Levels of Meprins and Meprin Targets in Patients with Diabetic Kidney Injury. Next, to identify new biomarkers of DKD and to potentially gain mechanistic insights into disease progression, we asked whether the levels of meprins A and B correlated with DKD. When compared to nondiabetic controls, Western blot analysis revealed detectable levels of both meprin A and meprin B in diabetic patients with DKD and some diabetic patients

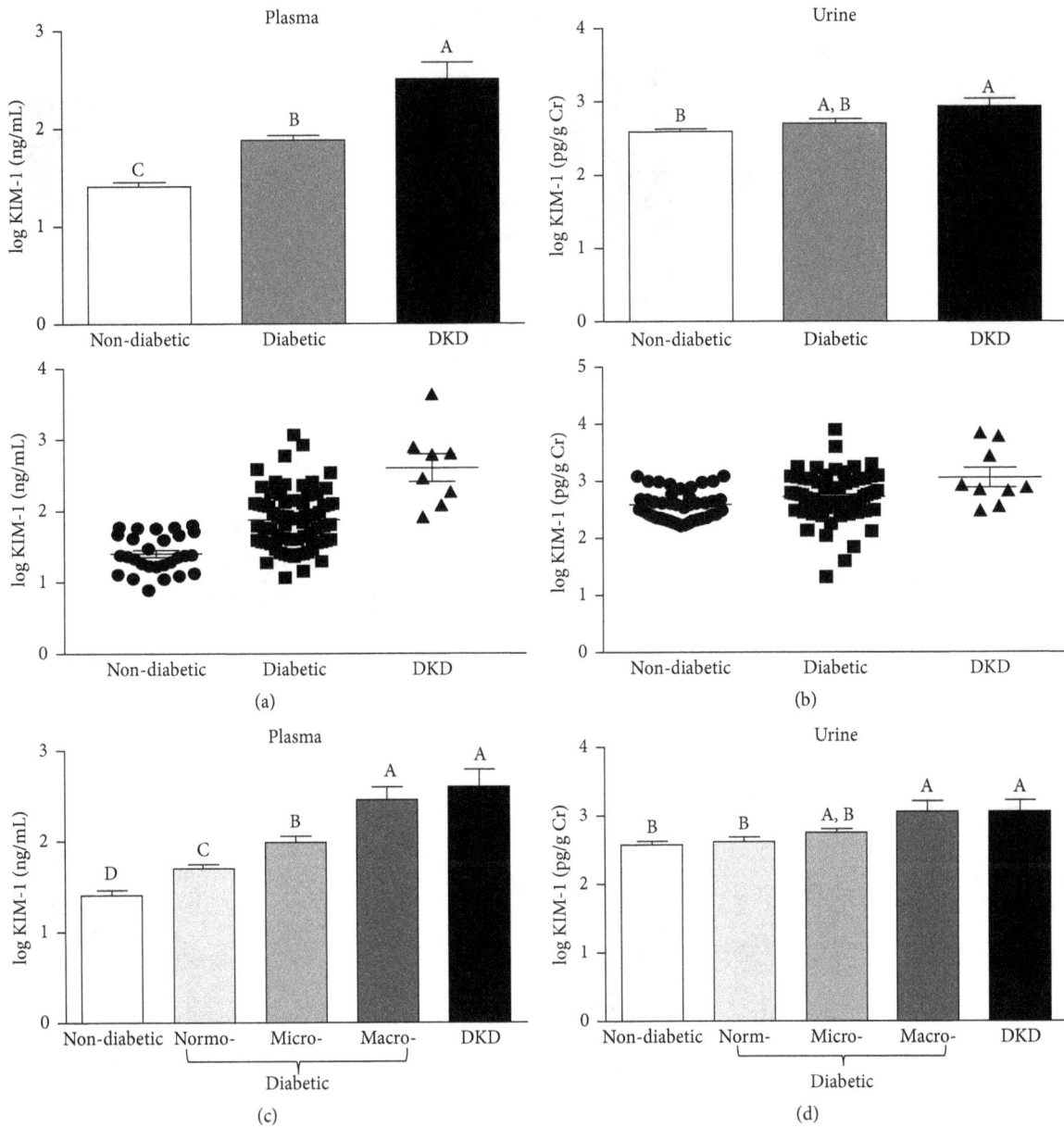

FIGURE 4: *Plasma and urinary kidney injury molecule-1 (KIM-1).* (a)-(b) Log-transformed plasma (a) and urinary (b) KIM-1 levels among nondiabetic subjects, diabetic patients with no known kidney disease (diabetic), and patients with diagnosed diabetic kidney disease (DKD). Urinary KIM-1 levels were normalized to creatinine to account for differences in urine concentration. Data are represented as both a bar chart showing mean log KIM-1 ± SEM within each group (top) and a scatter plot showing values for each individual within the group (bottom). (c)-(d) Log-transformed plasma (c) and urinary (d) KIM-1 levels among nondiabetic subjects, diabetic patients with normo-, micro, or macroalbuminuria, and patients with diagnosed diabetic kidney disease (DKD). Urinary KIM-1 was normalized to urinary creatinine. Data are represented as mean ± SEM. Labeled means without a common letter are significantly different from one another ($p < 0.05$) based on one-way ANOVA and Tukey's honest significant difference test.

without diagnosed kidney disease (Figure 7(a)). Importantly, similar to plasma KIM-1, the levels of urinary meprins were higher in patients with both micro- and macroalbuminuria, suggesting a positive correlation between urinary meprins and the severity of kidney injury (Figure 7(b)). The 90 kDa band corresponds to the expected size of shed monomeric meprins under reducing/denaturing conditions [41, 42]. To determine if the meprin levels were due to shedding or

general damage to the proximal tubules, we probed for villin, a cytoskeletal protein that is highly expressed in the BBM of proximal tubules. There were no detectable levels of villin in the urine from any of the groups evaluated (data not shown). We also demonstrated that patients with DKD exhibited relatively high levels of two meprin targets, nidogen-1 and MCP-1. For instance, while nidogen-1 was undetectable in patients with UACR ≤ 300 mg/g, the levels were much higher

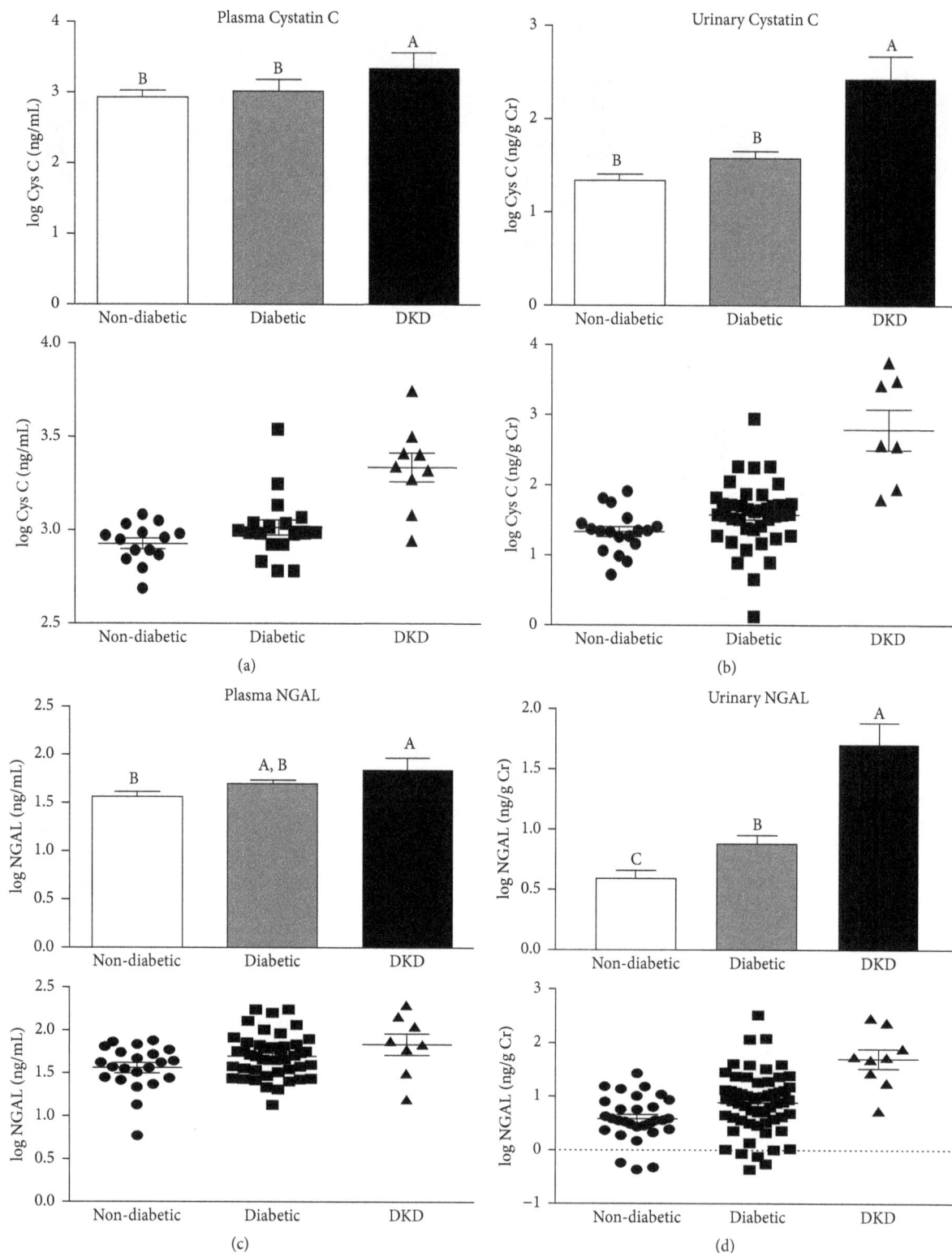

FIGURE 5: *Cystatin C and neutrophil gelatinase-associated lipocalin (NGAL) levels based on clinical diagnosis status.* (a)-(b) Log-transformed plasma (a) or urinary (b) cystatin C levels among nondiabetic subjects, diabetic patients with no known kidney disease (diabetic), and patients with diagnosed diabetic kidney disease (DKD). Urinary cystatin C levels were normalized to urinary creatinine to account for differences in urine concentration. Data are represented as both a bar chart showing mean log Cystatin C ± SEM within each group (top) and a scatter plot showing values for each individual within the group (bottom). (c)-(d) Log-transformed plasma (c) and (d) urinary NGAL levels among nondiabetic subjects, diabetic patients with no known kidney disease (diabetic), and patients with diagnosed diabetic kidney disease (DKD). Urinary NGAL levels were normalized to urinary creatinine to account for differences in urine concentration. Data are represented as both a bar chart showing mean log NGAL ± SEM within each group (top) and a scatter plot showing values for each individual within the group (bottom). Labeled means without a common letter are significantly different from one another ($p < 0.05$) based on one-way ANOVA and Tukey's honest significant difference test.

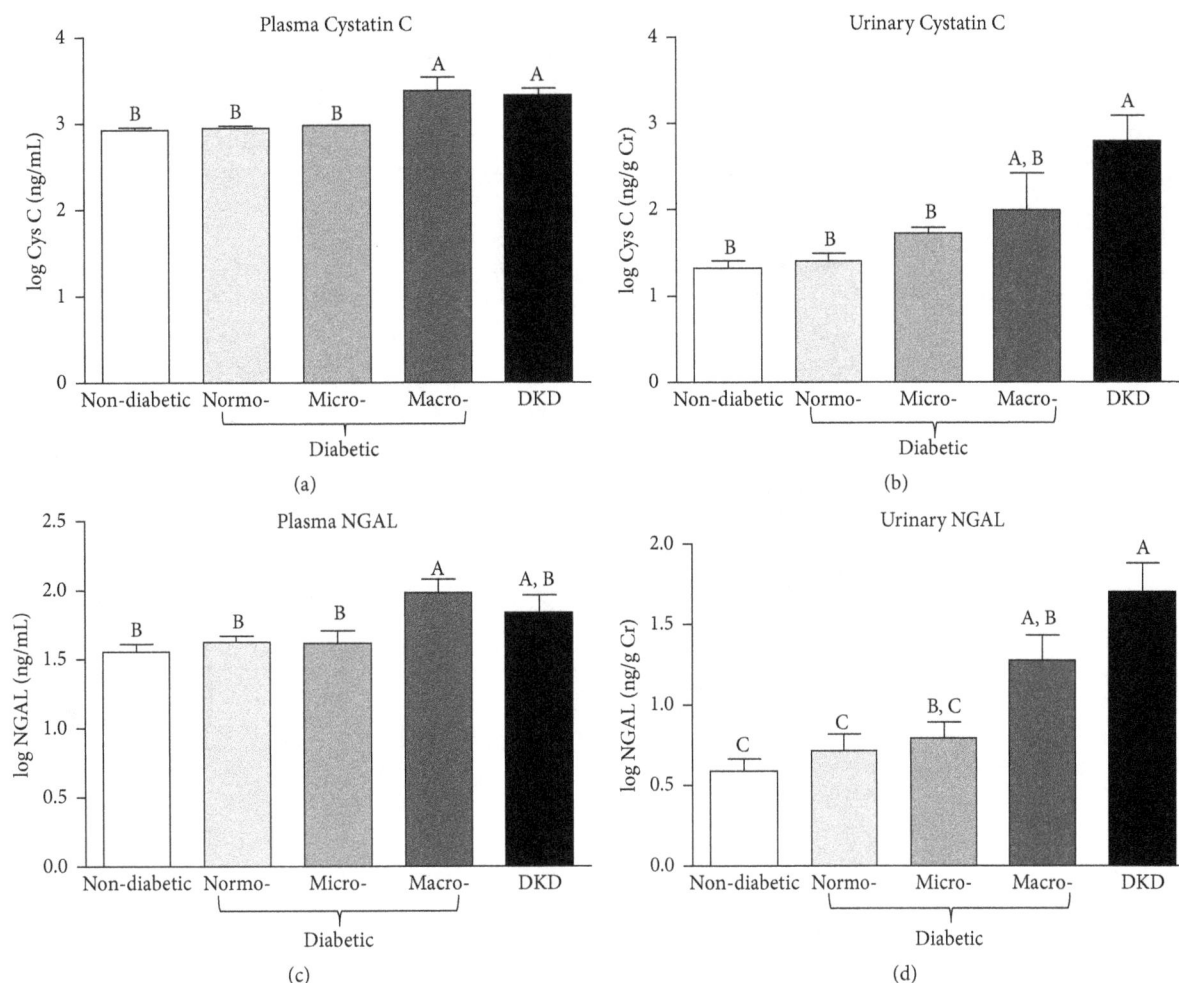

FIGURE 6: *Cystatin C and neutrophil gelatinase-associated lipocalin (NGAL) levels.* (a)-(b) Log-transformed plasma (a) or urinary (b) cystatin C levels among nondiabetic subjects, diabetic patients with normo-, micro- or macroalbuminuria, and diabetic patients with diagnosed kidney disease (DKD). Urinary cystatin C levels were normalized to urinary creatinine. (c)-(d) Log-transformed plasma (c) and urinary (d) NGAL levels among nondiabetic subjects, diabetic patients with normo-, micro- or macroalbuminuria, and diabetic patients with diagnosed kidney disease (DKD). Urinary NGAL levels were normalized to urinary creatinine. Data are represented as mean ± SEM. Labeled means without a common letter are significantly different from one another ($p < 0.05$) based on one-way ANOVA and Tukey's honest significant difference test.

in patients with UACR > 300 mg/g, increasing with severity of kidney injury (Figure 7(b)). Interestingly, a fragment of nidogen-1 migrating at ~50 kDa was also detectable in urine from diabetic patients with kidney injury as determined by UACR, perhaps corresponding to a cleavage product. A similar trend was also observed for urinary MCP-1, with levels being highest in patients with diagnosed DKD and diabetic patients with macroalbuminuria (Figures 7(c) and 8(a)). Interestingly, although both the normoalbuminuria and DKD groups are characterized by higher plasma MCP-1 levels than the nondiabetic group, there were no significant differences in plasma MCP-1 levels among the DKD and diabetic groups regardless of their UACR levels (Figures 7(d) and 8(b)). The observed increase in urinary MCP-1, but not plasma MCP-1, may suggest that the elevated urinary excretion of MCP-1 was caused by impaired kidney function.

4. Discussion

Diabetes is the leading cause of chronic kidney disease, a complication associated with high morbidity and high mortality rates [43]. Diabetic kidney disease (DKD) affects ~40% of diabetic patients and is the leading cause of ESRD. Treating DKD costs tens of billions of dollars each year and negatively impacts the quality of life for patients and their families. In the United States, minority ethnic groups (e.g., African Americans, Native Americans, and Hispanics) are disproportionately burdened by DKD [44]. Nearly all DKD in African Americans is caused by type 2 diabetes. In addition to environmental influences, type 2 diabetes has a strong genetic component [45–47]. Asymptomatic elevations in urinary albumin excretion and serum creatinine levels, key measures of DKD, are frequently present in diabetic siblings of

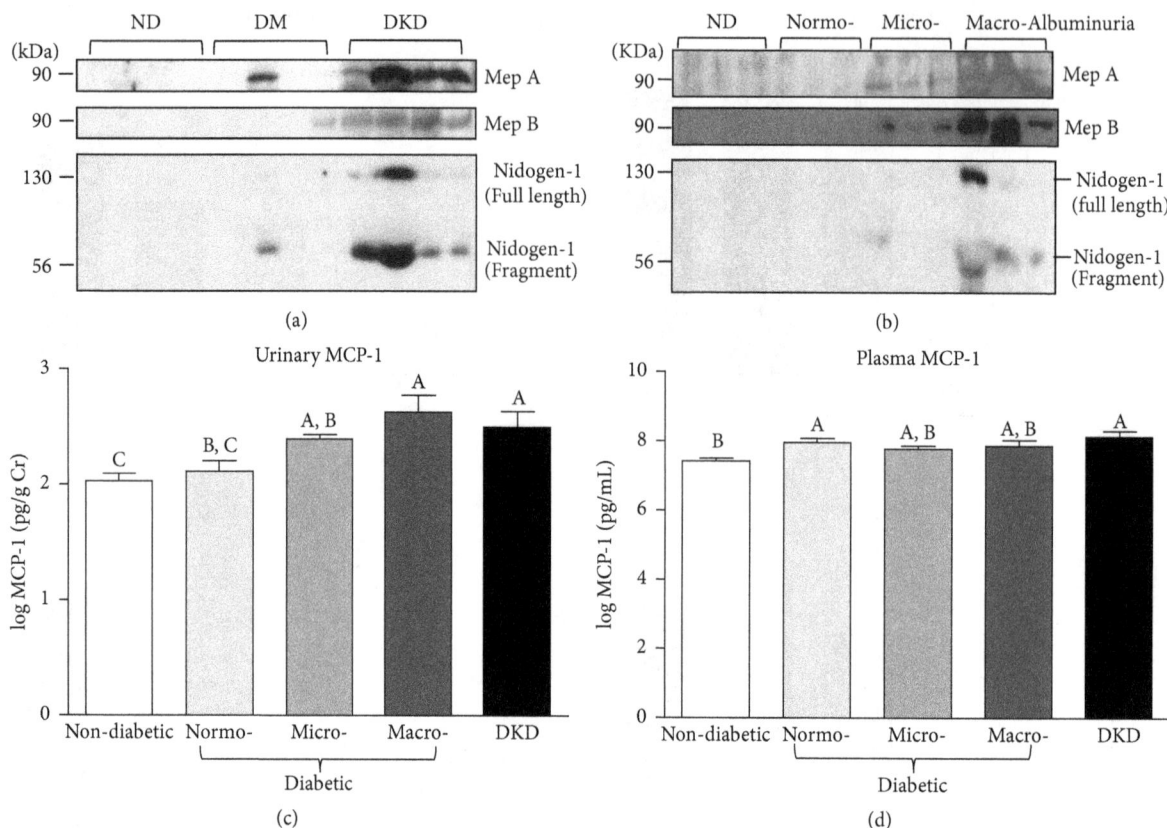

FIGURE 7: *Urinary meprin A, meprin B, nidogen-1, and monocyte chemoattractant protein-1 (MCP-1).* (a) Representative immunoblots for urinary meprin A, meprin B, and nidogen-1 grouped according to diabetes status; nondiabetic controls (ND), diabetic patients with no known kidney disease (DM), and patients with diagnosed diabetic kidney disease (DKD). (b) Representative immunoblots for meprin A, meprin B, and nidogen-1 in samples from nondiabetic controls (ND) and diabetic patients without known kidney disease grouped into normo-, micro-, and macroalbuminuria based on the UACR. (c)-(d) Log-transformed plasma (c) and urinary (d) MCP-1 levels among nondiabetic controls, diabetic patients with normo-, micro-, or macroalbuminuria, and patients with diagnosed diabetic kidney disease (DKD). Urinary MCP-1 was normalized to urinary creatinine. Data are represented as mean ± SEM. Labeled means without a common letter are significantly different from one another ($p < 0.05$) based on one-way ANOVA and Tukey's honest significant difference test.

African American individuals with overt type 2 diabetes [45]. Although DKD is highly prevalent among African American men, the diagnosis and management in this subpopulation has not been well studied. This is due, in part, to the fact that participation in biomedical research among African American men has traditionally been low. Moreover, even when there is equal access to care, diabetic African American men have a higher risk of ESRD than either their Caucasian counterparts or female African American diabetic patients [48]. Despite evidence that genetic factors play a role in the health disparities of DKD, data pertaining to the molecular mechanisms underlying diabetic kidney disease in African Americans—particularly African American men—is lacking. Gaining this information will be important if we are to provide patients with strategies for effective interventions. Proportional representation of all ethnic groups and genders during the analysis of biological samples used for the development of biomarkers of DKD ensures that those with diverse genetic backgrounds are included. This also ensures development of therapeutic targets and diagnostic tools that

are efficacious for all patients. Moreover, they may facilitate more targeted interventions in situations where predisposing genetic factors alter the pathology of disease. Previous studies showed that metabolic markers used for diagnosis of the metabolic syndrome, which is associated with a high risk for diabetes, have ethnic differences [49]. Although obesity, insulin resistance, diabetes, and hypertension are more common in African Americans than Caucasians, ethnic differences often lead to underdiagnosis of the metabolic syndrome among African American children and adults. Consequently, many African Americans who are at risk for type 2 diabetes and cardiovascular disease are not diagnosed in a timely manner, which delays the therapeutic interventions that could slow the progression of the disease.

The current study reveals undiagnosed kidney injury in a significant proportion of uninsured and underinsured diabetic African American men in Greensboro, NC (Table 2). Importantly, the data provide insights into a potential role of meprin metalloproteases in the progression of kidney injury in this population. The kidney injury assessment

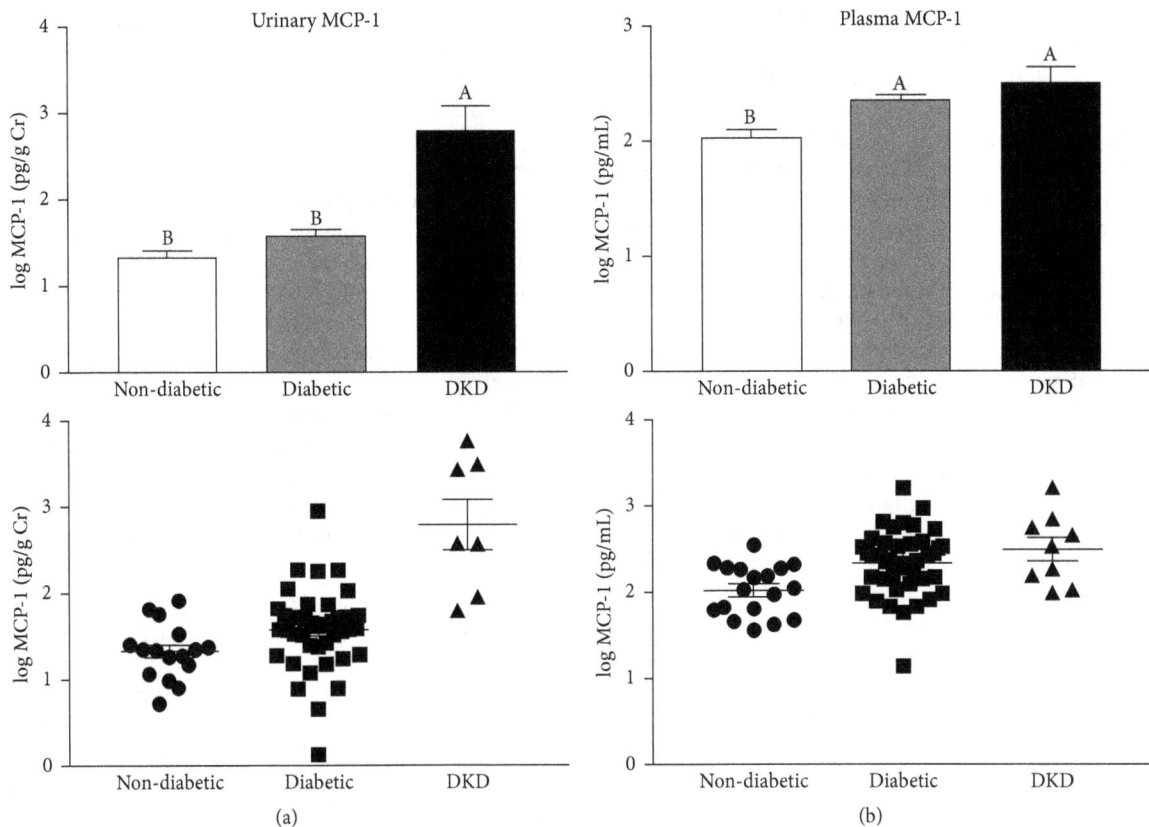

FIGURE 8: *Plasma and urinary monocyte chemoattractant protein-1 (MCP-1).* Log-transformed plasma (a) and urinary (b) MCP-1 levels among nondiabetic subjects, diabetic patients with no known kidney disease (diabetic), and patients with diagnosed diabetic kidney disease (DKD). Urinary MCP-1 levels were normalized to creatinine to account for differences in urine concentration. Data are represented as both a bar chart showing mean log MCP-1 ± SEM within each group (top) and a scatter plot showing values for each individual within the group (bottom). Labeled means without a common letter are significantly different from one another ($p < 0.05$) based on one-way ANOVA and Tukey's honest significant difference test.

utilized the UACR, which is the gold standard clinical test for DKD, together with a panel of three recently developed protein biomarkers of kidney injury that are not yet clinically available. Microalbuminuria, which occurs due to ultrastructural changes in the glomerular filtration barrier, is the earliest clinical sign of DKD and is positively correlated with age, hypertension, hyperglycemia, smoking, and male gender [50]. However, unlike the UACR, which confirms general kidney injury, the recently developed proteomic biomarkers have the potential to offer insights into the sites of kidney injury. KIM-1 is a type 1 transmembrane glycoprotein expressed in the proximal tubule [9]. Its ectodomain is shed from cells following kidney injury, allowing urinary KIM-1 concentrations to become detectable within 24 hours of tubular necrosis [51]. Urinary KIM-1 levels have been detected after exposure to a variety of nephrotoxic agents, even before the increase of serum creatinine concentrations [51]. For this reason, KIM-1 is considered a sensitive biomarker of acute kidney injury. *In vitro* studies demonstrated that release of soluble KIM-1 is mediated by a metalloprotease [52]. The current study shows that both urinary and plasma KIM-1 correlate with DKD, particularly among diabetic patients with macroalbuminuria. Interestingly, compared to levels

of urinary KIM-1, plasma KIM-1 levels appear to correlate with severity of kidney injury more closely (as determined by UACR range). Similarly, urinary NGAL levels correlated with DKD and were significantly elevated among diabetic patients with macroalbuminuria. NGAL is a 25 kDa protein expressed in neutrophils and certain epithelia, including those in the renal tubules. Renal NGAL is released into both urine and plasma and has been shown to be a sensitive biomarker that is predictive of tubular damage in both acute and chronic kidney injury [53, 54]. In fact, in some physiological contexts, NGAL may be a more promising early marker of kidney injury than UACR [55, 56]. In the current study, although we observed significant increases in urinary NGAL among patients already diagnosed with DKD, there were no significant differences between the DKD group and diabetic groups in terms of plasma NGAL levels. Likewise, both urinary and plasma NGAL levels were comparable to controls among patients whose UACR suggested early stages of kidney injury (i.e., microalbuminuria). Interestingly, however, a significant increase in plasma NGAL levels was observed in diabetic patients with macroalbuminuria. Finally, the cysteine-protease inhibitor, cystatin C, has been shown to be a good marker for assessing renal injuries. Urinary cystatin

C is considered to be a sensitive marker for the detection of DKD, with levels preceding histopathological changes. Importantly, in previous studies, the levels of cystatin C increased with the progression of renal damage, making it suitable for early detection of kidney injury and accurate assessment of DKD [8, 57]. In the current study, plasma cystatin C levels were significantly elevated in patients with DKD and diabetic patients with macroalbuminuria. Moreover, the elevation of urinary cystatin C levels in patients with DKD was significant ($p < 0.0001$) compared to all the other groups except for the macroalbuminuria subgroup.

This study also suggests that the meprin metalloproteases, meprin A and meprin B, and two kidney meprin targets, nidogen-1 and MCP-1, may play a role in the pathology of DKD in African American men. Previous studies have implicated meprins in the pathophysiology of acute and chronic kidney injury in humans and rodent models of DKD [10, 17]. For instance, single nucleotide polymorphisms (SNPs) in the meprin β gene were associated with diabetic kidney injury among the Pima Indians, a US ethnic group with extremely high incidence of type 2 diabetes and diabetic nephropathy [10]. Consistently, meprin expression and activity are decreased in rodents with diabetic kidney injury [16, 17]. In the current study, we detected ~90 kDa protein bands for both meprin A and B in the urine of patients with diabetic kidney injury. Other studies have identified 110 kDa species for meprins, corresponding to the monomeric protein forms [41, 58]. It is possible that the 90 kDa band represents a cleavage product released under pathological conditions. A cleaved meprin fragment of comparable size was reported in kidney proteins from mice subjected to ischemia/reperfusion-induced kidney injury [59]. The fact that meprin protein levels were significantly increased in patients with DKD suggests increased shedding of meprins in diabetic kidney injury. To our knowledge, this is the first study to report increased meprin shedding during human diabetic kidney injury. ADAM10-mediated shedding of meprin A was reported in ischemia/reperfusion and in small intestines [59, 60]. Furthermore, among diabetic patients, the levels of urinary meprins increased with progression from normo- to micro- and macroalbuminuria, suggesting the that meprins may have diagnostic value in detecting diabetic kidney injury. Moreover, increased shedding of meprins from the BBM could have negative pathological consequences in DKD. For instance, previous work from our group showed that meprin-deficient mice with STZ-induced type 1 diabetes had more severe kidney injury when compared to wild-type counterparts [17]. We also documented meprin expression in the glomeruli of diabetic mice, suggesting that they could play a role in both glomerular and tubulointerstitial renal pathology [34].

Knowledge about potential mechanisms by which meprins modulate the pathology of kidney disease is growing. Several studies have identified meprin targets in the kidney, which release proteolytic products into urine. Urinary meprins have previously been proposed as biomarkers of DKD [61]. The current study demonstrates that increased urinary levels for meprins A and B, as well as two meprin targets, nidogen-1 and MCP-1, correlate with progression

of DKD. Nidogen-1, an ECM protein, is an important component of the renal basement membrane. Nidogen-1 integrates other membrane components into the ECM and acts as a connecting element between collagen and laminin [62]. Meprins were shown to cleave nidogen-1 and release an approximately 50 kDa fragment in the urine of mice with cisplatin-induced nephrotoxicity [20]. Meanwhile, monocyte chemoattractant protein-1 (MCP-1) is a chemokine that contributes to inflammation by recruiting and trafficking of mononuclear immune cells to sites of inflammation [63]. In vitro studies have shown that both meprin A and meprin B proteolytically process and cause inactivation of MCP-1 [32]. The current study shows that urinary, but not plasma, levels of MCP-1 increase with kidney injury in diabetic African American men. Previous studies have shown that MCP-1 is a potential marker for predicting progression of DKD [64, 65]. Urinary MCP-1 levels were significantly elevated in patients with DKD and advanced tubulointerstitial lesions [66].

Together, these studies suggest that meprins and several meprin targets could serve as diagnostic tools for the identification of kidney injury in African American men. However, additional large-scale studies are needed to determine the efficacy of these proteins as biomarkers of DKD in this population. Likewise, the utility of meprins and their proteolytic products as diagnostic biomarkers of DKD in other ethnic groups has yet to be explored. Indeed, due to genetic factors contributing to disparities in DKD, new biomarkers are needed for early identification of patients who are prone to the development of DKD. In the age of precision medicine, the development of such biomarkers would facilitate early interventions and thus slow progression to ESRD. Importantly, participants for this study were recruited from a community health and wellness clinic run by Cone Health, the largest healthcare provider in the city of Greensboro, NC. Community clinics play a large role in providing healthcare for uninsured and underinsured patients. The outcomes from this study will enable us to plan community outreach programs that are relevant to African American men in North Carolina.

Disclosure

The content of this paper is solely the responsibility of the authors and does not necessarily represent the official views of the National Institutes of Health.

Acknowledgments

This study was supported by the Minority Men's Health Initiative (MMHI) through NIH/NIMHD Center Award no. U54MD008621 (CFDA 93.307) and Subawards nos. HU140400 (to Robert H. Newman and Elimelda Moige Ongeri) and HU150006 (to Elimelda Moige Ongeri and Scott H. Harrison) and the NIH/NIGMS Award no. SC3GM102049 to Elimelda Moige Ongeri. The authors thank Ronald Huntley and Rev. William J. Dingle and the staff of Manasseh Baptist church for their assistance in organizing outreach activities for participants that contributed to increased recruitment of patients. The authors are also grateful to Ms. Juanita Painter and Mrs. Carolyn Norford, as well as Mr. Dante Humphrey and the staff at the Cone Health Community Health and Wellness Center and Administrators at Cone Health, who worked on the logistics of this study.

References

[1] S. T. Miller, D. G. Schlundt, C. Larson et al., "Exploring ethnic disparities in diabetes, diabetes care, and lifestyle behaviors: the Nashville REACH 2010 community baseline survey," *Ethnicity & Disease*, vol. 14, 3 supplement 1, pp. S38–S45, 2014.

[2] C. M. Hales, *Prevalence of Obesity Among Adults and Youth: United States, 2015–2016*, United States, 2017.

[3] T. A. LaVeist, R. J. Thorpe Jr., J. E. Galarraga, K. M. Bower, and T. L. Gary-Webb, "Environmental and socio-economic factors as contributors to racial disparities in diabetes prevalence," *Journal of General Internal Medicine*, vol. 24, no. 10, pp. 1144–1148, 2009.

[4] M. O. Bachmann, J. Eachus, C. D. Hopper et al., "Socio-economic inequalities in diabetes complications, control, attitudes and health service use: a cross-sectional study," *Diabetic Medicine*, vol. 20, no. 11, pp. 921–929, 2003.

[5] G. Maskarinec, A. Grandinetti, G. Matsuura et al., "Diabetes prevalence and body mass index differ by ethnicity: the multiethnic cohort," *Ethnicity & Disease*, vol. 19, no. 1, pp. 49–55, 2009.

[6] K. Felix-Aaron, E. Moy, M. Kang, M. Patel, F. D. Chesley, and C. Clancy, "Variation in quality of men's health care by race/ethnicity and social class," *Medical Care*, vol. 43, no. 3, pp. I72–I81, 2005.

[7] D. Bolignano, A. Lacquaniti, G. Coppolino et al., "Neutrophil gelatinase-associated lipocalin as an early biomarker of nephropathy in diabetic patients," *Kidney and Blood Pressure Research*, vol. 32, no. 2, pp. 91–98, 2009.

[8] Y. K. Jeon, M. R. Kim, J. E. Huh et al., "Cystatin C as an early biomarker of nephropathy in patients with type 2 diabetes," *Journal of Korean Medical Science*, vol. 26, no. 2, pp. 258–263, 2011.

[9] W. K. Han, V. Bailly, R. Abichandani, R. Thadhani, and J. V. Bonventre, "Kidney Injury Molecule-1 (KIM-1): a novel biomarker for human renal proximal tubule injury," *Kidney International*, vol. 62, no. 1, pp. 237–244, 2002.

[10] A. R. Red Eagle, R. L. Hanson, W. Jiang et al., "Meprin β metalloprotease gene polymorphisms associated with diabetic nephropathy in the Pima Indians," *Human Genetics*, vol. 118, no. 1, pp. 12–22, 2005.

[11] B. Oneda, N. Lods, D. Lottaz et al., "Metalloprotease meprinβ in rat kidney: glomerular localization and differential expression in glomerulonephritis," *PLoS ONE*, vol. 3, no. 5, Article ID e2278, 2008.

[12] Q. Sun, H.-J. Jin, and J. S. Bond, "Disruption of the meprin α and β genes in mice alters homeostasis of monocytes and natural killer cells," *Experimental Hematology*, vol. 37, no. 3, pp. 346–356, 2009.

[13] J. S. Bond, K. Rojas, J. Overhauser, H. Y. Zoghbi, and W. Jiang, "The structural genes, MEP1A and MEP1B, for the α and β subunits of the metalloendopeptidase meprin map to human chromosomes 6p and 18q, respectively," *Genomics*, vol. 25, no. 1, pp. 300–303, 1995.

[14] W. Jiang, G. Dewald, E. Brundage et al., "Fine mapping of MEP1A, the gene encoding the α subunit of the metalloendopeptidase meprin, to human chromosome 6P21," *Biochemical and Biophysical Research Communications*, vol. 216, no. 2, pp. 630–635, 1995.

[15] J. F. Reckelhoffl, P. E. Butler, J. S. Bond, R. J. Beynon, and H. C. Passmore, "Mep-1, the gene regulating meprin activity, maps between Pgk-2 and Ce-2 on mouse chromosome 17," *Immunogenetics*, vol. 27, no. 4, pp. 298–300, 1988.

[16] R. Mathew, S. Futterweit, E. Valderrama et al., "Meprin-α in chronic diabetic nephropathy: interaction with, the renin-angiotensin axis," *American Journal of Physiology-Renal Physiology*, vol. 289, no. 4, pp. F911–F921, 2005.

[17] J. E. Bylander, F. Ahmed, S. M. Conley, J.-M. Mwiza, and E. M. Ongeri, "Meprin metalloprotease deficiency associated with higher mortality rates and more severe diabetic kidney injury in mice with STZ-induced type 1 diabetes," *Journal of Diabetes Research*, vol. 2017, Article ID 9035038, 11 pages, 2017.

[18] D. Köhler, M.-N. Kruse, W. Stöcker, and E. E. Sterchi, "Heterologously overexpressed, affinity-purified human meprin α is functionally active and cleaves components of the basement membrane in vitro," *FEBS Letters*, vol. 465, no. 1, pp. 2–7, 2000.

[19] M.-N. Kruse, C. Becker, D. Lottaz et al., "Human meprin α and β homo-oligomers: cleavage of basement membrane proteins and sensitivity to metalloprotease inhibitors," *Biochemical Journal*, vol. 378, part 2, pp. 383–389, 2004.

[20] C. Herzog, R. Marisiddaiah, R. S. Haun, and G. P. Kaushal, "Basement membrane protein nidogen-1 is a target of meprin β in cisplatin nephrotoxicity," *Toxicology Letters*, vol. 236, no. 2, pp. 110–116, 2015.

[21] P. D. Walker, G. P. Kaushal, and S. V. Shah, "Meprin A, the major matrix degrading enzyme in renal tubules, produces a novel nidogen fragment in vitro and in vivo," *Kidney International*, vol. 53, no. 6, pp. 1673–1680, 1998.

[22] D. Kronenberg, B. C. Bruns, C. Moali et al., "Processing of procollagen III by meprins: new players in extracellular matrix assembly," *Journal of Investigative Dermatology*, vol. 130, no. 12, pp. 2727–2735, 2010.

[23] R. Osterby, "Kidney structural abnormalities in early diabetes," *Advances in Metabolic Disorders*, vol. 2, 2, pp. 323–340, 1973.

[24] S. M. Mauer, M. W. Steffes, E. N. Ellis, D. E. Sutherland, D. M. Brown, and F. C. Goetz, "Structural-functional relationships in diabetic nephropathy," *The Journal of Clinical Investigation*, vol. 74, no. 4, pp. 1143–1155, 1984.

[25] M. W. Steffes, R. Østerby, B. Chavers, and S. M. Mauer, "Mesangial expansion as a central mechanism for loss of kidney function in diabetic patients," *Diabetes*, vol. 38, no. 9, pp. 1077–1081, 1989.

[26] P. H. Lane, M. W. Steffes, P. Fioretto, and S. M. Mauer, "Renal interstitial expansion in insulin-dependent diabetes mellitus," *Kidney International*, vol. 43, no. 3, pp. 661–667, 1993.

[27] P. Arnold, A. Otte, and C. Becker-Pauly, "Meprin metalloproteases: molecular regulation and function in inflammation and fibrosis," *Biochimica et Biophysica Acta (BBA)—Molecular Cell Research*, vol. 1864, no. 11, pp. 2096–2104, 2017.

[28] C. Herzog, R. S. Haun, V. Kaushal, P. R. Mayeux, S. V. Shah, and G. P. Kaushal, "Meprin A and meprin α generate biologically functional IL-1β from pro-IL-1β," *Biochemical and Biophysical Research Communications*, vol. 379, no. 4, pp. 904–908, 2009.

[29] C. Herzog, G. P. Kaushal, and R. S. Haun, "Generation of biologically active interleukin-1β by meprin B," *Cytokine*, vol. 31, no. 5, pp. 394–403, 2005.

[30] T. R. Keiffer and J. S. Bond, "Meprin metalloproteases inactivate interleukin 6," *The Journal of Biological Chemistry*, vol. 289, no. 11, pp. 7580–7588, 2014.

[31] S. Banerjee and J. S. Bond, "Prointerleukin-18 is activated by meprin β *in vitro* and *in vivo* in intestinal inflammation," *The Journal of Biological Chemistry*, vol. 283, no. 46, pp. 31371–31377, 2008.

[32] C. Herzog, R. S. Haun, S. V. Shah, and G. P. Kaushal, "Proteolytic processing and inactivation of CCL2/MCP-1 by meprins," *Biochemistry and Biophysics Reports*, vol. 8, pp. 146–150, 2016.

[33] N. Kumar, P. Nakagawa, B. Janic et al., "The anti-inflammatory peptide Ac-SDKP is released from thymosin-β4 by renal meprin-α and prolyl oligopeptidase," *American Journal of Physiology-Renal Physiology*, vol. 310, no. 10, pp. F1026–F1034, 2016.

[34] J.-M. V. Niyitegeka, A. C. Bastidas, R. H. Newman, S. S. Taylor, and E. M. Ongeri, "Isoform-specific interactions between meprin metalloproteases and the catalytic subunit of protein kinase a: significance in acute and chronic kidney injury," *American Journal of Physiology-Renal Physiology*, vol. 308, no. 1, pp. F56–F68, 2015.

[35] B. L. Martin, S. M. Conley, R. S. Harris, C. D. Stanley, J.-M. V. Niyitegeka, and E. M. Ongeri, "Hypoxia associated proteolytic processing of OS-9 by the metalloproteinase meprin β," *International Journal of Nephrology*, vol. 2016, Article ID 2851803, 11 pages, 2016.

[36] E. M. Ongeri, O. Anyanwu, W. B. Reeves, and J. S. Bond, "Villin and actin in the mouse kidney brush-border membrane bind to and are degraded by meprins, an interaction that contributes to injury in ischemia-reperfusion," *American Journal of Physiology-Renal Physiology*, vol. 301, no. 4, pp. F871–F882, 2011.

[37] J. V. Bonventre, "Kidney injury molecule-1 (KIM-1): a urinary biomarker and much more," *Nephrology Dialysis Transplantation*, vol. 24, no. 11, pp. 3265–3268, 2009.

[38] A. Wasilewska, K. Taranta-Janusz, W. Dębek, W. Zoch-Zwierz, and E. Kuroczycka-Saniutycz, "KIM-1 and NGAL: new markers of obstructive nephropathy," *Pediatric Nephrology*, vol. 26, no. 4, pp. 579–586, 2011.

[39] S. E. Nielsen, K. J. Schjoedt, and A. S. Astrup, "Neutrophil gelatinase-associated lipocalin (NGAL) and kidney injury molecule 1 (KIM1) in patients with diabetic nephropathy: a cross-sectional study and the effects of lisinopril," *Diabetic Medicine*, vol. 27, no. 10, pp. 1144–1150, 2010.

[40] S. M. Bagshaw and R. Bellomo, "Cystatin C in acute kidney injury," *Current Opinion in Critical Care*, vol. 16, no. 6, pp. 533–539, 2010.

[41] C. Becker-Pauly, M. Höwel, T. Walker et al., "The α and β subunits of the metalloprotease meprin are expressed in separate layers of human epidermis, revealing different functions in keratinocyte proliferation and differentiation," *Journal of Investigative Dermatology*, vol. 127, no. 5, pp. 1115–1125, 2007.

[42] F. T. Ishmael, M. T. Norcum, S. J. Benkovic, and J. S. Bond, "Multimeric structure of the secreted meprin a metalloproteinase and characterization of the functional protomer," *The Journal of Biological Chemistry*, vol. 276, no. 25, pp. 23207–23211, 2001.

[43] J. L. Gross, M. J. de Azevedo, S. P. Silveiro, L. H. Canani, M. L. Caramori, and T. Zelmanovitz, "Diabetic nephropathy: diagnosis, prevention, and treatment," *Diabetes Care*, vol. 28, no. 1, pp. 164–176, 2005.

[44] D. A. Price and E. D. Crook, "Kidney disease in African Americans: genetic considerations," *Journal of the National Medical Association*, vol. 94, 8, pp. 16S–27S, 2002.

[45] S. G. Satko, C. D. Langefeld, P. Daeihagh, D. W. Bowden, S. S. Rich, and B. I. Freedman, "Nephropathy in siblings of African Americans with overt type 2 diabetic nephropathy," *American Journal of Kidney Diseases*, vol. 40, no. 3, pp. 489–494, 2002.

[46] J. Gitter, C. D. Langefeld, S. S. Rich, C. F. Pedley, D. W. Bowden, and B. I. Freedman, "Prevalence of nephropathy in black patients with type 2 diabetes mellitus," *American Journal of Nephrology*, vol. 22, no. 1, pp. 35–41, 2002.

[47] A. Malhotra, R. P. Igo Jr., F. Thameem et al., "Genome-wide linkage scans for type 2 diabetes mellitus in four ethnically diverse populations—significant evidence for linkage on chromosome 4q in African Americans: the family investigation of nephropathy and diabetes research group," *Diabetes/Metabolism Research and Reviews*, vol. 25, no. 8, pp. 740–747, 2009.

[48] Y. Wang, P. T. Katzmarzyk, R. Horswell et al., "Racial disparities in diabetic complications in an underinsured population," *The Journal of Clinical Endocrinology & Metabolism*, vol. 97, no. 12, pp. 4446–4453, 2012.

[49] R. B. Ervin, "Prevalence of metabolic syndrome among adults 20 years of age and over, by sex, age, race and ethnicity, and body mass index: United States, 2003–2006," *National Health Statistics Reports*, no. 13, pp. 1–7, 2009.

[50] S. C. Satchell and J. E. Tooke, "What is the mechanism of microalbuminuria in diabetes: a role for the glomerular endothelium?" *Diabetologia*, vol. 51, no. 5, pp. 714–725, 2008.

[51] W. S. Waring and A. Moonie, "Earlier recognition of nephrotoxicity using novel biomarkers of acute kidney injury," *Clinical Toxicology*, vol. 49, no. 8, pp. 720–728, 2011.

[52] V. Bailly, Z. Zhang, W. Meier, R. Cate, M. Sanicola, and J. V. Bonventre, "Shedding of kidney injury molecule-1, a putative adhesion protein involved in renal regeneration," *The Journal of Biological Chemistry*, vol. 277, no. 42, pp. 39739–39748, 2002.

[53] J. Mishra, Q. Ma, C. Kelly et al., "Kidney NGAL is a novel early marker of acute injury following transplantation," *Pediatric Nephrology*, vol. 21, no. 6, pp. 856–863, 2006.

[54] M. M. Mitsnefes, T. S. Kathman, J. Mishra et al., "Serum neutrophil gelatinase-associated lipocalin as a marker of renal function in children with chronic kidney disease," *Pediatric Nephrology*, vol. 22, no. 1, pp. 101–108, 2007.

[55] W. Fu, S. Xiong, Y. Fang et al., "Urinary tubular biomarkers in short-term type 2 diabetes mellitus patients: a cross-sectional study," *Endocrine Journal*, vol. 41, no. 1, pp. 82–88, 2012.

[56] W. Fu, B. Li, S. Wang et al., "Changes of the tubular markers in type 2 diabetes mellitus with glomerular hyperfiltration," *Diabetes Research and Clinical Practice*, vol. 95, no. 1, pp. 105–109, 2012.

[57] Y. Togashi, Y. Sakaguchi, M. Miyamoto, and Y. Miyamoto, "Urinary cystatin C as a biomarker for acute kidney injury and its immunohistochemical localization in kidney in the CDDP-treated rats," *Experimental and Toxicologic Pathology*, vol. 64, no. 7-8, pp. 797–805, 2012.

[58] R. Wichert, A. Ermund, S. Schmidt et al., "Mucus detachment by host metalloprotease meprin β requires shedding of its inactive pro-form, which is abrogated by the pathogenic protease RgpB," *Cell Reports*, vol. 21, no. 8, pp. 2090–2103, 2017.

[59] C. Herzog, R. S. Haun, A. Ludwig, S. V. Shah, and G. P. Kaushal, "ADAM10 is the major sheddase responsible for the release of membrane-associated meprin A," *The Journal of Biological Chemistry*, vol. 289, no. 19, pp. 13308–13322, 2014.

[60] P. Arnold, I. Boll, M. Rothaug et al., "Meprin metalloproteases generate biologically active soluble interleukin-6 receptor to

induce trans-signaling," *Scientific Reports*, vol. 7, Article ID 44053, 2017.

[61] J. B. DeGuzman, P. W. Speiser, and H. Trachtman, "Urinary meprin-α: a potential marker of diabetic nephropathy," *Journal of Pediatric Endocrinology and Metabolism*, vol. 17, no. 12, pp. 1663–1666, 2004.

[62] J. W. Fox, U. Mayer, R. Nischt et al., "Recombinant nidogen consists of three globular domains and mediates binding of laminin to collagen type IV," *EMBO Journal*, vol. 10, no. 11, pp. 3137–3146, 1991.

[63] H. Haller, A. Bertram, F. Nadrowitz, and J. Menne, "Monocyte chemoattractant protein-1 and the kidney," *Current Opinion in Nephrology and Hypertension*, vol. 25, no. 1, pp. 42–49, 2016.

[64] F. W. K. Tam, B. L. Riser, K. Meeran, J. Rambow, C. D. Pusey, and A. H. Frankel, "Urinary monocyte chemoattractant protein-1 (MCP-1) and connective tissue growth factor (CCN2) as prognostic markers for progression of diabetic nephropathy," *Cytokine*, vol. 47, no. 1, pp. 37–42, 2009.

[65] S. M. Titan, J. M. Vieira Jr., W. V. Dominguez et al., "Urinary MCP-1 and RBP: independent predictors of renal outcome in macroalbuminuric diabetic nephropathy," *Journal of Diabetes and Its Complications*, vol. 26, no. 6, pp. 546–553, 2012.

[66] K. Tashiro, I. Koyanagi, and A. Saitoh, "Urinary levels of monocyte chemoattractant protein-1 (MCP-1) and interleukin-8 (IL-8), and renal injuries in patients with type 2 diabetic nephropathy," *Journal of Clinical Laboratory Analysis*, vol. 16, no. 1, pp. 1–4, 2002.

25

Murine Nephrotoxic Nephritis as a Model of Chronic Kidney Disease

M. K. E. Ougaard ⓘ,[1,2] **P. H. Kvist** ⓘ,[3] **H. E. Jensen,**[2] **C. Hess,**[1] **I. Rune** ⓘ,[1] and **H. Søndergaard**[1]

[1]*Department of Diabetes Complications Pharmacology, Novo Nordisk, Maaloev, Denmark*
[2]*Department of Veterinary and Animal Sciences, University of Copenhagen, Frederiksberg, Denmark*
[3]*Department of Histology and Bioimaging, Novo Nordisk, Maaloev, Denmark*

Correspondence should be addressed to M. K. E. Ougaard; moug@novonordisk.com

Academic Editor: Frank Park

Using the nonaccelerated murine nephrotoxic nephritis (NTN) as a model of chronic kidney disease (CKD) could provide an easily inducible model that enables a rapid test of treatments. Originally, the NTN model was developed as an acute model of glomerulonephritis, but in this study we evaluate the model as a CKD model and compare CD1 and C57BL/6 female and male mice. CD1 mice have previously showed an increased susceptibility to CKD in other CKD models. NTN was induced by injecting nephrotoxic serum (NTS) and evaluated by CKD parameters including albuminuria, glomerular filtration rate (GFR), mesangial expansion, and renal fibrosis. Both strains showed significant albuminuria on days 2-3 which remained significant until the last time point on days 36-37 supporting dysfunctional filtration also observed by a significantly declined GFR on days 5-6, 15–17, and 34–37. Both strains showed early progressive mesangial expansion and significant renal fibrosis within three weeks suggesting CKD development. CD1 and C57BL/6 females showed a similar disease progression, but female mice seemed more susceptible to NTS compared to male mice. The presence of albuminuria, GFR decline, mesangial expansion, and fibrosis showed that the NTN model is a relevant CKD model both in C57BL/6 and in CD1 mice.

1. Introduction

Animal models with clinical and pathological features of human chronic kidney disease (CKD) are highly warranted to advance novel therapies for CKD and would enable a deeper understanding of the pathogenesis and thereby more target-specific therapies. CKD is defined clinically by prolonged and progressive loss of kidney function measured by a declined glomerular filtration rate (GFR) and the presence of albuminuria with pathological findings of mesangial expansion, inflammation, and renal fibrosis [1].

Prior work has documented limitations of the classical murine models of CKD including the unilateral ureteral obstruction (UUO), 5/6 nephrectomy, and diabetic nephropathy models [2, 3]. The pathogenesis of the UUO and the 5/6 nephrectomy models is difficult to study. The unobstructed kidney in the UUO model compensates for the loss of function in the obstructed kidney [2]. In the 5/6 nephrectomy model, only a small amount of kidney tissue is available, and the model requires a difficult technical surgery making it difficult to reproduce [3–6]. Models of diabetic nephropathy also have their limitations as both the classical streptozotocin- (STZ-) induced model and the db/db model develop slowly and often only show mild signs of CKD [7].

The pathogenesis in the nonaccelerated nephrotoxic nephritis (NTN) model is initiated by anti-glomerular IgGs that impair the glomerular filtration barrier and induce proteinuria and inflammation. The NTN model is largely described as a model of acute glomerulonephritis, and the knowledge of the long-term pathogenesis and strain differences in the nonaccelerated murine NTN model is therefore limited [3, 8–10]. The standard of care for CKD has for many decades consisted of treatment with angiotensin-converting-enzyme inhibitors (ACE-I's) or angiotensin receptor blockers

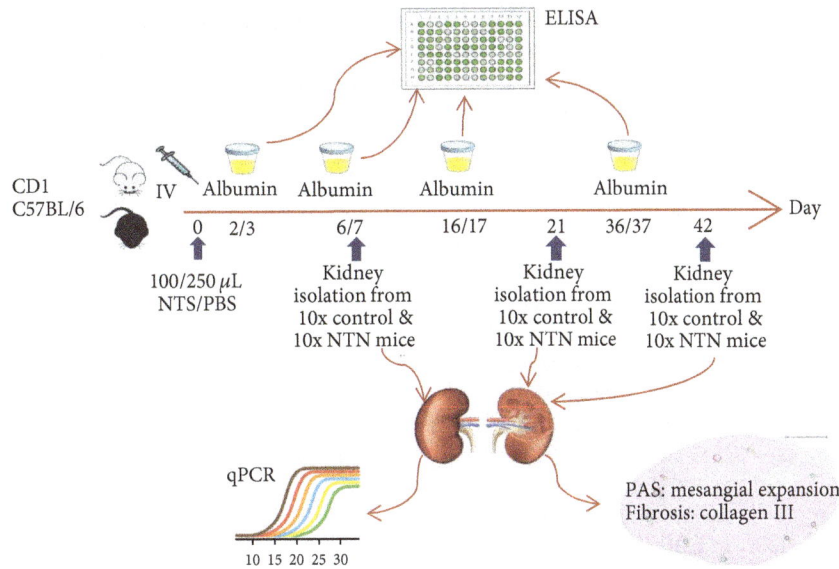

FIGURE 1: Study set up in C57BL/6 and CD1 mice.

that reduce albuminuria and slow down the disease progression [11]. A previous study in the NTN rat has demonstrated that ACE-Is reduce albuminuria and glomerular sclerosis indicating the NTN model is a suitable model of human CKD [12].

The murine C57BL/6 strain is the most commonly used genetic background of inbred strains in research. However, these strains are resistant to the development of CKD in the standard model; 5/6 nephrectomy unless hypertension is induced in addition [13]. Furthermore, the nephrectomy and the streptozotocin models show increased CKD severity in the outbred stock—CD1—compared to the C57BL/6 mice [14–16]. The influence of gender on CKD is still debated. However, the prevalence of CKD tends to be increased in women, but the CKD is more severe in men [17].

The murine model of NTN allows investigations of the immune mechanisms in rapidly progressive glomerulonephritis (GN). Few chronic experiments have evaluated the more chronic features of the induced kidney damage by testing therapeutic strategies for renal fibrosis in the accelerated NTN model with the use of immunisation and adjuvants [18, 19]. Therefore, we performed an in-depth time course study using both C57BL/6 and CD1 male and female mice in the nonaccelerated NTN model by measuring their acute and progressive chronic manifestations of CKD.

2. Materials and Methods

2.1. Experimental Animals and Study Design. C57BL/6 mice (8–10 weeks) were purchased from Taconic (Ry, Denmark) and CD1 mice (8–10 weeks) were purchased from Charles River (Germany). The mice were housed in a facility with a 12 h light/dark cycle with free access to water and Altromin chow. Before the study, the mice were acclimatised for one week. All animal experiments were approved by the Danish Animal Inspectorate and the Novo Nordisk ethical review

board. Mice were euthanised if they experienced >20% weight loss or compromised health.

Prior to termination, mice were induced with isoflurane, and the kidneys were perfused with 0.9% NaCl with Heparin (10 U/ml) before isolation and collection.

Initial dose titration studies were conducted to determine the optimal dose of NTS in both strains using 50–250 μl of NTS. The optimal doses were used in two parallel experiments conducted in C57BL/6 and CD1 mice to determine the time course of CKD disease development. Nonaccelerated NTN was induced by a single tail-vein injection of 250 μl (C57BL/6) and 100 μl (CD1) of sheep anti-rat NTS (Probetex, San Antonio, USA, PTX-001S lot#199-8). Control mice received PBS by same administration and volume. The study design followed a randomised block design with 30 mice in each group. At days 7, 21, and 42 ten mice per group were sacrificed, and plasma and kidneys were collected (Figure 1). The mice were weighed on day 0 just before NTS was injected and hereafter twice a week, and the percentage weight change was calculated throughout the study. The gender studies in CD1 and C57BL/6 are described in supplementary materials.

2.2. Urine and Plasma Analysis. Urine was collected by metabolic caging to measure the urinary albumin concentration and to calculate the urinary albumin excretion rate (UAER). Mice were single-housed in metabolic cages for 18 hours on days 2-3, 6-7, 16-17, and 36-37. Urinary markers were measured by ELISA: albumin (Bethyl Laboratories, cat.no. E90-134), Cystatin C (R&D systems, Minneapolis, MN Cat. number MSCTCO) and TNFR1 (R&D systems, Minneapolis MN Cat. number MRT10). Urinary creatinine was measured by high-performance liquid chromatography (HPLC). Creatinine was measured in serum by acetonitrile deproteinization, followed by isocratic, cation exchange HPLC as previously described [20].

Blood plasma was prepared from blood samples collected on days 7, 14, 21, 28, and 42. Serum Amyloid P (SAP) was measured by ELISA (Genway, San Diego, CA). Cystatin C was measured using ELISA (R&D systems, Minneapolis, MN Cat. number MSCTCO).

2.3. Glomerular Filtration Rate. The glomerular filtration rate (GFR) was measured in CD1 female mice (8–10 weeks) in an additional study with similar induction of NTN. The glomerular filtration rate (GFR) was measured on days 5-6, 15–17, and 34–37 by preclinical transdermal GFR monitors (Medibeacon GmBH, Mannheim, Germany) as previously described [21]. In short, a square of 2×2 centimetres fur on the back of the mice were depilated 24 hours prior to GFR measurements. A stock of FITC-sinistrin (Medibeacon GmBH, Mannheim, Germany) was prepared and stored in aliquots at $-20°C$. Prior to injection of FITC-sinistrin, the mice were lightly anaesthetised and the GFR monitor was adhered to the depilated area by adhesive tape. The mice were injected intravenously in the tail vein with 7.5 mg/100 g BW of FITC-sinistrin and placed in an enriched cage for one hour.

2.4. Kidney Gene Expression by Real-Time Quantitative PCR. Following euthanasia, one-half of the left kidney was snap frozen in liquid nitrogen and stored at $-80°C$. Frozen kidney tissue was homogenised in Qiazol reagent, RNA was isolated using the RNAeasy Mini kit as described by the suppliers (Qiagen, Mississauga, ON, Canada) and cDNA was generated using SuperScript VILO cDNA Synthesis kit (Life Technologies, Burlington, ON, Canada). Afterwards Real-Time Quantitative PCR (RT qPCR) was performed with Gene Expression Master Mix (Life Technologies) using a 7900HT Fast Real-Time PCR System. Specific gene expression was measured with the following Taqman assays (Life Technologies): C3 (Mm01232779_m1, C3), procollagen 3a1, (Mm01254476_m1, Col3a1), Fibronectin (Mm01256744_m1, Fn1), and PAI-1 (Mm00435858_m1, Serpine1). RT qPCR was performed in triplicate, and the values normalised to GAPDH and RPL27 as previously described [22].

2.5. Histological Analysis. Perfused kidneys were fixed in 4% paraformaldehyde for 30 h, processed by standard procedures through graded concentrations of alcohol and xylene and embedded in paraffin. Paraffin sections of 3 microns were stained with Periodic Acid-Schiff (PAS) and scanned using the Nanozoomer 2.0 (Hamamatsu Photonics K.K., Hamamatsu, Japan) at a magnification of ×40. The mesangial expansion was evaluated in a blinded fashion as 20 glomeruli of each kidney were assessed and graded into four categories: 0 (no mesangial expansion), 1 (mild mesangial expansion, mesangial matrix wide < 2 nucleus diameter), 2 (moderate mesangial expansion, mesangial matrix wide < 4 nucleus diameter), and 3 (severe mesangial expansion, > 4 nucleus diameter). The 20 glomeruli of each mouse were evaluated for metaplasia, segmental or global sclerosis. Furthermore, the kidneys were evaluated for the presence of protein casts. The tubular casts were visualised as solidification of protein in the lumen of the kidney tubules. The metaplasia was visualised as a change from flattened parietal epithelium to cuboidal

epithelium lining the glomerulus. The segmental glomerulosclerosis was visualised as glomeruli that showed scarring of small sections of the glomeruli, while global glomerulosclerosis was visualised as totally scarred glomeruli.

2.6. Immunohistochemistry. Immunohistochemical (IHC) staining of collagen III was performed to quantitate renal fibrosis. Paraffin-embedded sections were deparaffinised and hydrated followed by antigen retrieval with proteinase K (10 μg/ml) treatment for 10 minutes at $37°C$ and treated in TBS for 5 minutes. Endogenous peroxidase was blocked using 0.5% H_2O_2 in TBS for 20 minutes, and sections were incubated with avidin and biotin for 10 min each. Sections were incubated with TBS mixed with 7% donkey, 3% mouse serum, and 3% skimmed milk. Subsequently, sections were incubated overnight at $4°C$ with goat anticollagen III (Southern Biotech, Birmingham, USA) diluted in 7% donkey, 3% mouse serum, and 0.5% skimmed milk in TBS. The next day, the sections were incubated in biotinylated donkey anti-goat IgG (cat. number 705-065-147) diluted in 7% donkey, 3% mouse serum, and 0.5% skimmed milk in TBS and afterwards in vectastain ABC complex in TBS. Specific binding of antibodies was visualised by enzymatic conversion of the chromogenic substrate DAB into a brown precipitate by HRP activated by hydrogen peroxide. The slides were counterstained with haematoxylin.

2.7. Digital Image Analysis for Quantification of Fibrosis. All slides were scanned using the Nanozoomer 2.0 at an original magnification of ×40. The image analysis was performed using Visiopharm Integrator System software (VIS; Visiopharm, Hoersholm, Denmark). An automated tissue detection protocol was performed as previously published [23]. Evaluation of the collagen III staining was determined in a region of interest (ROI) restricted to the cortex region. Within the ROI a threshold (∞–70) analysis was performed using HDAB-DAB channel as previously published [23].

2.8. Statistics. Statistical analyses were performed using GraphPad Prism (v6.5; GraphPad Software, CA), and data were presented as the mean ± standard deviation (SD). D'Agistino-Pearson normality test was performed. Normally distributed data were analysed by one-way ANOVA multiple testing with Turkey's correction, and nonnormally distributed data were analysed using Kruskal-Wallis multiple testing with Dunn's correction. Two-way ANOVA was applied for comparing CD1 and C57BL/6 mice at different time points. A P value < 0.05 was accepted as statistically significant.

3. Results

3.1. CD1 Mice Display Increased Susceptibility to NTS Compared to C57BL/6 Mice. The initial dose titration studies showed that mice subjected to NTS developed albuminuria in a dose-dependent manner in both CD1 mice (Figure 2(a)) and C57BL/6 mice (Figure 2(b)). C57BL/6 mice subjected to 250 μl NTS showed an increased urinary albumin excretion rate (UAER) on days 9/10 compared to the groups subjected

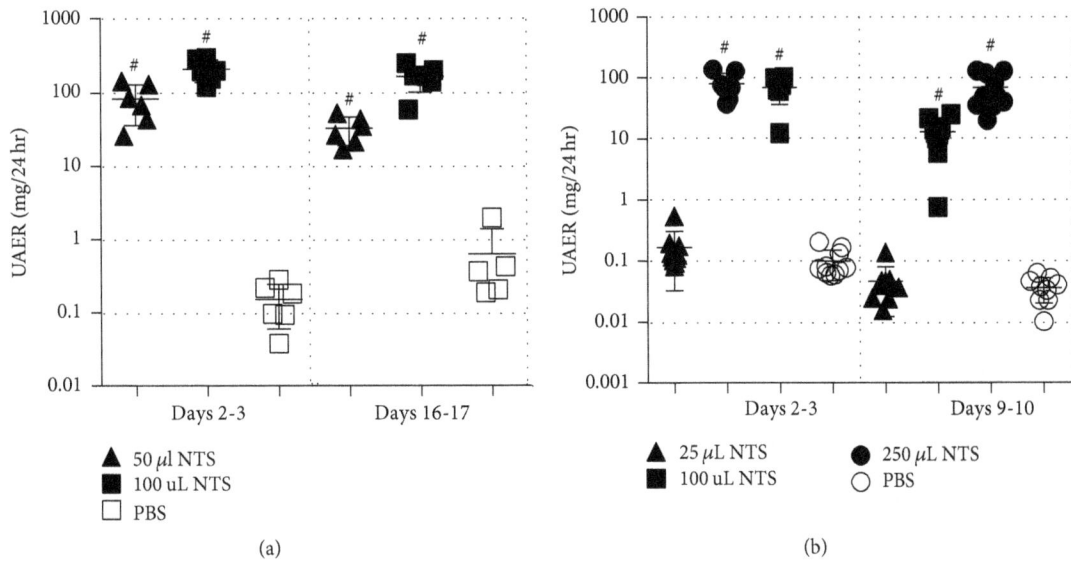

(a)

(b)

FIGURE 2: *CD1 mice are more susceptible to NTS measured by albuminuria compared to C57BL/6 mice.* (a) Scatter plot showing the 24 h urinary albumin excretion rate (UAER) of CD1 mice over time. (b) Scatter plot showing the 24 h urinary albumin excretion rate (UAER) of C57BL/6 mice over time. Data are shown as mean ± SD. $^{\#}P < 0.0001$ NTS groups ($n = 5$-6) versus PBS group ($n = 5$-6) by one-way ANOVA.

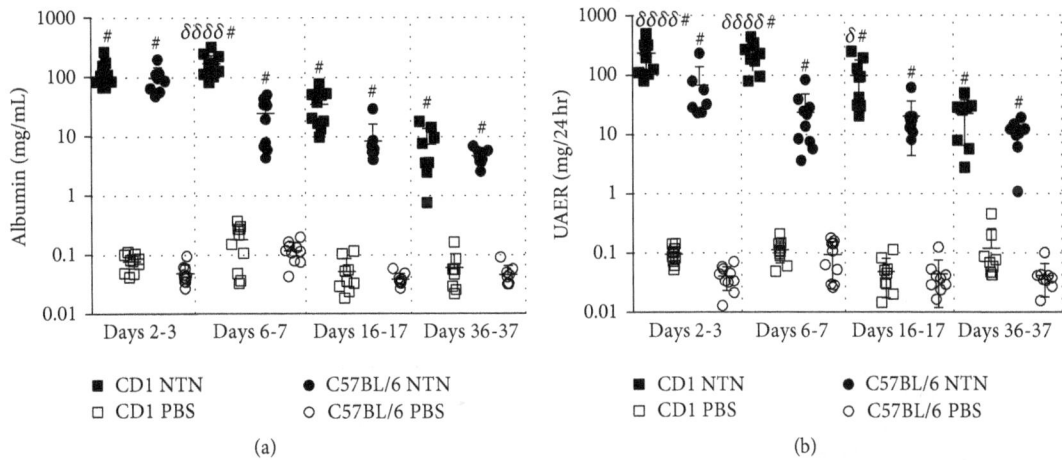

(a)

(b)

FIGURE 3: *NTS induces significant and chronic increase in UAER and urine albumin concentration.* (a) Scatter plot showing the 24 h urinary albumin excretion rate (UAER) on days 2-3, 6-7, 16-17, and 36-37. (b) Scatter plot showing urinary albumin concentration on days 2-3, 6-7, 16-17, and 36-37. Data are shown as mean ± SD. $^{\#}P < 0.0001$ NTN groups versus PBS groups and $^{\delta}P < 0.05$, $^{\delta\delta\delta\delta}P < 0.0001$ CD1 NTN versus B6 NTN groups by two-way ANOVA ($n = 10$).

to 25 or 100 μl NTS (Figure 2(b)). The dose of 250 μl NTS severely affected the welfare of the CD1 mice, and 65% of this group were euthanised shortly after study initiation due to severe weight loss and signs of compromised health. A gross pathological evaluation showed that these mice had severe glomerulonephritis, and consequently, this group was excluded. CD1 mice subjected to 100 μl NTS showed an increased UAER on days 16/17 compared to the group subjected to 50 μl NTS (Figure 2(a)).

Based on these results, 250 μl and 100 μl NTS were selected for subsequent experiments in C57BL/6 and CD1, respectively.

3.2. NTS Induces Albuminuria, GFR Decline, and Transient Weight Loss.
NTN induction in both strains resulted in significantly increased UAER compared to the healthy controls on days 2-3, 6-7, 16-17, and 36-37 after NTS injection (Figure 3(a)). Furthermore, the albumin concentrations of the NTN urine samples were significantly increased compared to the control urine samples at all-time points (Figure 3(b)). The CD1 NTN mice developed significantly increased UAER on days 2-3, 6-7, and 16-17 compared to C57BL/6 NTN mice (Figure 3(a)). No difference in UAER was observed between C57BL/6 male and female mice, but the female NTN mice showed a trend towards increased UAER ($P = 0.0708$ at

(a)

(b)

(c)

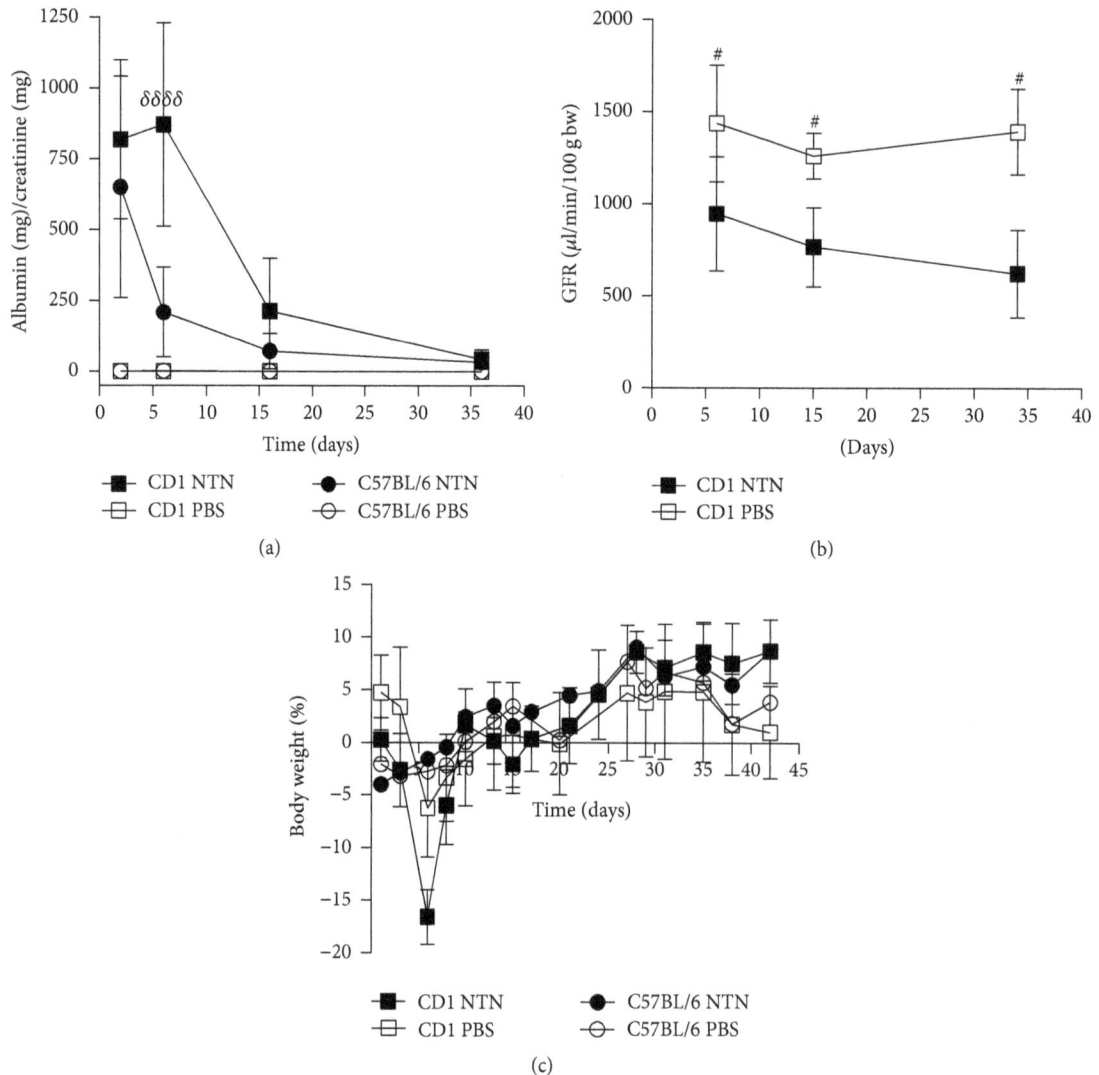

FIGURE 4: *NTS induces albuminuria, GFR decline, and transient weight loss.* (a) Graph showing the average urinary albumin/creatine ratio (mg/mg) on days 2-3, 6-7, 16-17, and 36-37. (b) Graph showing the mean glomerular filtration rate (μl/min/100 g body weight (bw)) in CD1 mice on days 5-6, 15-17, and 34-37. (c) Graph showing the average percentage change in body weight over time. Data are shown as mean ± SD. [#]$P < 0.05$ CD1 NTN versus CD1 PBS by one-way ANOVA ($n = 10$); [$\delta\delta\delta\delta$]$P < 0.0001$ CD1 NTN versus B6 NTN groups by two-way ANOVA ($n = 10$).

6 weeks and $P = 0.0746$ at 10 weeks, data not shown). However, CD1 NTN female mice developed significantly increased UAER compared to male NTN mice on days 35-36 (Supplementary material, Figure 1). The urinary albumin creatinine ratio (UACR) showed similar temporal dynamics as the UAER. The UACR peaked on days 6-7 and 2-3 in CD1 and C57BL/6 NTN mice, respectively (Figure 4(a)). The NTN induction caused a significant decrease in GFR on days 5-6, 15-17, and 34–37 in CD NTN mice compared to their controls. NTS induced transient body weight loss from day one until day 6; C57BL/6 NTN mice showed significantly greater weight loss (mean: −16,9%) compared to the CD1 NTN mice (mean: −6,3%). However, both CD1 and C57BL/6 NTN mice recovered to their initial body weight within 20 days and gained weight throughout the study (Figure 4(c)).

3.3. NTS Induces Significant Urinary Excretion of Cystatin C and Tumour Necrosis Factor Receptor 1. The urine analysis showed that the 24-hour urinary Cystatin C excretion was significantly increased on days 2-3, 6-7, and 16-17 in CD1 NTN mice and on days 2-3 and 6-7 in C57BL/6 NTN mice compared to control mice (Figure 5(a)). The 24-hour urinary excretion of tumour necrosis factor receptor 1 (TNFR1) was also significantly increased on days 2-3, 6-7, 16-17, and 36-37 in both strains (Figure 5(b)).

3.4. NTS Induces Systemic Inflammation and Elevation of a GFR Marker. The plasma levels, of the acute phase protein SAP, were significantly increased on day 7 in C57BL/6 mice and days 7 and 14 in CD1 mice injected with NTS (Figure 6(a)). Supporting this notion, Cystatin C, a marker

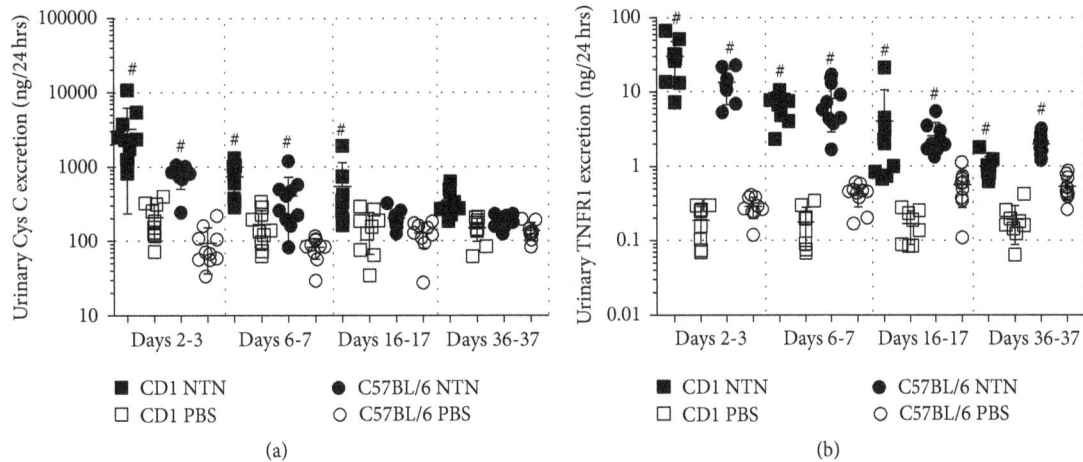

FIGURE 5: NTS induces significant urinary excretion of Cystatin C and TNFR1. (a) Scatter plot showing the 24 h urinary Cystatin C excretion rate over time measured by ELISA. (b) Scatter plot showing 24 h urinary TNFR1 excretion rate over time measured by ELISA. Data are shown as mean ± SD. $^{#}P < 0.01$ NTN groups versus PBS groups by two-way ANOVA ($n = 10$).

of inflammation and GFR, was also significantly increased on days 7 and 14 in both C57BL/6 and CD1 following NTS. In addition, Cystatin C was also significantly increased on days 21, 28, and 42 in both strains compared to control mice (Figure 6(b)). The inflammatory response was further investigated by complement involvement by looking at mRNA levels of C3. NTN induction significantly increased C3 gene expression in both strains on days 7, 21, and 42 (Figure 6(c)).

3.5. NTS Induces Chronic Kidney Injury with Mesangial Expansion and Renal Fibrosis. The mesangial expansion was observed in both CD1 and C57BL/6 NTN mice on days 7, 21, and 42 compared to their healthy controls (Figures 7(a) and 7(b)). The glomerular mesangial expansion progressed over time as it significantly increased from days 7 to 21 and from days 21 to 42 in both strains (Figure 7(b)). Both strains showed 20–22% segmentally sclerosed glomeruli on days 7, 21, and 42 and developed increased globally sclerosed glomeruli over time (2% on day 7 and 13% on day 42 (Table 1)). In addition, both strains developed metaplasia in 24–29% of the assessed glomeruli on days 7, 21, and 42. Tubular casts within cortex were present at all-time points (Table 1).

Moreover, hypercellular glomeruli, tubular proliferation, and dilatation were observed together with increasing immune cells accumulating in the tubulointerstitium and infiltrating the periglomerular space surrounding glomeruli.

NTS induced similar significantly increased collagen III accumulation, and thereby renal fibrosis was observed already on day 21 in both strains (Figures 8(a) and 8(b)) compared to healthy controls. Renal fibrosis remained significantly increased on day 42 compared to controls, but it did not progress from day 21 (Figure 8(b)). No difference in collagen III accumulation was observed between C57BL/6 male and female NTN mice. However, only the female C57BL/6 NTN mice developed significantly increased collagen III deposition compared to their healthy controls (Supplementary Material, Figure 2). The female NTN mice

developed significantly increased collagen III deposition compared to male CD1 NTN mice (Supplementary Material, Figure 1).

To further investigate the development of kidney fibrosis and matrix remodeling, mRNA levels of collagen type III (col III), fibronectin (fn1), and PAI-1 (Serpine1) were quantified. The NTN induction significantly increased the mRNA levels of collagen type III and PAI-1 in CD1 mice on days 7, 21, and 42 and in C57BL/6 mice on days 7 and 42 (Figures 8(c)–8(e)). The fibronectin mRNA levels were significantly increased in CD1 NTN mice on days 7 and 21 and in C57BL/6 mice on day 7 compared to control mice. In general, the CD1 female NTN mice showed increased mRNA levels on the profibrotic genes compared to C57BL/6 NTN mice, and in addition, C57BL/6 female NTN mice developed significantly increased collagen III mRNA levels compared to C57BL/6 male NTN mice (Supplementary Material, Figure 2).

4. Discussion

The nonaccelerated NTN model is a widely used model of acute GN, but no characterisation of the chronic progression of the disease is thoroughly described in mice. The nonaccelerated NTN model has previously been characterised in the rat, where NTN induces an autologous (acute) phase characterised by inflammation and severe proteinuria and a heterogeneous (chronic) phase characterised by glomerular lesions [24–26]. In this study we show that NTS injection in both CD1 and C57BL/6 mice induced not only an acute phase, as previously described, but also several hallmarks of CKD including albuminuria, GFR decline, mesangial expansion, inflammation, and renal fibrosis which were significantly present in the later stages of the induced NTS kidney damage.

The NTS induction significantly increased albuminuria, already on days 2-3 in both CD1 and C57BL/6 mice, suggesting an acute leakage of protein as soon as anti-GBM antibodies are deposited. The mean albuminuria declined around days 16-17, but significant elevation in UAER and

(a)

(b)

(c)

(d)

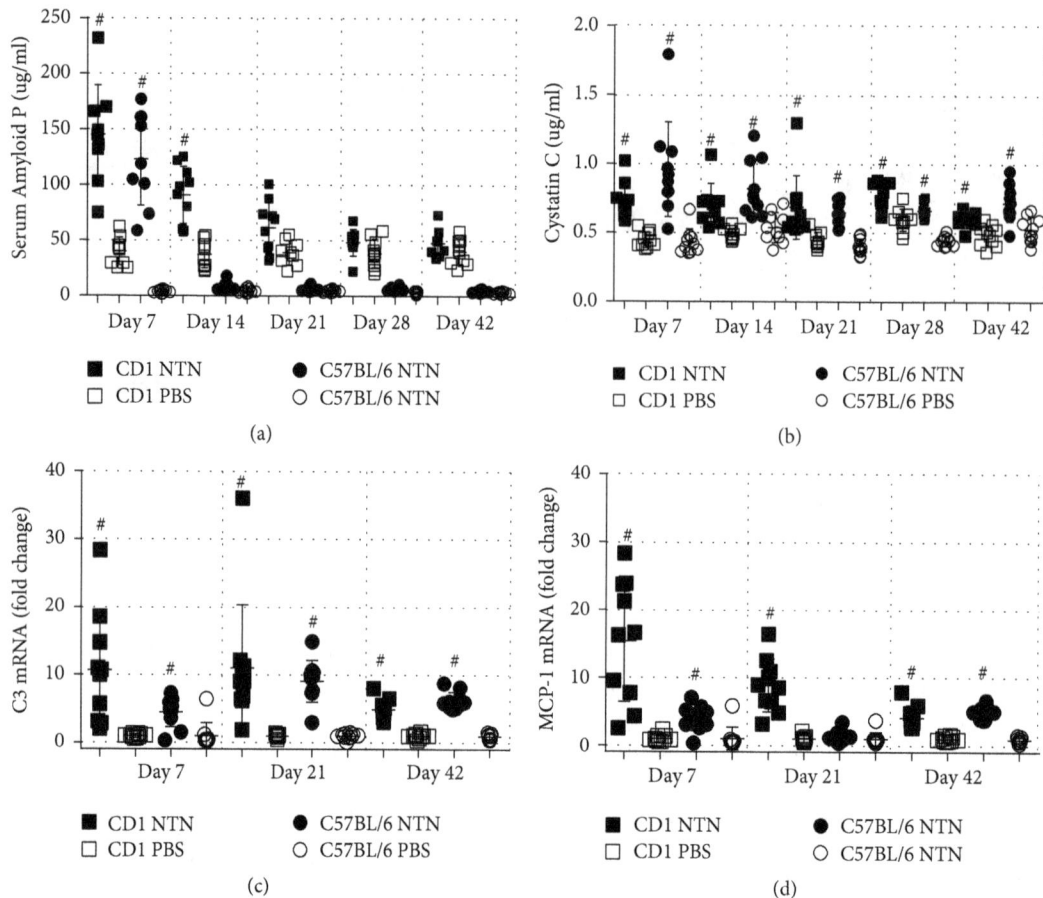

Figure 6: *NTS induces systemic inflammation and elevation of GFR marker.* (a) Scatter plot showing the SAP plasma concentration on days 7, 14, 21, 28, and 42 measured by ELISA. (b) Scatter plot of Cystatin C plasma concentration days 7, 14, 21, 28, and 42 measured by ELISA. (c) Scatter plot showing mRNA expression in whole kidney tissue of C3 and MCP-1 (CCL2) on days 7, 21, and 42, expressed as fold change. Data are shown as mean ± SD. #$P < 0.001$ NTN groups versus PBS groups by two-way ANOVA ($n = 10$).

urine albumin concentration remained at days 36-37 in both strains at approximately 2 logs above controls. At days 36-37 the ACR were still in the range of 33-43 mg/mg which is above the observed ACR of CKD models such as renal ablation models, UUO, and the STZ model supporting that the NTN model is a potential CKD model [27–29].

Decreased GFR is a hallmark of CKD and GFR is estimated or measured in patients for confirming diagnosis [30]. Thus, the observed GFR decline on days 5-6, 15–17, and 34–37 demonstrates that the NTN model resembles features of human CKD. The significantly increased urinary albumin concentration, UACR, UAER, and the GFR decline point towards glomerular impairment and thereby kidney dysfunction in the NTN mice [31]. Furthermore, the significant urinary excretion of Cystatin C indicates that NTN induction causes tubular dysfunction. Cystatin C is freely filtered by the glomerulus and is in healthy individuals almost 100% reabsorbed by the tubules and catabolised. On days 36-37 the urinary Cystatin C excretion in the NTN mice had returned to baseline levels which might be explained by increased reabsorption of the remaining functional nephrons or a resolution of the tubules.

The increased urinary excretion of TNFR1 might be explained by the phenomenon of shedding the receptors from membranes of TNF-α activated glomerular and tubular cells by a proteolytic process where the TNF-alpha converting enzyme (TACE) cleaves TNFR1 as an immunological response. On the other hand, Bemelmans et al. suggested that a continuous release of soluble TNFR1 occurs and the kidney clears it in healthy individuals [32]. The consistent levels of urinary TNFR1 excretion in the control mice support the hypothesis of a continuous release of TNFR1, and the significantly increased UAER at all-time points indicates a dysfunctional filtration barrier as both TNFR1 and albumin in healthy individuals are blocked by the glomerular filtration barrier by size and charge selectivity [33–35].

The pathological characterisation of human CKD is defined as the presence of kidney damage that progresses or remains over time and includes, in general, glomerular lesions and renal fibrosis [36–38]. The NTN model shows the presence of chronically progressing kidney damage detected by significant impairment of mesangial expansion and increased globally sclerosed glomeruli between each time point in both strains. Furthermore, the significant mesangial

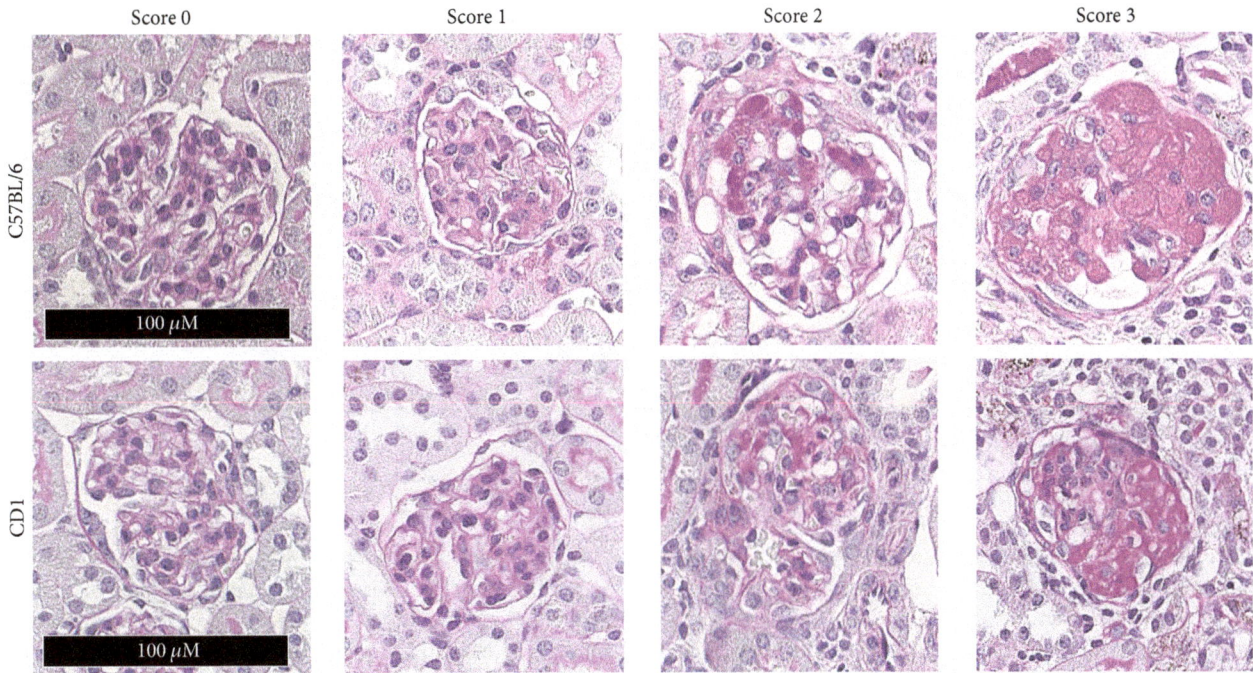

(a)

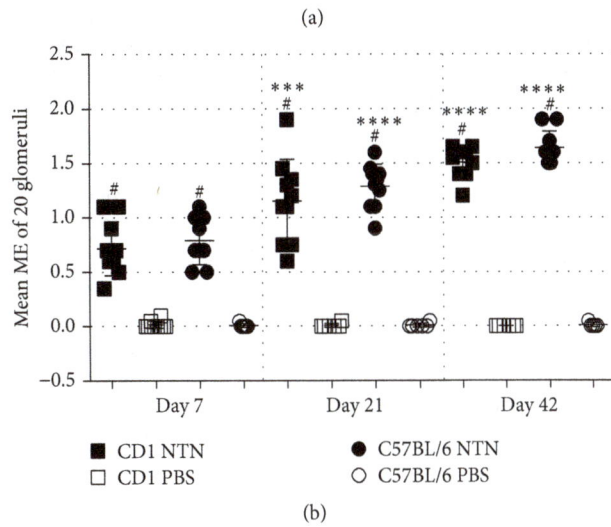

(b)

FIGURE 7: *NTS causes chronic and progressive glomerular mesangial expansion in C57BL/6 and CD1 mice.* (a) Representative glomeruli showing scores 0, 1, 2, and 3 of mesangial expansion. (b) Scatter plot showing the mean glomerular mesangial expansion (ME) score on days 7, 21, and 42. Data are shown as mean ± SD. [#]$P < 0.0001$ NTN groups versus PBS groups; [***]$P < 0.001$ NTN group day 7 versus NTN group day 21; [****]$P < 0.0001$ NTN group day 21 versus NTN group day 42 by two-way ANOVA and using Kruskal-Wallis multiple testing ($n = 10$).

expansion on day 7 indicates a fast disease development. The progressive mesangial expansion developing on day 42 shows that the NTS causes features of chronic and progressive disease development.

In human CKD, renal fibrosis is characterised by the deposition of extracellular matrix (ECM) components including collagen III and fibronectin [39]. During pathological conditions, PAI-1 contributes to the accumulation of ECM components as PAI-1 inhibits degradation of ECM proteins [39]. NTS induced significant renal fibrosis detected by collagen III deposition on day 21 and day 42 in both strains. However, in contrast to the mesangial expansion, the renal fibrosis did not progress from day 21, suggesting that the fibrotic response observed here could be linked to the resolution of the initial inflammatory reaction in the NTN model. Interestingly, the development of renal fibrosis was somewhat similar in CD1 and C57BL/6 mice, which contradicts previous studies describing CD1 mice with an increased susceptibility to renal fibrosis in the 5/6 nephrectomy and STZ models [13, 15, 16]. However, differences in model duration and insult could be the explanation.

The significantly increased mRNA levels of collagen III, fibronectin, and PAI-1 in both strains were reduced on day 42 compared to day 7 suggesting a continued but slowed

TABLE 1: *Histopathological lesions by mouse strains.* The tubular casts were visualised as solidification of protein in the lumen of the kidney tubules. The metaplasia was visualised as a change from flattened parietal epithelium to cuboidal epithelium lining the glomerulus. The segmental glomerulosclerosis was visualised as glomeruli that showed scarring of small sections of the glomeruli, while global glomerulosclerosis was visualised as totally scarred glomeruli.

Pathologic changes NTN mice	CD1 day 7 $n = 9$	%	B6 day 7 $n = 6$	%	CD1 day 21 $n = 10$	%	B6 day 21 $n = 6$	%	CD1 day 42 $n = 8$	%	B6 day 42 $n = 7$	%
Tubular casts (cortex)												
Present (yes/no)	9	100	6	100	9	90	6	100	7	86	6	86
Metaplasia												
	47	26	35	29	54	27	32	27	38	24	33	24
Glomerulosclerosis (segmental)												
	39	22	24	20	44	22	25	21	35	22	20	14
Glomerulosclerosis (global)												
	4	2	2	2	22	11	8	7	20	13	18	13

profibrotic activity which correlates with the discontinued progression of collagen III depositions from day 21.

Immune system activation and inflammation play a central role in the pathogenesis of acute kidney injury and CKD [40]. Following NTS injection both CD1 and C57BL/6 mice developed an acute phase inflammatory response evaluated by significantly elevated SAP in plasma on days 7–14. The baseline SAP levels of CD1 mice were significantly higher compared to C57BL/6 mice, which is consistent with literature describing strain differences in baseline SAP levels [41]. Cystatin C is described as being elevated during systemic inflammation [42], which could account for the elevation observed on days 7 and 14 consistently with the elevated plasma SAP. However, Cystatin C is not only increased due to inflammation as several studies describe Cystatin C as a superior marker of GFR [43, 44]. The observed decline in GFR on days 5-6, 15–17, and 34–37 in CD1 NTN mice strongly suggests that the increase in Cystatin C levels observed on days 7 and 14 is caused both by inflammation and by a decline in renal function. It is very likely that the elevated Cystatin C after day 14 is mainly a response to the declined GFR.

Activation of the complement system by immune complexes is known to occur in immune-mediated CKDs [45]. Complement 3 is synthesised by glomerular cells, and tubular cells and the local synthesised C3 has been demonstrated to play a role in the development of kidney disease [45, 46]. The upregulation of C3 mRNA levels in the NTN mice suggests that the injected anti-GBM antibodies activate the complement system which is in agreement with literature describing this phenomenon in the NTN model [47].

NTS induced a transient weight loss in both the CD1 and C57BL/6 NTN mice. The weight loss could be a response to NTS induced illness causing decreased diet and fluid intake. However, the recovered body weight after around day 10 indicates that the NTS doses are tolerated.

Comparing the nonaccelerated NTN model to other CKD models, the NTN model displays a technically easy and consistently inducible model with rapid disease progression when the optimal NTS dose is identified. We have shown that NTN mice develop a chronic stage of kidney disease within 21 days as seen by glomerulosclerosis, fibrosis, inflammation,

tubular damage, elevated systemic markers of kidney damage, and albuminuria, whereas, for example, classical diabetic nephropathy models develop mild signs of CKD within 15–18 weeks [7]. The NTN model displays morphological aspects as mesangial expansion as well as inflammatory and fibrotic responses. In contrast, the widely used UUO model which also develops rapid inflammation and renal fibrosis is limited by the unobstructed kidney compensating for the obstructed kidney making it impractical to study the pathogenesis [2]. The 5/6 nephrectomy model develops glomeruli sclerosis and renal fibrosis within 12 weeks, but it requires a technically difficult surgery making it difficult to reproduce [6, 48].

The inbred C57BL/6 and outbred CD1 mice showed similar kidney disease progression. However, the CD1 mice had significantly increased UAER and mRNA levels of profibrotic genes at several time points compared to C57BL/6 mice. In addition, the strains showed different susceptibility to NTS as the doses needed to induce similar kidney damage were 100 and 250 μl NTS, respectively. At present this difference is not well understood but is possibly related to their different genetic background, which could result in different binding properties of anti-GBM antibodies, different inflammatory response to antibody deposition, or different reactivity to other sheep serum components in the two strains. The C57Bl/6 mice showed only mild gender differences based on the significantly increased collagen III mRNA levels observed in NTN females compared to NTN males in week 10. Conversely, the CD1 NTN females showed significant UAER on days 35-36 and significantly increased collagen III deposition compared to NTN males indicating that the CD1 females are more susceptible to NTS compared to CD1 males.

In conclusion, we have shown that the nonaccelerated NTN model in addition to acute inflammatory kidney disease develops several chronic hallmarks of CKD such as albuminuria, GFR decline, progressive mesangial expansion, and renal fibrosis. C57BL/6 and CD1 mice showed similar disease manifestations making them both applicable to studies of the acute and chronic phases of kidney disease using the nonaccelerated NTN model. The CD1 mice did not display increased susceptibility to develop renal fibrosis as described in other CKD models. However, the CD1 mice, especially

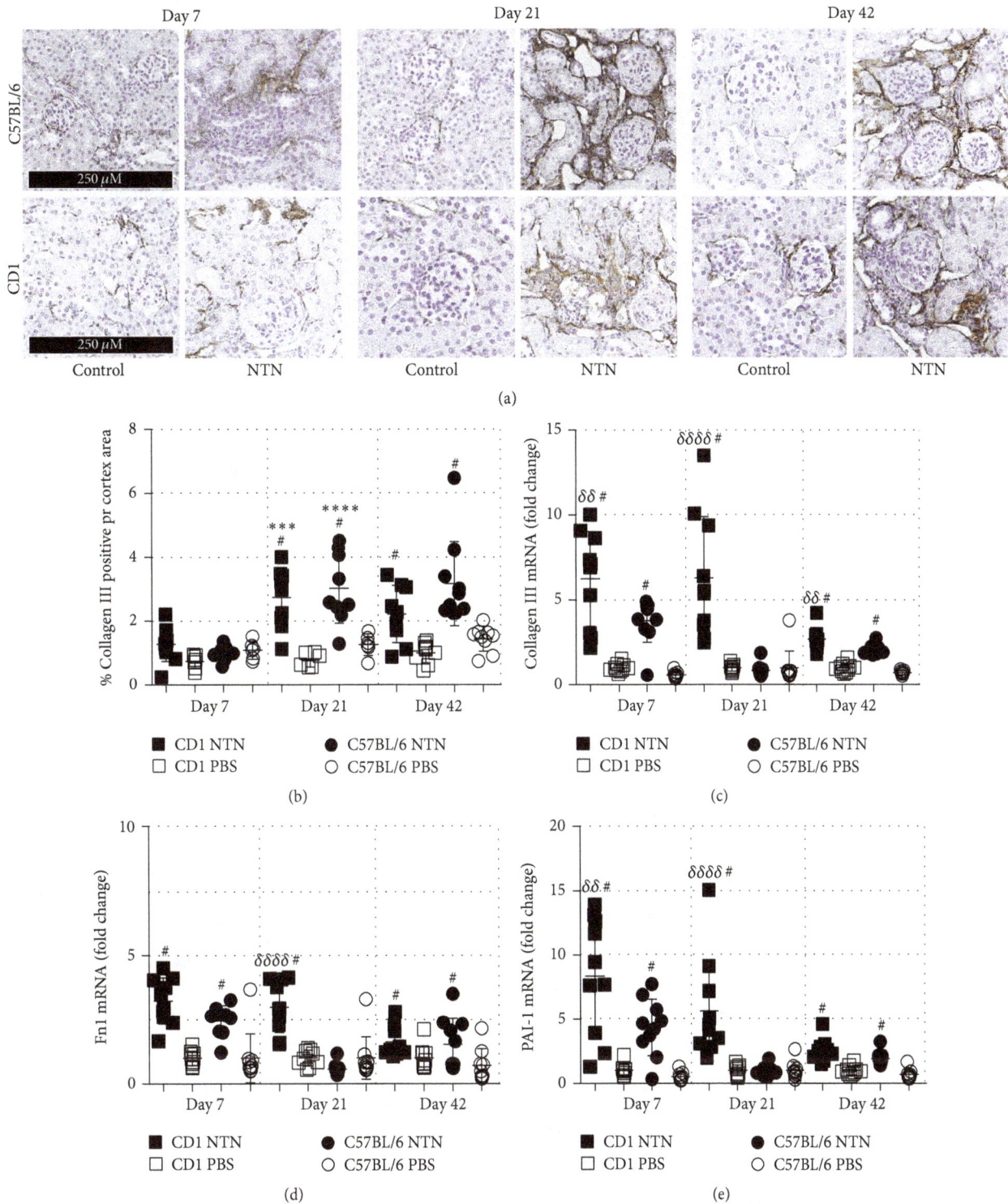

FIGURE 8: *NTS induces chronic renal fibrosis.* (a) Representative images of tubulointerstitial fibrotic area visualised by immunohistochemical collagen III staining. (b) Semiquantification of collagen III positive area of the cortex area. (c) Scatter plot showing mRNA expression in whole kidney tissue of Col3a1 as fold change. (d) Fibronectin (Fn1) mRNA expression as fold change. (e) PAI-1 (Serpine-1) mRNA expression as fold change. Data are shown as mean ± SD. $^{#}P < 0.0001$ NTN groups versus PBS groups; $^{***}P < 0.001$ NTN day 7 versus NTN day 21; $^{****}P < 0.0001$ NTN day 7 versus NTN day 21; and $^{\delta\delta}P < 0.01$, $^{\delta\delta\delta\delta}P < 0.0001$ CD1 NTN versus B6 NTN groups by two-way ANOVA ($n = 10$).

the CD1 female mice, did show a higher susceptibility to NTS which would possibly make them the more practical choice. The nonaccelerated NTN model quickly resembles hallmarks of acute and chronic CKD and its robustness and relatively simple NTS induction phase make it a valid alternative compared to other cumbersome models of CKD.

Acknowledgments

This project was supported by Novo Nordisk A/S and the Danish In Vivo Pharmacology PhD Program. The authors thank Anja Koustrup, Jette Mandelbaum, Helle Hvorup, Julie Dybdal Jensen, and Tina Lundager for outstanding technical support.

References

[1] A. B. Fogo, "Mechanisms of progression of chronic kidney disease," *Pediatric Nephrology*, vol. 22, no. 12, pp. 2011–2022, 2007.

[2] G. J. Becker and T. D. Hewitson, "Animal models of chronic kidney disease: useful but not perfect," *Nephrology Dialysis Transplantation* , vol. 28, no. 10, pp. 2432–2438, 2013.

[3] A. A. Eddy, J. M. López-Guisa, D. M. Okamura, and I. Yamaguchi, "Investigating mechanisms of chronic kidney disease in mouse models," *Pediatric Nephrology*, vol. 27, no. 8, pp. 1233–1247, 2012.

[4] A. B. Fogo, "Animal models of FSGS: Lessons for pathogenesis and treatment," *Seminars in Nephrology*, vol. 23, no. 2, pp. 161–171, 2003.

[5] L. Huang, A. Scarpellini, M. Funck, E. A. Verderio, and T. S. Johnson, "Development of a chronic kidney disease model in C57BL/6 mice with relevance to human pathology," *Nephron Extra*, vol. 3, no. 1, pp. 12–29, 2013.

[6] R. Waldherr and N. Gretz, "Natural course of the development of histological lesions after 5/6 nephrectomy," *Contributions to Nephrology*, vol. 60, pp. 64–72, 1988.

[7] C. E. Alpers and K. L. Hudkins, "Mouse models of diabetic nephropathy," *Current Opinion in Nephrology and Hypertension*, vol. 20, no. 3, pp. 278–284, 2011.

[8] Y. Kaneko, F. Nimmerjahn, M. P. Madaio, and J. V. Ravetch, "Pathology and protection in nephrotoxic nephritis is determined by selective engagement of specific Fc receptors," *The Journal of Experimental Medicine*, vol. 203, no. 3, pp. 789–797, 2006.

[9] H. Nagai, H. Yamada, and A. Koda, "The susceptibility of experimental glomerulonephritis in six different strains of mice," *Journal of Pharmacobio-Dynamics*, vol. 8, no. 7, pp. 586–589, 1985.

[10] C. Xie, R. Sharma, H. Wang, X. J. Zhou, and C. Mohan, "Strain distribution pattern of susceptibility to immune-mediated nephritis," *The Journal of Immunology*, vol. 172, no. 8, pp. 5047–5055, 2004.

[11] J. E. Pena-Polanco and L. F. Fried, "Established and emerging strategies in the treatment of chronic kidney disease," *Seminars in Nephrology*, vol. 36, no. 4, pp. 331–342, 2016.

[12] A. Ohno, C. Inagaki, K. Honda, and N. Sugino, "Comparison of converting enzyme inhibitor and calcium channel blocker in SHR with nephrotoxic serum nephritis," *The Japanese Journal of Nephrology*, vol. 34, no. 4, pp. 405–410, 1992.

[13] A. Leelahavanichkul, Q. Yan, X. Hu et al., "Angiotensin II overcomes strain-dependent resistance of rapid CKD progression in a new remnant kidney mouse model," *Kidney International*, vol. 78, no. 11, pp. 1136–1153, 2010.

[14] A. Leelahavanichkul, Q. Yan, X. Hu, C. Eisner, Y. Huang, R. Chen et al., "Rapid CKD progression in a new mouse kidney remnant model: strain-dependent resistance is overcome by angiotensin II," *Kidney International*, vol. 78, no. 11, pp. 1136–1153, 2010.

[15] H. Sugimoto, G. Grahovac, M. Zeisberg, and R. Kalluri, "Renal fibrosis and glomerulosclerosis in a new mouse model of diabetic nephropathy and its regression by bone morphogenic protein-7 and advanced glycation end product inhibitors," *Diabetes*, vol. 56, no. 7, pp. 1825–1833, 2007.

[16] L. Walkin, S. E. Herrick, A. Summers et al., "The role of mouse strain differences in the susceptibility to fibrosis: a systematic review," *Fibrogenesis & Tissue Repair*, vol. 6, no. 1, article 18, 2013.

[17] I. Goldberg and I. Krause, "The role of gender in chronic kidney disease," *Emergency Medicine Journal*, vol. 1, no. 2, pp. 58–64, 2016.

[18] M. Zeisberg, J.-I. Hanai, H. Sugimoto et al., "BMP-7 counteracts TGF-β1-induced epithelial-to-mesenchymal transition and reverses chronic renal injury," *Nature Medicine*, vol. 9, no. 7, pp. 964–968, 2003.

[19] H. Sugimoto, V. S. LeBleu, D. Bosukonda et al., "Activin-like kinase 3 is important for kidney regeneration and reversal of fibrosis," *Nature Medicine*, vol. 18, no. 3, pp. 396–404, 2012.

[20] P. S. T. Yuen, S. R. Dunn, T. Miyaji, H. Yasuda, K. Sharma, and R. A. Star, "A simplified method for HPLC determination of creatinine in mouse serum," *American Journal of Physiology-Renal Physiology*, vol. 286, no. 6, pp. F1116–F1119, 2004.

[21] S. J. Ellery, X. Cai, D. D. Walker, H. Dickinson, and M. M. Kett, "Transcutaneous measurement of glomerular filtration rate in small rodents: Through the skin for the win?" *Nephrology*, vol. 20, no. 3, pp. 117–123, 2015.

[22] J. Wen, Y. Xia, A. Stock et al., "Neuropsychiatric disease in murine lupus is dependent on the TWEAK/Fn14 pathway," *Journal of Autoimmunity*, vol. 43, no. 1, pp. 44–54, 2013.

[23] C. Soendergaard, O. H. Nielsen, K. Skak, M. A. Røpke, J. B. Seidelin, and P. H. Kvist, "Objective Quantification of Immune Cell Infiltrates and Epidermal Proliferation in Psoriatic Skin: A Comparison of Digital Image Analysis and Manual Counting," *Applied Immunohistochemistry & Molecular Morphology* , vol. 24, no. 6, pp. 453–458, 2016.

[24] A. A. Eddy, "Tubulointerstitial nephritis during the heterologous phase of nephrotoxic serum nephritis," *Nephron*, vol. 59, no. 2, pp. 304–313, 1991.

[25] T. Nishihara, Y. Kusuyama, E. Gen, N. Tamaki, and K. Saito, "Masugi nephritis produced by the antiserum to heterologous glomerular basement membrane. I. Results in mice," *Acta Pathologica Japonica*, vol. 31, no. 1, pp. 85–92, 1981.

[26] K. J. M. Assmann, M. M. Tangelder, W. P. J. Lange, G. Schrijver, and R. A. Koene, "Anti-GBM nephritis in the mouse: severe proteinuria in the heterologous phase," *Virchows Archiv A Pathological Anatomy and Histopathology*, vol. 406, no. 3, pp. 285–299, 1985.

[27] J. Norlin, L. N. Fink, P. H. Kvist, E. D. Galsgaard, and K. Coppieters, "Abatacept treatment does not preserve renal function in the streptozotocin-induced model of diabetic nephropathy," *PLoS ONE*, vol. 11, no. 4, Article ID e0152315, 2016.

[28] H. S. Min, J. E. Kim, M. H. Lee et al., "Dipeptidyl peptidase IV inhibitor protects against renal interstitial fibrosis in a mouse

model of ureteral obstruction," *Laboratory Investigation*, vol. 94, no. 6, pp. 598–607, 2014.

[29] A. Lehners, S. Lange, G. Niemann et al., "Myeloperoxidase deficiency ameliorates progression of chronic kidney disease in mice," *American Journal of Physiology-Renal Physiology*, vol. 307, no. 4, pp. F407–F417, 2014.

[30] M. Arici, "Clinical assessment of a patient with chronic kidney disease," in *Management of Chronic Kidney Disease: A Clinician's Guide*, Springer, Berlin, Germany, 2014.

[31] H. Birn and E. I. Christensen, "Renal albumin absorption in physiology and pathology," *Kidney International*, vol. 69, no. 3, pp. 440–449, 2006.

[32] M. H. A. Bemelmans, D. J. Gouma, and W. A. Buurman, "Tissue distribution and clearance of soluble murine TNF receptors in mice," *Cytokine*, vol. 6, no. 6, pp. 608–615, 1994.

[33] Y. S. Kanwar, "Biophysiology of glomerular filtration and proteinuria," *Laboratory Investigation*, vol. 51, no. 1, pp. 7–21, 1984.

[34] T. S. Larson, "Evaluation of proteinuria," *Mayo Clinic Proceedings*, vol. 69, no. 12, pp. 1154–1158, 1994.

[35] N. Neirynck, G. Glorieux, E. Schepers, F. Verbeke, and R. Vanholder, "Soluble tumor necrosis factor receptor 1 and 2 predict outcomes in advanced chronic kidney disease: A prospective cohort study," *PLoS ONE*, vol. 10, no. 3, Article ID e0122073, 2015.

[36] L. Lopez-Marin, Y. Chavez, X. A. Garcia, W. M. Flores, Y. M. Garcia, R. Herrera et al., "Histopathology of chronic kidney disease of unknown etiology in Salvadoran agricultural communities," *Medical Education Cooperation with Cuba*, vol. 16, no. 2, pp. 49–54, 2014.

[37] L. G. Fine and J. T. Norman, "Chronic hypoxia as a mechanism of progression of chronic kidney diseases: From hypothesis to novel therapeutics," *Kidney International*, vol. 74, no. 7, pp. 867–872, 2008.

[38] H. Jacobson, "Chronic renal failure: pathophysiology," *The Lancet*, vol. 338, no. 8764, pp. 419–423, 1991.

[39] A. K. Ghosh and D. E. Vaughan, "PAI-1 in tissue fibrosis," *Journal of Cellular Physiology*, vol. 227, no. 2, pp. 493–507, 2012.

[40] J. D. Imig and M. J. Ryan, "Immune and inflammatory role in renal disease," *Comprehensive Physiology*, vol. 3, no. 2, pp. 957–976, 2013.

[41] R. F. Mortensen, K. Beisel, N. J. Zeleznik, and P. T. Le, "Acute-phase reactants of mice. II. Strain dependence of serum amyloid P-component (SAP) levels and response to inflammation," *The Journal of Immunology*, vol. 130, no. 2, pp. 885–889, 1983.

[42] T. Okura, M. Jotoku, J. Irita et al., "Association between cystatin C and inflammation in patients with essential hypertension," *Clinical and Experimental Nephrology*, vol. 14, no. 6, pp. 584–588, 2010.

[43] D. J. Newman, H. Thakkar, R. G. Edwards et al., "Serum cystatin C measured by automated immunoassay: a more sensitive marker of changes in GFR than serum creatinine," *Kidney International*, vol. 47, no. 1, pp. 312–318, 1995.

[44] G. Filler, A. Bökenkamp, W. Hofmann, T. Le Bricon, C. Martínez-Brú, and A. Grubb, "Cystatin C as a marker of GFR—history, indications, and future research," *Clinical Biochemistry*, vol. 38, no. 1, pp. 1–8, 2005.

[45] A. Fearn and N. S. Sheerin, "Complement activation in progressive renal disease," *World Journal of Nephrology*, vol. 4, no. 1, pp. 31–40, 2015.

[46] M. Miyazaki, K. Abe, T. Koji, A. Furusu, Y. Ozono, T. Harada et al., "Intraglomerular C3 synthesis in human kidney detected by in situ hybridization," *Journal of the American Society of Nephrology*, vol. 7, no. 11, pp. 2428–2433, 1996.

[47] M.-J. Hébert, T. Takano, A. Papayianni et al., "Acute nephrotoxic serum nephritis in complement knockout mice: Relative roles of the classical and alternate pathways in neutrophil recruitment and proteinuria," *Nephrology Dialysis Transplantation*, vol. 13, no. 11, pp. 2799–2803, 1998.

[48] A. Nogueira, M. J. Pires, and P. A. Oliveira, "Pathophysiological mechanisms of renal fibrosis: A review of animal models and therapeutic strategies," *In Vivo*, vol. 31, no. 1, pp. 1–22, 2017.

26

Contrast-Induced Nephropathy: Update on the Use of Crystalloids and Pharmacological Measures

D. Patschan ⓘ, I. Buschmann, and O. Ritter

Innere Medizin I, Kardiologie, Angiologie, Nephrologie, Klinikum Brandenburg, Medizinische Hochschule Brandenburg, Brandenburg, Germany

Correspondence should be addressed to D. Patschan; d.patschan@klinikum-brandenburg.de

Academic Editor: Alejandro Ferreiro

Contrast-induced nephropathy (CIN) is a frequent and severe complication in subjects receiving iodinated contrast media for diagnostic or therapeutic purposes. Several preventive strategies were evaluated in the past. Recent clinical studies and meta-analyses delivered some new aspects on preventive measures used in the past and present. We will discuss all pharmacological and nonpharmacological procedures. Finally, we will suggest individualized recommendations for CIN prevention.

1. Introduction

Acute kidney injury frequently occurs in hospitalized patients. Approximately 15% of all European in-hospital patients develop AKI during the disease [1]. The prognosis has not substantially been improved in recent years. Among exogenously administered substances that may cause AKI, iodinated contrast media are particularly relevant since they are extensively in use for diagnostic purposes all over the world. They may induce intrarenal vasoconstriction and potentially exhibit toxic effects on tubular epithelial cells in a direct manner [2]. An average of 2–10% of all subjects receiving contrast media (CM) suffers from an acute decline of excretory kidney function after being exposed [3]. Typically, the kidney deteriorates 2-3 days later. Comparably to AKI in general, the preventive and therapeutic measures for avoiding and improving CIN are limited, to put it mildly. For many years, preventive hydration, performed intravenously, has been the strategy of first choice. Recent studies put this well-established concept in question. Also, some smaller studies indicate that oral fluid administration could serve as a reliable alternative for iv prophylaxis. Uncertainty exists, on whether N-Acetylcysteine is truly useful or not. Finally, two recent meta-analyses identified a potential role of statins in preventing AKI after CM administration. This article

is intended to discuss several newer investigations on the topic mainly. Finally, we will suggest recommendations for CIN prevention in the clinical practice. Nevertheless, we do not intend to replace current guidelines, for instance, the "KDIGO Clinical Practice Guidelines for Acute Kidney Injury" [4].

2. Risk

The individual risk for acquiring CIN depends on numerous exogenous and endogenous circumstances such as the type and volume of CM used, the type of diagnostic or therapeutic procedure applied, and specific comorbidities [5]. Diseases that are associated with reduced effective perfusion pressure typically increase the risk [6]. Among those are dehydration, heart failure, and low arterial blood pressure due to overdosing of antihypertensive drugs. A higher risk also evolves in individuals with preexisting chronic kidney disease, particularly in subjects with diabetic nephropathy [3]. Multiple myeloma patients are also at higher risk for CIN; numerous causes may be involved (dehydration, increased blood viscosity, and infections due to immunosuppression) [7]. In 2004, Mehran and colleagues [6] published a score for estimating the AKI probability after CM exposure. The following qualities were incorporated: hypotension, application

TABLE 1: Illustration of CIN risk qualities and scores assigned to each quality as proposed by Mehran and colleagues [6]. The risks for CIN and dialysis vary, depending on the cumulative score. Sixteen or more points are associated with an average CIN risk of 57.3% and a dialysis risk of 12.6% (see text).

Quality	Score
Hypotension	5
Intra-aortic ballon pump therapy	5
Chronic heart failure	5
Age > 75 years	4
Anemia	3
Diabetes	3
Contrast volume	Increasing with increasing volume
Serum creatinine > 1.5 mg/dL	4
eGFR < 60 ml/min/1.73 m^2	Increasing with decreasing eGFR

of intra-aortic balloon pump therapy, chronic heart failure, age > 75 years, anemia, diabetes, higher contrast volume, and preexisting CKD. Each quality was assigned an individual score (e.g., hypotension 5 points as opposed to diabetes with 3 points). Four categories were defined (≤5; 6 to 10; 11 to 16; and ≥16) with progressively increasing risks for CIN and dialysis, respectively (Table 1). More recent approaches also aimed to define the individual CIN risk during coronary intervention [8–10]. A 2017 published meta-analysis by Allen and colleagues identified 75 individual articles describing 74 models designed for CIN risk prediction [11]. Only three models were found to allow a generalizable risk estimation. Controversy still exists on the exact eGFR (estimated glomerular filtration rate) threshold that requires prophylactic measures. It has been accepted that preventive care is mandatory in subjects with an eGFR of below 30 ml/min; some authors even suggest initiating prophylaxis at <40 ml/min [12]. In general, the need for prevention in patients with eGFR values ranging from 30 to 60 ml/min is still being discussed. The latest "KDIGO Clinical Practice Guidelines for Acute Kidney Injury" also do not offer any specific recommendations in this respect [4]. Thus, the final decision must be made individually, concerning preexisting comorbidities, the procedure which requires CM administration, and the type and volume of CM needed.

3. Prevention Using Crystalloids

Since many years, intravenous volume expansion using crystalloids has been established as first choice-strategy for CIN prevention. The general concept behind the administration of crystalloids is to increase the tubular flow of glomerular filtrate, thus to minimize the effective contact period between CM and tubular epithelial cells. The most widely used crystalloid is saline (0.9%), followed by sodium bicarbonate.

The latter was particularly thought to additionally neutralize CM-derived reactive oxygen species by increasing the intratubular pH. We intend to firstly summarize currently available data on the effects of volume administration per se, since a newer study published in April 2017 doubted the efficacy of crystalloid prevention in general [27]. We will then summarize studies comparing sodium chloride with sodium bicarbonate. Finally, we will conclude with several remarks on oral versus intravenous hydration.

3.1. Crystalloids versus No Crystalloids. Since many years, intravenous administration of crystalloids has widely been used for CIN prevention all over the world. No study of the past evaluated the efficacy of hydration versus no hydration, most likely due to ethical reasons. Therefore, one may ask how exactly the concept of volume prevention was established. Comparisons between randomized controlled trials and historical control subjects that did not receive any prophylaxis at all suggested a clear benefit from the fluid administration [28]. A recent study put the "hydration concept" in question in general. The AMACING trial (prospective, randomized, phase 3, open-label, and noninferiority) compared prophylactic saline hydration with no hydration in a total number of 660 individuals with an estimated GFR ranging from 30 to 59 ml/min/1.73 m^2 [27]. The primary outcome was CIN incidence which was defined as a rise in serum creatinine of at least 45 μmol/l within 2–6 days. CIN incidences were 2.6% in nonhydrated and 2.7% in hydrated subjects. Nevertheless, no hydration was significantly associated with fewer side effects and lower costs. Though intriguing, the study has its limitations. The first surprising observation was the relatively small CIN frequency in general. Most studies performed in the past reported AKI to occur in more than 10% after CM exposure [2]. One may argue that CIN remained undiagnosed in several individuals, possibly a result of collecting not all serum samples between days 2 and 4 after procedure. Another reason for such low incidences may be attributable to one of the inclusion criteria: the estimated GFR was defined to range from 30 to 59 ml/min. Thus, patients at higher risk (eGFR < 30 ml/min) were not included. However, the study provided some new information in either case. It potentially helps to define more precisely whether a patient indeed requires aggressively prophylactic measures or not. To repeat the trial with a higher number of individuals has been discussed as unethical and should, also in our opinion, be avoided. Some of these issues have been addressed in a recent commentary by Sato et al. [29].

3.2. Sodium Chloride versus Sodium Bicarbonate. The first investigation comparing the two crystalloids was published in 2004 by Merten and colleagues [30]. It included a total of 260 individuals receiving either one of the two solutions. CIN incidences were 1.7% (sodium bicarbonate) versus 13.6% (sodium chloride) ($p = 0.02$). The study earned criticism, mostly due to the relatively low number of subjects enrolled, which did not allow excluding false positive results [28]. Numerous other trials were published since then [31–38]. As reviewed by Weisbord and colleagues [28], the literature, up to this point, did not allow concluding which solution was truly superior to the other. It needs to be mentioned that sample sizes in these and other studies varied between 59 and 502. Therefore, certain effects may have been the result of inadequately low numbers of subjects enrolled. The latest study on the topic was published in November 2017 [39]. The PRESERVE trial investigated the efficacy of sodium bicarbonate versus sodium chloride and N-Acetylcysteine (ACC) versus placebo. In a multicenter, prospective design, nearly 5.000 individuals receiving contrast media for diagnostic purposes were randomized into one of four groups. CIN incidence was defined as a secondary endpoint. Surprisingly, CIN occurred with comparable frequencies in all groups and in the placebo group. If objected prematurely, one may conclude that any of the three prophylactic procedures mentioned is avoidable at all. Nevertheless, several limitations must be considered. (I) The vast majority of the participants were males since the trial was performed in hospitals of the "Veterans Affairs Hospitals" organization. (II) The diagnosis of AKI was made by measuring serum creatinine once, exclusively between days 3 and 5 after CM exposure. Thus, a substantial number of individuals may have been missed. (III) CM was exclusively applied for diagnostic reasons. (IV) The cumulative volume administered prior to and after contrast media infusion was anything but comparable between subjects. The proposed dose-regimen for pre-CM administration, for instance, was 1–3 ml/kg/h, to be started between hours 2 and 12 before the procedure. Therefore, an individual weighting 100 kg could, in theory, have been infused with either 200 or 3.000 ml in total. These limitations do certainly not allow the conclusion that iv hydration using crystalloids is unnecessary. The study simply shows that sodium bicarbonate is most likely neither inferior nor superior to sodium chloride regarding AKI prevention in this particular cohort.

3.3. Oral versus Intravenous Volume Administration. Significantly fewer studies evaluated the role of oral crystalloid supplementation in comparison to iv infusion. A randomized, controlled single-center trial compared three protocols using either iv sodium bicarbonate ($n = 43$) or oral sodium citrate ($n = 43$) or oral nonspecific hydration ($n = 44$) [40]. CIN incidences did not significantly differ between the groups (7.0% versus 11.6% versus 9.1%). The authors concluded that oral hydration is as safe and effective as intravenous prophylaxis. Akyuz and colleagues [41] exclusively included subjects with normal or moderately impaired kidney function (CKD stages 1-2). All subjects had at least one CIN high risk factor such as higher age, diabetes, heart failure, and anemia. CIN occurred with comparable frequencies in both groups [41]. Although oral hydration may appear as a more feasible option, at first sight, several questions remain unanswered. So far, no analyses have been performed in subjects at very high CIN risk (eGFR < 30 ml/min). Also, in the studies mentioned above only limited patient numbers were included, respectively ($n = 130$ and $n = 225$). Larger investigations must be performed to confirm or falsify these preliminary observations.

4. N-Acetylcysteine (ACC)

The rationale behind the use of ACC in the past was to neutralize reactive, CM-driven oxygen species in the kidney. A first prospective trial was published in 2000 [42]. Tepel and colleagues included 83 patients at risk for CIN who were injected with a nonionic, low-osmolality contrast agent for computed tomography. Subjects received either 0.45% sodium chloride alone or the crystalloid in combination with ACC. One out of 41 individuals in the ACC$^+$ group versus 9 out of 42 in the ACC- group showed an increase in serum creatinine of 44 μmol/l or higher at 48 hours after CM exposure. In 2013, Weisbord et al. [28] reviewed the literature and listed 15 studies revealing positive effects and 21 investigations showing negative impacts of ACC prophylaxis. The "KDIGO Clinical Practice Guidelines for Acute Kidney Injury" suggested the use of ACC "together with i.v. isotonic crystalloids, in patients at increased risk of CIN" [4]. The recommendation was graded with "2D." The PRESERVE trial (see Sodium Chloride versus Sodium Bicarbonate) also evaluated one subgroup of patients undergoing ACC prophylaxis [39]. Keeping in mind the limitations of the study, no differences in CIN incidences were observed between any of the four groups. The data from this prospective, controlled multicenter study put the concept of ACC prevention in question in general. On the other hand, Su and colleagues published a large meta-analysis in January 2017 [19]. Herein, the authors analyzed a total of 150 trials with 31.631 subjects included. The following pharmacological measures for CIN prevention were investigated: N-acetylcysteine, theophylline, fenoldopam, iloprost, alprostadil, prostaglandin E 1, statins, statins plus ACC, bicarbonate sodium, bicarbonate sodium plus ACC, ascorbic acid (vitamin C), tocopherol (vitamin E), alpha-lipoic acid, atrial natriuretic peptide, B-type natriuretic peptide, and carperitide. They identified the following interventions as the most effective measures: high-dose statins plus hydration with or without ACC. The limitations of the analysis were discussed in detail; most importantly, event rates were comparably low, and the distribution of participants among treatment strategies was quite heterogenous. Li and colleagues finally published another meta-analysis in August 2017 [43]. A total number of 19 clinical trials with more than 4.000 individuals was evaluated, concluding that ACC is not an effective strategy for CIN prophylaxis.

Regarding the heterogenous literature, it is impossible to recommend or deny the use of ACC for CIN prevention. However, since the substance is by no means expensive, it may be applied optionally but always in addition to other drugs/substances such as sodium chloride/bicarbonate and possibly high-dose statins.

5. Other Drugs

Several pharmacological measures have been evaluated in the past including ascorbic acid, fenoldopam, prostaglandins, probucol, statins, theophylline, tocopherol, and trimetazidine (Table 2). Some essential information shall be given about each drug.

TABLE 2: Summary of clinical trials related to CIN protective effects of different pharmacological strategies.

Substance	CIN protection	No CIN protection
Ascorbic acid	Meta-analysis of nine RCTs, 33% lower CIN risk if compared to either placebo or to alternative pharmacological regimen (risk ratio by random-effects model: 0.672; 95% confidence interval, 0.466 to 0.969; $p = 0.034$) [13]	Meta-analysis of multiple substances including ascorbic acid, no superiority as compared to saline (odds ratio active treatment versus saline: 1.84; 95% confidence interval: 0.16 to 24.98) [14]
Fenoldopam	None	(i) Prospective, placebo-controlled, double-blind, multicenter RCT, CIN incidences in fenoldopam versus placebo: 33.6 versus 30.1%; $p = 0.61$ [15] (ii) Prospective, randomized trial, CIN incidences in saline versus saline + fenoldopam versus saline + ACC: 15.3 versus 15.7 versus 17.1%; $p = 0.9$ [16]
Probucol	(i) Prospective, randomized trial, CIN incidences in probucol + hydration versus hydration alone: 4 versus 10.9%; p value significant [17] (ii) Meta-analysis of multiple substances including probucol, further odds ratio reduction with probucol odds ratio active treatment versus saline 0.27; 95% confidence interval: 0.09 to 0.79 [14]	None
Prostaglandins	Two meta-analyses indicated beneficial effects of different types of prostaglandins in CIN prevention [14, 18]	None
Statins	(i) Benefit of combined administration of high-dose statins and saline [19] (ii) Meta-analysis published by Liang et al.: diabetic subjects benefit from moderate or high-dose rosuvastatin [20]	None
Theophylline	Beneficial effects in three trials [21–23]	None
Tocopherol	(i) Rezaei et al. [24]: additional administration of tocopherol prior to elective coronary intervention lowered CIN risk further (ii) Benefit in two other randomized controlled trials [25, 26]	None
Trimetazidine	Meta-analysis published by Ye and colleagues [18]: 6 randomized controlled trials indicate additional CIN protection by the substance	None

As a vitamin, ascorbic acid exhibits antioxidative effects. Two meta-analyses evaluated the efficacy of the substance in CIN prevention. The first analysis was published by Sadat and colleagues [13]. It included 9 randomized controlled trials and showed a 33% lower CIN risk in comparison to either placebo or other pharmacological strategies. A second meta-analysis, published in 2017 [14], failed to show additional benefit from administration of ascorbic acid; the substance was not superior to saline.

Fenoldopam, though beneficial in theory, is not recommended for CIN prevention [4]. It antagonizes intrarenal dopamine A1 receptors in a selective manner and was therefore hypothesized to act renoprotectively by increasing the medullary blood-flow. However, two prospective studies failed to show different AKI incidences after CM administration [15, 16]. Thus, this approach was not evaluated further since.

As a vasodilatory substance, Alprostadil has been applied in clinical studies for CIN prevention. A meta-analysis of studies in diabetic subjects, published by Ye et al., came to the conclusion that, in comparison to conventional hydration, the prostaglandins lower CIN incidences without significantly causing unwanted side effects [44]. Navarese and colleagues reported a substantial CIN odds ratio reduction under prostaglandins [14] and comparable conclusions were drawn by Kassis et al. who analyzed a total number of 8 clinical trials [45].

Probucol was initially designed as lipid-lowering drug but was never established in the clinic since it also exhibits HDL-lowering effects. In a randomized controlled trial published this year, Fu et al. compared probucol plus hydration with hydration alone in subjects with coronary heart disease undergoing percutaneous coronary intervention [17]. CIN incidences were 4 versus 10.9%. This observation is in line with the results of the meta-analysis by Navarese and colleagues [14] who found a substantial CIN odds ratio reduction under the drug.

The KDIGO guidelines [4], published in 2012, did not reliably recommend the prophylactic use of statins in CM exposed individuals. However, some newer aspects must be considered. A 2017 published meta-analysis by Su and colleagues [19] identified high-dose statins (if combined with hydration) of definite benefit. The same effects were not observed under low-dose statins (dose categories: high-dose statin category: simvastatin, 40 to 80 mg; rosuvastatin, 20 to 40 mg; and atorvastatin, 40 to 80 mg; low-dose statin category: simvastatin, 10 to 20 mg; rosuvastatin, 10 mg; and atorvastatin, 10 to 20 mg). Comparable conclusions were drawn from a meta-analysis of Liang et al. [20]. Fifteen trials were included showing that moderate- or high-dose rosuvastatin reduced CIN incidences after coronary angiography and particularly in diabetic subjects.

The administration of theophylline in clinical trials has been motivated by its adenosine-antagonistic effects. Adenosine has been documented to increase in serum and urine after CM exposure [46]. Although the substance is not regularly in clinical use for CIN prevention, the literature indicates some beneficial effects under defined circumstances. Huber et al. [21] compared the effectiveness of theophylline, ACC, and both substances combined in 91 individuals with at least one CIN risk factor treated at the ICU and receiving CM. Peak creatinine levels were significantly higher in the "ACC alone" than in the "theophylline" or the "ACC + theophylline" group(s), indicating a substantial role for the drug in CIN prevention. A more recent study from 2009 confirmed such effects [22]. Baskurt and colleagues randomized 217 subjects (estimated GFR 30–60 ml/min) to receive either isotonic saline alone or isotonic saline + ACC or the two latter substances combined with oral theophylline. No single individual from group 3 developed CIN after coronary angiography. It needs to be mentioned that the total number of AKI events in this investigations was comparably low ($n = 12$). A third study from 2010 further confirmed beneficial effects of theophylline [23]. However, the substance has not been established as CIN preventive strategy, most likely due to its proarrhythmogenic effects and the numerous pharmacological interactions. The latest KDIGO guidelines summarize these aspects in detail [4].

Two further drugs shall finally be mentioned: tocopherol (vitamin E) and trimetazidine. Tocopherol also acts antioxidatively. Rezaei et al. [24] compared CIN preventive treatment with tocopherol plus hydration with hydration alone. The vitamin was applied with 600 mg at hour 12 before and with 400 mg at hour 2 before elective coronary angiography. Subjects suffered from preexisting chronic kidney disease (CKD, eGFR < 60 ml/min/1.73 m^2) and controls received placebo instead of tocopherol. CIN incidences were 6.7 versus 14.1% (tocopherol versus placebo). These observations were confirmed by two randomized controlled studies from 2009 and 2013 [25, 26]. Trimetazidine finally was developed as anticancer agent. A more recent study from 2017 [47]

compared the additional (+hydration) administration of the drug with hydration alone and found lower CIN incidences: 10 versus 26%. Nevertheless, the mean contrast media volume was higher in CIN patients. In a meta-analysis from the same year (2017), Ye et al. [18] included 6 randomized controlled trials with evidence for additional protective effects of the substance in CIN prevention.

6. Dialysis

Dialysis for CM elimination cannot be recommended as CIN preventive measure. One study showed beneficial effects of hemofiltration if started 6 hours before CM exposure and continued until hours 18–24 after infusion [48]. However, such an approach is accompanied by enormous logistic difficulties and may therefore not be suitable for the clinical practice. Other studies failed to show any clear benefit of dialysis [49, 50]. A general problem that occurs with renal replacement therapy is the limited diagnostic value of serum creatinine since the procedure eliminates the substance naturally.

7. Recommendations

The following recommendations reflect, to some extent, individual conclusions made by the authors. This is not intended to revise official recommendations as given in the KDIGO guidelines [4] or other guidelines published so far.

(i) We recommend prophylactic hydration of patients at risk for CIN.

(ii) Hydration should be performed intravenously; either sodium chloride or sodium bicarbonate may be applied.

(iii) The individual risk must be quantified. Prophylactic measures should be initiated in subjects with an eGFR of lower than 30 ml/min. In subjects with an eGFR of 30–60 ml/min, additional risk factors should be considered.

(iv) ACC may be administered additionally.

(v) High-dose statins may be administered additionally.

(vi) Probucol, prostaglandins, tocopherol, and trimetazidine are new candidates in the management of CIN. Definite recommendations cannot be made at the moment.

(vii) Ascorbic acid, theophylline, and fenoldopam are obsolete.

(viii) Peri-/postprocedure dialysis is obsolete.

Figure 1 summarizes CIN risk factors and preventive strategies.

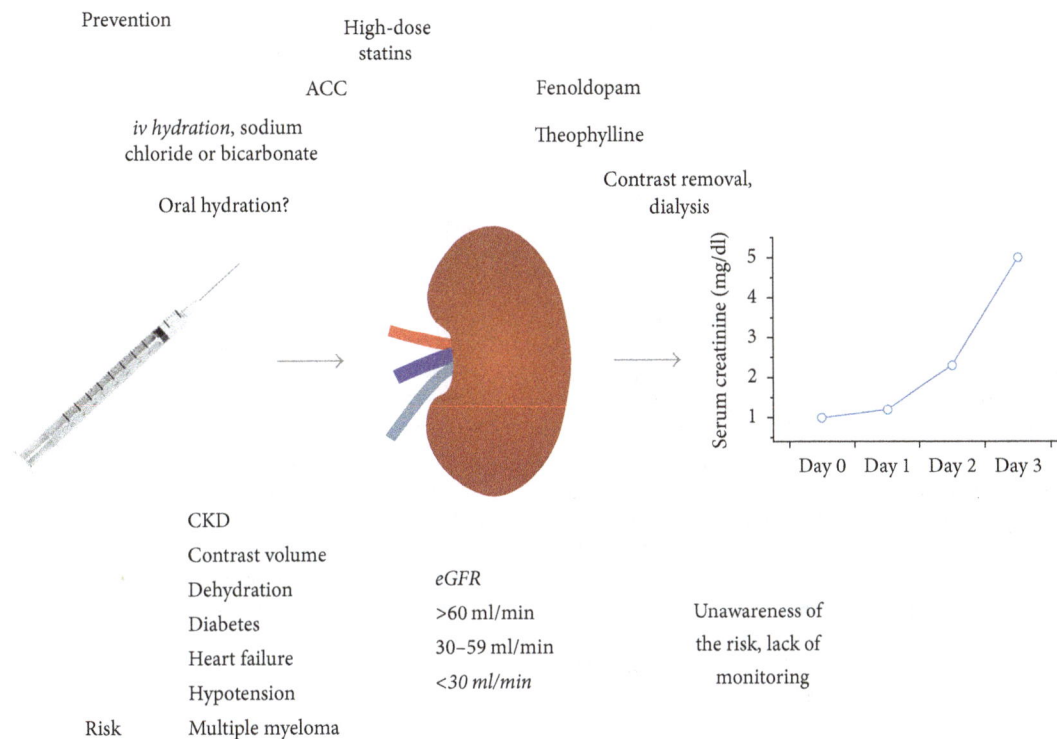

FIGURE 1: CIN risk factors and preventive measures. Risk: multiple comorbidities may increase the vulnerability of the kidney. It has widely been accepted that subjects with an eGFR of <30 ml/min are at very high risk for acquiring CIN (red and italic). Prevention: the concept of iv hydration is the basis of all preventive interventions (green and italic). Measures without proven benefit or with uncertain risk-benefit ratio are put in grey.

References

[1] A. Bienholz, B. Wilde, and A. Kribben, "From the nephrologist's point of view: diversity of causes and clinical features of acute kidney injury," *Clinical Kidney Journal*, vol. 8, no. 4, pp. 405–414, 2015.

[2] K. Modi and S. C. Dulebohn, *Contrast-Induced Nephropathy*, StatPearls Publishing, Treasure Island, Florida, Fla, USA, 2017, http://www.ncbi.nlm.nih.gov/books/NBK448066/.

[3] S. Ozkok and A. Ozkok, "Contrast-induced acute kidney injury: a review of practical points," *World Journal of Nephrology*, vol. 6, no. 3, pp. 86–99, 2017.

[4] A. Khwaja, *KDIGO Clinical Practice Guidelines for Acute Kidney Injury*, Karger Publishers, Berlin, Germany, 2012.

[5] J. L. Wichmann, R. W. Katzberg, S. E. Litwin et al., "Contrast-induced nephropathy," *Circulation*, vol. 132, no. 20, pp. 1931–1936, 2015.

[6] R. Mehran, E. D. Aymong, E. Nikolsky et al., "A simple risk score for prediction of contrast-induced nephropathy after percutaneous coronary intervention: development and initial validation," *Journal of the American College of Cardiology*, vol. 44, no. 7, pp. 1393–1399, 2004.

[7] M. Mussap and G. Merlini, "Pathogenesis of renal failure in multiple myeloma: any role of contrast media?" *BioMed Research International*, vol. 2014, Article ID 167125, 10 pages, 2014.

[8] X. Hu, X.-D. Zhuang, Y. Li et al., "A nomogram to predict contrast induced nephropathy in patients undergoing percuta-neous coronary intervention: Is the "anti-aging" agent klotho a candidate predictor?" *International Heart Journal*, vol. 58, no. 2, pp. 191–196, 2017.

[9] K.-Y. Lin, W.-P. Zheng, W.-J. Bei et al., "A novel risk score model for prediction of contrast-induced nephropathy after emergent percutaneous coronary intervention," *International Journal of Cardiology*, vol. 230, pp. 402–412, 2017.

[10] L. Ji, X. Su, W. Qin et al., "Novel risk score of contrast-induced nephropathy after percutaneous coronary interven-tion," *Nephrology*, vol. 20, no. 8, pp. 544–551, 2015.

[11] D. W. Allen, B. Ma, K. C. Leung et al., "Risk prediction models for contrast-induced acute kidney injury accompanying cardiac catheterization: systematic review and meta-analysis," *Canadian Journal of Cardiology*, vol. 33, no. 6, pp. 724–736, 2017.

[12] R. K. Gupta and T. J. Bang, "Prevention of contrast-induced nephropathy (CIN) in interventional radiology practice," *Seminars in Interventional Radiology*, vol. 27, no. 4, pp. 348–359, 2010.

[13] U. Sadat, A. Usman, J. H. Gillard, and J. R. Boyle, "Does ascorbic acid protect against contrast-induced acute kidney injury in patients undergoing coronary angiography: a systematic review with meta-analysis of randomized, controlled trials," *Journal of the American College of Cardiology*, vol. 62, no. 23, pp. 2167–2175, 2013.

[14] E. P. Navarese, P. A. Gurbel, F. Andreotti et al., "Prevention of contrast-induced acute kidney injury in patients undergoing cardiovascular procedures-A systematic review and network meta-Analysis," *PLoS ONE*, vol. 12, no. 2, Article ID e0168726, 2017.

[15] G. W. Stone, P. A. McCullough, J. A. Tumlin et al., "Fenoldopam mesylate for the prevention of contrast-induced nephropathy: a randomized controlled trial," *Journal of the American Medical Association*, vol. 290, no. 17, pp. 2284–2291, 2003.

[16] S. Allaqaband, R. Tumuluri, A. M. Malik et al., "Prospective randomized study of N-acetylcysteine, fenoldopam, and saline for prevention of radiocontrast-induced nephropathy," *Catheterization and Cardiovascular Interventions*, vol. 57, no. 3, pp. 279–283, 2002.

[17] N. Fu, S. Yang, J. Zhang, P. Zhang, M. Liang, and H. Cong, "The efficacy of probucol combined with hydration in preventing contrast-induced nephropathy in patients with coronary heart disease undergoing percutaneous coronary intervention: a multicenter, prospective, randomized controlled study," *International Urology and Nephrology*, vol. 50, no. 1, pp. 105–112, 2018.

[18] Z. Ye, H. Lu, Q. Su et al., "Clinical effect of trimetazidine on prevention of contrast-induced nephropathy in patients with renal insufficiency: An updated systematic review and meta-analysis," *Medicine (United States)*, vol. 96, no. 9, Article ID e6059, 2017.

[19] X. Su, X. Xie, L. Liu et al., "Comparative effectiveness of 12 treatment strategies for preventing contrast-induced acute kidney injury: a systematic review and bayesian network meta-analysis," *American Journal of Kidney Diseases*, vol. 69, no. 1, pp. 69–77, 2017.

[20] M. Liang, S. Yang, and N. Fu, "Efficacy of short-term moderate or high-dose rosuvastatin in preventing contrast-induced nephropathy: a meta-analysis of 15 randomized controlled trials," *Medicine*, vol. 96, no. 27, Article ID e7384, 2017.

[21] W. Huber, F. Eckel, M. Hennig et al., "Prophylaxis of contrast material-induced nephropathy in patients in intensive care: acetylcysteine, theophylline, or both? A randomized study," *Radiology*, vol. 239, no. 3, pp. 793–804, 2006.

[22] M. Baskurt, B. Okcun, O. Abaci et al., "N-acetylcysteine versus N-acetylcysteine + theophylline for the prevention of contrast nephropathy," *European Journal of Clinical Investigation*, vol. 39, no. 9, pp. 793–799, 2009.

[23] M. Malhis, S. Al-Bitar, and K. A. Zaiat, "The role of theophylline in prevention of radiocontrast media-induced nephropathy," *Saudi Journal of Kidney Diseases and Transplantation*, vol. 21, no. 2, pp. 276–283, 2010.

[24] Y. Rezaei, K. Khademvatani, B. Rahimi, M. Khoshfetrat, N. Arjmand, and M.-H. Seyyed-Mohammadzad, "Short-term high-dose vitamin e to prevent contrast medium-induced acute kidney injury in patients with chronic kidney disease undergoing elective coronary angiography: a randomized placebo-controlled trial," *Journal of the American Heart Association*, vol. 5, no. 3, Article ID e002919, 2016.

[25] A. Tasanarong, D. Piyayotai, and S. Thitiarchakul, "Protection of radiocontrast induced nephropathy by vitamin E (alpha tocopherol): a randomized controlled pilot study," *Journal of the Medical Association of Thailand*, vol. 92, no. 10, pp. 1273–1281, 2009.

[26] A. Tasanarong, A. Vohakiat, P. Hutayanon, and D. Piyayotai, "New strategy of α-and γ-tocopherol to prevent contrast-induced acute kidney injury in chronic kidney disease patients undergoing elective coronary procedures," *Nephrology Dialysis Transplantation*, vol. 28, no. 2, pp. 337–344, 2013.

[27] E. C. Nijssen, R. J. Rennenberg, P. J. Nelemans et al., "Prophylactic hydration to protect renal function from intravascular iodinated contrast material in patients at high risk of contrast-induced nephropathy (AMACING): a prospective, randomised, phase 3, controlled, open-label, non-inferiority trial," *The Lancet*, vol. 389, no. 10076, pp. 1312–1322, 2017.

[28] S. D. Weisbord, M. Gallagher, J. Kaufman et al., "Prevention of contrast-induced AKI: A review of published trials and the design of the prevention of serious adverse events following angiography (PRESERVE) trial," *Clinical Journal of the American Society of Nephrology*, vol. 8, no. 9, pp. 1618–1631, 2013.

[29] A. Sato, T. Hoshi, and K. Aonuma, "No prophylaxis is non-inferior and cost-saving to prophylactic intravenous hydration in preventing contrast-induced nephropathy on requiring iodinated contrast material administration," *Journal of Thoracic Disease*, vol. 9, no. 6, pp. 1440–1442, 2017.

[30] G. J. Merten, W. P. Burgess, L. V. Gray et al., "Prevention of contrast-induced nephropathy with sodium bicarbonate: a randomized controlled trial," *Journal of the American Medical Association*, vol. 291, no. 19, pp. 2328–2334, 2004.

[31] C. Briguori, F. Airoldi, D. D'Andrea et al., "Renal insufficiency following contrast media administration trial (REMEDIAL): a randomized comparison of 3 preventive strategies," *Circulation*, vol. 115, no. 10, pp. 1211–1217, 2007.

[32] M. Masuda, T. Yamada, T. Mine et al., "Comparison of usefulness of sodium bicarbonate versus sodium chloride to prevent contrast-induced nephropathy in patients undergoing an emergent coronary procedure," *American Journal of Cardiology*, vol. 100, no. 5, pp. 781–786, 2007.

[33] M. Motohiro, H. Kamihata, S. Tsujimoto et al., "A new protocol using sodium bicarbonate for the prevention of contrast-induced nephropathy in patients undergoing coronary angiography," *American Journal of Cardiology*, vol. 107, no. 11, pp. 1604–1608, 2011.

[34] E. E. Ozcan, S. Guneri, B. Akdeniz et al., "Sodium bicarbonate, *N*-acetylcysteine, and saline for prevention of radiocontrast-induced nephropathy. A comparison of 3 regimens for protecting contrast-induced nephropathy in patients undergoing coronary procedures. A single-center prospective controlled trial," *American Heart Journal*, vol. 154, no. 3, pp. 539–544, 2007.

[35] M. Pakfetrat, M. H. Nikoo, L. Malekmakan et al., "A comparison of sodium bicarbonate infusion versus normal saline infusion and its combination with oral acetazolamide for prevention of contrast-induced nephropathy: a randomized, double-blind trial," *International Urology and Nephrology*, vol. 41, no. 3, pp. 629–634, 2009.

[36] A. Recio-Mayoral, M. Chaparro, B. Prado et al., "The renoprotective effect of hydration with sodium bicarbonate plus N-acetylcysteine in patients undergoing emergency percutaneous coronary intervention: the RENO Study," *Journal of the American College of Cardiology*, vol. 49, no. 12, pp. 1283–1288, 2007.

[37] M. Maioli, A. Toso, M. Leoncini et al., "Sodium bicarbonate versus saline for the prevention of contrast-induced nephropathy in patients with renal dysfunction undergoing coronary angiography or intervention," *Journal of the American College of Cardiology*, vol. 52, no. 8, pp. 599–604, 2008.

[38] E. Adolph, B. Holdt-Lehmann, T. Chatterjee et al., "Renal insufficiency following radiocontrast exposure trial (REINFORCE): a randomized comparison of sodium bicarbonate versus sodium chloride hydration for the prevention of contrast-induced nephropathy," *Coronary Artery Disease*, vol. 19, no. 6, pp. 413–419, 2008.

[39] S. D. Weisbord, M. Gallagher, H. Jneid, S. Garcia, A. Cass, and S.-S. Thwin, "Outcomes after angiography with sodium bicarbonate and acetylcysteine," *The New England Journal of Medicine*, 2017.

[40] P. L. Martin-Moreno, N. Varo, E. Martínez-Ansó et al., "Comparison of intravenous and oral hydration in the prevention of contrast-induced acute kidney injury in low-risk patients: a randomized trial," *Nephron*, vol. 131, no. 1, pp. 51–58, 2015.

[41] S. Akyuz, M. Karaca, T. Kemaloglu Oz et al., "Efficacy of oral hydration in the prevention of contrast-induced acute kidney injury in patients undergoing coronary angiography or intervention," *Nephron Clinical Practice*, vol. 128, no. 1-2, pp. 95–100, 2014.

[42] M. Tepel, M. van der Giet, C. Schwarzfeld, U. Laufer, D. Liermann, and W. Zidek, "Prevention of radiographic-contrast-agent-induced reductions in renal function by acetylcysteine," *The New England Journal of Medicine*, vol. 343, no. 3, pp. 180–184, 2000.

[43] J.-X. Li, E.-Z. Jin, L.-H. Yu et al., "Oral N-acetylcysteine for prophylaxis of contrast-induced nephropathy in patients following coronary angioplasty: a meta-analysis," *Experimental and Therapeutic Medicine*, vol. 14, no. 2, pp. 1568–1576, 2017.

[44] Z. Ye, H. Lu, W. Guo et al., "The effect of alprostadil on preventing contrast-induced nephropathy for percutaneous coronary intervention in diabetic patients: a systematic review and meta-analysis," *Medicine*, vol. 95, article e5306, no. 46, 2016.

[45] H. M. Kassis, K. D. Minsinger, P. A. McCullough, C. A. Block, M. S. Sidhu, and J. R. Brown, "A review of the use of iloprost, a synthetic prostacyclin, in the prevention of radiocontrast nephropathy in patients undergoing coronary angiography and intervention," *Clinical Cardiology*, vol. 38, no. 8, pp. 492–498, 2015.

[46] L. J. Arend, G. L. Bakris, J. C. Burnett, C. Megerian, and W. S. Spielman, "Role for intrarenal adenosine in the renal hemodynamic response to contrast media," *Journal of Laboratory and Clinical Medicine*, vol. 110, no. 4, pp. 406–411, 1987.

[47] T. A. Ibrahim, R. H. El-Mawardy, A. S. El-Serafy, and E. M. El-Fekky, "Trimetazidine in the prevention of contrast-induced nephropathy in chronic kidney disease," *Cardiovascular Revascularization Medicine*, vol. 18, no. 5, pp. 315–319, 2017.

[48] G. Marenzi, G. Lauri, J. Campodonico et al., "Comparison of two hemofiltration protocols for prevention of contrast-induced nephropathy in high-risk patients," *American Journal of Medicine*, vol. 119, no. 2, pp. 155–162, 2006.

[49] G. Deray, "Dialysis and iodinated contrast media," *Kidney International*, vol. 69, no. 100, pp. S25–S29, 2006.

[50] B. Vogt, P. Ferrari, C. Schönholzer et al., "Prophylactic hemodialysis after radiocontrast media in patients with renal insufficiency is potentially harmful," *American Journal of Medicine*, vol. 111, no. 9, pp. 692–698, 2001.

27

Prevalence of Microalbuminuria in Adult Patients with Sickle Cell Disease in Eastern Saudi Arabia

Ahmed M. Alkhunaizi ⓘ,[1] Adil A. Al-Khatti,[2] and Mansour A. Alkhunaizi[3]

[1]*Nephrology Unit, Specialty Medicine Department, Johns Hopkins Aramco Healthcare, Dhahran, Saudi Arabia*
[2]*Hematology Unit, Cancer Institute, Johns Hopkins Aramco Healthcare, Dhahran, Saudi Arabia*
[3]*Royal College of Surgeons in Ireland, Dublin, Ireland*

Correspondence should be addressed to Ahmed M. Alkhunaizi; aalkhunaizi@gmail.com

Academic Editor: David B. Kershaw

Background. Proteinuria is a common feature of sickle cell nephropathy (SCN) that can progress to renal insufficiency and end stage renal disease. Microalbuminuria (MA) is the earliest manifestation of SCN and precedes the development of overt proteinuria. In addition to the renal consequences, MA is linked to cardiovascular complications. Periodic screening and early detection of MA allow early intervention that may reduce the risk of progression to advanced renal failure and cardiovascular diseases. *Objective.* The aim of this study was to investigate the prevalence of MA in patients with SCD in the eastern region of Saudi Arabia. *Methods.* A prospective cross-sectional observational study was conducted at Johns Hopkins Aramco Healthcare (JHAH). Urine samples of SCD patients 18 years old and older were tested for the presence of MA using urinary albumin over creatinine ratio (ACR). Correlation was tested with multiple variables including age, gender, body mass index (BMI), hemoglobin level, blood pressure, blood transfusion history, pain episodes, and use of hydroxyurea. *Results.* Urine samples were tested on 72 patients. The mean age of the study cohort was 35 ± 16.9 years. Microalbuminuria was detected in 18 patients (25%). No correlation was found with any of the tested variables. *Conclusion.* Microalbuminuria is a common finding in patients with SCD in eastern Saudi Arabia. Patients with SCD should be screened for MA, and those with positive tests should probably be treated with antiproteinuric agents that may slow the progression to advanced stages of renal failure and decrease the risk of cardiovascular diseases.

1. Introduction

Sickle cell disease (SCD) is prevalent in the eastern region of Saudi Arabia (SA). Proteinuria is a common feature of sickle cell nephropathy (SCN) that can progress to renal insufficiency and end stage renal disease (ESRD) [1–3]. Prior to the development of overt proteinuria, patients with SCD manifest with microalbuminuria (MA) that is believed to be a result of hyperfiltration and early glomerular dysfunction [4]. In addition, MA is predictive of all cause and cardiovascular mortality among patients with diabetes mellitus, hypertension, and the general population [5]. The prevalence of MA among patients with SCD in eastern SA has not been previously determined. The objective of this study was to investigate the prevalence of MA and to establish clinical characteristics associated with MA among patients with SCD in this part of the world who have a less severe disease compared to other populations. Early intervention, when MA is present, using antiproteinuric measures such as blockade of the renin angiotensin system or use of hydroxyurea, may slow the progression to overt proteinuria and advanced chronic kidney disease (CKD) [6]. Treatment of MA may also affect mortality and morbidity associated with cardiovascular diseases.

2. Methods

A prospective cross-sectional observational study was carried out at Johns Hopkins Aramco Healthcare (JHAH) in Dhahran, eastern SA, between July 2014 and October 2016. Consecutive patients with SCD, 18 years and older, who attended the hematology clinic for routine follow-up at the Cancer Institute of JHAH were enrolled after they gave an informed consent. The diagnosis of SCD was

TABLE 1: Patients' demographics.

Total	Male (%)	Female (%)	Age Years	BMI Kg/m^2	SBP mmHg	DBP mmHg	Pain crisis	eGFR ml/min	Hb g/dL	HbF%	HU (%)
72	35 (49)	37 (51)	35 ± 16.9	24.2 ± 4.19	118 ± 13	76 ± 24	2	127 ± 40	10.5 ± 1.6	17.6 ± 7.1	70 (97)

BMI: body mass index; SBP: systolic blood pressure; DBP: diastolic blood pressure; eGFR: estimated glomerular filtration rate; Hb: hemoglobin; HbF: fetal hemoglobin; HU: hydroxyurea.

confirmed using hemoglobin electrophoresis. The two geno-types encountered and considered as having SCD were homozygous SS and compound heterozygous sickle-beta zero thalassemia. Patients with diabetes mellitus, essential hypertension, patients who had positive proteinuria by urine dipstick, patients with preexisting renal disease with or without proteinuria, and those who had an acute illness, fever, or SCD crisis in the preceding two weeks were excluded. Pregnant women were also excluded. Patients were instructed to submit early morning urine samples for measurement of MA. In addition to urine samples, blood was collected for measurement of serum creatinine. Estimated glomerular filtration rate (eGFR) was calculated from serum creatinine, age, weight, and gender, using the Cockroft-Gault formula [7]. Data about patients' weight, body mass index (BMI), blood pressure (BP), hospitalization, blood transfusion history, and use of hydroxyurea were collected by reviewing the electronic medical records and reflected the most recent measurements. Baseline fetal hemoglobin (HbF) prior to initiation of hydroxyurea and glucose-6-phosphate dehydro-genase status (G6PD) were also assessed. Cut-offs of the independent variables were determined based on the recognized normal values for BP, BMI, eGFR, and hemoglobin. The mean of three resting systolic and diastolic BP measurements during routine clinic visits was used. Microalbuminuria was determined by measuring the albumin/creatinine ratio (ACR) on an early morning spot urine sample using rate nephelometry. Level of >24.9 mg albumin/g creatinine was considered abnormal. Correlation was made with various variables including age, sex, BP, BMI, level of hemoglobin, use of hydroxyurea, and hospitalization for pain crises. Patients' parameters were divided into age < 30 and ≥30 years; BMI < 25 and ≥ 25 kg/m^2; SBP < 120 and ≥ 120 mmHg; DBP < 80 and ≥ 80 mmHg; pain crisis < 2 and ≥ 2 episodes/year; Hb < 10 and ≥ 10 g/dL.

The study was approved by the institutional review board at JHAH before it began.

2.1. Statistical Analysis. Data were entered into Microsoft Excel 2013 and then uploaded into Statistical Package for Social Sciences (SPSS) 21 for analysis. Association between the independent variables and MA was assessed by bivariate and multivariate analyses using Chi square test (χ^2) for independence and logistic regression analysis. *T*-test was used to compare the mean values. Means were expressed as ±1 standard deviation (SD). Odds ratios (OR) were expressed together with 95% confidence interval (CI) and associated *P* values. A *P* value of < 0.05 was considered significant.

3. Results

One hundred and two patients were recruited, of whom 72 submitted urine and blood samples for analysis and were included in the final analysis. The remaining 30 patients (29%) failed to submit urine and or blood samples and were excluded. Out of the 72 patients who were included in the analysis, 37 patients were females (51%) and 35 were males (49%) with a female : male ratio of 1.06 : 1. The vast majority of patients are expected to have the Arab-Indian (AI) beta-globin gene (HBB) cluster haplotype as previously determined [8–10]. The mean age of the study population was 35 ± 16.9 years. The mean BMI of the cohort was 24 ± 4.19 kg/m^2. The mean SBP and DBP were 118 ± 13 and 72 ± 24 mm Hg, respectively. The mean Hb was 10.5 ± 1.6 g/dL. The mean eGFR was 127 ± 40 ml/min. Seventy (97%) patients were receiving hydroxyurea at the time of enrolment. None of the patients received treatment with angiotensin converting enzyme inhibitors or angiotensin receptor blockers at time of enrolment. The demographics of patients are shown in Table 1.

Increased MA was found in 18 patients (25%). In a multivariate logistic regression model of MA, there was no correlation between the presence of MA and any of the variables including age, sex, BP, BMI, level of Hb, number of hospitalizations for pain crisis, and eGFR as shown in Tables 2 and 3. The mean baseline HbF was 18.4 ± 6.3% of total Hb (range 7–39%) in patients with normal albumin excretion compared to 15.4 ± 9.0% (3.5–33%) in those with MA, *P* = 0.138. In addition, in a post hoc analysis we found no correlation between G6PD status and the development of MA.

4. Discussion

Sickle cell nephropathy may develop early in the course of patients with SCD and can have a variety of manifestations such as hyposthenuria, hematuria, proteinuria, abnormal urinary acidification, and renal failure [1, 4, 11]. Microalbuminuria is an early manifestation of SCN which is believed to be a consequence of glomerular hyperfiltration [12]. Glomerular hyperfiltration has been implicated in the pathogenesis of glomerular hypertrophy and glomerular sclerosis which is the predominant glomerular lesion found in renal biopsy of patients with SCN [12, 13].

In SA, SCD is found mainly in the eastern, southwestern, and northwestern regions [8, 9]. Patients in the eastern region have less severe disease, attributed to the presence of the

TABLE 2: Study variables in association with microalbuminuria.

Variable	Abnormal ACR N = 18 (25%) No (%)	Normal ACR N = 54 (75%) No (%)	χ^2 value	P value
Sex				
Male	10 (28.6)	25 (71.4)	0.463	0.496
Female	8 (21.6)	29 (78.4)		
Age (years)				
<30	9 (26.5)	25 (73.5)	0.074	0.785
≥30	9 (23.7)	29 (76.3)		
BMI (kg/m^2)				
<25	10 (26.3)	28 (73.7)	0.074	0.785
≥25	8 (23.5)	26 (76.5)		
SBP (mm Hg)				
<120	9 (21.4)	33 (78.6)	0.686	0.408
≥120	9 (30)	21 (70)		
DBP (mm Hg)				
<80	14 (22.6)	48 (77.4)	1.394	0.238
≥80	4 (40)	6 (60)		
Pain crisis				
<2	9 (20.9)	34 (79.1)	0.943	0.331
≥2	9 (31)	20 (69)		
Hb (gm/dL)				
<10	7 (31.8)	15 (68.2)	0.785	0.375
≥10	11 (22)	39 (78)		
eGFR (ml/min)				
<100	6 (33.3)	12 (66.7)	0.889	0.346
≥100	12 (22.2)	42 (77.8)		

ACR: albumin/creatinine ratio; BMI: body mass index; SBP: systolic blood pressure; DBP: diastolic blood pressure; Hb: hemoglobin; eGFR: estimated glomerular filtration rate.

TABLE 3: Logistic regression analysis of study variables in association with microalbuminuria.

Variable	OR	95% CI	P value
Sex			
Male versus female	0.402	0.10–1.64	0.204
Age (years)			
<30 versus ≥30	1.618	0.41–6.41	0.494
BMI (kg/m^2)			
<25 versus ≥25	1.139	0.33–4.00	0.838
SBP (mm Hg)			
<120 versus ≥120	0.858	0.22–3.40	0.827
DBP (mm Hg)			
<80 versus ≥80	0.471	0.09–2.56	0.383
Pain crisis			
<2 versus ≥2	0.467	0.14–1.58	0.219
Hb (gm/dL)			
<10 versus ≥10	2.072	0.52–8.30	0.304
eGFR (ml/min)			
<100 versus ≥100	0.300	0.06–1.63	0.163

OR: odds ratio; CI: confidence interval; BMI: body mass index; SBP: systolic blood pressure; DBP: diastolic blood pressure; Hb: hemoglobin; eGFR: estimated glomerular filtration rate.

AI beta-globin haplotype that results in a much higher HbF level, as compared with those in the south western and north western regions, who have the Benin haplotype [10, 14, 15]. We have previously determined the prevalence of overt proteinuria among patients with SCD in the eastern region of SA which was less than what had been reported in other populations in the United States and Africa [16–18]. We also have studied the course of patients with SCD who developed ESRD and were started on renal replacement therapy (RRT) at two large centers in eastern SA [19]. Among 942 patients with SCD who were followed up at our center between 2003 and 2016, only 11 patients developed ESRD and required RRT [19]. Therefore, we believe that renal involvement is less common and less severe in this patients' population. However, with the prevalence of MA, the early manifestation of SCN in this patients' population has not been previously determined.

The aim of this study was to determine the prevalence of MA in SCD patients in eastern SA and to define the clinical and hematologic correlates of the disease. Microalbuminuria is an important marker of early renal complication, and is a predictor of cardiovascular disease not only among diabetic and hypertensive patients but also in the general population [5].

Unlike many studies that have looked at the prevalence of MA in children with SCD, our cohort included adults above the age of 18 years. We found that the overall prevalence of MA among adult patients with SCD was 25%. In comparison, we have previously determined the prevalence of overt proteinuria (macroalbuminuria) in the same patients' population to be 8.4% [16]. Microalbuminuria cannot be detected by simple urine dipstick testing, and the presence of abnormal albumin excretion should be performed using more sensitive methods such as nephelometry. Adding the prevalence of macroalbuminuria found in our previous study to the current prevalence of MA, we can conclude that the overall prevalence of abnormal albumin excretion among SCD patients in this geographic area approximates 30%. We did not find a correlation between MA and any of the variables studied including age, gender, BMI, BP, level of Hb, frequency of pain episodes, and eGFR. Similarly there was no correlation between the development of MA and the G6PD status, a condition that predisposes to episodic hemolysis among affected individuals. In addition, there was no difference in the level of HbF between patients with MA and those with normal albumin excretion. The relatively small size of the study population may have contributed to the lack of correlation.

The mean eGFR in our cohort is relatively high and is likely to be an overestimate of the true GFR. We used the Cockcroft-Gault formula to estimate GFR which was derived from estimation of creatinine production based on gender, age, and weight [7]. Cockcroft-Gault formula may overestimate creatinine production in patients with SCD who have low muscle mass. In addition, proximal tubular excretion of creatinine in patients with SCD is believed to be elevated, averaging 40% even in the presence of normal renal function which may lead to over estimation of GFR [20]. Other methods to measure GFR such as inulin and iothalamate clearance are more accurate albeit cumbersome and not practical to use in every day practice.

Other studies have shown a higher prevalence of albuminuria among African American patients with SCD. In an earlier study in African American children, Dhrnidharka et al. found MA in 46% of children between 10 and 18 years of age [21]. There was a correlation with age but no correlation with pain frequency, hospitalization, frequency of blood transfusion, ferritin level, and creatinine clearance. Guasch et al. investigated the prevalence of albuminuria (micro- and macroalbuminuria) among African American adults with SCD [17]. In hemoglobin SS disease, increased albuminuria occurred in 68% of adult patients, and macroalbuminuria occurred in 26%. At the age of 40 years, 40% of patients with SS disease had macroalbuminuria. The prevalence of albuminuria was more common in SS disease compared with other sickling disorders. Albuminuria correlated with age and serum creatinine in SS disease but not with BP or hemoglobin levels. In a more recent study, MA was found in 44% of adults with HbSS as compared to 23% in patients with HbSC [22].

Other investigators found MA in 40% of teenagers and adults with SCD in Brazil with no correlation between MA and age, creatinine clearance, and Hb level [23]. In a cohort study in Jamaica, MA was found in 26% of subjects with SCD between the ages of 18 and 23 years. There was a positive correlation with GFR and BP and a negative correlation with Hb [24].

In our cohort, the great majority of the patients were receiving hydroxyurea at the time of enrolment. Whether treatment with hydroxyurea has affected the course of patients and lowered the prevalence of MA is not known. The data about the role of hydroxyurea in modifying the renal abnormalities associated with SCD are conflicting. McKie et al. have shown that microalbumin excretion normalized in 44% of patients with SCD treated with hydroxyurea [6]. In a more recent study, Aygun et al. reported that, after three years of treatment with hydroxyurea, there was a decrease in hyperfiltration, and the GFR dropped from 167 to 145 ml/min; however, there was no change in urine microalbumin excretion [25]. Similarly, the BABY HUG clinical trial for infants with SCD showed that treatment with hydroxyurea for 24 months did not influence GFR in young children with SCD. However, hydroxyurea was associated with better urine concentrating ability and less renal enlargement [26]. Considering the good safety profile of hydroxyurea and the benefits in patients with SCD in general, we believe that all patients with SCD who have MA should be treated with hydroxyurea in addition to blockers of the renin angiotensin system. Treatment with captopril was shown in a small study of 22 patients to be effective in reducing albuminuria associated with SCD [27]. Similarly, in a phase-2 multicenter trial, losartan decreased urinary albumin excretion in SCD patients with albuminuria, especially in those with MA [28]. More recently, losartan was shown to decrease albuminuria in 20 patients with SCD who were treated with hydroxyurea [29]. A larger prospective randomized study will be required to document the effectiveness of renin angiotensin system inhibitors to decrease MA in this patients' population.

In conclusion, MA is an early manifestation of SCN and is a common finding in patients with SCD in eastern SA. All patients with SCD should be screened periodically for MA and those who test positive may benefit from treatment with antiproteinuric agents in addition to hydroxyurea.

Disclosure

Opinions expressed in this article are those of the authors and not necessarily of JHAH.

Acknowledgments

The authors would like to thank Amalraj Antony, Ph.D., from the Division of Epidemiology at JHAH for performing the statistical analysis of this study. The authors acknowledge the use of JHAH facilities for research data used in this article.

References

[1] P.-T. T. Pham, P.-C. T. Pham, A. H. Wilkinson, and S. Q. Lew, "Renal abnormalities in sickle cell disease," *Kidney International*, vol. 57, no. 1, pp. 1–8, 2000.

[2] M. Airy and G. Eknoyan, "The kidney in sickle hemoglobinopathies," *Clinical Nephrology*, vol. 87, no. 2, pp. 55–68, 2017.

[3] M. Asnani, G. Serjeant, T. Royal-Thomas, and M. Reid, "Predictors of renal function progression in adults with homozygous sickle cell disease," *British Journal of Haematology*, vol. 173, no. 3, pp. 461–468, 2016.

[4] F. Schmitt, F. Martinez, G. Brillet et al., "Early glomerular dysfunction in patients with sickle cell anemia," *American Journal of Kidney Diseases*, vol. 32, no. 2, pp. 208–214, 1998.

[5] M. R. Weir, "Microalbuminuria and cardiovascular disease," *Clinical Journal of the American Society of Nephrology*, vol. 2, no. 3, pp. 581–590, 2007.

[6] K. T. McKie, C. D. Hanevold, C. Hernandez, J. L. Waller, L. Ortiz, and K. M. McKie, "Prevalence, prevention, and treatment of microalbuminuria and proteinuria in children with sickle cell disease," *Journal of Pediatric Hematology/Oncology*, vol. 29, no. 3, pp. 140–144, 2007.

[7] D. W. Cockcroft and M. H. Gault, "Prediction of creatinine clearance from serum creatinine," *Nephron*, vol. 16, no. 1, pp. 31–41, 1976.

[8] H. Lehmann, G. Maranjian, and A. E. Mourant, "Distribution of sickle-cell hæmoglobin in Saudi Arabia," *Nature*, vol. 198, no. 4879, pp. 492-493, 1963.

[9] M. M. Al-Qurashi, M. I. El-Mouzan, A. S. Al-Herbish, A. A. Al-Salloum, and A. A. Al-Omar, "The prevalence of sickle cell disease in Saudi children and adolescents. A community-based survey," *Saudi Medical Journal*, vol. 29, no. 10, pp. 1480–1483, 2008.

[10] M. A. Padmos, K. Sackey, G. T. Roberts et al., "Two different forms of homozygous sickle cell disease occur in Saudi Arabia," *British Journal of Haematology*, vol. 79, no. 1, pp. 93–98, 1991.

[11] J. R. Stallworth, A. Tripathi, and J. M. Jerrell, "Prevalence, treatment, and outcomes of renal conditions in pediatric sickle cell disease," *Southern Medical Journal*, vol. 104, no. 11, pp. 752–756, 2011.

[12] M. Allon, "Renal abnormalities in sickle cell disease," *JAMA Internal Medicine*, vol. 150, no. 3, pp. 501–504, 1990.

[13] R. J. Falk, J. Scheinman, G. Phillips, E. Orringer, A. Johnson, and J. C. Jennette, "Prevalence and pathologic features of sickle cell nephropathy and response to inhibition of angiotensin-converting enzyme," *The New England Journal of Medicine*, vol. 326, no. 14, pp. 910–915, 1992.

[14] I. Akinsheye, A. Alsultan, N. Solovieff et al., "Fetal hemoglobin in sickle cell anemia," *Blood*, vol. 118, no. 1, pp. 19–27, 2011.

[15] D. Ngo, H. Bae, M. H. Steinberg, P. Sebastiani, N. Solovieff, C. T. Baldwin et al., "Fetal hemoglobin in sickle cell anemia: genetic studies of the Arab-Indian haplotype," *Blood Cells, Molecules and Diseases*, vol. 51, pp. 22–26, 2013.

[16] A. Alkhunaizi and A. Al-Khatti, "Proteinuria in patients with sickle cell disease," *Saudi Journal of Kidney Diseases and Transplantation*, vol. 25, no. 5, pp. 1038–1041, 2014.

[17] A. Guasch, J. Navarrete, K. Nass, and C. F. Zayas, "Glomerular involvement in adults with sickle cell hemoglobinopathies: Prevalence and clinical correlates of progressive renal failure," *Journal of the American Society of Nephrology*, vol. 17, no. 8, pp. 2228–2235, 2006.

[18] C. T. Osei-Yeboah and O. Rodrigues, "Renal status of children with sickle cell disease in Accra, Ghana.," *Ghana Medical Journal*, vol. 45, no. 4, pp. 155–160, 2011.

[19] A. M. Alkhunaizi, A. A. Al-Khatti, S. H. Al-Mueilo, A. Amir, and B. Yousif, "End-stage renal disease in patients with sickle cell disease," *Saudi Journal of Kidney Diseases and Transplantation*, vol. 28, no. 4, pp. 751–757, 2017.

[20] A. Guasch, M. Cua, and W. E. Mitch, "Early detection and the course of glomerular injury in patients with sickle cell anemia," *Kidney International*, vol. 49, no. 3, pp. 786–791, 1996.

[21] V. R. Dharnidharka, S. Dabbagh, B. Atiyeh, P. Simpson, and S. Sarnaik, "Prevalence of microalbuminuria in children with sickle cell disease," *Pediatric Nephrology*, vol. 12, no. 6, pp. 475–478, 1998.

[22] P. Drawz, S. Ayyappan, M. Nouraie et al., "Kidney disease among patients with sickle cell disease, hemoglobin SS and SC," *Clinical Journal of the American Society of Nephrology*, vol. 11, no. 2, pp. 207–215, 2016.

[23] R. Y. Aoki and S. T. Saad, "Microalbuminuria in sickle cell disease," *Brazilian Journal of Medical and Biological Research*, vol. 23, no. 11, pp. 1103–1106, 1990.

[24] J. Thompson, M. Reid, I. Hambleton, and G. R. Serjeant, "Albuminuria and renal function in homozygous sickle cell disease: Observations from a Cohort Study," *JAMA Internal Medicine*, vol. 167, no. 7, pp. 701–708, 2007.

[25] B. Aygun, N. A. Mortier, M. P. Smeltzer, B. L. Shulkin, J. S. Hankins, and R. E. Ware, "Hydroxyurea treatment decreases glomerular hyperfiltration in children with sickle cell anemia," *American Journal of Hematology*, vol. 88, no. 2, pp. 116–119, 2013.

[26] O. Alvarez, S. T. Miller, W. C. Wang et al., "Effect of hydroxyurea treatment on renal function parameters: Results from the multicenter placebo-controlled BABY HUG clinical trial for infants with sickle cell anemia," *Pediatric Blood & Cancer*, vol. 59, no. 4, pp. 668–674, 2012.

[27] L. Foucan, "A randomized trial of captopril for microalbuminuria in normotensive adults with sickle cell anemia," *American Journal of Medicine*, vol. 104, no. 4, pp. 339–342, 1998.

28

Matrix Metalloproteinases and Subclinical Atherosclerosis in Chronic Kidney Disease

Andreas Kousios,[1] Panayiotis Kouis,[2] and Andrie G. Panayiotou[2]

[1]*Department of Nephrology, Nicosia General Hospital, 2230 Nicosia, Cyprus*
[2]*Cyprus International Institute for Environmental & Public Health in Association with Harvard T. H. Chan School of Public Health, Cyprus University of Technology, 3041 Limassol, Cyprus*

Correspondence should be addressed to Andrie G. Panayiotou; andrie.panayiotou@cut.ac.cy

Academic Editor: Hermann Haller

Background. Cardiovascular disease (CVD) remains a significant problem in Chronic Kidney Disease (CKD). Subclinical atherosclerosis identified by noninvasive methods could improve CVD risk prediction in CKD but these methods are often unavailable. We therefore systematically reviewed whether circulating levels of Matrix Metalloproteinases (MMPs) and tissue inhibitors (TIMPs) are associated with subclinical atherosclerosis in CKD, as this would support their use as biomarkers or pharmacologic targets. *Methods.* All major electronic databases were systematically searched from inception until May 2015 using appropriate terms. Studies involving CKD patients with data on circulating MMPs levels and atherosclerosis were considered and subjected to quality assessment. *Results.* Overall, 16 studies were identified for qualitative synthesis and 9 studies were included in quantitative synthesis. MMP-2 and TIMP-1 were most frequently studied while most studies assessed carotid Intima-Media Thickness (cIMT) as a measure of subclinical atherosclerosis. Only MMP-2 demonstrated a consistent positive association with cIMT. Considerable variability in cIMT measurement methodology and poor plaque assessment was found. *Conclusions.* Although MMPs demonstrate great potential as biomarkers of subclinical atherosclerosis, they are understudied in CKD and not enough data existed for meta-analysis. Larger studies involving several MMPs, with more homogenized approaches in determining the atherosclerotic burden in CKD, are needed.

1. Introduction

Cardiovascular disease (CVD) burden is substantially higher in Chronic Kidney Disease (CKD) compared to non-CKD patients [1]. In the End-Stage Renal Disease (ESRD) population, cardiovascular mortality is the leading cause of death, and despite the recently reported improvement in survival rates, CVD in this group remains unacceptably high [2]. The increase in cardiovascular risk starts early on in CKD, with a lower estimated Glomerular Filtration Rate (eGFR) shown to be independently associated with increased cardiovascular risk [3] even at the stage of microalbuminuria [4]. CKD patients are therefore justifiably considered in the highest-risk group classification for CVD [5] and, in fact, their risk of dying from a cardiac cause actually exceeds the risk of reaching ESRD [1].

Atheromatosis and arteriosclerosis are the main underlying pathologic processes in arterial disease in CKD [6]. They are attributed to a rather complex interplay of uremia-associated risk factors that are superimposed, as the disease progresses, on the already high burden of CVD traditional factors that characterizes the CKD population [7]. Subclinical atherosclerosis, as measured by noninvasive methods such as ultrasonically determined carotid Intima-Media Thickness (cIMT), is a valid predictor of coronary heart disease and vascular events in asymptomatic individuals [8]. This is particularly important in the CKD group where the classic cardiovascular risk score approach underestimates the atherosclerotic burden [9]. Measuring subclinical atherosclerosis in CKD may significantly improve CVD risk prediction [10]. Additionally, novel early atherosclerosis biomarkers, as well as possible therapeutic targets, are greatly needed in

CKD patients. Matrix Metalloproteinases (MMPs) may fall into this category of both useful markers and targets in CKD disease.

MMPs are a large family of endopeptidases that function under tight control, remodeling the extracellular matrix (ECM) and regulating the activity of many important non-ECM molecules including adhesion molecules, cytokines, and growth factors. They are classified according to their substrate specificity, sequence similarity, and domain organization into six groups: collagenases (MMP-1, MMP-8, MMP-13, and MMP-18), gelatinases (MMP-2, MMP-9), stromelysins (MMP-3, MMP-10), matrilysins (MMP-7, MMP-26), membrane-type MMPs (MMP-14, MMP-15, MMP-16, MMP-24, MMP-17, and MMP-25), and other MMPs (MMP-12, MMP-19, MMP-20, MMP-21, MMP-23, MMP-27, and MMP-28) [11]. Their proteolytic activity is regulated at transcriptional and posttranslational levels but also at the tissue level by endogenous inhibitors, known as tissue inhibitors of metalloproteinases (TIMPs 1–4) [12]. In vascular physiology and pathophysiology, they hold a prominent role by remodeling the ECM scaffold of the vessel wall and as regulators of the biological activity of nonmatrix molecules, including angiotensin-I, endothelin, TNF-α, and others [13–15]. Based on the emerging role of MMPs in vascular remodeling and their increased expression and activation under inflammatory and oxidative stress conditions, many studies have shown MMPs imbalance to be a key event in atherosclerosis, arterial aneurysmal formation, and plaque instability [15]. Circulating levels of various MMPs have been associated with both clinical manifestations of CVD [16, 17] and subclinical atherosclerosis [18–20] or even as predictors of outcomes following revascularization [21, 22]. Additionally, increased expression of MMPs was observed at tissue level, in human carotid, coronary, and aortic atherosclerotic lesions [23–25]. Currently, the focus is on clarifying their exact role in the disease state [26] and exploiting them in innovative diagnostic and research methodologies [27], as well as using them for prevention and therapy of vascular disease [28–30].

In CKD, a plethora of underlying factors, with preeminent toxic uremic milieu and the increased levels of proinflammatory cytokines, oxidative stress, and acidosis, maintain a state of persistent low-grade inflammation, especially in ESRD, with the addition of dialysis-related factors [31, 32]. Although this state of chronic inflammation in CKD renders MMPs attractive candidates for studies in this population and despite the mounting evidence of their role in CVD, the association between MMPs and subclinical atherosclerosis in CKD patients has not been systematically studied. To this effect, we performed a systematic literature review and evaluation of the evidence associating circulating levels of MMPs with subclinical atherosclerosis outcomes in CKD patients.

2. Subjects and Methods

2.1. Search Strategy and Selection Criteria. The electronic databases SCOPUS, PubMed, and Google Scholar were searched from inception until May 2015 using the keywords: "atherosclerosis", "metalloproteinases", "kidney diseases", and "hemodialysis" either in the title or the abstract or using Medical Subject Headings (MeSH) terms. The references of eligible studies were also screened for missing articles. Inclusion criteria were CKD cohort or case-control studies involving CKD patients, reporting as one of the outcomes of interest, the relationship of circulating measurement of MMPs or their tissue inhibitors (TIMPs), and markers of atherosclerosis (i.e., IMT, plaque number, or similar atherosclerotic outcomes). The electronic search was limited to articles in the English language. The included studies were identified after two reviewers (Andreas Kousios, Panayiotis Kouis) independently screened the title and abstract of the obtained electronic search results and final selection was based on full text evaluation. A third researcher (Andrie G. Panayiotou) resolved any discrepancies.

2.2. Data Extraction and Quality Assessment. Two reviewers (Andreas Kousios, Panayiotis Kouis) independently extracted data regarding the studies' design, characteristics of the included CKD population, methodology for circulating MMPs levels determination, and assessment of atherosclerosis outcomes. The direction and magnitude of the association were recorded, as well as additional information such as method of statistical analysis and adjustment for potential confounders. The Newcastle-Ottawa scale for observational studies [33], which evaluates the selection of participants, the comparability of different groups, and ascertainment of exposure and outcome of interest, was utilized for the quality assessment of the included studies. In addition, a more detailed quality assessment was carried out regarding the methodology of atherosclerosis outcome evaluation based on the Mannheim Consensus criteria for carotid Intima-Media Thickness and plaque assessment [34].

3. Results

3.1. Eligible Studies. The online search retrieved 6324 items. Of them, 6218 items were excluded from further analysis based on title and abstract, while the remaining 106 were retrieved for full text assessment. Studies with overlapping populations were cross-checked and final selection was based on the number of CKD participants. Among the reports assessed in full text, 32 were literature reviews, 6 were commentaries or editorials, and another 4 were animal studies. Additionally, 12 studies did not provide data on serum concentrations of MMPs or their tissue inhibitors, 31 studies did not provide evidence on atherosclerosis related outcomes while 4 studies did not comprise a CKD population, and another one involved an overlapping population with another study. In summary, out of the total 106 reports retrieved, 16 reports were included in the qualitative synthesis and, among these, a total of 9 studies provided enough data to be included in the quantitative synthesis (Figure 1, Prisma diagram). The studies that were excluded at the last step prior to quantitative synthesis and the reason for their exclusion are presented in Supplementary Table 1 (in Supplementary Material available online at http://dx.doi.org/10.1155/2016/9498013).

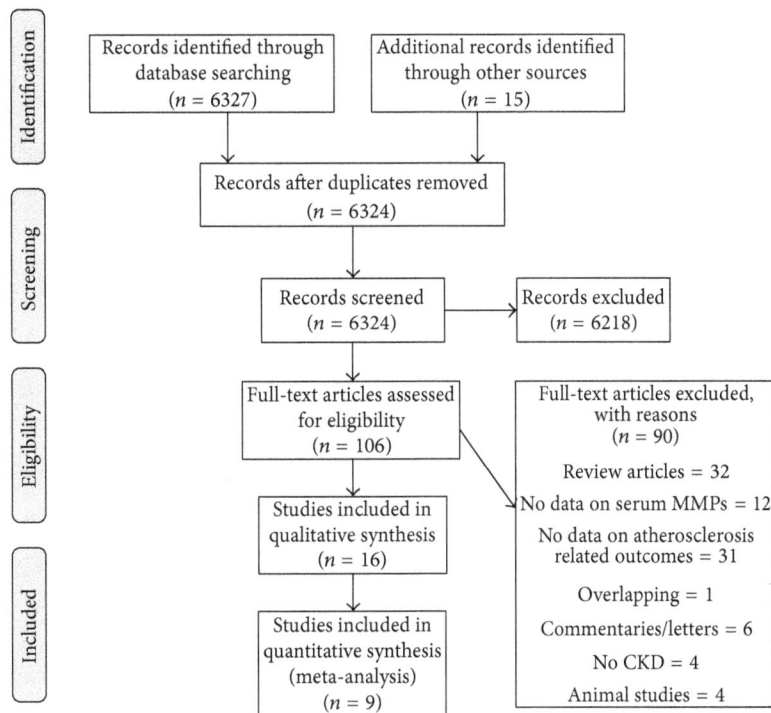

FIGURE 1: Prisma diagram for the search strategy and selected studies.

3.2. Study Characteristics. Descriptive characteristics of the studies that were included are presented in Table 1. Four studies were carried out in Europe while the remaining studies were performed in the USA (two), Africa (two), and Asia (one). All the studies were observational and the majority of them included a CKD subgroup of participants along with age-matched healthy controls. Weber et al. evaluated the association of MMPs with atherosclerosis outcomes only in CKD stages III and IV [35] while Sánchez-Escuredo et al. evaluated MMPs and cIMT in CKD patients awaiting renal transplantation [36].

Overall, the nine studies reviewed here involved a total of 1061 participants, of whom 858 were CKD patients and 203 were healthy controls. Of the CKD patients, 450 were CKD patients already undergoing hemodialysis (HD).

The association between MMP-2 and TIMP-1 with atherosclerosis was the most frequently assessed (four studies) with MMP-9 also assessed in three. MMP-10, TIMP-2, and PAPP-A were assessed in two studies. Seven studies used cIMT as the atherosclerosis outcome and two of them also used an Atherosclerosis Score and carotid plaque number [37, 38]. The two studies included that did not measure cIMT provided data on the relationship between MMPs or their tissue inhibitors and aortic and coronary artery calcification [35] and carotid plaque presence [36]. Characteristics of studies, including atherosclerotic outcome assessed, are shown in Table 1.

MMP-2 was found to have a positive association with cIMT even after adjustment for multiple confounders in three studies [39–41] and a positive association with abdominal

aortic calcification but not with coronary artery and thoracic aortic calcification [35].

The relationship of TIMP-1 with cIMT was less consistent as only one of the three studies evaluating this relationship reported a statistically significant positive association; however, it did not account for different confounders [38]. Similarly, Weber et al., who evaluated the relationship between TIMP-1 and calcification at coronary and aortic sites and included adjustment for multiple confounders, reported no statistically significant association either.

MMP-9 was found to be positively and strongly associated with cIMT, Atherosclerosis Score, and number of carotid plaques in a CKD population by Addabbo et al. [37] but this relationship was not confirmed in two additional studies evaluating MMP-9 and cIMT [39, 40]. MMP-10 was only assessed in two studies and both of them reported a positive association with cIMT in HD subgroups [38, 42] but only one of them reported a similar association in a non-HD, CKD subgroup.

Sánchez-Escuredo et al. evaluated the relationship of PAPP-A with plaque presence and reported a significant positive association in a population of HD patients awaiting kidney transplant (OR: 4.45; CI: 1.22–16.2; *P* value: 0.023) [36]. However, PAPP-A was not found to be associated with cIMT in a more recent study also involving HD patients [43].

Among the tissue inhibitors of MMPs evaluated in this review (i.e., TIMP-1 and TIMP-2), only TIMP-2 showed some evidence of a negative association with atherosclerosis as Pawlak et al. reported a negative association after adjusting for confounders between TIMP-2 and cIMT [39], although

TABLE 1: Characteristics of included studies.

Number	Author, country (Year)	Participants (n)	Age	Evaluated MMPs	IMT	Plaque/other	Association in CKD/HD patients	P	Direction
1	Pawlak et al. [39] Poland (2004)	Total: 58 HD: 38 Controls: 20	HD: 59 ± 15 C: —	MMP-2 MMP-9 TIMP-1 TIMP-2	✓	—	*cIMT* MMP-2: β = 0.596 (0.278) (adjusted) MMP-9: r : = −0.135 (unadjusted) TIMP-1: β = −0.312 (0.238) (adjusted) TIMP-2: β = −0.767 (0.276) (adjusted)	0.04 NR 0.20 0.010	↑ ↕ ↕ ↓
2	Addabbo et al. [37] USA (2007)	Total: 108 CKD: 75 Controls: 33	CKD: 52 ± 16	MMP-9	✓	✓	*cIMT* MMP-9: r = 0.30 (unadjusted) *Plaque number* MMP-9: r = 0.30 (unadjusted) *Atherosclerosis Score* MMP-9: r = 0.37 (unadjusted)	0.009 0.009 0.001	↑ ↑ ↑
3	Pawlak et al. [40] Poland (2008)	Total: 62 HD: 42 Controls: 20	HD: 59 ± 18 C: 53 ± 15	MMP-2 MMP-9 TIMP-2 TIMP-1	✓	—	*cIMT in HD* MMP-2: 0.402 (0.143) (adjusted) MMP-9: NR TIMP-1: 0.097 (−0.175) (adjusted) TIMP-2: r = 0.248 (unadjusted)	0.012 — 0.59 NR	↑ — ↕ ↕
4	Nagano et al. [41] Japan (2009)	Total: 129 CKD: 99 Controls: 30	CKD: 58.3 ± 17.9 C: 56 ± 5.5	MMP-2	✓	—	*cIMT* MMP-2: β = 0.240 (adjusted)	0.04	↑
5	Coll et al. [38] Spain (2010)	Total: 378 HD: 217 CKD I–III: 43 CKD IV–V: 68 Controls: 50	HD: 64.7 ± 12 CKD I–III: 59.6 ± 11 CKD IV–V: 69.2 ± 12 C: 64.9 ± 3	MMP-8 MMP-10 TIMP-1	✓	✓	*cIMT in HD* MMP-8: NR (unadjusted) MMP-10: r = 0.16 (unadjusted) TIMP-1: NR (unadjusted) *cIMT in CKD* MMP-8: NR (unadjusted) MMP-10: NR (unadjusted) TIMP-1: r = 0.32 (unadjusted) *Atherosclerosis Score* MMP-8: 1.15 (0.77–1.73) MMP-10: 1.57 (1.06–2.32) TIMP-1: 1.00 (0.65–1.54)	NR 0.01 NR NR NR 0.03 0.02 0.47 0.97	↕ ↑ ↕ — — ↑ ↑ ↕ ↕
6	Sánchez-Escuredo et al. [36] Spain (2010)	Total: 93 RT: 93	RT: 54 ± 12	PAPP-A	—	✓	*Plaque presence* PAPP-A: OR: 4.45 (1.22–16.2) (adjusted)	0.02	↑
7	Belal et al. [42] Egypt (2014)	Total: 60 CKD: 20 HD: 20 Controls: 20	CKD: 49 ± 6.6 HD: 52 ± 6.7 C: 49 ± 6.5	MMP-10	✓	—	*cIMT in CKD* MMP-10: r = 0.697 (unadjusted) *cIMT in HD* MMP-10: r = 0.836 (unadjusted)	<0.001 <0.001	↑ ↑

TABLE 1: Continued.

Number	Author, country (Year)	Participants (n)	Age	Evaluated MMPs	Outcome IMT	Outcome Plaque/other	Association in CKD/HD patients	P	Direction
8	Weber et al. [35] USA (2014)	Total: 103 CKD III: 56 CKD IV: 47	CKD III: 66.1 (12) CKD IV: 68.0 (9.3)	MMP-2 TIMP-1	—	✓	*Abdominal aortic calcification*		
							MMP-2: β = NR (adjusted)	0.02	↑
							TIMP-1: β = NR (adjusted)	0.06	↕
							Coronary artery calcification		
							MMP-2: β = NR (adjusted)	0.90	↕
							TIMP-1: β = NR (adjusted)	0.27	↕
							Thoracic aortic calcification		
							MMP-2: β = NR (adjusted)	0.18	↕
							TIMP-1: β = NR (adjusted)	0.16	↕
9	Issac et al. [43] Egypt (2014)	Total: 70 HD: 40 Control: 30	HD: 45 (30.5–55.8) C: 36.5 (28.8–46.8)	PAPP-A	✓	—	*cIMT* PAPP-A: No association	NR	↕

CKD: Chronic Kidney Disease, HD: hemodialysis, C: controls, MMP: Metalloproteinases, IMT: Intima-Media Thickness, NR: not reported, RT: renal transplant.

TABLE 2: Quality assessment of the included studies (Newcastle-Ottawa scale).

Number	Author	Year	Newcastle-Ottawa scale scores			
			Selection	Comparability	Exposure	Summary
1	Pawlak et al. [39]	2004	4	2	2	8
2	Addabbo et al. [37]	2007	4	2	2	8
3	Pawlak et al. [40]	2008	4	2	2	8
4	Nagano et al. [41]	2009	3	2	3	8
5	Coll et al. [9]	2010	4	2	2	8
6	Sánchez-Escuredo et al. [36]	2010	2	2	2	6
7	Belal et al. [42]	2014	3	1	2	6
8	Weber et al. [35]	2014	2	2	3	7
9	Isaac et al. [43]	2014	3	1	2	6

Selection criteria (4): adequate case definition, representativeness of cases, selection of controls, and definition of controls. Comparability criteria (2): control for factor A and an additional factor B on the basis of the design or analysis. Exposure criteria (3): ascertainment of exposure, the same method for cases and controls, and nonresponse rate.

in a more recent study by the same group this finding was not repeated [40].

3.3. Quality Assessment.

The quality assessment of the included studies was performed according to the Newcastle-Ottawa scale and the results are presented in Table 2. Overall, the included studies were characterized by good methodology and this offers some reassurance that the results presented have not been substantially influenced by bias. However, due to the substantial variability in the methodology and equipment used for the evaluation of atherosclerosis outcome, an additional table was constructed with particular emphasis on the modalities and the measurement and reporting methods used by each study (Table 3). In concordance with the Mannheim Consensus [34], most studies assessed atherosclerosis in longitudinal view on the far wall and common carotid artery (CCA) was the most commonly used anatomical site followed by carotid bulb (CB) and the internal carotid artery (ICA). However, few studies reported whether measurements were obtained at the end of diastole or whether measurement was obtained in a blinded fashion.

4. Discussion

This systematic review evaluated the published evidence on the association between circulating levels of MMPs and subclinical atherosclerosis in CKD patients. We identified only nine observational studies that adequately addressed this relationship. Furthermore, the vast majority of studies were also characterized by a small sample size as most of them included less than 100 CKD patients. cIMT was the main measure of subclinical atherosclerosis reported and MMP-2 and TIMP-1 were the most commonly assessed metalloproteinases.

Although the number of studies providing the same data on MMP-2 was too small for a formal meta-analysis, the overall consistent direction and magnitude of the association of MMP-2 with cIMT reported in the different studies suggest that this is positively associated with subclinical atherosclerosis in CKD patients. It is however important to note that two out of the four studies reporting on MMP-2 were in hemodialysis patients only. On the contrary, most of the studies that evaluated TIMP-1 and subclinical atherosclerosis did not find any significant relationship, while for the remaining MMPs, the low number of studies identified does not allow for any inferences regarding their association with subclinical atherosclerosis.

Studies involving CKD patients that did not use atherosclerosis measures as an outcome were excluded at the last step, prior to quantitative synthesis, in order to limit the results of this study to objective atherosclerosis measures as opposed to clinical or self-reported measures such as "history of CVD." Notably, in these studies, circulating levels of MMP-2 were associated with previous history of CVD in a non-HD CKD population [44] and in a Peritoneal Dialysis (PD) population [45], providing further supporting evidence for MMP-2 association with CVD in CKD (Supplementary Table 1). For consistency, we also excluded studies that had measured MMP expression in vessel tissue instead of circulating concentrations. Although tissue expression level is a direct evidence of MMP implication in the pathophysiology of atherosclerosis, it is not easily transferrable in the clinical setting as a biomarker. Furthermore, studies that involved pediatric CKD patients instead of adults were also excluded. Interestingly, only one study was found to report an association between serum measurements of MMPs and atherosclerosis markers in pediatric CKD patients, making a separate review of these findings not possible [46]. Overall, although this approach limits the number of informative studies reviewed here, it allowed us to answer the more precise question on the association between circulating MMPs and subclinical atherosclerosis in adult CKD patients.

Regulation of MMPs expression and activity in physiological or pathological vascular remodeling is induced by hemodynamics, injury, inflammation, and oxidative stress [15, 47, 48]. In CKD, a condition where these processes are enhanced, it is expected that MMP dysregulation is intensified, particularly in late CKD stages and HD. Persistent, low-grade inflammation in CKD is attributed to the production of proinflammatory cytokines combined with their decreased renal

TABLE 3: Subclinical atherosclerosis assessment of the included studies based on the Manheim Consensus.

Number	Author (Year)	Tools	Angle	Anatomical site	Walls used	cIMT or IMTmax	Plaques assessed separately	Measurements	Quantitative measures of plaques	Measurement during end diastole	Single observer/blinded
1	Pawlak et al. [39] (2004)	NR	L	CCA (B)	FW	NR	No	Mean of 2 measurements per site	No	NR	NR NR
2	Addabbo et al. [37] (2007)	NR	NR	CCA (B) CB (B) ICA (B)	FW	cIMT	Yes	Mean of 6 measurements per site DCCA	Number of plaques	Yes	Single/blinded
3	Pawlak et al. [40] (2008)	NR	L	CCA (B)	FW	cIMT	No	Mean of 2 measurements per site	No	NR	Single/blinded
4	Nagano et al. [41] (2009)	NR	L	CCA	LW MW	NR	NR	Mean of 6 measurements of CCA	No	Yes	Single/blinded
5	Coll et al. [38] (2010)	SA	L	CCA (B) CB (B) ICA (B)	FW	cIMT	Yes	NR	No	Manheim Consensus	NR Blinded
6	Sánchez-Escuredo et al. [36] (2010)	NR	NR	CCA (B) CB (B) ICA (B)	FW	cIMT	If IMT > 1,2 mm	Mean of 6 measurements per site	No	Yes	Single/NR
7	Belal et al. [42] (2014)	A	L	CCA (B)	FW	cIMT	Yes	Maximum of 2 measurements per site	No	NR	NR NR
8	Weber et al. [35] (2014)	—	—	—	—	—	—	—	—	—	—
9	Issac et al. [43] (2014)	NR	L, T	NR	NR	NR	No	IMT (B), CSA (B)	No	NR	NR NR

NR: not reported.
A: automated, SA: semiautomated.
L: longitudinal, T: transverse, and CS: cross-sectional.
CCA: common carotid artery, CB: carotid bulb, ICA: internal carotid artery, and B: bilateral.
FW: far wall, NW: near wall, LW: lateral wall, and MW: medial wall.
CSA: cross-sectional area, DCCA: internal diameter of the common carotid artery.

clearance, the CKD-associated metabolic acidosis, the uremic milieu induced oxidative and carbonyl stress, the chronic or frequent recurrent infections, and thrombotic events [32]. In addition, dialysis-related factors, such as membrane biocompatibility, water and dialysate purity, and microbiological quality, further contribute and sustain inflammation in ESRD [31]. This uremia-inflammation interplay in CKD underlies the accelerated atherosclerosis and increased IMT, the arterial stiffening, and increased vascular calcification of both intima and media and impairs the vascular repair process with the detrimental consequences of neointimal hyperplasia [49]. Moreover, plaque morphology, composition, and vulnerability differ in CKD, as coronary and carotid plaques of CKD patients were shown to be more calcified, more unstable, and frequently ruptured and containing less fibrous tissue [50–52]. Central to the pathogenesis of these processes and plaque formation are the endothelial cell (EC) dysfunction and vascular smooth muscle cell (VSMC) migration and their phenotypic shift to a more proliferative and secretory state [49, 53].

Activated MMPs participate in both early and late stages in atherosclerosis progression. Their cleaving of ECM and non-ECM molecules induces the pathogenic phenotypic shift of ECs and VSMCs and facilitates increased endothelial inflammation and permeability, intimal-medial thickening, fibrosis, calcification, and stiffening [26, 54]. MMPs 1, 2, 8, 9, and 12 are mostly implicated in these processes with MMP-2 and MMP-9 having a prominent role [26]. In later stages of atherosclerosis, MMPs contribute to reducing the atherosclerotic plaques' fibrous cap, [55] thus rendering plaques more unstable and prone to rupture [56]. In CKD patients, only few studies have examined the levels of circulating MMPs compared to controls demonstrating increased circulating MMP levels in CKD, particularly those of MMP-2, MMP-9, and MMP-10 [57, 58]. Additionally, MMP-2 and MMP-9 were shown to be upregulated focally in uremic vessels in two studies by Chung et al. [59, 60]. MMP-2 was upregulated in arteries of ESRD patients and activated MMP-2 was strongly correlated with arterial stiffness in dialyzed patients [60] (Supplementary Table 1). MMP-2 and MMP-9 were upregulated in diabetic CKD arteries and correlated with stiffening and endothelial dysfunction [59] (Supplementary Table 1).

As research is ongoing on the development of cardiovascular risk markers in CKD patients [7], MMPs stand to serve as potential biomarkers for atherosclerosis and cardiovascular risk assessment in this high risk group. In order for a potential biomarker to be approved for clinical use, it needs to be confirmed through rigorous testing of multiple subjects and testing should be characterized by reproducibility, good sensitivity, and specificity [61]. The limited number of studies identified in this review reflects the fact that the level of evidence is still quite low for use of MMPs as biomarkers for atherosclerosis in CKD patients, although the accessibility and relatively low cost of circulating MMPs measurements along with knowledge of the disease mechanisms argue about the benefit of additional and larger studies involving CKD patients. Moreover, such studies would provide further insight into their contribution to the higher CVD burden in

CKD and, more importantly, would pave the way for their use in therapeutic interventions [30] or even their targeted and specific inhibition [62].

Although the majority of the studies reviewed here are characterized by good overall methodology according to the Newcastle-Ottawa scale criteria, we have identified additional parameters relating to the performance of atherosclerosis assessment that vary between studies and may introduce additional variability in the estimated relationship between circulating MMPs and subclinical atherosclerosis. As most of the studies used cIMT and plaque measurements as surrogates for subclinical atherosclerosis, it is important to highlight the necessity of a homogenized approach for image acquisition, data analysis, and reporting methods, as well as the use of unified criteria to distinguish early atherosclerotic plaques from increased IMT [34]. With regards to IMT measurement, the Manheim Carotid Intima-Media Thickness and Plaque Consensus report proposes the site of measurement to be the far wall of the CCA. Mean IMT values across the CCA may be less susceptible to errors compared to maximum values and composite measures of IMT and plaque should be avoided. Plaque assessment should include the location, thickness and area, and plaque number and should be scanned in longitudinal and cross sections [34]. In most of the reviewed studies, although IMT was measured in the far wall of CCA, there was considerable variability in methodology and poor plaque assessment. Furthermore, circulating levels of MMPs are influenced by environmental, genetic, disease, and drug related factors and although evaluating each of these factors individually is beyond the scope of this review; they need to be carefully examined in future study designs involving CKD populations [63]. Additionally, variations in sample collection methodology and preanalytical care have been found to significantly affect MMPs levels with serum samples reported to have higher mean values compared to plasma samples [64, 65]. The majority of the included studies in this review had measured MMPs levels in serum [36, 38–43], with only two studies using plasma [35, 37]. Although we cannot exclude the possibility of such discrepancies in explaining part of the heterogeneity in the results, it seems unlikely that they would explain all of it as similar heterogeneity exists in the results obtained from studies that used serum. Also, variations in MMPs levels could arise from the status of recruited patients as it is suggested that hemodialysis may affect MMP levels, especially MMP-2, MMP-9, and their inhibitors [66, 67]. Additionally, all studies included patients with a history of CVD. However, only six out of the nine studies reported the prevalence of CVD history in their patients groups which ranged between ~8% and 80%, while the cross-sectional design of the studies further limits the causal inferences that could be made. Finally, none of the studies performed a priori power analysis in order to estimate the appropriate sample size and the possibility of publication bias cannot be excluded as almost no study included in this review reported only a negative association between MMPs levels and subclinical atherosclerosis.

Despite the extensive study of MMPs and their role in the atherosclerotic process in both animal models [68] and human studies, there are disproportionately fewer published studies of the atherogenic effects of MMPs in patients with CKD. This is in keeping with a well described phenomenon of underrepresentation of CKD patients in cardiovascular disease studies [69] despite the growing global burden of kidney disease [70] and the high prevalence of CKD among CVD patients [71]. Nonetheless, based on their central role in arterial wall remodeling, MMPs demonstrate great potential for further studies in CKD, a condition where the main drivers for MMP dysregulation, such as inflammation and oxidative stress, are intensified. Their linkage to early atherosclerotic change, reflected in established but often not easily accessible subclinical atherosclerosis markers, provides the basis for MMPs use as biomarkers or even as pharmacological targets of cardiovascular disease in CKD patients.

To this effect, we have systematically reviewed the literature and critically appraised all studies addressing the association of various MMPs with subclinical atherosclerosis in CKD patients. We aimed to help structure the knowledge derived from human studies in the field and identify potential candidate MMPs for further research. Moreover, several methodological caveats were identified with regard to IMT measurement and sampling. Future research initiatives in this field are thus urgently needed and would benefit by addressing the methodological issues identified in this review, during the study design process. Overall, these findings are highly relevant in view of the undiminished interest in MMPs and the need for novel approaches to address the significant problem of CVD in Chronic Kidney Disease.

5. Conclusions

In summary, the published evidence reviewed here demonstrates that circulating MMPs levels could potentially be of use as biomarkers of subclinical atherosclerosis in adult CKD populations. MMP-2 shows the greatest promise although most of the other MMPs or their tissue inhibitors are mostly understudied in the CKD population and no inferences about their potential can be made. Studies characterized by larger and well defined CKD populations and involving several MMPs and a consistent and homogenized assessment of different measures of subclinical atherosclerosis such as IMT and plaque burden are urgently needed.

Authors' Contribution

Andreas Kousios and Panayiotis Kouis contributed equally to this work. Andreas Kousios and Panayiotis Kouis performed the search and extraction of information from the papers, organized the material, and prepared the first draft of the paper. Andrie G. Panayiotou provided advice on the methodology of the search and selection of the papers, contributed to the interpretation of the findings, critically revised the paper, and contributed towards the final version of the paper.

Acknowledgments

This work was performed at the Cyprus International Institute for Environmental and Public Health in association with Harvard T. H. Chan School of Public Health, Cyprus University of Technology, Limassol, Cyprus.

References

[1] R. N. Foley, A. M. Murray, S. Li et al., "Chronic kidney disease and the risk for cardiovascular disease, renal replacement, and death in the United States medicare population, 1998 to 1999," *Journal of the American Society of Nephrology*, vol. 16, no. 2, pp. 489–495, 2005.

[2] R. Saran, Y. Li, B. Robinson et al., "US renal data system 2014 annual data report: epidemiology of kidney disease in the United States," *American Journal of Kidney Diseases*, vol. 66, supplement 1, article A7, no. 1, 2015.

[3] C. Daly, "Is early chronic kidney disease an important risk factor for cardiovascular disease? A background paper prepared for the UK Consensus Conference on early chronic kidney disease," *Nephrology Dialysis Transplantation*, vol. 22, supplement 9, pp. ix19–ix25, 2007.

[4] H. C. Gerstein, J. F. E. Mann, Q. Yi et al., "Albuminuria and risk of cardiovascular events, death, and heart failure in diabetic and nondiabetic individuals," *The Journal of the American Medical Association*, vol. 286, no. 4, pp. 421–426, 2001.

[5] M. J. Sarnak, A. S. Levey, A. C. Schoolwerth et al., "Kidney disease as a risk factor for development of cardiovascular disease: a statement from the American Heart Association Councils on Kidney in Cardiovascular Disease, High Blood Pressure Research, Clinical Cardiology, and Epidemiology and Prevention," *Circulation*, vol. 108, no. 17, pp. 2154–2169, 2003.

[6] U. Schwarz, M. Buzello, E. Ritz et al., "Morphology of coronary atherosclerotic lesions in patients with end-stage renal failure," *Nephrology Dialysis Transplantation*, vol. 15, no. 2, pp. 218–223, 2000.

[7] P. Stenvinkel, J. J. Carrero, J. Axelsson, B. Lindholm, O. Heimbürger, and Z. Massy, "Emerging biomarkers for evaluating cardiovascular risk in the chronic kidney disease patient: how do new pieces fit into the uremic puzzle?" *Clinical Journal of the American Society of Nephrology*, vol. 3, no. 2, pp. 505–521, 2008.

[8] M. W. Lorenz, H. S. Markus, M. L. Bots, M. Rosvall, and M. Sitzer, "Prediction of clinical cardiovascular events with carotid intima-media thickness: a systematic review and meta-analysis," *Circulation*, vol. 115, no. 4, pp. 459–467, 2007.

[9] B. Coll, Á. Betriu, M. Martínez-Alonso et al., "Cardiovascular risk factors underestimate atherosclerotic burden in chronic kidney disease: usefulness of non-invasive tests in cardiovascular assessment," *Nephrology Dialysis Transplantation*, vol. 25, no. 9, pp. 3017–3025, 2010.

[10] K. Matsushita, Y. Sang, S. H. Ballew et al., "Subclinical atherosclerosis measures for cardiovascular prediction in CKD," *Journal of the American Society of Nephrology*, vol. 26, no. 2, pp. 439–447, 2015.

[11] R. Visse and H. Nagase, "Matrix metalloproteinases and tissue inhibitors of metalloproteinases: structure, function, and biochemistry," *Circulation Research*, vol. 92, no. 8, pp. 827–839, 2003.

[12] R. J. Tan and Y. Liu, "Matrix metalloproteinases in kidney homeostasis and diseases," *The American Journal of Physiology—Renal Physiology*, vol. 302, no. 11, pp. F1351–F1361, 2012.

[13] T. H. Vu and Z. Werb, "Matrix metalloproteinases: effectors of development and normal physiology," *Genes and Development*, vol. 14, no. 17, pp. 2123–2133, 2000.

[14] D. Rodríguez, C. J. Morrison, and C. M. Overall, "Matrix metalloproteinases: what do they not do? New substrates and biological roles identified by murine models and proteomics," *Biochimica et Biophysica Acta (BBA)—Molecular Cell Research*, vol. 1803, no. 1, pp. 39–54, 2010.

[15] Z. S. Galis and J. J. Khatri, "Matrix metalloproteinases in vascular remodeling and atherogenesis: the good, the bad, and the ugly," *Circulation Research*, vol. 90, no. 3, pp. 251–262, 2002.

[16] D. Fukuda, K. Shimada, A. Tanaka et al., "Comparison of levels of serum matrix metalloproteinase-9 in patients with acute myocardial infarction versus unstable angina pectoris versus stable angina pectoris," *American Journal of Cardiology*, vol. 97, no. 2, pp. 175–180, 2006.

[17] B. Alvarez, C. Ruiz, P. Chacón, J. Alvarez-Sabin, and M. Matas, "Serum values of metalloproteinase-2 and metalloproteinase-9 as related to unstable plaque and inflammatory cells in patients with greater than 70% carotid artery stenosis," *Journal of Vascular Surgery*, vol. 40, no. 3, pp. 469–475, 2004.

[18] J. Orbe, I. Montero, J. A. Rodríguez, O. Beloqui, C. Roncal, and J. A. Páramo, "Independent association of matrix metalloproteinase-10, cardiovascular risk factors and subclinical atherosclerosis," *Journal of Thrombosis and Haemostasis*, vol. 5, no. 1, pp. 91–97, 2007.

[19] C. Tan, Y. Liu, W. Li et al., "Associations of matrix metalloproteinase-9 and monocyte chemoattractant protein-1 concentrations with carotid atherosclerosis, based on measurements of plaque and intima-media thickness," *Atherosclerosis*, vol. 232, no. 1, pp. 199–203, 2014.

[20] I. Goncalves, E. Bengtsson, H. M. Colhoun et al., "Elevated plasma levels of MMP-12 are associated with atherosclerotic burden and symptomatic cardiovascular disease in subjects with type 2 diabetes," *Arteriosclerosis, Thrombosis, and Vascular Biology*, vol. 35, no. 7, pp. 1723–1731, 2015.

[21] P. Sapienza, V. Borrelli, L. di Marzo, and A. Cavallaro, "MMP and TIMP alterations in asymptomatic and symptomatic severe recurrent carotid artery stenosis," *European Journal of Vascular and Endovascular Surgery*, vol. 37, no. 5, pp. 525–530, 2009.

[22] K.-F. Wang, P.-H. Huang, C.-H. Chiang et al., "Usefulness of plasma matrix metalloproteinase-9 level in predicting future coronary revascularization in patients after acute myocardial infarction," *Coronary Artery Disease*, vol. 24, no. 1, pp. 23–28, 2013.

[23] K. J. Molloy, M. M. Thompson, J. L. Jones et al., "Unstable carotid plaques exhibit raised matrix metalloproteinase-8 activity," *Circulation*, vol. 110, no. 3, pp. 337–343, 2004.

[24] N. Fiotti, N. Altamura, C. Orlando et al., "Metalloproteinases-2, -9 and TIMP-1 expression in stable and unstable coronary plaques undergoing PCI," *International Journal of Cardiology*, vol. 127, no. 3, pp. 350–357, 2008.

[25] Z. Li, L. Li, H. R. Zielke et al., "Increased expression of 72-kd type IV collagenase (MMP-2) in human aortic atherosclerotic lesions," *The American Journal of Pathology*, vol. 148, no. 1, pp. 121–128, 1996.

[26] M. Wang, S. H. Kim, R. E. Monticone, and E. G. Lakatta, "Matrix metalloproteinases promote arterial remodeling in aging, hypertension, and atherosclerosis," *Hypertension*, vol. 65, no. 4, pp. 698–703, 2015.

[27] S. Lenglet, A. Thomas, P. Chaurand, K. Galan, F. Mach, and F. Montecucco, "Molecular imaging of matrix metalloproteinases in atherosclerotic plaques," *Thrombosis and Haemostasis*, vol. 107, no. 3, pp. 409–416, 2012.

[28] R. E. Vandenbroucke and C. Libert, "Is there new hope for therapeutic matrix metalloproteinase inhibition?" *Nature Reviews Drug Discovery*, vol. 13, pp. 904–927, 2014.

[29] A. C. Newby, "Metalloproteinases promote plaque rupture and myocardial infarction: a persuasive concept waiting for clinical translation," *Matrix Biology*, vol. 44–46, pp. 157–166, 2015.

[30] G. Cerisano, P. Buonamici, A. M. Gori et al., "Matrix metalloproteinases and their tissue inhibitor after reperfused ST-elevation myocardial infarction treated with doxycycline. Insights from the TIPTOP trial," *International Journal of Cardiology*, vol. 197, pp. 147–153, 2015.

[31] J. J. Carrero and P. Stenvinkel, "Inflammation in end-stage renal disease-what have we learned in 10 years?" *Seminars in Dialysis*, vol. 23, no. 5, pp. 498–509, 2010.

[32] O. M. Akchurin and F. Kaskel, "Update on inflammation in chronic kidney disease," *Blood Purification*, vol. 39, no. 1–3, pp. 84–92, 2015.

[33] G. Wells, B. Shea, D. O'connell et al., *The Newcastle-Ottawa Scale (NOS) for Assessing the Quality of Nonrandomised Studies in Meta-Analyses*, Ottawa Hospital Research Institute, Ottawa, Canada, 2000, http://www.ohri.ca/programs/clinical_epidemiology/oxford.htm.

[34] P.-J. Touboul, M. G. Hennerici, S. Meairs et al., "Mannheim carotid intima-media thickness and plaque consensus (2004–2006–2011). An update on behalf of the advisory board of the 3rd, 4th and 5th watching the risk symposia, at the 13th, 15th and 20th European Stroke Conferences, Mannheim, Germany, 2004, Brussels, Belgium, 2006, and Hamburg, Germany, 2011," *Cerebrovascular Diseases*, vol. 34, no. 4, pp. 290–296, 2012.

[35] C. I. K. Weber, G. Duchateau-Nguyen, C. Solier et al., "Cardiovascular risk markers associated with arterial calcification in patients with chronic kidney disease Stages 3 and 4," *Clinical Kidney Journal*, vol. 7, no. 2, pp. 167–173, 2014.

[36] A. Sánchez-Escuredo, M. C. Pastor, B. Bayés et al., "Inflammation, metalloproteinases, and growth factors in the development of carotid atherosclerosis in renal transplant patients," *Transplantation Proceedings*, vol. 42, no. 8, pp. 2905–2907, 2010.

[37] F. Addabbo, F. Mallamaci, D. Leonardis et al., "Searching for biomarker patterns characterizing carotid atherosclerotic burden in patients with reduced renal function," *Nephrology Dialysis Transplantation*, vol. 22, no. 12, pp. 3521–3526, 2007.

[38] B. Coll, J. A. Rodríguez, L. Craver et al., "Serum levels of matrix metalloproteinase-10 are associated with the severity of atherosclerosis in patients with chronic kidney disease," *Kidney International*, vol. 78, no. 12, pp. 1275–1280, 2010.

[39] K. Pawlak, D. Pawlak, and M. Mysliwiec, "Extrinsic coagulation pathway activation and metalloproteinase-2/TIMPs system are related to oxidative stress and atherosclerosis in hemodialysis patients," *Thrombosis and Haemostasis*, vol. 92, no. 3, pp. 646–653, 2004.

[40] K. Pawlak, D. Pawlak, and M. Myśliwiec, "Urokinase-type plasminogen activator and metalloproteinase-2 are independently related to the carotid atherosclerosis in haemodialysis patients," *Thrombosis Research*, vol. 121, no. 4, pp. 543–548, 2008.

[41] M. Nagano, K. Fukami, S.-I. Yamagishi et al., "Circulating matrix metalloproteinase-2 is an independent correlate of

proteinuria in patients with chronic kidney disease," *American Journal of Nephrology*, vol. 29, no. 2, pp. 109–115, 2009.

[42] D. Belal, M. El Deeb, N. Adly, M. Mostafa, K. Kaffas, and N. Mohammed, "The relationship between Matrix Metalloproteinase-10 (MMP-10) and atherosclerosis in patients with chronic kidney disease," *International Journal of Advanced Research*, vol. 2, no. 10, pp. 409–430, 2014.

[43] M. S. M. Issac, A. Afif, N. A. Gohar et al., "Association of E-selectin gene polymorphism and serum PAPP-A with carotid atherosclerosis in end-stage renal disease," *Molecular Diagnosis & Therapy*, vol. 18, no. 2, pp. 243–252, 2014.

[44] M. Peiskerová, M. Kalousová, M. Kratochvílová et al., "Fibroblast growth factor 23 and matrix-metalloproteinases in patients with chronic kidney disease: are they associated with cardiovascular disease?" *Kidney and Blood Pressure Research*, vol. 32, no. 4, pp. 276–283, 2009.

[45] K. Pawlak, J. Tankiewicz, M. Mysliwiec, and D. Pawlak, "Systemic levels of MMP2/TIMP2 and cardiovascular risk in CAPD patients," *Nephron Clinical Practice*, vol. 115, no. 4, pp. c251–c258, 2010.

[46] K. Musiał and D. Zwolińska, "Matrix metalloproteinases (MMP-2,9) and their tissue inhibitors (TIMP-1,2) as novel markers of stress response and atherogenesis in children with chronic kidney disease (CKD) on conservative treatment," *Cell Stress and Chaperones*, vol. 16, no. 1, pp. 97–103, 2011.

[47] G. Siasos, D. Tousoulis, S. Kioufis et al., "Inflammatory mechanisms in atherosclerosis: the impact of matrix metalloproteinases," *Current Topics in Medicinal Chemistry*, vol. 12, no. 10, pp. 1132–1148, 2012.

[48] M. Amin, S. Pushpakumar, N. Muradashvili, S. Kundu, S. C. Tyagi, and U. Sen, "Regulation and involvement of matrix metalloproteinases in vascular diseases," *Frontiers in Bioscience*, vol. 21, pp. 89–118, 2016.

[49] P. Brunet, B. Gondouin, A. Duval-Sabatier et al., "Does uremia cause vascular dysfunction?" *Kidney and Blood Pressure Research*, vol. 34, no. 4, pp. 284–290, 2011.

[50] J. Pelisek, I. N. Hahntow, H.-H. Eckstein et al., "Impact of chronic kidney disease on carotid plaque vulnerability," *Journal of Vascular Surgery*, vol. 54, no. 6, pp. 1643–1649, 2011.

[51] U. Baber, G. W. Stone, G. Weisz et al., "Coronary plaque composition, morphology, and outcomes in patients with and without chronic kidney disease presenting with acute coronary syndromes," *JACC: Cardiovascular Imaging*, vol. 5, no. 3, pp. S53–S61, 2012.

[52] K. Kono, H. Fujii, K. Nakai et al., "Composition and plaque patterns of coronary culprit lesions and clinical characteristics of patients with chronic kidney disease," *Kidney International*, vol. 82, no. 3, pp. 344–351, 2012.

[53] S. Lim and S. Park, "Role of vascular smooth muscle cell in the inflammation of atherosclerosis," *BMB Reports*, vol. 47, no. 1, pp. 1–7, 2014.

[54] A. C. Newby, "Matrix metalloproteinases regulate migration, proliferation, and death of vascular smooth muscle cells by degrading matrix and non-matrix substrates," *Cardiovascular Research*, vol. 69, no. 3, pp. 614–624, 2006.

[55] A. C. Newby, "Dual role of matrix metalloproteinases (matrixins) in intimal thickening and atherosclerotic plaque rupture," *Physiological Reviews*, vol. 85, no. 1, pp. 1–31, 2005.

[56] P. Libby, "Collagenases and cracks in the plaque," *Journal of Clinical Investigation*, vol. 123, no. 8, pp. 3201–3203, 2013.

[57] K. Pawlak, M. Mysliwiec, and D. Pawlak, "Peripheral blood level alterations of MMP-2 and MMP-9 in patients with chronic kidney disease on conservative treatment and on hemodialysis," *Clinical Biochemistry*, vol. 44, no. 10-11, pp. 838–843, 2011.

[58] R. S. Friese, F. Rao, S. Khandrika et al., "Matrix metalloproteinases: discrete elevations in essential hypertension and hypertensive end-stage renal disease," *Clinical and Experimental Hypertension*, vol. 31, no. 7, pp. 521–533, 2009.

[59] A. W. Y. Chung, H. H. Clarice Yang, J. M. Kim et al., "Upregulation of matrix metalloproteinase-2 in the arterial vasculature contributes to stiffening and vasomotor dysfunction in patients with chronic kidney disease," *Circulation*, vol. 120, no. 9, pp. 792–801, 2009.

[60] A. W. Y. Chung, H. H. C. Yang, M. K. Sigrist et al., "Matrix metalloproteinase-2 and-9 exacerbate arterial stiffening and angiogenesis in diabetes and chronic kidney disease," *Cardiovascular Research*, vol. 84, no. 3, pp. 494–504, 2009.

[61] E. Drucker and K. Krapfenbauer, "Pitfalls and limitations in translation from biomarker discovery to clinical utility in predictive and personalised medicine," *EPMA Journal*, vol. 4, no. 1, p. 7, 2013.

[62] G. B. Fields, "New strategies for targeting matrix metalloproteinases," *Matrix Biology*, vol. 44–46, pp. 239–246, 2015.

[63] A. Papazafiropoulou and N. Tentolouris, "Matrix metalloproteinases and cardiovascular diseases," *Hippokratia*, vol. 13, no. 2, pp. 76–82, 2009.

[64] K. Jung, C. Laube, M. Lein et al., "Kind of sample as preanalytical determinant of matrix metalloproteinases 2 and 9 and tissue inhibitor of metalloproteinase 2 in blood," *Clinical Chemistry*, vol. 44, no. 5, pp. 1060–1062, 1998.

[65] K. Jung, S. Klotzek, C. Stephan, F. Mannello, and M. Lein, "Impact of blood sampling on the circulating matrix metalloproteinases 1, 2, 3, 7, 8, and 9," *Clinical Chemistry*, vol. 54, no. 4, pp. 772–773, 2008.

[66] J. Rysz, M. Banach, R. A. Stolarek et al., "Serum metalloproteinases MMP-2, MMP-9 and metalloproteinase tissue inhibitors TIMP-1 and TIMP-2 in patients on hemodialysis," *International Urology and Nephrology*, vol. 43, no. 2, pp. 491–498, 2011.

[67] F.-P. Chou, S.-C. Chu, M.-C. Cheng et al., "Effect of hemodialysis on the plasma level of type IV collagenases and their inhibitors," *Clinical Biochemistry*, vol. 35, no. 5, pp. 383–388, 2002.

[68] S. Janssens and H. R. Lijnen, "What has been learned about the cardiovascular effects of matrix metalloproteinases from mouse models?" *Cardiovascular Research*, vol. 69, no. 3, pp. 585–594, 2006.

[69] I. Konstantinidis, G. N. Nadkarni, R. Yacoub et al., "Representation of patients with kidney disease in trials of cardiovascular interventions: an updated systematic review," *JAMA Internal Medicine*, vol. 176, no. 1, pp. 121–124, 2016.

[70] V. Jha, G. Garcia-Garcia, K. Iseki et al., "Chronic kidney disease: global dimension and perspectives," *The Lancet*, vol. 382, no. 9888, pp. 260–272, 2013.

[71] C. S. Fox, P. Muntner, A. Y. Chen et al., "Use of evidence-based therapies in short-term outcomes of ST-segment elevation myocardial infarction and non-ST-segment elevation myocardial infarction in patients with chronic kidney disease: a report from the national cardiovascular data acute coronary treatment and intervention outcomes network registry," *Circulation*, vol. 121, no. 3, pp. 357–365, 2010.

29

Dialysate White Blood Cell Change after Initial Antibiotic Treatment Represented the Patterns of Response in Peritoneal Dialysis-Related Peritonitis

Pichaya Tantiyavarong,[1,2] **Opas Traitanon,**[2] **Piyatida Chuengsaman,**[3] **Jayanton Patumanond,**[1] **and Adis Tasanarong**[2]

[1]*Division of Clinical Epidemiology, Faculty of Medicine, Thammasat University, Rangsit Campus, Pathum Thani, Thailand*
[2]*Division of Nephrology, Department of Medicine, Thammasat University Hospital, Pathum Thani, Thailand*
[3]*Banphaeo Hospital, Prommitr Branch, Bangkok, Thailand*

Correspondence should be addressed to Pichaya Tantiyavarong; ball.tanti@gmail.com

Academic Editor: Francesca Mallamaci

Background. Patients with peritoneal dialysis-related peritonitis usually have different responses to initial antibiotic treatment. This study aimed to explore the patterns of response by using the changes of dialysate white blood cell count on the first five days of the initial antibiotic treatment. *Materials and Methods.* A retrospective cohort study was conducted. All peritoneal dialysis-related peritonitis episodes from January 2014 to December 2015 were reviewed. We categorized the patterns of antibiotic response into 3 groups: early response, delayed response, and failure group. The changes of dialysate white blood cell count for each pattern were determined by multilevel regression analysis. *Results.* There were 644 episodes in 455 patients: 378 (58.7%) of early response, 122 (18.9%) of delayed response, and 144 (22.3%) of failure episodes. The patterns of early, delayed, and failure groups were represented by the average rate reduction per day of dialysate WBC of 68.4%, 34.0%, and 14.2%, respectively (p value < 0.001 for all comparisons). *Conclusion.* Three patterns, which were categorized by types of responses, have variable rates of WBC declining. Clinicians should focus on the delayed response and failure patterns in order to make a decision whether to continue medical therapies or to aggressively remove the peritoneal catheter.

1. Introduction

Peritoneal dialysis-related peritonitis is a common complication in end stage renal disease patients treated with continuous ambulatory peritoneal dialysis (CAPD) [1]. The nationwide prevalence was one episode every 17.1 to 25.8 months [2–5]. Bacteria are the most causative organism; thus initial antibiotics should be started immediately after the diagnosis is made [6]. Delayed treatment may lead to undesirable events such as prolonged hospitalization, higher rate of treatment failure, long-term peritoneal membrane dysfunction, and increased mortality.

Physicians usually use clinical parameters such as abdominal pain and dialysate white blood cells (WBC) to monitor treatment response. Numerous studies demonstrated that if dialysate WBC are more than 100 cells/mm^3 at day 5 after treatment, the chance of treatment failure is high [7–9]. Consequently, the International Society of Peritoneal Dialysis (ISPD) defined the term "refractory peritonitis" as failure of dialysate WBC clearance after five days of antibiotic treatment and recommended removing the peritoneal catheter and stopping dialysis therapy in order to prevent morbidity and mortality associated with treatment failure [10, 11]. However, in some places where the hemodialysis resource is limited or the dialysis catheter is not readily removable, clinicians might choose to continue antibiotic treatment in selected patients who may have a delayed response to the treatment even though the target of dialysate WBC after the fifth day was not reached. Moreover, some of these patients were later recovered from peritonitis even without catheter removal. In our practice, we usually observe that dialysate WBC reduction in each patient is quite different; some have rapidly declined WBC in a few days, but some have a slow pattern of WBC reduction or increasing WBC. We then hypothesized that the pattern of response to antibiotic treatment varies individually. Therefore we designed this study to explore the pattern of response to initial antibiotic treatment by categorizing patients into early response, delayed response, and failure groups according to the rate of dialysate WBC change and we also explored the factors associated with treatment response.

2. Materials and Methods

2.1. Study Design and Setting. This was a retrospective cohort study which was jointly conducted at Banphaeo Hospital and Thammasat University Hospital, Thailand. Consecutive episodes of CAPD peritonitis in adult patients between January 2014 and December 2015 were included. The study was approved by the human research ethics committee of Thammasat University (Faculty of Medicine).

2.2. Participants. The patients included in this study were over 18 years old with a diagnosis of peritoneal dialysis-related peritonitis, defined by at least 2 out of 3 following criteria: (1) abdominal pain or cloudy peritoneal fluid, (2) amount of dialysate WBC greater than 100 cells/mm^3, and (3) the organism being identified by Gram stain or microbiological culture [6]. Episodes were excluded if medical records were not found or held incomplete records of dialysate WBC at the time of peritonitis diagnosis or contained less than three time records of dialysate WBC in the first five days after treatment.

Standard care was applied to all peritoneal dialysis patients. A Tenckhoff catheter was placed on the abdominal wall and the dialysate was a lactated-buffered glucose solution in a twin-bag connecting system (Baxter Healthcare or Fresenius Medical Care). Training programs were introduced when CAPD was starting. All patients ran 3–5 cycles of CAPD. Since patients' caregivers or the patients themselves had suspected an incident of peritonitis, they would contact a nurse by phone and come to the hospital as soon as possible. After assessment by CAPD nurses and doctors, dialysate would be collected and sent to a laboratory for WBC counts (5 mL in EDTA tube) and bacterial culture (10 mL in two blood culture bottles and 5 mL centrifuged sediment for solid media). Antibiotics and other treatments were prescribed following the current ISPD guideline and the duration of treatment was mostly between 14 and 21 days depending on the clinician's judgments. Clinical symptoms and dialysate WBC counts were routinely monitored once a day or every other day to assess the treatment response. Specific antibiotics were prescribed according to the culture result. If there was no clinical improvement or dialysate WBC was persistently high, the clinician would make a decision whether to use a salvage antibiotic regimen, such as carbapenem and vancomycin, or to remove the Tenckhoff catheter.

We categorized outcomes of treatment into 3 groups: early response, delayed response, and failure. Early response was defined by clinical improvement with dialysate WBC counts at less than 100 cells/mm^3 within 5 days of antibiotic treatment. Delayed response was determined if the dialysate WBC gradually decreased but still persisted more than 100 cells/mm^3 after 5 days of antibiotic treatment with success at the end of treatment. The failure group was patients who were not cured by antibiotics and changed to hemodialysis either temporarily or permanently. Patients who died due to peritonitis would be classified into failure group as well.

2.3. Patterns of Response Assessment. The primary outcome was the WBC changing patterns in five days after administration of antibiotics for all groups. Dialysate WBC were counted and differentiated by using an automatic machine. Data recorded included age, gender, diabetes status, HIV status, primary kidney disease, peritoneal dialysis vintage, episodes of peritonitis, body temperature, types of empirical antibiotics, microbiology, and outcomes of treatment.

2.4. Statistical Analysis. The characteristics of the early response, delayed response, and failure groups were profiled. Descriptive statistics were used depending on the types of variables. Continuous data were expressed by mean and standard deviation if their distributions were normal. Median and range were applied for skewed data. Continuous variables were compared by one-way analysis of variance or the Kruskal-Wallis H test as appropriate. Exact probability test and Chi-square test were used for categorical variables comparison. Furthermore, subgroups by types of organism were shown.

Serial measurements of dialysate WBC were plotted graphically for each group. Due to the right skewed distribution of peritoneal WBC in each day, we used natural logarithm transformation for normalizing this particular data. The linear patterns of WBC in logarithm scale were found over the time of treatment. To combat the disproportionate effect of individual patients with repeated peritonitis, we used the multilevel regression for numerical data to explore the slope of WBC change. Multiple comparison with Bonferroni adjustment for p value was used to demonstrate the statistical difference of each pattern. The constant rate of WBC reduction per day was achieved by applying the exponential function of the Beta coefficient in the model. Finally, the ratio was internally validated using a bootstrapping procedure with 1,000 random samples with replacement.

All statistical tests were two-sided. We considered p value of less than 0.05 to point out the level of significance. All statistical analyses and graphics were performed with Stata software version 14.0 (StataCorp).

3. Results

3.1. Characteristics. A total of 727 episodes of peritonitis were recorded between January 2014 and December 2015. Six hundred and forty-four episodes (from 455 patients) were included for analysis: 378 of early response (58.7%), 122 of

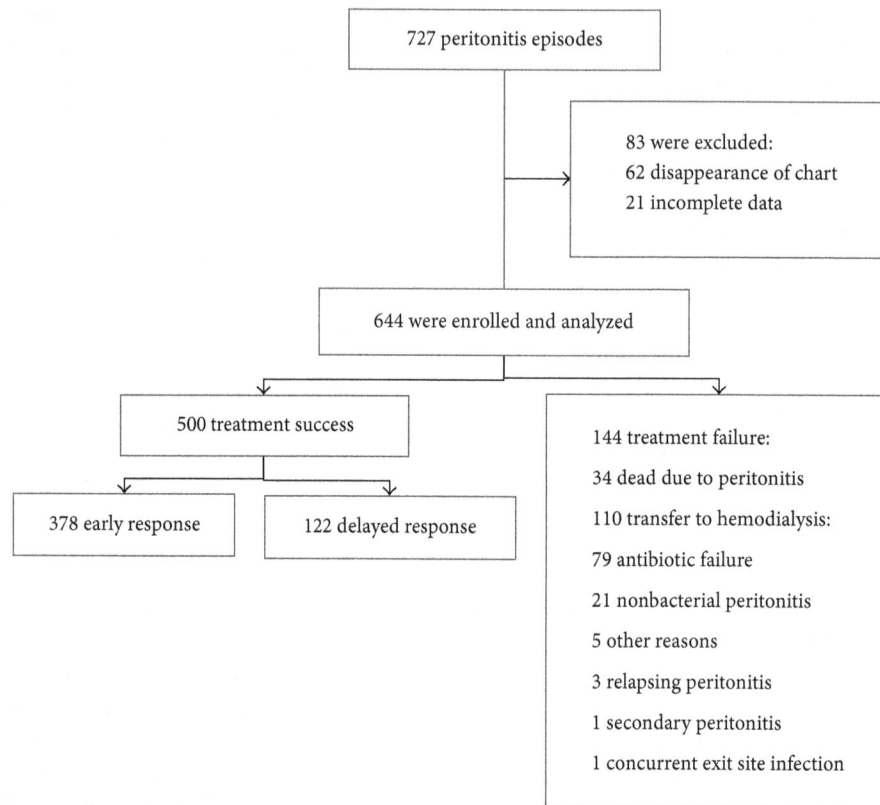

FIGURE 1: Study flow.

delayed response (18.9%), and 144 of failure groups (22.3%). Thirty-four patients died due to peritonitis (mortality rate 5.3%) and the major causes of peritoneal dialysis termination were antibiotic failure (79 episodes) and nonbacterial peritonitis (21 episodes) (Figure 1).

Clinical characteristics were categorized by whether episodes of peritonitis had early response, delayed response, or treatment failure (Table 1). Two-thirds of our patients had diabetes. The failure group showed a higher median duration of peritoneal dialysis (19.8 months) and a lower percentage of the first episode of peritonitis (49.3%) but no statistical significance when compared with other groups. The usual empirical antibiotic regimen in our centers was intraperitoneal cefazolin (88.7%) and ceftazidime (89.9%). The rate of culture negative peritonitis which was about 30% in this cohort and types of organism differ significantly among the 3 groups (p value < 0.001). Gram-negative organism was found less in the early response group when compared with the delayed response group (24% versus 36.9%). Moreover, mixed organism and nonbacterial peritonitis appeared more frequently in the failure group. Empirical antibiotic success, defined as successful treatment without changing to any salvage antibiotic regimens, was found in all early response groups and 48.7 percent in delayed response groups in culture negative cases.

3.2. Types of Organism. Subgroup analysis was done according to the types of organism (Table 2). We found 75.6%

of early response pattern in 213 episodes of single Gram-positive infection. This result suggested that, in general, if a Gram-positive organism was the causative pathogen, the response to initial antibiotic was usually good except for *Staphylococcus aureus* or methicillin-resistant *Staphylococcus aureus* (MRSA) infection (38.1% and 14.3%, resp.). In cases of single Gram-negative infection, the early response pattern was found only 52% in average. Delayed response pattern was accounted for one-fourth of single Gram-negative infection. Extended-Spectrum Beta-Lactamase- (ESBL-) producing *Escherichia coli* had the worst response to antibiotics: 23.5% of early response, 29.4% of delayed response, and 47.1% of failure pattern. The percentage of failure was highest in mycobacterium and fungal infection, followed by *Escherichia coli* (ESBL), MRSA, mixed organism, *Pseudomonas* species, and *Enterobacter* species.

3.3. Dialysate WBC Change. We presented the amounts of dialysate WBC five days after treatment in a boxplot graph due to the right skewed distribution of WBC (Figure 2). Log-transformed WBC was used to calculate a geometric mean and also standard error which were $2{,}202 \pm 348$ cells/mm^3 in early response, $3{,}024 \pm 603$ cells/mm^3 in delayed response, and $2{,}195 \pm 452$ cells/mm^3 in failure group on the first day of treatment (Table 3). A constant trend in all groups was a reduction of dialysate WBC over time of treatment (Figure 3). We used multilevel linear regression,

TABLE 1: Clinical characteristics of peritoneal episodes, categorized by early response, delayed response, and failure groups (455 patients; 644 episodes).

Characteristics	Early response ($N = 378$)	Delayed response ($N = 122$)	Failure ($N = 144$)	p value
Male, n (%)	192 (50.8)	58 (47.5)	70 (48.6)	0.789
Age, year	62.1 ± 12.0	60.2 ± 13.5	59.3 ± 13.1	0.051
Diabetes, n (%)	246 (65.1)	79 (64.8)	97 (67.4)	0.871
HIV, n (%)	4 (1.1)	0	3 (2.1)	0.275
Primary kidney disease, n (%)				
Diabetic nephropathy	245 (64.8)	78 (63.9)	96 (66.7)	0.890
Glomerulonephritis	3 (0.8)	1 (0.8)	2 (1.4)	
Nephrosclerosis	60 (15.9)	15 (12.3)	21 (14.6)	
Obstructive uropathy	3 (0.8)	0	1 (0.7)	
Others	18 (4.8)	9 (7.4)	9 (6.3)	
Unknown	49 (13.0)	19 (15.6)	15 (12.9)	
Dialysis vintage, month				
Median [min–max]	16.8 [0–87.6]	15.0 [0–76.8]	19.8 [0–81.6]	0.309
First episode of peritonitis	218 (57.7)	64 (52.5)	71 (49.3)	0.190
Episode of peritonitis				
Median [min–max]	1 [1–8]	1 [1–8]	2 [1–9]	0.494
Body temperature, Celsius	37.1 ± 0.9	37.0 ± 0.9	37.0 ± 1.0	0.520
Empirical antibiotic regimen				
Cefazolin	333 (88.1)	111 (91.0)	127 (88.2)	0.701
Vancomycin	17 (4.5)	5 (4.1)	8 (5.6)	0.869
Ceftazidime	335 (88.6)	113 (92.6)	131 (91.0)	0.423
Gentamicin/amikacin	12 (3.2)	1 (0.8)	1 (0.7)	0.167
Meropenem	6 (1.6)	2 (1.6)	6 (4.2)	0.222
Cefepime	23 (6.1)	5 (4.1)	4 (2.8)	0.284
Organism				
Culture negative	106 (28.0)	39 (32.0)	46 (31.9)	<0.001
Gram-positive	161 (42.6)	33 (27.1)	19 (13.2)	
Gram-negative	92 (24.3)	45 (36.9)	40 (27.8)	
Mixed organism	19 (5.0)	4 (3.3)	14 (9.7)	
Tuberculosis	0	0	9 (6.3)	
Fungus	0	1 (0.8)	16 (11.1)	
Empirical antibiotic success*				
In total cases	375 (99.2)	36 (29.5)	0	<0.001
In culture negative cases	106/106 (100)	19/39 (48.7)	0	<0.001

*Empirical antibiotic success; success in treatment without changing to any salvage antibiotic regimens.

which had been adjusted for baseline white blood cells, to explore the average rate reduction per day in all three groups (early response, delayed response, and failure) which were 68.4% (95% CI, 67.4–69.3%), 34.0% (95% CI, 30.7–37.0%), and 14.2% (95% CI, 9.8–18.3%), respectively (p value < 0.001 for all comparisons) (Table 2). Internal validation using bootstrapping technique also revealed similar rate reduction in all groups (68.1% (95% CI, 67.5–68.7%) in early response, 30.8% (95% CI, 28.7–32.9%) in delayed response, and 12.9% (95% CI, 10.1–15.1%) in failure groups).

4. Discussion

This was the study exploring the change of dialysate WBC in order to represent the patterns of response to initial antibiotic treatment. We categorized episodes of peritonitis into 3 groups (early response, delayed response, and failure) and our data can confirm the definite patterns, which was derived from the mathematic model of log-transformed WBC counts over the treatment time. Each pattern showed the gradual decline of dialysate WBC, but with varying rates. By using

TABLE 2: Predictive value of early response, delayed response, and failure groups according to types of organism.

Type of organism	Number of episodes	Early response (N = 378)	Delayed response (N = 122)	Failure (N = 144)
Culture negative	191	106 (55.5)	39 (20.4)	46 (24.1)
Gram-positive organism	213	161 (75.6)	33 (15.5)	19 (8.9)
Staphylococcus epidermidis	70	52 (74.3)	10 (14.3)	8 (11.4)
Staphylococcus aureus	21	8 (38.1)	9 (42.9)	4 (19.1)
MRSA	7	1 (14.3)	3 (42.9)	3 (42.9)
Other *Staphylococcus*	5	5 (100)	0	0
Streptococcus viridan	21	20 (95.2)	1 (4.8)	0
Streptococcus group D	42	38 (90.5)	4 (9.5)	0
Enterococcus	9	6 (66.7)	2 (22.2)	1 (11.1)
Other *Streptococcus*	35	29 (82.9)	3 (8.6)	3 (8.6)
Other Gram-positive organisms	3	2 (66.7)	1 (33.3)	0
Gram-negative organism	177	92 (52.0)	45 (25.4)	40 (22.6)
Escherichia coli	57	34 (59.7)	15 (26.3)	8 (14.0)
Escherichia coli (ESBL)	17	4 (23.5)	5 (29.4)	8 (47.1)
Klebsiella species	40	23 (57.5)	11 (27.5)	6 (15.0)
Pseudomonas aeruginosa/spp.	15	7 (46.7)	3 (20.0)	5 (33.3)
Acinetobacter baumannii/spp.	18	8 (44.4)	5 (27.8)	5 (27.8)
Enterobacter spp.	15	6 (40.0)	4 (26.7)	5 (33.3)
Other Gram-negative organisms	15	10 (66.7)	2 (13.3)	3 (20.0)
Mixed organism	37	19 (51.2)	4 (10.8)	14 (37.8)
Tuberculosis	9	0	0	9 (100)
Fungus	17	0	1 (5.9)	16 (94.1)

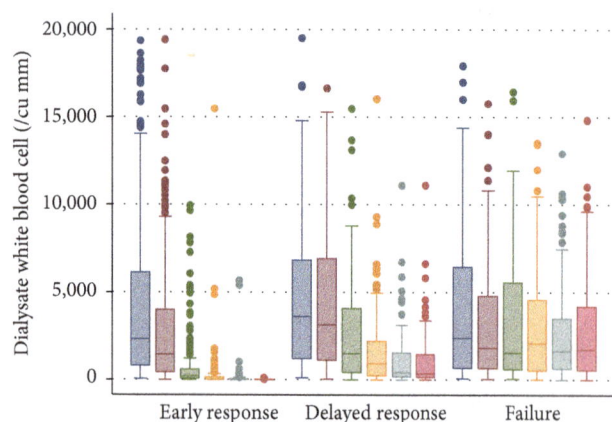

FIGURE 2: Boxplot of dialysate white blood cells in days 0–5 after antibiotic treatment, categorized by early response, delayed response, and failure groups.

these patterns, clinicians can predict whether each treatment episode will be success or failure.

Our patterns of WBC change are practical and match with the real clinical practice. We developed this model based on the first 5 days after antibiotic treatment because it represents the effectiveness of the empirical therapy and

clinicians can use this information to guide further treatment. There were two previous reports exploring the pattern of dialysate WBC change. First, Dong et al. [12] categorized dialysate WBC patterns over the seven days of treatment into four groups based on a disease severity score [13], which was calculated by the sum of points for abdominal pain and fever at the time of diagnosis of dialysate-related peritonitis. One point increase in the disease severity score at baseline was correlated with higher number of WBC when compared between groups. Unfortunately, these patterns failed to predict either peritonitis-related death or transfer to hemodialysis. One year later, the same group presented additional data of WBC count patterns which categorized peritonitis episodes by the trend of WBC change in five days into four groups: group A (WBC count persistently declined), group B (WBC count declined after a transient increase), group C (WBC count increased after a transient decline), and group D (WBC count persistently increased). This report showed that WBC change does not always change in one direction. They found that the causative organisms were statistically different between groups. Gram-positive infection was found the most in group A but Gram-negative infection was rare. Groups A and B had a lower risk of treatment failure (11.8 and 16.4%, resp.); on the other hand groups C and D had higher failure rate (66.7 and 50%, resp.). The limitation of this report was a small sample size and excluded a large

TABLE 3: Dialysate white blood cell count five days after antibiotics treatment, categorized by early response, delayed response, and failure groups.

Day of treatment	Dialysate WBC, cell/mm^3 (geometric mean ± SE)		
	Early response ($N = 378$)	Delayed response ($N = 122$)	Failure ($N = 144$)
Day 0	2202 ± 348	3024 ± 603	2195 ± 452
Day 1	1174 ± 220	2650 ± 476	1633 ± 403
Day 2	164 ± 72	1028 ± 307	1494 ± 340
Day 3	27 ± 54	613 ± 295	1264 ± 278
Day 4	9 ± 25	409 ± 164	1004 ± 255
Day 5	3 ± 1	345 ± 151	895 ± 274
% reduction (developed model)*	68.4 [67.4, 69.3]	34.0 [30.7, 37.0]	14.2 [9.8, 18.2]
% reduction (bootstrapping model)*	68.1 [67.5, 68.7]	30.8 [28.7, 32.9]	12.9 [10.1, 15.1]

WBC: white blood cells; % reduction presented in average rate per day [95% confident interval].
* p value < 0.001 for all comparisons by multiple comparison under multilevel modeling.

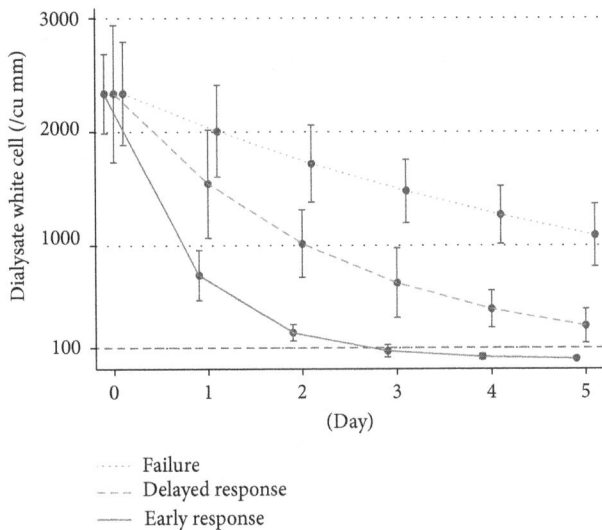

FIGURE 3: Pattern of dialysate white blood cell change, geometric mean of white blood cells, and standard error bar, categorized by early response, delayed response, and failure groups (parametric plot adjusted for baseline white blood cells). Red dashed line refers to the response level of dialysate white cell.

number of patients due to missing data that may not be able to extrapolate to other settings. Unlike the previous studies, our data categorized patterns by using a different approach because we did the analysis based on the outcomes of therapy and we use the mathematic model to calculate the average trend of WBC change without considering the fluctuation of WBC. Our study confirmed the association between the pattern of response and the type of causative microorganism. Gram-negative bacteria were found more in the delayed response group whereas mixed organisms, tuberculosis, and fungus appeared with a higher frequency in the failure group.

Gram-positive organism remains the major causative pathogen of peritoneal dialysis-related peritonitis in several studies [7, 9, 14, 15]. Staphylococcus epidermidis was the most common causative organism but the virulence of this organism is low. On the contrary, Staphylococcus aureus either methicillin-sensitive or methicillin-resistant often caused severe episodes of peritonitis [16]. One study showed that MRSA increased the failure rate of peritoneal dialysis and also hospitalization rate by double when compared to other Gram-positive organisms [17]. Our study revealed the same findings. The onset of response in our study could represent the severity of each organism. We found that most episodes of Staphylococcus epidermidis and other Staphylococcus (not Staphylococcus aureus), Streptococcus viridan, and Streptococcus group D (non-Enterococcus) had the early response pattern. Conversely, the delayed response and failure patterns were found more in Staphylococcus aureus and Enterococcus infection. These data were similar to the study of O'Shea et al. [18] and Edey et al. [19] data.

Pseudomonas species is a group of the Gram-negative bacteria that lead to severe peritoneal dialysis-related peritonitis. Szeto et al. [20] found that the primary response rate, which was defined as resolution of abdominal pain and dialysate neutrophil count of less than 100 cell/mm^3 on day 10 with antibiotic, was 60.6% and complete cure rate, which was defined as complete cure with antibiotic alone within 120 days, was 22.1% in Pseudomonas peritonitis. There were 14 cases that had Tenckhoff catheter removed immediately when primary response could not be achieved and 10 of 20 cases with delayed Tenckhoff catheter removal after salvage antibiotics. Siva et al. [21] also found the rate of peritoneal catheter removal of 44% in Pseudomonas peritonitis, compared to 20% of non-Pseudomonas peritonitis. In the same way, our study showed that failure pattern was greater in Gram-negative infection especially in Pseudomonas aeruginosa and also in Escherichia coli (ESBL), Acinetobacter baumannii, and Enterobacter species infection.

From our point of view, the pattern of response will be helpful in 2 situations. First, when symptoms of patients relieve, but the dialysate WBC still persists more than 100 cells/mm^3 on day 5 after antibiotic treatment and clinicians believe that those patients are in the delayed response group. If the rate of dialysate WBC reduction is about 34%

(95% CI, 30.7–37), clinicians can wait and see instead of immediate removal of Tenckhoff catheter, whereas when the rate of dialysate WBC decline is less than 14.2%, it would suggest the failure of antibiotic treatment and a further management decision should be planned. Second, when the causative organism cannot be identified, the pattern of WBC change may help to predict the type of causative organism. We found that delayed pattern of response was associated with unique pathogens such as *Staphylococcus aureus*, *Pseudomonas aeruginosa*, *Enterobacter* species, and some drug-resistant organisms. Clinicians should combine these information with local prevalence of responsible organism and prescribe the appropriate salvage antibiotics. However, close follow-up is also important to help identify the patients who may have to stop peritoneal dialysis if the failure pattern occurs or another indication is present.

The strength of our report was large sample sizes and we classified the groups that matched with routine clinical practice. Furthermore, we used the multilevel mixed effect model to cope with serial measurement of dialysate WBC and repeated episodes of peritonitis in the same patients and we also had internal validation of these patterns which help make a more accurate conclusion. Nevertheless, there were some limitations. First, we excluded 83 medical records (11.4%) due to incomplete data. But we thought our sample was adequate to explore the patterns of WBC with less selection bias. Second, the percent reduction of WBC in each group could only be interpreted as an average trend of change. We suggested using the pattern with clinical correlation. Third, this study focused on the pattern of dialysate WBC in aspect of short term outcomes. Long-term follow-up in each pattern would be done and reported in further studies. Finally, the retrospective nature of this study needs to be considered when interpreting these results. We believed that this study will generate the idea of how important WBC patterns are. Prospective study should be done to confirm our hypothesis.

5. Conclusion

In conclusion, our study determined the patterns of WBC response after empirical antibiotic therapy in peritoneal dialysis-related peritonitis patients which could be categorized into early response, delayed response, and failure groups. These findings may guide clinicians to decide a proper treatment whether to continue medical therapies or to aggressively remove the peritoneal catheter.

Acknowledgments

This study has been supported by operating grants from the Thammasat University under the TU Research Scholar and The Kidney Foundation of Thailand.

References

[1] B. Piraino, "Peritonitis as a complication of peritoneal dialysis," *Journal of the American Society of Nephrology*, vol. 9, no. 10, pp. 1956–1964, 1998.

[2] T. N. Oo, T. L. Roberts, and A. J. Collins, "A comparison of peritonitis rates from the United States Renal Data System database: CAPD versus continuous cycling peritoneal dialysis patients," *American Journal of Kidney Diseases*, vol. 45, no. 2, pp. 372–380, 2005.

[3] M. C. Brown, K. Simpson, J. J. Kerssens, and R. A. Mactier, "Peritoneal dialysis-associated peritonitis rates and outcomes in a national cohort are not improving in the post-millennium (2000–2007)," *Peritoneal Dialysis International*, vol. 31, no. 6, pp. 639–650, 2011.

[4] P. Dhanakijcharoen, D. Sirivongs, S. Aruyapitipan, P. Chuengsaman, and A. Lumpaopong, "The 'PD First' policy in Thailand: three-years experiences (2008–2011)," *Journal of the Medical Association of Thailand*, vol. 94, supplement 4, pp. S153–S161, 2011.

[5] Y. Cho, S. V. Badve, C. M. Hawley et al., "Seasonal variation in peritoneal dialysis-associated peritonitis: a multi-centre registry study," *Nephrology, Dialysis, Transplantation*, vol. 27, no. 5, pp. 2028–2036, 2012.

[6] B. Piraino, G. R. Bailie, J. Bernardini et al., "Peritoneal dialysis-related infections recommendations: 2005 update," *Peritoneal Dialysis International*, vol. 25, no. 2, pp. 107–131, 2005.

[7] M. Krishnan, E. Thodis, D. Ikonomopoulos et al., "Predictors of outcome following bacterial peritonitis in peritoneal dialysis," *Peritoneal Dialysis International*, vol. 22, no. 5, pp. 573–581, 2002.

[8] C.-C. Szeto, K.-M. Chow, T. Y.-H. Wong et al., "Feasibility of resuming peritoneal dialysis after severe peritonitis and Tenckhoff catheter removal," *Journal of the American Society of Nephrology*, vol. 13, no. 4, pp. 1040–1045, 2002.

[9] K. M. Chow, C. C. Szeto, K. K.-T. Cheung et al., "Predictive value of dialysate cell counts in peritonitis complicating peritoneal dialysis," *Clinical Journal of the American Society of Nephrology*, vol. 1, no. 4, pp. 768–773, 2006.

[10] P. K.-T. Li, C. C. Szeto, B. Piraino et al., "Peritoneal dialysis-related infections recommendations: 2010 update," *Peritoneal Dialysis International*, vol. 30, no. 4, pp. 393–423, 2010.

[11] G. E. Digenis, G. Abraham, E. Savin et al., "Peritonitis-related deaths in continuous ambulatory peritoneal dialysis (CAPD) patients," *Peritoneal Dialysis International*, vol. 10, no. 1, pp. 45–47, 1990.

[12] J. Dong, Z. Li, R. Xu, Y. Chen, S. Luo, and Y. Li, "Disease severity score could not predict the outcomes in peritoneal dialysis-associated peritonitis," *Nephrology Dialysis Transplantation*, vol. 27, no. 6, pp. 2496–2501, 2012.

[13] F. Scharfer, G. Klaus, D. E. Müller-Wiefel, and O. Mehls, "Intermittent versus continuous intraperitoneal glycopeptide/ceftazidime treatment in children with peritoneal dialysis-associated peritonitis. The Mid-European Pediatric Peritoneal Dialysis Study Group (MEPPS)," *Journal of the American Society of Nephrology*, vol. 10, no. 1, pp. 136–145, 1999.

[14] R. Xu, Y. Chen, S. Luo et al., "Clinical characteristics and outcomes of peritoneal dialysis-related peritonitis with different trends of change in effluent white cell count: A Longitudinal Study," *Peritoneal Dialysis International*, vol. 33, no. 4, pp. 436–444, 2013.

[15] J. A. Quintanar Lartundo, R. Palomar, A. Dominguez-Diez et al., "Microbiological profile of peritoneal dialysis peritonitis and predictors of hospitalization," *Advances in Peritoneal Dialysis*, vol. 27, pp. 38–42, 2011.

[16] C.-C. Szeto, K.-M. Chow, B. C.-H. Kwan et al., "*Staphylococcus aureus* peritonitis complicates peritoneal dialysis: review of 245 consecutive cases," *Clinical Journal of the American Society of Nephrology*, vol. 2, no. 2, pp. 245–251, 2007.

[17] S. Govindarajulu, C. M. Hawley, S. P. Mcdonald et al., "Staphylococcus Aureus peritonitis in Australian peritoneal dialysis patients: predictors, treatment, and outcomes in 503 cases," *Peritoneal Dialysis International*, vol. 30, no. 3, pp. 311–319, 2010.

[18] S. O'Shea, C. M. Hawley, S. P. McDonald et al., "Streptococcal peritonitis in Australian peritoneal dialysis patients: predictors, treatment and outcomes in 287 cases," *BMC Nephrology*, vol. 10, no. 1, article 19, 2009.

[19] M. Edey, C. M. Hawley, S. P. McDonald et al., "Enterococcal peritonitis in Australian peritoneal dialysis patients: predictors, treatment and outcomes in 116 cases," *Nephrology Dialysis Transplantation*, vol. 25, no. 4, pp. 1272–1278, 2010.

[20] C.-C. Szeto, K.-M. Chow, C.-B. Leung et al., "Clinical course of peritonitis due to Pseudomonas species complicating peritoneal dialysis: a review of 104 cases," *Kidney International*, vol. 59, no. 6, pp. 2309–2315, 2001.

[21] B. Siva, C. M. Hawley, S. P. McDonald et al., "*Pseudomonas* peritonitis in Australia: predictors, treatment, and outcomes in 191 cases," *Clinical Journal of the American Society of Nephrology*, vol. 4, no. 5, pp. 957–964, 2009.

Permissions

All chapters in this book were first published in IJN, by Hindawi Publishing Corporation; hereby published with permission under the Creative Commons Attribution License or equivalent. Every chapter published in this book has been scrutinized by our experts. Their significance has been extensively debated. The topics covered herein carry significant findings which will fuel the growth of the discipline. They may even be implemented as practical applications or may be referred to as a beginning point for another development.

The contributors of this book come from diverse backgrounds, making this book a truly international effort. This book will bring forth new frontiers with its revolutionizing research information and detailed analysis of the nascent developments around the world.

We would like to thank all the contributing authors for lending their expertise to make the book truly unique. They have played a crucial role in the development of this book. Without their invaluable contributions this book wouldn't have been possible. They have made vital efforts to compile up to date information on the varied aspects of this subject to make this book a valuable addition to the collection of many professionals and students.

This book was conceptualized with the vision of imparting up-to-date information and advanced data in this field. To ensure the same, a matchless editorial board was set up. Every individual on the board went through rigorous rounds of assessment to prove their worth. After which they invested a large part of their time researching and compiling the most relevant data for our readers.

The editorial board has been involved in producing this book since its inception. They have spent rigorous hours researching and exploring the diverse topics which have resulted in the successful publishing of this book. They have passed on their knowledge of decades through this book. To expedite this challenging task, the publisher supported the team at every step. A small team of assistant editors was also appointed to further simplify the editing procedure and attain best results for the readers.

Apart from the editorial board, the designing team has also invested a significant amount of their time in understanding the subject and creating the most relevant covers. They scrutinized every image to scout for the most suitable representation of the subject and create an appropriate cover for the book.

The publishing team has been an ardent support to the editorial, designing and production team. Their endless efforts to recruit the best for this project, has resulted in the accomplishment of this book. They are a veteran in the field of academics and their pool of knowledge is as vast as their experience in printing. Their expertise and guidance has proved useful at every step. Their uncompromising quality standards have made this book an exceptional effort. Their encouragement from time to time has been an inspiration for everyone.

The publisher and the editorial board hope that this book will prove to be a valuable piece of knowledge for researchers, students, practitioners and scholars across the globe.

List of Contributors

Michael A. Mao, YiFan Wu, Vickram Tejwani, Myriam Vela-Ortiz and Qi Qian
Division of Nephrology and Hypertension, Department of Medicine, Mayo Clinic College of Medicine, Rochester, MN 55905, USA

Charat Thongprayoon
Division of Anesthesiology, Mayo Clinic College of Medicine, Rochester, MN 55905, USA

Joseph Dearani
Department of Surgery, Mayo Clinic College of Medicine, Rochester, MN 55905, USA

Mohamad Adam Bujang, Tassha Hilda Adnan, Nadiah Hanis Hashim and Kirubashni Mohan
National Clinical Research Centre, Kuala Lumpur, Malaysia

Ang Kim Liong,
Clinical Research Centre, Serdang Hospital, Kajang, Malaysia

Goh Bak Leong
Clinical Research Centre, Serdang Hospital, Kajang, Malaysia
Department of Nephrology, Serdang Hospital, Kajang, Malaysia

Ghazali Ahmad and Sunita Bavanandan
Department of Nephrology, Kuala Lumpur Hospital, Kuala Lumpur, Malaysia

Jamaiyah Haniff
Malaysian Health Performance Unit, Ministry of Health, Kuala Lumpur, Malaysia

Ramya Bhargava, Paul Brenchley and Alastair Hutchison
Institute of Cardio-Vascular Sciences, Faculty of Medical and Human Sciences, University of Manchester, Manchester M13 9PL, UK
Manchester Royal Infirmary, Central Manchester University Hospitals NHS Foundation Trust, Manchester Academic Health Science Centre, Manchester M13 9WL, UK

Helen Hurst
Manchester Royal Infirmary, Central Manchester University Hospitals NHS Foundation Trust, Manchester Academic Health Science Centre, Manchester M13 9WL, UK

Philip A. Kalra
Salford Royal Hospitals NHS Foundation Trust, Salford M6 8HD, UK
Institute of Population Studies, Faculty of Medical and Human Sciences, University of Manchester, Manchester M13 9PL, UK

Juan José Bollain-y-Goytia, Mariela Arellano-Rodríguez, Felipe de Jesús Torres-Del-Muro, Esperanza Avalos-Díaz and Rafael Herrera-Esparza
Laboratorios de Inmunología y Biología Molecular, UA Ciencias Biológicas, Universidad Autónoma de Zacatecas, 98040 Zacatecas, ZAC, Mexico

Leonel Daza-Benítez
Unidad Médica de Alta Especialidad (UMAE) HPGNo. 48, InstitutoMexicano del Seguro Social (IMSS), 37320 Léon, GTO, Mexico

José FranciscoMuñoz-Valle
Instituto de Investigacíon en Ciencias Biomédicas, Centro Universitario de Ciencias de la Salud, Universidad de Guadalajara, 45178 Guadalajara, JAL, Mexico

Livia Victorino de Souza, Vanessa Oliveira, Aline Oliveira Laurindo, Luciana de Santis Feltran, José Osmar Medina-Pestana and Maria do Carmo Franco
Nephrology Division, School of Medicine, Federal University of São Paulo, São Paulo, SP, Brazil

DelmaRegına Gomes Huarachı and Paulo Cesar Koch Nogueira
PediatricsDepartment, School of Medicine, Federal University of São Paulo, São Paulo, SP, Brazil

Taiwo Augustina Ladapo, Christopher Imokhuede Esezobor and Foluso Ebun Lesi
Department of Paediatrics, College of Medicine, University of Lagos, PMB 12003, Lagos, Nigeria
Department of Paediatrics, Lagos University Teaching Hospital, Idi-Araba, PMB 12003, Lagos, Nigeria

Maisarah Jalalonmuhali, Ng Kok Peng and Lim Soo Kun
University Malaya Medical Centre, 59100 Kuala Lumpur, Malaysia

Monika Tooulou
Laboratory of Experimental Nephrology, Department of Biochemistry, Faculty of Medicine, Université Libre de Bruxelles (ULB), 1070 Brussels, Belgium

Joëlle L. Nortier and Agnieszka A. Pozdzik
Laboratory of Experimental Nephrology, Department of Biochemistry, Faculty of Medicine, Université Libre de Bruxelles (ULB), 1070 Brussels, Belgium
Department of Nephrology, Cliniques Universitaires de Bruxelles (CUB), Erasme Hospital, Université Libre de Bruxelles (ULB), 1070 Brussels, Belgium

Pieter Demetter
Department of Pathology, Cliniques Universitaires de Bruxelles (CUB), Erasme Hospital, Université Libre de Bruxelles (ULB), 1070 Brussels, Belgium

Anwar Hamade
Department of Nephrology, Cliniques Universitaires de Bruxelles (CUB), Erasme Hospital, Université Libre de Bruxelles (ULB), 1070 Brussels, Belgium

Caroline Keyzer
Department of Radiology, Cliniques Universitaires de Bruxelles (CUB), Erasme Hospital, Université Libre de Bruxelles (ULB), 1070 Brussels, Belgium

Belayneh Kefale
Department of Pharmacy, College of Medicine and Health Science, Ambo University, Ambo, Ethiopia

Yewondwossen Tadesse
Department of Internal Medicine, School of Medicine, College of Health Sciences, Addis Ababa University, Addis Ababa, Ethiopia

Minyahil Alebachew and Ephrem Engidawork
Department of Pharmacology and Clinical Pharmacy, School of Pharmacy, College of Health Sciences, Addis Ababa University, Addis Ababa, Ethiopia

Ayse Karaaslan, Eda Kepenekli Kadayifci, Serkan Atici, Gulsen Akkoc, Nurhayat Yakut, Sevliya Öcal Demir, Ahmet Soysal and Mustafa Bakir
Department of Pediatric Infectious Diseases, Marmara University School of Medicine, 34890 Istanbul, Turkey

Cristina García
CASMU Arrhythmia Service, 8 de Octubre 3310, 11600 Montevideo, Uruguay

Gabriel Vanerio
CASMU Arrhythmia Service, 8 de Octubre 3310, 11600 Montevideo, Uruguay
British Hospital, Avenida Italia 2420, 11600 Montevideo, Uruguay

Carlota González
CASMU Arrhythmia Service, 8 de Octubre 3310, 11600 Montevideo, Uruguay
Uruguayan Registry of Dialysis, Uruguay

Alejandro Ferreiro
CASMU Arrhythmia Service, 8 de Octubre 3310, 11600 Montevideo, Uruguay
Uruguayan Registry of Dialysis, Uruguay
Nephrology Clinic, Hospital de Clinicas, Faculty of Medicine, The University of the Republic, Avenida Italia s/n, 11600 Montevideo, Uruguay

Shahbaz Mehmood, Raouf Seyam and Waleed Mohammad Altaweel
Department of Urology, King Faisal Specialist Hospital and Research Centre, Riyadh 11211, Saudi Arabia

Sadia Firdous
Fatima Jinnah Medical University, Lahore, Pakistan

Sandra Wray
Favaloro University (AIDUF-CONICET), Sol´is 453, C1078AAI Buenos Aires, Argentina

Edmundo Cabrera Fischer and Cintia Galli
Favaloro University (AIDUF-CONICET), Sol´is 453, C1078AAI Buenos Aires, Argentina
Technological National University, C1179AAQ Buenos Aires, Argentina

Yanina Zócalo and Daniel Bia
Physiology Department, School of Medicine, CUiiDARTE, Republic University, 11800 Montevideo, Uruguay

Danielle Creme and Kieran McCafferty
Royal London Hospital, Whitechapel Road, London E1 1BB, UK

Bennur Esen
Department of Internal Medicine and Nephrology, Bagcilar Education and Research Hospital, Istanbul, Turkey

Irfan Sahin
Department of Cardiology, Bagcilar Education and Research Hospital, Istanbul, Turkey

Ahmet Engin Atay and Emel Saglam Gokmen
Department of Internal Medicine, Bagcilar Education and Research Hospital, Istanbul, Turkey

Ozlem Harmankaya Kaptanogullari and Mürvet Yılmaz
Department of Internal Medicine and Nephrology, Bakırkoy Sadi Konuk Education and Research Hospital, Istanbul, Turkey

Suat Hayri Kucuk
Department of Biochemistry, Bagcilar Education and Research Hospital, Istanbul, Turkey

Serdar Kahvecioglu
Department of Internal Medicine and Nephrology, Sevket Yılmaz Education and Research Hospital, Bursa, Turkey

Nurhan Seyahi
Department of Internal Medicine and Nephrology, Cerrahpasa School of Medicine, Istanbul University, Istanbul, Turkey

Katia Bravo-Jaimes
University of Rochester Medical Center, 601 Elmwood Avenue, Box MED, Rochester, NY 14642, USA
Facultad de Medicina de San Fernando, Universidad Nacional Mayor de San Marcos (UNMSM), Lima, Peru

Alvaro Whittembury and Vilma Santivañez
Facultad de Medicina de San Fernando, Universidad Nacional Mayor de San Marcos (UNMSM), Lima, Peru

U. E. Ekrikpo, E. E. Akpan and A. S. Obot
University of Uyo and University of Uyo Teaching Hospital, Uyo, Nigeria

E. E. Effa
University of Calabar, Calabar, Nigeria

S. Kadiri
University College Hospital, Ibadan, Nigeria

Basil Alnasrallah and John F. Collins,
Department ofNephrology, Auckland City Hospital, 2 Park Drive, Grafton, Auckland 1023, New Zealand

L. Jonathan Zwi
Department of Pathology, Auckland City Hospital, 2 Park Drive, Grafton, Auckland 1023, New Zealand

Ramya Hettiarachchi
Community Medicine, Postgraduate Institute of Medicine, University of Colombo, Colombo, Sri Lanka

Chrishantha Abeysena
Department of Public Health, Faculty of Medicine, University of Kelaniya, Colombo, Sri Lanka

D. Patschan and G. A. Müller
Clinic of Nephrology and Rheumatology, University Hospital of Göttingen, Göttingen, Germany

Attilio Losito and Loretta Pittavini
Renal Unit, Santa Maria Della Misericordia Hospital, Perugia, Italy

Ivano Zampi
Institute of Geriatrics and Gerontology, Department of Clinical and Experimental Medicine, University of Perugia, Ospedale S. Maria della Misericordia, Perugia, Italy

Elena Zampi
Department of Medicine, Hospital of Pantalla, Todi, Italy

Vinod Krishnappa and Shivani Kwatra
Akron Nephrology Associates/Akron General Cleveland Clinic, Akron, OH, USA

Mohit Gupta
Department of Internal Medicine, Akron General Cleveland Clinic, Akron, OH, USA

Gurusidda Manu
Onco-Hospitalist, Beth Israel Deaconness Medical Center, Boston, MA, USA

Osei-Tutu Owus
Department Hematology/Medical Oncology, Akron General Cleveland Clinic, Akron, OH, USA

Rupesh Raina
Department of Nephrology/Internal Medicine, Akron General Cleveland Clinic, Akron, OH, USA

Cristin D. W. Kaspar, Megan Lo and Timothy E. Bunchman
Virginia Commonwealth University, Children's Hospital of Richmond, Pediatric Nephrology, Virginia, USA

Keia Sanderson
University of North Carolina, Department of Medicine-Nephrology, North Carolina, USA

Seza Ozen
Hacettepe University, Department of Pediatrics, Turkey

Priya S. Verghese
University of Minnesota, Division of Pediatric Nephrology, Minnesota, USA

Scott E. Wenderfer
Baylor College of Medicine, Pediatrics-Renal, Texas, USA

Jason Kidd
Virginia Commonwealth University, Internal Medicine Nephrology, Virginia, USA

Lei Cao, Rashin Sedighi, Ava Boston, Lakmini Premadasa, George E. Crawford, Scott H. Harrison, Robert H. Newman and Elimelda Moige Ongeri
Department of Biology, North Carolina A&T State University, Greensboro, NC 27411, USA

Jamilla Pinder and Olugbemiga E. Jegede
Cone Health Community Health andWellness Center, Greensboro, NC 27401, USA

C. Hess, I. Rune and H. Søndergaard
Department of Diabetes Complications Pharmacology, Novo Nordisk, Maaloev, Denmark

M. K. E. Ougaard
Department of Diabetes Complications Pharmacology, Novo Nordisk, Maaloev, Denmark
Department of Veterinary and Animal Sciences, University of Copenhagen, Frederiksberg, Denmark

H. E. Jensen
Department of Veterinary and Animal Sciences, University of Copenhagen, Frederiksberg, Denmark

P. H. Kvist
Department of Histology and Bioimaging, Novo Nordisk, Maaloev, Denmark

D. Patschan, I. Buschmann and O. Ritter
Innere Medizin I, Kardiologie, Angiologie, Nephrologie, Klinikum Brandenburg, Medizinische Hochschule Brandenburg, Brandenburg, Germany

Ahmed M. Alkhunaizi
Nephrology Unit, Specialty Medicine Department, Johns Hopkins Aramco Healthcare, Dhahran, Saudi Arabia

Adil A. Al-Khatti
Hematology Unit, Cancer Institute, Johns Hopkins Aramco Healthcare, Dhahran, Saudi Arabia

Mansour A. Alkhunaizi
Royal College of Surgeons in Ireland, Dublin, Ireland

Andreas Kousios
Department of Nephrology, Nicosia General Hospital, 2230 Nicosia, Cyprus

Panayiotis Kouis and Andrie G. Panayiotou
Cyprus International Institute for Environmental and Public Health in Association withHarvard T. H. Chan School of Public Health, Cyprus University of Technology, 3041 Limassol, Cyprus

Jayanton Patumanond
Division of Clinical Epidemiology, Faculty of Medicine, Thammasat University, Rangsit Campus, Pathum Thani, Thailand

Pichaya Tantiyavarong
Division of Clinical Epidemiology, Faculty of Medicine, Thammasat University, Rangsit Campus, Pathum Thani, Thailand
Division of Nephrology, Department of Medicine, Thammasat University Hospital, PathumThani, Thailand

Opas Traitanon and Adis Tasanarong
Division of Nephrology, Department of Medicine, Thammasat University Hospital, PathumThani, Thailand

Piyatida Chuengsaman
Banphaeo Hospital, Prommitr Branch, Bangkok, Thailand

Index

A

Acute Kidney Injury, 1-2, 7-8, 56, 64, 67, 146, 151-152, 159, 162, 164, 166-170, 194, 204, 208-209, 213-215

Acute Renal Failure, 7, 148, 151-152, 154, 168-170

Adipocytes, 56-59, 61-64

Augmentation Cystoplasty, 93-94, 99

Azotemia, 66

B

Baseline Serum Creatinine, 2

Blood Pressure, 14, 36-39, 42, 44, 47, 101-103, 108, 113, 115, 117, 126-127, 157-158, 181, 184-185, 193, 208, 216, 218, 229, 231

Bone Marrow Failure, 159, 167

C

Cardiovascular Disease, 25, 42, 49, 67, 69, 72, 76, 78, 85, 89, 100, 107, 111-112, 118-121, 123, 151, 153, 157-158, 190, 219-221, 229-230

Cerebrovascular Disease, 119-122

Childhood Nephrotic Syndrome, 43, 45, 47-48

Chronic Kidney Disease, 2, 7, 10-11, 13, 15, 24-25, 37-40, 42, 45, 47, 55, 57, 66, 85, 94, 101, 104, 106, 112, 123-125, 140, 145, 154, 168, 180, 189, 194, 196, 212, 221

Chronic Renal Failure, 36, 123, 131, 207

Cloacal Exstrophy, 93

Contrast-induced Nephropathy, 146, 151, 208, 213-215

Crystalloids, 208-210

D

Diabetes Mellitus, 13, 25, 42, 49, 66, 72, 75-76, 79, 108, 125-128, 130-131, 146-148, 151, 153, 162, 184, 193-194, 216

Diabetic Kidney Disease, 180, 184, 186-191

Diabetic Nephropathy, 40, 86, 107, 125-126, 128-132, 146-147, 149-152, 162, 180, 193-195, 206, 208, 235

Diabetic Tubulopathy, 129-130

Dialysis Treatment, 9-10, 13, 15, 147

Dialysis-related Peritonitis, 232, 237-238

Diastolic Dysfunction, 116-117, 119-124

Dysplastic Kidneys, 93-95

E

Encapsulating Peritoneal Sclerosis, 56, 59-65

End-stage Renal Disease, 9-10, 15, 25, 41, 49, 78-79, 85, 91-93, 100, 106, 112, 123, 130-131, 145-146, 171-172, 177, 220-221, 231

Endothelial-to-mesenchymal Transition, 56

Enterobacteriaceae, 81-84

G

Glomerular Filtration Barrier, 41, 191, 196

Glomerular Filtration Rate, 36, 38, 41-42, 44, 49, 55, 71, 76, 78, 93, 126, 131, 147, 153, 158, 196, 198, 200, 206, 218, 221

Glomerulonephritis, 26, 35, 37-38, 44-45, 47, 59, 120, 138-139, 171-172, 176, 178, 193, 196, 206, 235

Glycated Albumin, 110, 112

Graft-versus-host Disease, 135, 159-160, 164, 169-170

Granulomatosis With Polyangiitis, 171, 178

H

Haemodialysis, 9-10, 13, 15-16, 21, 24, 59, 78-79, 105-107, 112, 124, 230

Heart Valve Replacement Surgery, 1, 7

Hematopoietic Stem Cell Transplantation, 159, 168-170

Hepatic Sinusoidal Obstruction Syndrome, 159, 165

Hypertension, 1-2, 9-10, 13, 26, 36-42, 44, 46, 55, 66, 69, 72, 75-76, 79-80, 88-89, 105-106, 112, 120-122, 125, 127-130, 147, 154-158, 165, 167, 185, 190-191, 195, 197, 207, 230-231

I

Idiopathic Nephrotic Syndrome, 43, 47-48

Immunohistochemistry, 26, 28, 32, 56-58, 198, 206

Inflammatory Cytokines, 37, 41, 111, 163

Interventricular Septal Hypertrophy, 113, 115

K

Kidney Dysfunction, 153, 155-157

L

Lower Urinary Tract Dysfunction, 93-94

Lupus Nephritis, 26, 28-30, 32, 34-35, 45

Lymphoproliferative Disorders, 159, 167

M

Marrow Infusion Toxicity, 159, 163, 166, 168

Matrix Metalloproteinases, 35, 221-222, 229-231

Membranous Nephropathy, 45, 133-134, 138-139

Meprin Metalloproteases, 180, 190, 194

Mesangial Expansion, 196-198, 201-204

Microalbuminuria, 40, 125-126, 128-131, 182-185, 191, 216, 218-221

Murine Nephrotoxic Nephritis, 196

N

Neoplasia, 133

Nephrectomy, 94-95, 196-197, 203, 206

Nephrotic Syndrome, 43-48, 133, 138

O

Obesity, 10, 66, 114, 117, 122, 124, 129-130, 147, 149, 180, 182, 190, 193

P

Pediatric Nephrology, 41-42, 47-48, 99, 131, 171-173, 178, 194, 206, 220

Pediatric Rheumatology, 171-173, 178

Peritoneal Biopsies, 56-58, 60-61

Peritoneal Dialysis, 9-10, 38, 41, 56-57, 59, 64-65, 100, 102-106, 113-114, 118, 120, 123, 178, 226, 232-234, 237-239

Permanent Cardiac Pacing, 85

Phosphate, 14-18, 21-25, 28, 44, 73, 76, 80, 104, 108-109, 163, 166

Posterior Urethral Valve, 93, 95

Primary Renal Disorders, 66

Proteinuria, 13, 26-31, 33, 44, 72, 104, 106, 126, 131, 134-135, 137, 147, 176, 196, 201, 206-207, 216, 219-220, 231

Pulse Wave Velocity, 100, 102-106

R

Renal Biopsy, 26, 126, 134-138, 175

Renal Fibrosis, 181, 196-197, 201-205, 207

Renal Replacement Therapy, 2, 10, 41, 64, 72, 85, 94, 100-101, 103-105, 107, 113, 125, 130, 146-147, 219

Renal Transplantation, 36-37, 41-42, 57, 59, 98, 103, 120, 140, 176, 179

Renin Angiotensin Aldosterone System, 67, 76

S

Serum Endocan, 36-38, 40, 42

Serum Phosphate, 14-17, 21-23

Sickle Cell Nephropathy, 216

Soluble Fas, 26-28, 30, 33-35

Subclinical Atherosclerosis, 221-222, 226, 228-229

Systemic Lupus Erythematosus, 26, 29, 33-35, 42, 44, 118, 135, 176

T

Thrombotic Microangiopathy, 163-164, 166, 169-170

Tumor Lysis Syndrome, 159, 163, 166-168, 170

Type 2 Diabetes Mellitus, 25, 42, 72, 79, 151, 153, 194

U

Uremia, 61, 65-66, 105-106, 228, 231, 268

Urinary Albumin Concentration, 125, 127-128, 197

Urinary Tract Infections, 38, 81, 83-84

V

Valvular Calcification, 113, 116